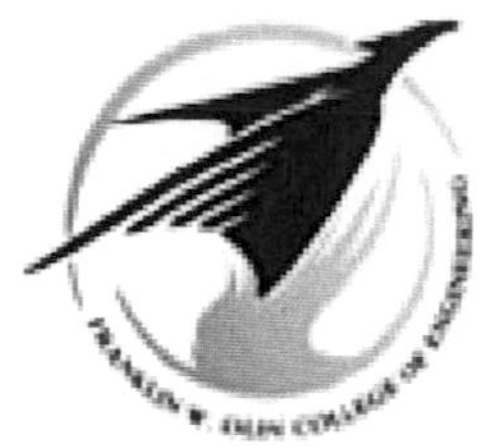

SAFETY OF SILICONE BREAST IMPLANTS

Stuart Bondurant, Virginia Ernster, and Roger Herdman, *Editors*

Committee on the Safety of Silicone Breast Implants

Division of Health Promotion and Disease Prevention

INSTITUTE OF MEDICINE

NATIONAL ACADEMY PRESS
Washington, D.C.

NATIONAL ACADEMY PRESS • 2101 Constitution Avenue, N.W. • Washington, D.C. 20418

NOTICE: The project that is the subject of this report was approved by the Governing Board of the National Research Council, whose members are drawn from the councils of the National Academy of Sciences, the National Academy of Engineering, and the Institute of Medicine. The members of the committee responsible for the report were chosen for their special competences and with regard for appropriate balance.

Support for this study was provided by the National Institute of Arthritis and Musculoskeletal and Skin Diseases of the National Institutes of Health under Task Order No. 36, Contract No. N01-OD-4-2139.

Library of Congress Cataloging-in-Publication Data

Safety of silicone breast implants / Stuart Bondurant, Virginia Ernster, and Roger Herdman, editors ; Committee on the Safety of Silicone Breast Implants, Division of Health Promotion and Disease Prevention, Institute of Medicine.

p. cm.

Includes bibliographical references and index.

ISBN 0-309-06532-1 (hardcover)

1. Breast implants—Complications. 2. Silicones—Toxicology. 3. Mammaplasty. I. Bondurant, Stuart. II. Ernster, Virginia L. III. Herdman, Roger. IV. Institute of Medicine (U.S.). Committee on the Safety of Silicone Breast Implants.

[DNLM: 1. Breast Implants—adverse effects. 2. Safety. 3. Silicones—adverse effects. WP 910 S128 1999]

RD539.8 .S24 1999

618.1'90592—dc21

99-040812

Safety of Silicone Breast Implants is available for sale from the National Academy Press, 2101 Constitution Avenue, N.W., Box 285, Washington, DC 20055. Call 800-624-6242 or 202-334-3313 (in the Washington Metropolitan Area). The full text of this publication is available on-line at **www.nap.edu.**

For more information about the Institute of Medicine, visit the IOM home page at **www.nas.edu/ iom.**

Printed in the United States of America.

The serpent has been a symbol of long life, healing, and knowledge among almost all cultures and religions since the beginning of recorded history. The image adopted as a logotype by the Institute of Medicine is based on a relief carving from ancient Greece, now held by the Staatliche Museen in Berlin.

THE NATIONAL ACADEMIES

National Academy of Sciences
National Academy of Engineering
Institute of Medicine
National Research Council

The **National Academy of Sciences** is a private, nonprofit, self-perpetuating society of distinguished scholars engaged in scientific and engineering research, dedicated to the furtherance of science and technology and to their use for the general welfare. Upon the authority of the charter granted to it by the Congress in 1863, the Academy has a mandate that requires it to advise the federal government on scientific and technical matters. Dr. Bruce M. Alberts is president of the National Academy of Sciences.

The **National Academy of Engineering** was established in 1964, under the charter of the National Academy of Sciences, as a parallel organization of outstanding engineers. It is autonomous in its administration and in the selection of its members, sharing with the National Academy of Sciences the responsibility for advising the federal government. The National Academy of Engineering also sponsors engineering programs aimed at meeting national needs, encourages education and research, and recognizes the superior achievements of engineers. Dr. William A. Wulf is president of the National Academy of Engineering.

The **Institute of Medicine** was established in 1970 by the National Academy of Sciences to secure the services of eminent members of appropriate professions in the examination of policy matters pertaining to the health of the public. The Institute acts under the responsibility given to the National Academy of Sciences by its congressional charter to be an adviser to the federal government and, upon its own initiative, to identify issues of medical care, research, and education. Dr. Kenneth I. Shine is president of the Institute of Medicine.

The **National Research Council** was organized by the National Academy of Sciences in 1916 to associate the broad community of science and technology with the Academy's purposes of furthering knowledge and advising the federal government. Functioning in accordance with general policies determined by the Academy, the Council has become the principal operating agency of both the National Academy of Sciences and the National Academy of Engineering in providing services to the government, the public, and the scientific and engineering communities. The Council is administered jointly by both Academies and the Institute of Medicine. Dr. Bruce M. Alberts and Dr. William A. Wulf are chairman and vice chairman, respectively, of the National Research Council.

COMMITTEE ON THE SAFETY OF SILICONE BREAST IMPLANTS

STUART BONDURANT, M.D. (*Chair*), Professor of Medicine, University of North Carolina at Chapel Hill

VIRGINIA L. ERNSTER, Ph.D. (*Vice Chair*), Professor and Vice Chair, Department of Epidemiology and Biostatistics, School of Medicine, University of California at San Francisco

MARGIT L. BLEECKER, M.D., Ph.D., Director, Center for Occupational and Environmental Neurology, Baltimore, Maryland

DIANE V. DADO, M.D., Associate Professor of Surgery and Pediatrics, Loyola University Medical Center

CARL J. D'ORSI, M.D., Professor and Vice Chairman, Department of Radiology, University of Massachusetts Medical Center, Worchester

JOANN G. ELMORE, M.D., M.P.H., Associate Professor of Medicine and Adjunct Professor of Epidemiology, Division of General Internal Medicine, University of Washington

THOMAS J. FAHEY, Jr., M.D., Senior Vice President for Clinical Program Development, Memorial Sloan-Kettering Cancer Center, New York City

BRIAN E. HENDERSON, M.D., Professor of Medicine, Department of Preventive Medicine, Norris Comprehensive Cancer Center, University of Southern California

ARTHUR C. MARTELLOCK, Ph.D., Consultant, Pittsford, New York

CHRIS D. PLATSOUCAS, M.D., Chairman, Department of Microbiology and Immunology, and Laura H. Carnell Professor of Medicine, Temple University School of Medicine

NAOMI F. ROTHFIELD, M.D., Professor of Medicine, Chief, Division of Rheumatic Diseases, University of Connecticut School of Medicine

DIANA TAYLOR, R.N., N.P., Ph.D., FAAN, Associate Professor, Department of Family Health Care Nursing, CoDirector, University of California at San Francisco, and Center for Collaborative Innovation in Primary Care, San Francisco

RALPH C. WILLIAMS, Jr., M.D., Professor Emeritus, Department of Medicine, University of Florida

IOM Staff

ROGER HERDMAN, Study Director
ANNICE HIRT, Research Associate
STACEY PATMORE, Research Associate
PATRICIA J. SPAULDING, Project Assistant

MICAH MILTON, Intern
KATHLEEN R. STRATTON, Director, Division of Health Promotion and Disease Prevention
DONNA D. THOMPSON, Division Assistant
SHARON GALLOWAY, Financial Associate

Staff Consultants

WESTLEY REEVES, Associate Professor, Department of Medicine, University of North Carolina at Chapel Hill
HANSPETER WITSCHI, Professor of Toxicology, Department of Molecular Biosciences, School of Veterinary Medicine, University of California at Davis

Reviewers

This report has been reviewed in draft form by individuals chosen for their diverse perspectives and technical expertise, in accordance with procedures approved by the National Research Council's Report Review Committee. The purpose of this independent review is to provide candid and critical comments that will assist the Institute of Medicine in making the published report as sound as possible and to ensure that the report meets institutional standards for objectivity, evidence, and responsiveness to the study charge. The review comments and draft manuscript remain confidential to protect the integrity of the deliberative process. The committee wishes to thank the following individuals for their participation in the review of this report:

GRACIELLA ALARCON, M.D., M.P.H., School of Medicine, University of Alabama, Birmingham;
J. CLAUDE BENNETT , M.D., BioCryst Pharmaceuticals, Inc., Birmingham, Alabama;
DONALD H. BERRY, Ph.D., Department of Chemistry, University of Pennsylvania;
JOHN DOULL, M.D., Department of Pharmacology, Toxicology, and Therapeutics, University of Kansas;
HAROLD J. FALLON, M.D., School of Medicine, University of Alabama, Birmingham;
SUZANNE W. FLETCHER, M.D., Department of Ambulatory Care and Prevention, Harvard Medical School;

RUTH T. GROSS, M.D., Stanford Univerity;
WALTER PETERS, M.D., Wellesley Central Hospital, Toronto, Ontario, Canada;
EDWARD A. SICKLES, M.D., Department of Radiology, University of California at San Francisco;
ROBERT WEST, Ph.D., University of Wisconsin; and
NANCY FUGATE WOODS, Ph.D., R.N., School of Nursing, University of Washington.

While the individuals listed above have provided constructive comments and suggestions, it must be emphasized that responsibility for the final content of this report rests entirely with the authoring committee and the Institute of Medicine.

Preface

To begin, we reflect that the need for this report and the oft-cited deficiencies of the research relevant to silicone breast implants both derive from the fact that silicone breast implants were widely used before there was any requirement for premarket assessment of toxicity and complications or any form of prior approval or licensing for all medical devices. For many years there were no requirements to document the composition of implants or the specific model that was implanted in a particular individual. Further, there was no systematic, comprehensive, postmarketing surveillance of the long-term positive and negative consequences of silicone breast implantation. In the absence of structured requirements for risk assessment before 1992, much of the literature on aspects of silicone breast implants is anecdotal, lacking in appropriate controls, or otherwise of little value in establishing risk. This report stands as strong evidence of the need for thorough and systematic assessment of medical devices prior to their utilization and for continuing assessment after widespread utilization to discover any rare complications that premarketing studies of feasible size might not demonstrate. In the judgment of the committee, however, there have now been sufficient studies of quality to reach a number of well-based conclusions.

Several important events have occurred since this study was initiated. A major class action litigation, brought on behalf of women with silicone breast implants, was settled with a substantial award to the plaintiffs. Meanwhile, a court turned to a panel of experts for advice on specific issues before the court concerning health consequences of silicone breast implants. The report of the National Science Panel, described in Appendix C, is a substantial work that sets forth clearly and definitively the strong scientific evidence not always available in the past to courts with jurisdiction over breast implant litigation. The report of the National Science Panel is a model of the provision to the courts of the best available scientific advice in a matter in which balanced and informed scientific information and judgment are essential.

The committee considered whether various known disease-related conditions occur more frequently in women with silicone breast implants than in women in the general population and also whether there might be a novel disease syndrome or syndromes in women with silicone breast implants. To date, proposals for the latter possibility have been based on criteria that are inadequate for scientific evaluation or confirmation. The proposed syndromes often involve ill-defined subjective symptoms that occur with substantial frequency in the general population. Absent a marker or set of markers to confer specificity, the existence of such a syndrome cannot be proven or used to exclude or include any individual or group.

The committee heard directly and indirectly from many women who suffer severe systemic illnesses that they firmly believe are due to their silicone breast implants. Many of these women are seriously ill, and the committee was moved by their suffering. However, the committee is convinced that in most instances the silicone breast implants are not causally related to these illnesses since such illnesses appear to occur at about the same frequency in women with silicone breast implants and in women without implants.

On the other hand, the committee was impressed by what appear to be the relatively high frequencies of local complications (such as rupture and contracture) that are unique to women with silicone breast implants. Although they are not life-threatening, these local complications may result in discomfort, inconvenience, disfigurement, pain, and other morbidity and when further corrective procedures are necessary, in additional expense.

Many women with silicone breast implants feel strongly that they were not provided with adequate information as a basis for consenting to have these implants. The committee is aware that recall by patients of the specific conditions and terms of medical consent is imperfect, and it is aware that several medical organizations have worked diligently to improve the quality of informed consent of patients with silicone breast implants. The committee believes, however, that more consistent and higher quality informed consent is possible and, among its recommendations, urges the development and testing of model processes and systems for ensuring fully informed consent for future recipients of silicone breast implants. A successful system may be applicable to other implantable devices in the future.

In addition to the acknowledgment in Chapter 1 that many individuals and groups helped in the committee's work, the committee wishes to express especially its respect and appreciation for the extraordinary work of Dr. Roger Herdman in serving as director of this study. Dr. Herdman oversaw the collection of the world's English language literature on silicone breast implants, and he personally mastered most of it. His database and the good and important help of his expert assistants, first Annice Hirt and subsequently Stacey Patmore, made this literature easily available to the committee. Dr. Herdman's reasoned, systematic, and fact-based approach earned him the respect and trust of the committee and of interested parties. Patricia Spaulding did an outstanding job of orchestrating the flow of information and arranging for meetings. The committee thanks Dr. Herdman and his staff for all they have contributed to this report.

Stuart Bondurant, M.D.
Chair

Virginia L. Ernster, Ph.D.
Vice Chair

Contents

Safety of Silicone Breast Implants

Executive Summary

In House Report 104-659, which accompanied a 1997 appropriations bill, Congress asked the U.S. Department of Health and Human Services (DHHS) to sponsor a study of the safety of silicone breast implants by the Institute of Medicine (IOM) of the National Academy of Sciences. Funds were committed from several sources in DHHS, and the National Institute of Arthritis and Musculoskeletal and Skin Diseases (NIAMS) was designated as the lead agency. In late 1997, the IOM agreed to carry out a comprehensive evaluation of the evidence for the association of silicone breast implants, both gel and saline filled, with human health conditions, assemble a comprehensive list of scientific references on this subject, and to consider recommendations for further research.

Chapter 1 recounts this history and the steps taken by the IOM to form the committee on the Safety of Silicone Breast Implants and to arrange for the preparation of a report with national public and scientific input, standards for evaluating evidence, and appropriate committee deliberations. Data and evidence for an association or for no association of a health condition with breast implants were ranked as either conclusive/convincing, limited/suggestive, insufficient, flawed or lacking. A finding of insufficient or absent data was not meant to imply that more information was needed. When this was desirable, and only then, the committee so noted. Chapter 1 also includes a brief description of the history of cosmetic breast surgery, cosmetic silicone injections, and the early development of silicone implants and continues with a discussion of women's satisfaction with breast implants.

Satisfaction is important, both inherently and because women's tolerance for complications influences their demand for medical and surgical interventions to correct implant problems, which in turn has safety implications. Yet surveys of satisfaction are often administered by plastic surgeons, which may bias results and influence women's reporting, and surveys are also often carried out before the likely appearance of some complications. The response rate itself may be influenced by the degree of satisfaction or other personal considerations.

The committee arrived at an estimate of 1.5 million to 1.8 million U.S. women with breast implants in 1997, the year the IOM study began. The committee estimates that about 70% of these implants were performed for augmentation, (i.e., enlarging or changing the appearance of the breast), and 30% for reconstruction, (i.e., restoring the form of the breast after mastectomy for cancer, fibrocystic disease, or other indications). The committee also noted that more than 10 million persons in the United States have some type of implant, such as finger joints or pacemakers, and many of these implants are made, at least in part, from silicone. A short review of regulation by the Food and Drug Administration (FDA) explains why current breast implantation is primarily with saline-filled implants, and describes the effects of government actions on gel-filled, polyurethane-coated, and other implants and on the companies that manufactured them.

Silicon is a semimetallic element, and silicone is a family of silicon-based organic compounds, of which the poly(dimethylsiloxanes) (PDMS) are prominent members. PDMS compounds are polymers, and the length and cross-linking of the polymer chain(s) affect the physical properties of these substances. Implant shells are made from an elastomer, that is, a high molecular weight, cross-linked rubbery substance, and they are filled with silicone gel, a less cross-linked spongy substance permeated with lower molecular weight silicone fluids. Other fillers are possible and include primarily saline. Chapter 2 describes in summary fashion the chemical steps in the manufacture of breast implants; Chapters 2 and 4 discuss the extensive presence of, and wide exposure of citizens in developed countries to silicones in foods, cosmetics, lubricants for machinery, hypodermic syringes and other products, insulators, and a wide array of consumer products.

Many kinds of implants with very different characteristics, made by various manufacturers, are described in Chapter 3. The committee was struck by the great number of changes in silicone breast implants since they were introduced in 1962. These changes have created different "generations" of gel-filled implants, which may have very different effects. The changes were introduced with little or no pretesting for biological or clinical effects as far as the committee could determine. Varying control of the diffusion of silicone fluid through gel implant shells, shell strength, and therefore durability of both gel- and saline-filled implants, and polyurethane coating were among the changes that affected the clinical performance of silicone breast implants in ways that were not predicted in many instances. The history and implications of polyurethane coating of breast implants were reviewed, although polyurethane implants have not been available from U.S. manufacturers since 1991. On the other hand, changes have been made that have improved implants, as plastic surgeons and manufacturers have learned from reports of problems with existing implant models. Barrier shells, texturing, better valves in saline implants, and stronger shells that are more resistant to rupture or deflation have been some of these changes.

Study of the toxicology of silicones began in the 1940s. Although these studies were consistent with the standards of the day, in hindsight they fall short of current regulatory requirements; in particular, more chronic, long-term studies would have been desirable. As would be expected for any large family of organic compounds, some silicones have toxic or biologic effects, but PDMS fluids, gels, and elastomers were generally well tolerated on injection or implantation. Like other polymers, silicone can induce "solid state" carcinogenesis in rodents, but there is no evidence that this occurs in humans. Studies of the reproductive toxicology of PDMS have been negative. Several studies of the distribution of silicones from depots of experimental gel implantation or fluid injection have shown that silicones remain localized where deposited and that low molecular weight silicones which may be mobile to a small extent, are cleared from the body after relatively short half-lives.

Since the evidence is lacking or flawed that amorphous silica in breast implant shells is available to, or found in tissues of experimental animals or humans, or that crystalline silica is formed or present at any time in women with implants, the toxicology of silica has not been reviewed, although literature on silica is included in the references. Some investigators have asserted that platinum catalysts in breast implants may diffuse through the implant shell, be present in multivalent states, and provoke toxic reactions. The evidence currently available suggests that platinum is present only in the zero valence elemental state. Evidence does not suggest there are high concentrations in implants, significant diffusion of platinum out of implants, or platinum toxicity in humans. In general, the committee has concluded that a review of the toxicology studies of silicones known to be used in breast implants does not provide a basis for concern at expected exposures.

Local complications and reoperations have significant implications for the safety of silicone breast implants, because they may involve risks themselves and may lead to medical and surgical interventions that have risks. Local complications were not extensively reviewed in other recent, important reports such as those of the Independent Review Group in the United Kingdom or the National Science Panel appointed by the court to examine systemic diseases and silicone breast implants. The committee considered local complications an important aspect of the story of breast implantation—historically, now, and in the future—for women considering these implants.

Chapter 5 approaches local complications both from the standpoint of overall reoperation and complication frequency and during reconstruction and augmentation. It then examines specific complications. In general, the committee concludes that complications are frequent. Specific complications discussed include implant rupture and deflation, contracture of the fibrous tissue capsule around implants, and elevated silicone concentrations in peri-implant tissues. Results with saline versus gel implants, barrier implants, textured implants, steroid-treated implants and implants in different positions are discussed. The infections, hematomas, and pain that may accompany implants are also considered.

A number of factors affect the integrity of the silicone elastomer implant shell. These include: shell thickness and strength which can vary considerably; untoward events such as needle sticks and other trauma associated with the vagaries of daily life, including closed capsulotomies, which the committee concludes should be abandoned; and the abrasion and wear of the implant shell in the body enhanced by wrinkling and fold flaws. Precise frequencies of the rupture of gel-filled, or the deflation of saline-filled, implants are not available. The properties of these devices that can affect rupture or deflation have changed markedly over time, and particularly in the case of gel implants, it has not been possible to reliably diagnose and study rupture in an unbiased cross section of implanted women. It is safe to say however that, like any device, breast implants have a finite life span. Rupture frequencies, in the past, have been considerable, and the rupture rate of current models has yet to be measured over the relevant periods of time. The deflation of saline implants is more easily diagnosed, but 100% discovery of deflations does not occur, and deflation frequencies of current models remain to be measured reliably.

Breast implants, like any foreign body, incite a surrounding fibrous tissue reaction. This fibrous capsule may contract, distorting the appearance of the implanted breast and causing pain. Contracture may be apparent as early as a few months after implantation, and the committee finds that it most likely continues over prolonged periods of time. As with any biologic reaction, some variation in contracture may be expected. The severity of contracture can differ in the breasts of the same woman. The exact frequency of contracture is not known because it has varied from 100% with pre-silicone implants to much lower prevalences, depending on a number of factors, as modern silicone implants have evolved. Few studies that have measured contracture have controlled all except one study variable.

Silicon or silicone levels are elevated in capsular and sometimes breast tissue around implants, and this may contribute to capsular contracture. The committee has found suggestive evidence that contracture frequency is lessened by saline implants and barrier shells that, among other things, diminish the exposure of peri-implant breast tissue to silicone. Construction of an implant shell with projections, known as texturing, also appears to control contracture. The committee reviewed the evidence on the effects of adrenal corticosteroids on capsular contracture. Although some data suggest that they may reduce contractures, steroids also cause damage to surrounding breast tissue, are not an FDA approved or manufacturer-recommended usage, and may weaken elastomer implant shells.

A number of studies have shown that bacteria can be cultured from normal breast tissue, even at some depth below the surface of the skin. These bacteria are skin flora that reside in the lactiferous ducts of the normal breast, and often can be cultured from implants, where they may contribute from time to time to infections. There is suggestive evidence that the presence of bacteria correlates with contracture. A few investigators have reported finding an association between the presence of bacteria around implants and systemic symptoms or breast pain, although this evidence is limited. Hematomas, or collections of blood around implants, have also been proposed as causes of contracture. Evidence for this is insufficient. Significant contractures are reported considerably more frequently than clinically observable hematomas. Pain is also a problem in some women with implants. A number of studies report pain that has resulted in considerable discomfort and led to the removal of implants.

The committee reached three major general conclusions regarding local and perioperative complications. First, these complications occur frequently enough to be a cause for concern and to justify the conclusion that they are the primary safety issue with silicone breast implants. Among others, these include overall reoperations, ruptures or deflations, contractures, infections, hematomas, and pain. Second, risks accumulate over the lifetime of the implant, but quantitative data on this point are lacking for modern implants and are deficient historically for a number of reasons that have been noted in this report. Among these are lack of data from representative samples of the population, lack of information on implant characteristics that affect complications, and lack of precise and reliable detection of complications. Third, information concerning the nature and relatively high frequency of local complications and reoperations is an essential element of adequate informed consent for women undergoing breast implantation.

Chapters 6 through 8 evaluate the immunology of silicone, the relationship of antinuclear and other autoantibodies to breast implants, and the association of breast implants with classic connective tissue disease, undifferentiated connective tissue disease, and proposed new signs, symptoms, or novel disease. Studies in experimental animals have reported modest adjuvant effects of silicone gel and some silicone fluids, but no clinical implications of adjuvant effects have been discovered. Human adjuvant disease is not a defined disease, and the term should be abandoned. Other animal studies have not elucidated a role for silicone in immune disease. Cytokine assays have not provided conclusive evidence of immune activation. Evidence for silicone as a superantigen is insufficient. Modest decreases in natural killer cell activity have been reported after exposure to silicone, but no clinical roles or biological effects on resistance to infection, tumor surveillance or immune responses have been demonstrated in these studies.

Evidence for a particular HLA (human lymphocyte antigen) class I or class II haplotype associated with symptomatic women with silicone breast implants, or for specific T-cell activation or delayed hypersensitivity to silicone is insufficient and often flawed, and there is limited evidence that HLA haplotypes of symptomatic women with implants resemble those of symptomatic women without implants and that there is no T-cell activation or delayed hypersensitivity from silicone. Studies addressing these issues are limited and technical problems substantial, providing the committee with no support for a role of silicone as a T-cell antigen or in creating T-cell autoantigens. The committee also finds no evidence for antisilicone antibodies. The clinical significance of a recently described antipolymer antibody test is unclear, although the polymer in question is not silicone or silicon containing, and it is extremely unlikely that it measures an antisilicone antibody. The committee also noted several reports suggesting that women with breast implants might have elevated serum immunoglobulin levels. A few case reports also suggested that there might be an increased frequency of multiple myeloma in women with breast implants. These data are insufficient and a number of current epidemiological studies do not report an increase in immunoglobulin levels or multiple myeloma in such women.

Reports of antinuclear antibodies and epidemiological studies of classical and atypical connective tissue or rheumatic disease in women with breast implants also do not provide any support for immunologic or autoimmune responses or diseases associated with silicone breast implants. The committee reviewed 30 studies of antinuclear antibodies and other autoantibodies in women with silicone (primarily gel-filled) breast implants. These reports were often conflicting; many used differing technologies to assay antinuclear antibodies or differing criteria to determine a positive test. Lack of controls and other design problems hampered the interpretation of some studies. No pattern of association of antinuclear antibodies with silicone breast implants emerged from these data. Several epidemiological studies suggested support for the conclusion that there is no association of antinuclear or other autoantibodies with breast implants.

A review of 17 epidemiological reports of connective tissue disease in women with breast implants was remarkable for the consistency in finding no elevated relative risk or odds ratio for an association of implants with disease. Studies of breast implants and undifferentiated connective tissue disease or atypical signs and symptoms were much fewer in number. Several high-quality studies of classical connective tissue disease in women with implants were available, but this was not the case with atypical signs and symptoms or unusual presentations. Nevertheless, many of the studies focusing on classical disease had also collected data on rheumatic and related signs and symptoms, and in general, no association with implants was found.

A novel syndrome or disease associated with silicone breast implants has been proposed. Evidence for this proposed disease rests on case reports and is insufficient or flawed. The disease definition includes, as a precondition, the presence of silicone breast implants, so it cannot be studied as an independent health problem. The committee finds that the diagnosis of this condition could depend on the presence of a number of symptoms that are nonspecific and common in the general population. Thus, there does not appear to be even suggestive evidence for the existence of a novel syndrome in women with breast implants. In fact, epidemiological evidence suggests that there is no novel syndrome.

Silicone like many polymers (and other substances) can cause solid state carcinogenesis. Implantation of a material formulated with appropriate size, shape, and surface characteristics causes infrequently metastasizing sarcomas in susceptible rodent species. This phenomenon is not believed to occur in humans, and no increases in human breast sarcomas have been observed. Epidemiological studies have not found elevated relative risks for breast cancer in women with implants. In fact, some of these studies, now evaluating women two decades or more after implantation, have found fewer breast cancers than expected, and some animal studies have suggested that breast implants might be associated with lower frequencies of breast cancer. The committee cannot find that evidence for a lower risk of breast cancer in women with breast implants is conclusive, but the committee does conclude that there is no increase in primary or recurrent breast cancer in these women.

Occasional reports of cancer occurring in the breasts of women injected with silicone for breast augmentation have been noted (see Chapter 1), but these are uncontrolled case reports or anecdotes, and do not constitute useful evidence of any carcinogenic effect of silicone in humans. Several cohort studies have examined the risk for all cancers combined in women with breast implants, and all have reported numbers of cases similar to or lower than the number expected based on rates in the general population. The committee concludes that evidence is lacking for a relationship of breast implants to any specific cancers.

Neurologic disease, symptoms, and pathological and physical findings have been reported in case series of women with breast implants by a few groups. Other investigators have not found neurological problems and have criticized the experimental design used in reports of such an association. Experimental animal studies do not lend support to silicone as a cause of neurologic disease. Some case reports describe silicone gel deposits that migrate from ruptured breast implants, causing scarring and constriction around peripheral nerves. However, reports that silicone might be associated with autoantibodies to nerve components, that silica might be present in the nerves of women with implants, or that multiple sclerosis-like or other neurologic syndromes might be associated with implants have been found to have design and methodological problems that limited any conclusions. Two epidemiological studies of neurologic disease in women with implants provide limited support for a conclusion that there is no elevated relative risk for any association, and the committee concludes that with the exception of local problems caused by the migration of gel from ruptured implants, evidence that silicone breast implants cause neurologic signs, symptoms, or disease is lacking or flawed.

In an overall consideration of the epidemiological evidence, the committee noted that because there are more than 1.5 million adult women of all ages in the United States with silicone breast implants, some of these women would be expected to develop connective tissue diseases, cancer, neurological diseases, or other systemic complaints or conditions. Evidence suggests that such diseases or conditions are no more common in women with breast implants than in women without implants.

A few investigators have proposed that women with silicone breast implants might transmit silicone or some immunological factor via breast milk or across the placenta to their children. There is limited evidence that implantation, especially through a periareolar incision, may interfere with lactation and breast feeding, but no differences are observed in milk or blood silicon (and thus presumably silicone) levels in lactating women with implants compared to lactating control women without implants. Much higher levels of silicon have been measured in cows' milk at the retail level and commercially available infant formula. It is likely that some of this silicon is organic. Infants are also exposed to other sources of silicone, for example, pacifiers, nipples, and widely available drops for colic. Antinuclear antibodies are reported in normal women without implants, and no untoward effects on their children have been observed. The committee can find no evidence of elevated silicone in breast milk or of any other substance that would be deleterious to infants. Because there is conclusive evidence that breast feeding is beneficial to infants, the committee strongly recommends a trial of breast feeding by mothers with implants.

A single group of investigators examined children at about 5 years of age who had been breast fed by mothers with implants and reported abnormalities of esophageal motility that they hypothesized might have been caused by exposure to silicone. These investigators did not carry out any silicon or silicone measurements in either the children or their mothers. A number of problems with the reports of this group have been identified, and an epidemiological study of esophageal disease in the children of mothers with implants found no elevated relative risk for esophageal disease. As noted, breast milk silicon concentrations in implanted women are normal. Also, an experimental animal study found no esophageal silicone or abnormalities in rat pups breast-fed by mothers with silicone implants, and toxicological studies of the reproductive and teratologic effects of silicone (PDMS) reviewed in Chapter 4 were negative. The committee concludes that evidence for health effects in children related to maternal breast implants is insufficient or flawed.

Breast implants interfere with diagnostic and screening imaging examinations of the breast by compressing and distorting breast tissue, by making compression of the breast in a mammographic examination difficult and obligating special views, and by interposing (particularly with gel-filled implants) a radiopaque mass in the middle of the breast that obscures some breast tissue. These problems are fewer with submuscular placement of the implant and can be at least partially overcome with special views. Data on whether cancer detection is impaired by implants do not allow definite conclusions, but no studies have shown increases in cancer mortality in women with implants because of diagnostic delays. Mammographic screening for cancer in women with implants under the same conditions as recommended for women without implants should be encouraged. The imaging techniques described in Chapter 12 have varying sensitivities and specificities for the diagnosis of implant rupture and varying advantages or disadvantages. Magnetic resonance imaging is the most sensitive and specific technology for rupture diagnosis. The committee did not find direct evidence on the cost/benefit of screening for rupture, however. Relevant screening data and analysis might allow a firmer conclusion on screening in general or in women with implants with known high prevalence of rupture or in other specific circumstances. Only if such data showed reduced morbidity as a result of screening and a screening driven intervention, would routine screening of the general population of asymptomatic women with breast implants be justified.

Appendix A describes a scientific workshop sponsored by the IOM to bring presentations and discussions of the work and experiences of academic, governmental, and industry physicians and scientists to the committee. Appendix B describes a public meeting sponsored by the Institute of Medicine primarily to hear the experiences of women with breast implants, although other interested parties spoke as well. Appendix C reviews two recent important, related reports from the Independent Review Group of the United Kingdom and the National Science Panel appointed by the judge for the U.S. multidistrict litigation.

CONCLUSIONS AND RESEARCH RECOMMENDATIONS

The committee wishes to highlight the following conclusions from this Summary:

- There is extensive presence of, and wide exposure of citizens of developed countries to silicones in foods, cosmetics, lubricants for machinery, hypodermic syringes and other products, insulators and a wide array of consumer products.
- The committee concludes that a review of the toxicology studies of silicones and other substances known to be in breast implants does not provide a basis for health concerns.

The committee has reached three major conclusions regarding local and perioperative complications. First, reoperations and local and perioperative complications are frequent enough to be a cause for concern and to justify the conclusion that they are the primary safety issue with silicone breast implants. Complications may have risks themselves, such as pain, disfigurement and serious infection and they may lead to medical and surgical interventions, such as reoperations, that have risks. Second, risks accumulate over the lifetime of the implant, but quantitative data on this point are lacking for modern implants and deficient historically. Third, information concerning the nature and the relatively high frequency of local complications and reoperations is an essential element of adequate informed consent for women undergoing breast implantation.

The committee has also come to the following conclusions:

- Studies addressing the immunology of silicones are limited and technical problems substantial, providing the committee with no support for an immunologic role of silicone.
- A novel syndrome or disease associated with silicone breast im-

plants has been proposed by a small group of physicians. Evidence for this proposed disease rests on case reports and is insufficient and flawed. The disease definition includes, as a precondition, the presence of silicone gel breast implants, so it cannot be studied as an independent health problem. The committee finds that the diagnosis of this condition could depend on the presence of a number of symptoms that are nonspecific and common in the general population. Thus, there does not appear to be even suggestive evidence of a novel syndrome in women with breast implants. In fact, epidemiological evidence suggests that there is no novel syndrome.

- There is no increase in primary or recurrent breast cancer in implanted women.
- In an overall consideration of the epidemiological evidence, the committee noted that because there are more than 1.5 million adult women of all ages in the United States with silicone breast implants, some of these women would be expected to develop connective tissue diseases, cancer, neurological diseases or other systemic complaints or conditions. Evidence suggests that such diseases or conditions are no more common in women with breast implants than in women without implants.
- The committee finds no evidence of elevated silicone in breast milk or any other substance that would be deleterious to infants; the committee strongly concludes that all mothers with implants should attempt breast feeding.
- The committee concludes that evidence for health effects in children related to maternal breast implants is insufficient or flawed.

RECOMMENDATIONS FOR RESEARCH

1. Reliable techniques for the measuring of silicone concentrations in body fluids and tissues are needed to provide established, agreed-upon values and ranges of silicone concentrations in body fluids and tissues with or without exposure to silicone from an implanted medical device. Such developments could improve the study of silicones and silicone distribution in humans, could help with regulatory requirements, and might in some circumstances resolve questions by providing quantitative data on the presence or absence of silicones.
2. Ongoing surveillance of recipients of silicone breast implants should be carried out for representative groups of women, including long-term outcomes and local complications, with attention to, or definition of the following:

- implant physical and chemical characteristics,
- tracking identified individual implants,

• using appropriate, standardized, and validated technologies for detecting and defining outcomes,

• carrying out associated toxicology studies by standards consistent with accepted toxicological standards for other devices; and

• ensuring representative samples, appropriate controls and randomization in any specific studies, as required by good experimental design.

3. The development of a national model of informed consent for women undergoing breast implantation should be encouraged, and the continuing effectiveness of such a model should be monitored.

1

Introduction

LEGISLATIVE AND EXECUTIVE BRANCH HISTORY OF THIS REPORT

House Report 104-659 accompanying the Labor, Health and Human Services, and Education and Related Agencies Appropriations Bill of 1997 expressed concern "with the fragmentation of research on the safety of silicone breast implants and the relationship, or lack thereof, between silicone gel breast implants and connective tissue disease, classic autoimmune symptoms and other serious diseases." The Appropriations Committee believed an independent study was needed and instructed the Department of Health and Human Services (DHHS) "to enter into a contract with the Institute of Medicine of the National Academy of Sciences to conduct a general review of past and ongoing research on silicone breast implants." Departmental involvement in this controversial subject stretched back over more than a decade and involved a significant number of organizational units. Prominent among these were the Food and Drug Administration (FDA), the Centers for Disease Control and Prevention (CDC), and several institutes of the National Institutes of Health (NIH). Important meetings of the FDA General and Plastic Surgery Devices Panel, other meetings and workshops under the auspices of NIH, and studies and notices from CDC had informed and advanced the regulation and science of silicone breast implants. Nevertheless, the regulatory process had not come to a satisfactory conclusion nor had the many scientific questions been resolved. Although this Institute of Medicine

(IOM) report is not about the legal issues; all involved are aware that a vigorous struggle has been taking place in American courts. This struggle, involving major U.S. corporations and hundreds of thousands of breast implant patients with billions of dollars at stake, could not fail to be an important influence on silicone breast implant-related activities and how they were perceived by Congress.

EARLY HISTORY OF THE INSTITUTE OF MEDICINE STUDY

Within this context, DHHS approached the IOM in the summer of 1997 to discuss a study of the scientific issues. The National Institute of Arthritis and Musculoskeletal and Skin Disease (NIAMS) was designated the lead agency, although funds were committed from a number of other departmental sources, including the Office of Women's Health at the FDA, the Office of Research on Women's Health at NIH, the National Cancer Institute, the National Institute of Allergy and Infectious Diseases, the Office of Women's Health at the CDC, and the Office of the Assistant Secretary for Planning and Evaluation and Office of Public Health and Science at DHHS. The original proposal contemplated a study of modest funding which would begin in October 1997 and would deliver a prepublication report to the sponsor in November 1998. As the magnitude of this project became clear to the IOM, its Committee on the Safety of Silicone Breast Implants and the sponsors, the proposal was later expanded to roughly double the financial support and to extend the delivery date to July 1999. At no time did the IOM receive other than DHHS funds in support of this study.

The scope of this study was defined in the contract with NIAMS and further refined in an address by NIAMS Director Stephen I. Katz to the committee on the occasion of its first meeting in April 1998. Important contractual items included a scientific workshop, held on July 22, 1998, which provided the committee with information on a number of scientific matters from researchers in the federal government and academia and offered former and current major silicone breast implant manufacturers—Dow Corning, Mentor, and McGhan—an opportunity to present data from clinical observational and other research studies. Also included was a public meeting held on July 24, 1998, at which more than 60 women formerly or currently with silicone breast implants, professional association representatives, scientists of all perspectives, consumer group representatives, and others addressed the committee. In addition, the committee was asked to comment on other important reports that became available during the time of its deliberations, specifically those of the United Kingdom's Independent Review Group and the multidistrict-litigation (MDL) National Science Panel.

This report is a general review of past and ongoing research on silicone breast implants, including (1) what associations between breast implants and various diseases, if any, are suggested by existing experimental, clinical, and epidemiological studies; (2) the nature and relative strength of these associations, (3) the quality of the studies; (4) the existence of plausible biological mechanisms to explain suggested associations between breast implants and disease; (5) the uncertainties associated with these kinds of analyses; and (6) suggestions for future research to fill in critical gaps. This report covers breast implants with a silicone shell, whether smooth, modified, or coated, and a gel or saline filler; local and systemic complications and manifestations of disease; and effects on mammographic screening and diagnosis and on the offspring of patients with breasts implants. In summarizing the purpose of the study at the committee's first meeting, Dr. Katz noted that it should be "a comprehensive survey and rigorous assessment of the scientific literature and scientific works related to the biological and health-related effects of silicone breast implants and their components. While the emphasis is on safety, we hope that areas of gaps in knowledge as well as scientific opportunity for future research will be identified." Such a report would serve as a resource for scientists and an educational tool for the public. It would also serve NIH and other components of DHHS as they develop policy and plan future research and prevention activities.

THE IOM COMMITTEE ON THE SAFETY OF SILICONE BREAST IMPLANTS

The Committee on the Safety of Silicone Breast Implants was assembled by the IOM to include expertise in preventive and internal medicine, nursing, family and women's health, rheumatology, clinical and basic research, epidemiology, immunology, neurology, silicone chemistry, toxicology, breast and other cancer, plastic surgery, and radiology or mammography. Committee members are listed at the front of this report. Because of the often polarized and controversial nature of the many issues involved, the IOM took active steps to avoid conflict of interest in constituting the committee in accordance with the Institute's rigorous bias and conflicts of interest procedures. Given the importance of the subject matter to women's health, it was desirable that women make up a substantial portion of the committee. Six of its thirteen members, including the vice chair, are women, and most of them are particularly interested in women's health issues. The committee's medical experts in breast cancer, rheumatology, radiology, and family medicine have, in the course of their practice, provided medical care to women who may have had breast implants in addition to their cancer, rheumatologic problems, mammography, or general health care needs. These experiences were deemed valuable. The committee's plastic surgery expert, on the other hand, does not perform breast implant surgery in her practice of pediatric plastic surgery.

In addition to the first committee meeting in April and the scientific workshop and public meeting (summarized in the appendixes), the committee had five days in three separate meetings to discuss and review the issues together over the course of the 15 months between its selection and the delivery of this report. During this time, with help from IOM staff and an immunological and toxicological consultant, members of the committee spent many additional days, individually and as a group, reviewing the studies listed in the references, discussing and evaluating the evidence, and preparing this report. The committee also accepted all offers of information that could be made public and received material and assistance from a number of individuals, companies, attorneys, associations, and organizations. The committee acknowledges this assistance with gratitude.

COLLECTION AND EVALUATION OF EVIDENCE

Since anecdote and isolated personal experience cannot, in themselves, be subject to scientific review (although they can provide a basis for the design of scientific studies), the committee decided to focus on evidence reported in the peer-reviewed, published scientific literature. A great deal of information was also provided by breast implant patients, manufacturers, involved scientists, and others, in the form of industry technical reports, prepublications, medical histories, and private or personal submissions of various kinds. The IOM, as a nongovernment entity carrying out an independent review, is generally not in a position to accept and preserve confidential business or personal information; the information presented to the committee is made available to the public. The committee recognized the selectivity involved, but was open to the receipt of such material nevertheless. Many of these items are included in the reference list and comprise a useful resource. However, the committee did not consider them of equal weight to the peer-reviewed literature, and an attempt has made to divide the reference list into two sections to recognize peer reviewed scientific literature and other informational material. About 80% of the almost 1,200 references cited in the text of this report are from the first, peer-reviewed list. The references in the second list were considered useful but clearly less so than those in the first or primary list.

Because this project involved the assessment of a large number of scientific studies, the committee reviewed ways in which these reports

BOX 1-1
Austin Bradford Hill Criteria for Determining Association as Causation

1. Strength of the association between an exposure and illness (e.g., relative risk)
2. Consistency of the association observed by different people, under different circumstances, in different ways
3. Specificity of the association: it uniquely affects certain people with certain illnesses
4. Temporality of the association: the exposure precedes the illness
5. Biological gradient: the frequency and severity of the illness are directly related to the frequency and severity of the exposure
6. Plausibility of the association in terms of the biological reasonableness
7. Coherence of the association with other knowledge of the exposure and the illness
8. Experimentation: manipulation of the exposure affects the illness
9. Analogy: the association is analogous to another known associations

and their data might be evaluated and ranked. When appropriate in reviewing epidemiological studies, the grading of evidence suggested by the U.S. Preventive Services Task Force—from well-designed, properly randomized clinical trials; to nonrandomized controlled trials; to well-designed cohort or case control studies; to multiple time series with or without the intervention; to expert opinion—was considered reasonable if an appropriate epidemiological set was being reviewed. Some suggestions from the Agency for Health Care Policy and Research (AHCPR)—for example, giving most weight to conclusions supported by multiple relevant and high-quality scientific studies and lesser weight to those based on fewer and lower-quality studies, were considered. Sir Austin Bradford Hill proposed criteria for evaluating relationships between sickness and environmental conditions (see Box 1-1) that were also useful (Hill, 1965).

The committee also considered oral and written communications that recorded many women's individual medical histories and experiences with breast implants. Although individual reports of personal experiences cannot be confirmed and are anecdotal and therefore not scientifically definitive, this human element, which is after all a part of medical care and medical science, provided an important context to the committee's deliberations.

A review of the reference lists at the end of this report indicates that much of the literature available to and considered relevant by the committee, did not consist of full, peer-reviewed, published scientific reports but was in the form of letters, position papers, abstracts, industry reports, and opinion pieces; these are found in the second of the two reference lists. Furthermore, review of the first reference list indicates that some of this material, although in peer-reviewed scientific publications, consisted of case reports, reviews, and other forms that the committee did not consider strong evidence. Case reports or case series reports are often essentially anecdotes or uncontrolled observational studies, which, lacking appropriate comparison or control groups, may not be helpful in determining rates of occurrence or accepting or rejecting causation. Controlled observational studies—that is, studies based on a cohort or case control design—offer stronger evidence because they provide information on relative risks or rates. Some controlled clinical trials were found by the committee, and this very strong kind of evidence was useful when available. In all of these studies, the committee was aware of the importance of randomization, that is, the assembly of unbiased, representative study groups (Stratton et al., 1994).

In summary, the committee found it useful to consider the varying strength and quality of the evidence. Although some reports had design limitations or problems in implementation, other excellent reports were available, and the committee has tried to point out the strengths and weakness of various studies in this report. Overall, the committee was impressed with the substantial amount of useful information and, in particular, with the marked improvement in the 1990s in the quantity and quality of studies relevant to its charge. A number of strong, well-designed epidemiological studies involving large numbers of women and clear results have been published since the early 1990s. These have allowed the committee to take firm conclusions on many of the important issues. To communicate this firmness, the committee adopted a ranking of evidence or data as: conclusive or convincing of an association or of no association; limited or suggestive of an association or of no association; or, in the committee's judgment, insufficient, flawed in terms of methodology, or lacking in support of the various evaluations of the safety of silicone breast implants. The modifiers in the last group were used to indicate that when evidence for an association or for no association was not conclusive or suggestive, it could fail to support a conclusion because it was: a.) insufficient in quality or quantity; b.) not perceived to present helpful evidence because the committee noted methodological flaws; or c.) simply lacking or absent. On occasion, evidence failed to support a proposed conclusion of an association because it supported a conclusion of *no association*; these circumstances were expressed more explicitly by simply noting that the evidence supported some other conclusion, not the proposed conclusion. These rankings allowed the committee to take many firm decisions. They are not meant to imply, as some might, that the committee means to support further research or studies, for example, when data are insufficient. If more information and analysis would be desirable, and only in such instances, the committee has indicated this in the text of this report.

COSMETIC BREAST SURGERY AND THE HISTORICAL CONTEXT OF THIS REPORT

Perspectives of Women with Breast Implants

Although estimates of the current number of U.S. women who have had breast implants vary, it is probably somewhere between 1.5 million and 2 million, as discussed later in this chapter. Many of these women have reported symptoms that they believe are associated with their breast implants. The symptoms reported involve many organ systems and bodily functions and are often associated with a compromised quality of life. The concerns of these women and their loved ones were a major factor leading to this IOM review. Women with breast implants as well as their spouses and children spoke to the committee. They advised that this is more than "a women's issue, but one that affects husbands, families, taxpayers and society." Some related how they were "young and vibrant" and are now ill and disabled. They reported feeling scorned and patronized or ignored as they searched for medical solutions. In many instances they did not think they had been informed of known complications. They were frequently told that the implants "would last a lifetime," but instead had experienced complications and repeated surgeries with associated pain and expense (see Appendix B).

Case reports from individual women can be used to generate hypotheses about disease and symptoms that may be associated with silicone breast implants. Whether such symptoms are causally associated with breast implants will be determined by comparing the occurrence of symptoms in women with implants and without implants and meeting other conditions for determining causality. Nevertheless, it was the burden of the personal vignettes that prompted the IOM to invite women with implants, as well as health care providers, scientists, and other interested parties, to make formal presentations to the committee and to submit written comments for the committee's deliberations (see appendixes). The committee heard from individual women about their experiences with both breast augmentation and breast reconstruction, and from representatives of many patient groups from throughout the United States. Their written statements were distributed to all committee members and also made available to the public.

Committee members were impressed by the thoughtful and detailed comments provided by women with implants, not only for the sake of their own health but also out of concern for other women who are considering breast implants. Many women support the continued availability of breast implants for those who want them for either augmentation or reconstruction, with the proviso that adequate information regarding potential complications and long-term safety is available to them for informed decision making. The commitment of these women to the scientific process and to partnering with scientists in future studies was clear and very much appreciated by committee members. Although the committee's mandate focuses primarily on peer-reviewed scientific evidence, the contributions of women with breast implants provided an extremely valuable context for its deliberations.

History of Cosmetic Breast Surgery

To varying degrees, people are concerned about the appearance of their bodies, and cosmetic surgery is a response to such concern. In a recent discussion of this, Sarwer et al. (1998a) noted that 34% of U.S. women were dissatisfied with their breasts, and more than half of breast augmentation patients reported having frequently checked the appearance of their breasts and camouflaging them. The literature also describes surgical interventions and the results of efforts to change natural breast dimensions over at least the past hundred years. Augmentation with modern silicone implants can variably affect the shape and size of the female breast; on average, an increase of two brassiere sizes (cup or cup and chest circumference; circumference increases in 1 inch or 2.5 cm increments) is achieved (Young et al., 1994).

Reconstruction after mastectomy for cancer, fibrocystic disease, or other reasons such as prevention in women at high risk for breast cancer is believed to provide a sense of having overcome disease (Bard and Sutherland, 1955). Especially when performed soon after mastectomy, breast reconstruction is reported to relieve or prevent a perception of loss, dissatisfaction with an external prosthesis, depression, and feelings of diminished sexual attractiveness (Schain et al., 1985; Stevens et al., 1984).

These powerful motivations may explain the continuing acceptance by many women and health professionals of evolving cosmetic surgical breast procedures despite complications, high incidence of hardness, and often globular or otherwise less than natural-looking breasts.

Autogenous Tissue

The modern history of cosmetic breast surgery began in the late 1800s. It has involved the use of both autogenous tissue (which is not the subject of this report) and alloplastic implants, culminating in the variously filled silicone shell implants for augmentation and reconstruction, which constitute the subject of this report. The use of autogenous tissue is reported to have begun in 1887 with part of a healthy breast transferred on a pedicle to reconstruct the other breast (Verneuil, 1887) and continued in 1895 with the transplantation of a lipoma from the hip to repair a surgical defect in the breast (Czerny, 1895). A pectoral muscle flap for immediate reconstruction and a latissimus dorsi flap were described shortly thereafter (Ombredanne, 1906; Tansini, 1906). Since transfer of fat alone is usually unsuccessful (Hinderer and Escalona, 1990) because it is substantially reabsorbed unless injected in quite small quantities (Bircoll and Novack, 1987), efforts continued with pedicle or dermis flaps or dermis–fat–fascia grafts (Bames, 1950, 1953; Berson, 1944; Watson, 1959). These early efforts were reviewed by Watson (1976) who described the tendency to long-term shrinkage of the dermis-fat grafts. Continued development culminated in musculocutaneous flaps, primarily from the abdomen (transverse rectus abdominis musculocutaneous [TRAM] flaps) but also from other sites (e.g., the latissimus dorsi or superior and inferior gluteus muscles, among others), and microsurgical free flaps. These events were reviewed in Kincaid (1984) in a chronological listing of surgical advances with citations to the literature and in 1995 by Wickman. About one-third of modern breast reconstructions are performed using autogenous tissue. Such reconstructions are performed more and more frequently and are often combined with implants (ASPRS, 1996, 1997; Trabulsy et al., 1994).

Alloplastic Implants

Also since the late 1800s, foreign substances have been injected or implanted to augment or reconstruct the breast, although sporadic efforts of this kind apparently date back centuries. Gersuny reported experimentation with paraffin injections beginning in 1889 (Gersuny, 1900). Although paraffin enjoyed some early acceptance, others later described disastrous results such as fistulas, granulomas, pulmonary emboli, and tissue necrosis (Letterman and Schurter, 1978). Subsequently, in the early to mid-1900s, a number of other substances were tried, including ivory, glass balls, ground rubber, ox cartilage, Terylene wool, gutta percha, Dicora, polyethylene chips, polyvinyl alcohol–formaldehyde polymer sponge (Ivalon), Ivalon in a polyethylene sac, polyether foam sponge (Etheron), polyethylene tape (Polystan) or strips wound into a ball, polyester (polyurethane foam sponge) Silastic rubber, and teflon–silicone prostheses (Broadbent and Woolf, 1967; Brown et al., 1960a,b; Edgerton et al., 1961; Edwards, 1963; Letterman and Schurter, 1978; Lewis, 1965; Lilla and Vistnes, 1976; Liu and Truong, 1996; Smahel et al., 1977). These early implants were unsuccessful and were not pursued seriously. The later efforts with so-called open-pore polymer sponge implants such as Ivalon or Etheron led to hard, unnatural-looking breasts and other complications (Broadbent and Woolf, 1967). Thousands of women had these implants, which made up about a third of implantations in the 1960s according to one large international survey (De Cholnoky, 1970).

Injections

During the decades after the Second World War an array of liquid substances were injected, often illegally by unlicensed practitioners, to augment the breast (and other sites; see e.g., Christ and Askew, 1982). These are cited in reports from Japan, the Far East, and domestic plastic surgeons. They include paraffin; other poorly defined, more radiolucent hydrocarbons called "Organogen" and "Bioplaxm" (Yamazaki et al., 1977) and some forms of petroleum jelly such as Vaseline (Ohtake et al., 1989). Adulterated silicone oil (e.g., the "Sakurai" formula) was also commonly used. It was believed to have been adulterated with 1% ricinoleic acid (Pearl et al., 1978); 1% animal and vegetable fatty acids (Kagan, 1963); or 1% mineral and vegetable (perhaps castor) oil (Chaplin, 1969), 1% olive oil (Tinkler et al., 1993), or to contain croton oil, peanut oil, concentrated vitamin D, snake venom, talc and paraffins (Kopf, 1966; Rapaport et al., 1996). Use of a variety of unknown oils has been reported, some with silicone of mostly unknown origins (Ortiz-Monasterio et al., 1972), as well as beeswax, shellac, glaziers' putty, epoxy resin (Symmers, 1968), and industrial silicone fluids. Medical-grade silicone fluid, including Dow Corning 200, 350, and MDX 44011 (Ashley et al., 1967); silicone (Elicon-Kogen Kogyo Co. Ltd.) gel (Boo-Chai, 1969); and silicone Silastic S-5392 RTV (room temperature vulcanized) fluid with a stannous octoate catalyst to form a silicone rubber within the breast tissue were also used for breast augmentation and other plastic surgical purposes with positive early reports (Ashley et al., 1967; Conway and Goulian, 1963; Freeman et al., 1966; Harris, 1965). Substantial amounts of these substances were injected on occasion, as much as 2 liters for breast augmentation and body contouring in a single patient (Kagan, 1963) or half a liter of fluid and catalyst per breast (Conway and Goulian, 1963).

Results with other than medical-grade silicone were poor, and included loss of both breasts and death (see references below). Dow Corning Medical Grade 360 fluid, which according to Vinnik (1991) was used extensively in Las Vegas, also resulted in complications, but the silicone mentioned in many reports was undoubtedly adulterated in the misguided hope that an adulterant would inhibit fluid migration and give better results. Sakurai personally reported 72,648 cases injected, including the breast among other sites (Kagan, 1963). At least 12,000 women (some have estimated as many as 40,000 women) had breast injections in Las Vegas by 1976 when the practice became a felony under Nevada State law. Practitioners reportedly charged $800 to $2,000 for a series of injections in 1966 (Kopf, 1966; Kopf et al., 1976; Vinnik, 1991), and domestic reports continue from there and elsewhere (Leibman and Sybers, 1994; Morgenstern et al., 1985; Sánchez-Guerrero et al., 1995a,b).

Soft-tissue (excluding breast) augmentation by injection with medical-grade silicone was approved for experimental use in the United States under an FDA investigational new drug (IND) exemption to Dow Corning for use by six, and later seven, plastic surgeons and one dermatologist for about a decade, 1965–1975 (Ashley et al., 1967; Braley, 1971; Wustrack and Zarem, 1979). Although this material broke up into "innumerable droplets" on injection and tended to spread out from the injection site, results appeared promising at first (Ashley et al., 1965; Rees et al., 1970). After a few to as many as 28 years, however, problems began to appear (Rapaport et al., 1996). As with paraffin earlier, initial enthusiasm was tempered by the appearance of complications. The question of systemic effects is discussed in Chapter 8 of this report. Among the more clear-cut effects associated with silicone breast injection (as noted, not an FDA-approved use as part of the Dow Corning IND) have been pain, skin discoloration, edema, ulceration and necrosis, calcification, granulomas, migration of the fluid, infection, cysts, axillary adenopathy, disfigurement and loss of the breast, liver granulomas and dysfunction, acute pneumonitis or adult respiratory distress syndrome, pulmonary embolism, coma, and death (Baker, 1992; Boo-Chai, 1969; Brozena et al., 1988; Celli et al., 1978; Chastre et al., 1983a, 1987; Chen, 1995; Chen et al., 1993; Cruz et al., 1985; Edgerton and Wells, 1976; Ellenbogen and Rubin, 1975; Inoue et al., 1983; Ko et al., 1995; Koide and Katayama, 1979; Lai et al., 1994; McCurdy and Solomons, 1977; Parsons and Thering, 1977; Perry et al., 1985; Piechotta, 1979; Rodriguez et al., 1989; Solomons and Jones, 1975; Symmers, 1968; Truong et al., 1988; Vinnik, 1978; Winer et al., 1964). Some of these complications occurred instantly, such as acute pneumonitis with findings of substantial deposition of silicone in the lung, which was probably due to pulmonary embolism from inadvertent intravenous injection or other circulatory access of the silicone fluid (Solomons and Jones, 1975). More often, complications were noticed after a few years. Various reports cited a complication rate of 1% of patients per year (Kopf et al., 1976), a prevalence of 50% at five years after injection (Vinnik, 1976a,b), the onset of disturbing problems at two or three to five or six years (Ohtake et al., 1989; Wustrack and Zarem, 1979), or the average occurrence of problems at about nine years (Parsons and Thering, 1977). Presumably because medical-grade silicone is a "mild irritant" as opposed to adulterated silicone or other substances, which are irritating to a greater extent, complications were noted in one study only after many years and differed according to individual patient reactions (Rapaport et al., 1996). Other surgeons reported complications after considerable delay, and these tended to be relentlessly progressive (Wustrack and Zarem, 1979). One author noted that "trying to provide an accurate timetable for these changes has proved futile" (Vinnik, 1978).

There are only anecdotal reports of breast malignancy in silicone-injected breasts (Ko et al., 1995; Kobayashi et al., 1988; Lewis, 1980; Maddox et al., 1993; Morgenstern et al., 1985; Okubo et al., 1992; Ortiz-Monasterio and Trigos, 1972; Pennisi, 1984; Smith et al., 1999; Suster et al., 1987; Talmor et al., 1995; Timberlake and Looney, 1986; see also Chapter 9 of this report). Although no epidemiological studies of the incidence of cancer in women with silicone-injected breasts have been reported, and thus there is no evidence of an elevated relative risk, case control studies of the frequency of breast implants in women with breast cancer indicate, if anything, a decreased odds ratio (Brinton et al., 1996; Glasser et al., 1989). Injected silicone clearly may handicap the diagnosis of breast cancer. Injected breasts are full of lumpy, radiopaque deposits of silicone that interfere with breast self-examination, physical examination, and mammography. Better visualization with magnetic resonance imaging (MRI) is helpful, but does not resolve this problem because MRI is not considered a screening technology and is used only when there is an indication for this more resource intensive modality (Helbich et al., 1997; Leibman and Sybers, 1994; Lewis, 1980; Maddox et al., 1993; Morgenstern et al., 1985; Okubo et al., 1992; Talmor et al., 1995; Timberlake and Looney, 1986; see Chapter 12). Although silicone injection for breast augmentation (or any cosmetic use) is not approved by the FDA, there are a number of reports advocating medical-grade silicone injection in other sites such as the face, using careful technique and small amounts—from a fraction of a milliliter to a few milliliters per treatment depending on location (Ashley et al., 1973; Hinderer and Escalona, 1990; Rees and Ashley, 1966; Rees et al., 1973a; Selmanowitz and Orentreich, 1977). Duffy (1990) reviewed thousands of such cases and himself reported more than 2,000 injections of 350-centistoke silicone fluid with good results, although his follow-up was limited to six years. The American Academy of Cosmetic Surgery (AACS) reported 7,170 women receiving such non-breast silicone injections from its members in 1994. Nevertheless, "FDA has not approved the marketing of liquid silicone for injection for any cosmetic purpose, including the treatment of facial defects or wrinkles…" (FDA, 1991). The history of silicone injection is relevant to the safety of silicone breast implants because of the possible analogy to silicone gel fluid diffusion through implant shells into breast tissue or the deposition of silicone gel (and gel fluid) in the breast on rupture of gel-filled implants.

SILICONE IMPLANTS

A successful silicone (urethral) implantation was reported in 1950 (De Nicola, 1950); subsequently silicone use for shunts and joints was proposed (Marzoni et al., 1959), and many such shunts, joints, and other devices were developed and used in medical practice. These clinical experiences, animal experiments, and early work on tissue reaction to silicone (Child et al., 1951; Kern et al., 1949; Rees and Ashley, 1966; Rowe et al., 1948; see also Chapter 4) provided a context and encouragement for the consideration of this technology in cosmetic breast surgery. The disappointing results with other technologies for breast augmentation or reconstruction provided an opportunity and an unmet need. The response to this need was the introduction of the silicone breast implant in 1962 and its continued development through the 1990s, as described in Chapter 3. The specific experimental basis for the clinical introduction of this device was the work reported by Cronin and Gerow (1963) on implantation of silicone shells (four to six per animal) filled with either dextran or electrolyte solution in each of 12 dogs for periods of a few days to 18 months without signs of toxicity or other complications.

Silicone Implants and Patient Satisfaction—Its Importance and Effect on Demand

Although the silicone implant was considered an improvement, it was not problem-free. Some implant complications such as small areas of epidermolysis or necrosis and small, isolated seromas are minor, although they might require medical attention; other complications, infections, implant ruptures, and severe fibrous capsule contractures are of greater import. Complications are less frequent in augmentation than in reconstruction, but as noted in Chapter 5, they still occur with considerable frequency. The more serious risks of reconstruction with implants, especially immediate reconstruction (Spear and Majidian, 1998), must be balanced against the psychological benefits (Stevens et al., 1984; Wellisch et al., 1985). Implants for augmentation are placed in healthy women who would otherwise not be operated on and incur such risks. Placement of a breast implant for either augmentation or reconstruction does not treat the physical component of human disease or disordered physiology. It is, in this sense, elective and therefore warranted only if it is relatively safe and provides patient satisfaction.

Satisfaction has an effect on the demand for interventions to manage or relieve complications and thus on the implications of complications for the safety of silicone breast implants. The high overall level of satisfaction of women in medical reports, if accurate and lasting, implies a low level of concern or at least a willingness to tolerate some complications. This may have an important moderating effect on the reported incidence of further operative or medical interventions. The committee believes that published reports of satisfaction may be misleading, however. Most surveys of satisfaction are carried out by plastic surgeons or others associated with the surgery or care of women with implants. This arguably introduces a possible bias or distortion of patients' responses.

Long-term satisfaction is an important test of the aesthetic results of cosmetic surgery. Many surveys were carried out immediately or shortly after surgery, and the degree of satisfaction may change with time and the occurrence of untoward events. Some surveys include small numbers of women and lack precise details on procedure, type of implant, timing, or other factors that might be important to results. Finally, almost all of these reports are based on women communicating an overall satisfaction level in general terms. Women may have specific problems or suffer from a particular dissatisfying aspect of the results of implantation; this may not be expressed clearly or at all in a report that focuses on satisfaction in a general way and not on problems.

When women with complications requiring secondary surgery such as deflation, contracture, and asymmetry ($N = 58$) from a large cohort ($N = 292$) surveyed by Strom et al. (1997) were compared with those who did not require additional surgery ($N = 234$), there was no significant difference in reporting of satisfaction on the Likert 1–5 scale. This may be because the end result was important enough to these women that they were prepared to put up with inconvenience and discomfort. Similarly, the Karolinska group (Sweden) has consistently found that, up to seven years after surgery, women were satisfied with, or tolerant of, severe (Class III or IV; see breast augmentation classification in Appendix D) implant capsular contractures. In 1989, this group found that 77% of women in its operative series were satisfied, although 79% had Class III or IV contractures. In 1990, the same group reported that 85% of women were satisfied, although 35% had severe contractures (Gylbert et al., 1989 and 1990a). In other instances, women may prefer a complication, such as Class III contractures with smooth shell implants, to the more ready detection by palpation of a textured implant even though such an implant produces a softer breast (Burkhardt and Demas, 1994). This could be a significant factor since 30% of submuscular textured saline and 47% of gel implants have been reported to be readily detected by palpation (Opitz and Young, 1998). In a study comparing women with submuscular and submammary (see definition in Appendix D) implants, patient satisfaction was not always proportional to the severity of contracture (Mahler and Hauben, 1981). Other surveys, however, have found substantial differences in satisfaction when women had significant contractures and waning satisfaction over time due perhaps to the accumulation of complications (Beale et al., 1985; Fiala et al., 1993).

In the group of 100 women implanted by van Heerden et al. (1987) 85% would recommend implant reconstruction to other women, and 73% rated it 6–10 on a scale of 1–10 (32 women rated it a 10). However, this questionnaire was administered by the operating service during the postoperative period. Spear and Majidian (1998) asked patients to express their degree of satisfaction, and 98% of 42 consecutive women rated themselves somewhat to completely satisfied with their breast implants. Again, this rating was carried out by the operating team, presumably shortly after surgery. A survey by Francel et al. (1993) of 197 implant reconstruction patients, with a 50% response rate, found that 100% of women who had been reconstructed immediately would try it again and 90% of them were satisfied. Of women who had undergone delayed reconstruction with implants, 90% would try it again and 80% were satisfied. This is another example of a survey performed by the surgical group after an unspecified, but clearly short, postoperative interval.

In a questionnaire administered by the medical team to an unspecified subset of 216 women who underwent implant and autologous reconstructions, results of autologous tissue ranked significantly better (Eberlein et al., 1993). Better cosmetic results of autologous compared to alloplastic reconstruction were also reported in the small survey by Mansel et al. (1986). In 1991, a survey by the Van Nuys Breast Center (Handel et al., 1993a) of patients augmented with polyurethane and other gel implants over the previous 12 years generated only a 32% (85 out of 321 patients) response rate. Of these, 66% were satisfied before exposure to negative publicity about breast implants and 61% after such exposure. The authors of this report felt that satisfaction was related inversely to complication rates (Handel et al., 1993a). In another study of 174 women who had double-lumen implants for breast reconstruction, 68% were satisfied or completely satisfied when rating postoperatively. After the occurrence of additional complications several years later, satisfaction waned (Fee-Fulkerson et al., 1996). In 1990, a survey by the American Society of Plastic and Reconstructive Surgeons (ASPRS) of representative U.S. households and a group of women from a medical devices registry found 93% of 592 responding women satisfied with the results of breast surgery and 82% prepared to undergo it again (ASPRS, 1990; Iverson, 1990), Park et al. (1996a) reported 84% of augmented women satisfied to very satisfied, as were 91% of implant-reconstructed women in a survey carried out at least one to ten years postoperatively by plastic surgeons.

Very high satisfaction rates (88%–96%) were reported by Hetter (1979, 1991) from a questionnaire of 165 women (a response rate of 69% of the series) augmented with gel and saline implants. Of 100 women with silicone implants for reconstruction who were interviewed by a plastic surgeon other than the operating surgeon, 96% reported that the reconstruction was important to them (Asplund and Körloff , 1984). In a multicenter survey of 504 women, 93.8% of whom had saline-filled implants for augmentation, Gutowski et al. (1997) reported a 94.2% satisfaction rate. In a survey of 292 women from a cohort who were augmented with saline implants and followed up at an average of seven years, Strom et al. (1997) reported that 80.2% were very satisfied (rating 1 or 2 on a 5 point Likert scale). A group of 20 women augmented with submammary silicone gel-filled implants and their husbands were asked about psychosocial and sexual benefits. They reported 70%–75% favorable results (Mahler and Hauben, 1981).

Many other reports describe significant psychosocial benefits and improvement in life functioning after augmentation or reconstruction (e.g., Beale et al., 1985; Corsten et al., 1992; Dean et al., 1983; Goin and Goin, 1981, 1982; Goldberg et al., 1984; Hetter, 1979, 1991; Jonsson et al., 1984; Reaby et al., 1994; Schain et al., 1984; Sihm et al., 1978). If putting in breast implants can confer psychosocial benefit, the loss of them may, as might be expected, be detrimental to overall body satisfaction and appearance-related cognition (Walden et al., 1997). On the other hand, the removal of implants in women who fear silicone-related health problems, although sometimes reported to be helpful, was also reported in other studies (carried out at a time of adverse publicity about implants) to do little for psychological distress and symptoms of somatization, depression, and anxiety (Roberts et al., 1997; Svahn et al., 1996; Wells et al., 1995, 1997).

National Perspectives and FDA Data on Satisfaction

Merkatz et al. (1993) and Brown et al. (1998) provide descriptions of national data on satisfaction and adverse implant events. The committee notes that all these data are based on self-reported or unconfirmed reports. These also are numerator data only, that is, raw numbers of events reported to have occurred in a population or group of unknown size, which depending on the time may to an unknown extent be distorted by publicity of changing focus and intensity. Some events are overreported due to manufacturer and plastic surgeon concerns for compliance with reporting requirements and organized letter writing campaigns, whereas in other instances, personal considerations or lack of systematic follow-up may cause underreporting of adverse events. These reports cover a distinct minority of the 1 million to 1.5 million U.S. women with breast implants in the early 1990s. Although they constitute the only national source, and provide expanded details on patient satisfaction from a somewhat different perspective than the plastic surgery reports of high levels of satisfaction, they do not establish an increased frequency of any disease in women with implants except for the direct complications of surgery.

In a qualitative analysis of national experience with women's self-reports to the FDA during January 1992, Merkatz et al. (1993) noted that a distinct minority of women were dissatisfied with their implants, reporting both local complications such as rupture and contracture and disabling general health conditions. A further analysis of FDA adverse events reporting cited 94,120 mandatory (i.e., required by law from manufacturers and importers) adverse events reported from the end of 1984 through 1995, with a peak of 83, 069 in 1992–94 and a marked decrease in 1995. The majority of these reports cited local and perioperative complications, particularly contracture and implant rupture, except in 1992 when general health complaints were temporarily more common. Reporting of deaths ($N = 70$) was so poorly characterized that a definite diagnosis could not be made except in a few cases of cancer ($N = 8$), specific connective tissue disease ($N = 3$), and operative mortality ($N = 2$). As noted earlier, the events reported tended to vary with the level of national publicity. The FDA received 4,303 voluntary reports. Some of these were from women with implants who were described by Merkatz et al. (1993). These peaked in 1992–1994 and decreased markedly in 1995 (Brown et al., 1998). Early reports from 1973 through January 15, 1992, from the FDA Product Problem Reporting System, which were voluntary reports from consumers and health professionals, numbered 379 and were concerned primarily with pain and contractures. FDA and National Cancer Institute (NCI) staff with some collaborators reported a follow-up in 1994 of 1,167 of these reports of local or systemic problems with implants with a survey requesting information on physician diagnoses. Of the original cohort, 820 completed the interview; 28% of these reported a physician diagnosis of a connective tissue disease and 43% reported multiple implant surgery. These self-reports were not independently verified, and this group was highly selected (Coleman et al., 1994).

Several conclusions seem to follow from these data on women's satisfaction or dissatisfaction with breast implants. Many women are satisfied with their implants, but it is not safe to assume that satisfaction is, and remains, at the levels often reported in the plastic surgery literature, given conflicting results and the possible biases and problems of some of these reports. Satisfaction is often surveyed by the operating service and shortly after implantation when some complications have yet to occur. Reports of satisfaction do not necessarily mean that complications have not occurred or that they are not troubling to many women. Women seem to accept trade offs, as noted earlier, and some are very dissatisfied. Some who are dissatisfied report obstacles to paying for implant removal, whereas others elect to tolerate distress for the perceived benefits of the implants. The improvements in the results of implantation, noted in the short history in this chapter and suggested later in this report, and in women's appreciation of these results have sustained the demand for breast implants, as the prevalence data below suggest. These complex and varied levels of satisfaction also appear to affect the demand for medical or surgical interventions to address complications. Since these interventions carry risks they are relevant to the safety of silicone breast implants (see Chapter 5).

Regulatory Controls

As noted earlier, the Food and Drug Administration exercised jurisdiction over silicone for injection under investigational new drug provisions of the Food, Drug and Cosmetic Act. However, the FDA did not have a statutory basis for oversight of silicone breast (or other) implants until the enactment in 1976 of the Medical Devices Amendments to the Food, Drug and Cosmetics Act (Public Law 94-295). At the time, on the advice of its independent General and Plastic Surgery Devices Panel, the FDA placed implants in a category requiring general controls and performance standards. No testing or applications for marketing were required. As time passed, more and more women received silicone implants, more than 90% of which were silicone gel-filled, for augmentation. In the 1980s, more women wanted, and more surgeons were willing to use, implants for reconstruction after cancer surgery (Freeman and Wiemer, 1979; Georgiade et al., 1982, 1985; Gilliland et al., 1983; Hartwell et al., 1976; Hueston and McKenzie, 1970; Noone et al., 1985). With increasing experience, more reports accumulated in the plastic surgery literature of implant rupture, silicone gel fluid diffusion through the implant shell, and severe contracture of the fibrous capsule surrounding the implant (see Chapter 5). The changing characteristics of implants, thinner shells—and more compliant gels in the 1970s and early 1980s (so-called second generation implants; see Chapter 3), contributed to some of this increased frequency of complications. Concerns surfaced that silicones might be associated with cancer, and reports of connective tissue diseases and less well defined systemic complications, perhaps of an immune nature, in women with silicone injections and implants began to appear (see Chapters 6, 7, and 8). As a result, in 1982, the FDA proposed and, on June 24, 1988, formally implemented a classification of silicone breast implants in a category (Class III) requiring stringent safety and effectiveness controls. In a critical series of actions from 1989 through 1991, the FDA required pre-market approval (PMA) applications from implant manufacturers (April 10, 1991), questioned specifically the safety of polyurethane-coated implants and required additional study of them, determined that PMA applications for silicone gel breast implants were insufficient when they were submitted by the manufacturers (August 22, 1991), and required dissemination of information on implant risks to patients (September 26, 1991). In 1992 and 1993, citing the absence of data on safety and effectiveness (Kessler, 1992), the FDA restricted the use of silicone gel-filled implants to participants in a clinical observational study, most of whom received implants for reconstruction (January 6, 1992); called for safety and effectiveness data on saline-filled silicone implants (April 16, 1992); issued a proposed rule to require PMA applications for saline implants (January 8, 1993); and designated gel and saline implants subject to device tracking rules (August 26, 1993). By this time, all U.S. companies (as noted in Chapter 3 of this report) except Mentor Corporation and McGhan Medical Corporation had withdrawn from the market (March 20, 1992), and polyurethane-coated implants were no longer in domestic production. At the time of issuance of this report, all companies who wished to remain in the U.S. silicone breast implant market will have attempted to carry out the observational and other studies required by the FDA as specified in 1996 and will have submitted PMA applications (FDA, 1998). Whatever the regulatory outcome and the real or hypothetical problems reported with these devices, the substantial, steady increases in their use for augmentation since 1992 after the dramatic drop in the early 1990s (see below), and the striking increase in implantation for reconstruction after mastectomy since the early 1980s, speak to the important interest of American women in cosmetic breast surgery.

Prevalence of Silicone Breast Implants

Implantation of silicone shell devices began from a small base, gradually replacing other breast alloplastic devices listed earlier in this chapter and slowly increasing in numbers. Early reports estimated that somewhat more than 50,000 women received implants between 1962 and 1970, and 98% of these were for augmentation (de Cholnoky, 1970; Braley, 1972; Robertson and Braley, 1973). The number of women who received implants rose annually until 1979, at which time it began to plateau. The number implanted after mastectomy, which had been low and stable, began to increase in about 1975 (Gabriel et al., 1995) as surgeons and oncologists started to appreciate that this was not only possible, but might be desirable (August et al., 1994; Bailey et al., 1989; Barreau-Pouhaer et al., 1992; Berrino et al., 1987; Dowden, 1983; Feller et al., 1986; Francel et al., 1993; Handel et al., 1990; Noone et al., 1982; Patel et al., 1993; Schain et al., 1985) and could be done immediately (Trabulsy et al., 1994; Van Heerden et al., 1987; Yule et al., 1996). In 1983, 3% of women received breast implants for reconstruction after mastectomy; in 1992, more than 25% received these implants (Edney, 1996). Local insurance data from 1988–1990 indicated that 5.9% of mastectomies were followed by reconstruction with implants (Francel et al., 1993), and a similar frequency (8%) was reported in Holland about that time (Houpt et al., 1988). Reconstruction after prophylactic mastectomy was recommended earlier and performed on a higher proportion of patients than after cancer surgery (Freeman, 1967; Jarrett et al., 1978; Kelly et al., 1966).

It is not possible to be sure of the division between augmentation and reconstruction at any given time in the total cohort of U.S. women receiving breast implants. There has been substantial variation. The general consensus has been that augmentation is the reason for about 80% of all breast implants. Two recent studies, however, report that 70%–71% of implants were placed for augmentation (Gabriel et al., 1995; Nemecek and Young, 1993). Also, a national survey reported 63% (R.R. Cook et al., 1995), and a study of a very large cohort of professional women reported 50%, of implant placements for augmentation (Sánchez-Guerrero et al., 1995a,b). As noted earlier, almost all implant placements from the 1960s to mid-1970s were for augmentation. The fraction for reconstruction increased steadily through the 1980s. During the early 1990s, almost 40% of breast implantation was for reconstruction. Most recently, reconstruction was the indication for less than 20% of implants, in part because approximately 35% of reconstructive procedures are now limited to autogenous tissue (ASPRS, 1996, 1997). Surveys of other than national cohorts of women may be misleading due to the variation in the frequency of augmentation relative to reconstruction in different parts of the country (R.R. Cook et al., 1995). For use in the calculation of modern prevalence (see below), the committee assumed that 30% of implants were for reconstruction as a midpoint in a range of 25%–35%. These are admittedly somewhat speculative estimates of reconstruction frequency from values found in the record review and surveys of Gabriel et al. (1995); R.R. Cook et al. (1995) and Sánchez-Guerrero et al. (1995a,b); the 30% figure used by Terry et al. (1995), and the oft-repeated 20% figure cited in most other reports. The committee also considered premature mortality in cancer patients that decreases the surviving cohort of women with reconstructions much more than the normal mortality of augmentation patients decreases the surviving cohort of women with implants for this purpose. This factor becomes more meaningful in estimating the percentage of women alive with implants for augmentation or reconstruction in long-term follow-up of studies from 1988.

Estimates of the number of women receiving breast implants in 1982 were 100,000, 22% for reconstruction, (Szycher and Poirier, 1984), 130,000 in 1988 (Lorentzen, 1988) 120,000–150,000 in 1990 (an estimate by the Inamed Corporation) and 130,000 in 1990 (Zones, 1992). Additional data collected from plastic surgeons by the ASPRS before 1992 are said by the society to be inconsistent with its modern surveys and are no longer released. The estimates cited here and the occasional annual estimates of new implants in the range of 100,000 or more reported in the literature by plastic surgeons are consistent with modern estimates, however.

An analysis of data from the 1988 National Health Interview Survey, which reported 11 million persons in the United States with implants of all kinds (Moss et al., 1991; see Chapter 2 for a partial list of silicone containing devices) suggested 304,000 women at least 18 years of age with silicone breast implants (95% confidence interval [CI], 239,000–369,000) or 0.33% of all women aged 18 to 75 years in 1988, of whom 73% were between ages 18 and 44 and 24% between ages 45 and 64 (Bright et al., 1993). As confirmation of the rising popularity of this procedure, only 30% of implantations had occurred before 1981 and 70% in the 1981–1988 interval. This report referred to market data suggesting 1,030,000 women with breast implants in 1988. Bright et al. (1993) observed that the design of the National Health Interview Survey (e.g., which asked for medical rather than cosmetic implants or allowed reporting by a family member) could have resulted in underreporting. On the other hand, market-based data could suffer from the vagaries of inventories, returns, breakage, and other factors that might have influenced their accuracy. In remarks to an FDA panel (FDA, 1992a) Bright recalculated the prevalence using supplemented market data with adjustments for mortality and replacements among others, and she provided an FDA estimate of 1,000,000 women with breast implants at the end of 1991.

A household survey carried out by Dow Corning Corp. identified 0.808% of women over age 14 years with implants, or 815,700 (95% CI, 715,757–924,729) women nationally in late 1989 (Cook and Perkins, 1996; Cook et al., 1995). Augmentation was the indication in 63.5% of those surveyed. This survey, in agreement with other studies and reports, identified higher prevalence in the southern and western regions of the country (three-times that in the eastern and midwestern regions) and over-representation of white (95%) and higher-income women. In low prevalence regions of the country, implantation for reconstruction was actually more common than for augmentation. A small CDC survey mentioned in this report found 0.25% of U.S. women with implants in 1983. This might be a reasonable approximation given the lower numbers of implants in the early years.

Another survey, using New York records to identify women who received implants for cosmetic reasons only, concluded that about 890,000 U.S. women (data simulations generated estimates ranging from 437,602 to 2,035,783, 95% of which were less than 1,205,820) had breast augmentation between 1963 and 1988. Assuming that reconstructions comprised

30% of total implantations, the authors adjusted this figure to about 1,270,000 U.S. women with implants for both augmentation and reconstruction in 1988 (Terry et al., 1995).

A record review carried out in a single Minnesota county of women over 14 years of age identified 749 women with implants. Their average age was 34 years (range 15–79), and augmentation, as noted earlier, was the indication in only 71%. Prevalence as of January 1, 1992 was estimated to be about 1%, which would extrapolate to about 1,000,000 women nationally (Gabriel et al., 1995). A number of other large cohorts were reviewed for the prevalence of women with implants in the course of carrying out other epidemiological studies. These cohorts either were from specific parts of the country (Brinton et al., 1996—2.2% of women, Seattle, Atlanta, and central New Jersey; Burns et al., 1996—1.18% of women, upper Midwest; Hochberg et al., 1993—1.24% of women, San Diego, Baltimore, and Pittsburgh); were characterized by a low response rate and self-reporting, which may have produced artificially high results (Hennekens et al., 1996, 2.74% of women), or were not a representative cross section of all ages of adult females (Brinton et al., 1996; Sánchez-Guerrero et al., 1995a,b, 1.35%). Nevertheless, given the number of adult women in the population, these values cluster around 1.2 million to 1.3 million U.S. women with breast implants in the early 1990s, which is consistent with other estimates (see below). Additionally, there is general agreement across reports examining the demographic characteristics of implant recipients that augmentation is carried out on average in women about 30–35 years of age and reconstruction in women about 40–55 years of age (including ages 48–49 after cancer and 40–41 years for prophylaxis and revision) (see also August et al., 1994; Birtchnell and Lacey, 1988; Cook et al., 1995; Gabriel et al., 1997; McGhan Medical Corporation, undated; Shipley et al., 1977; Wickman and Jurell, 1997; Winer et al., 1993).

All of the reported estimates of breast implant prevalence suffer from problems that affect their accuracy, as the authors themselves often point out. These problems include partial responses to questionnaires, varying accuracy and completeness of reporting, differing assumptions in projecting samples nationwide, small numbers, and noncomparable samples (among others noted above). A rough estimate of the current or near current number of women with breast implants can be made by assuming a reasonable range from among the estimates for 1988 with an upper bound of the estimate (1.27 million) based on actual record reviews (Terry et al., 1995), and projecting this range (1 million to 1.27 million, see below) forward using annual estimates and ASPRS and AACS survey data for ensuing years.

Of course, the estimated numbers after 1988 are also subject to error. Some are educated guesses. The ASPRS sample, based on a membership that does 70–80% of the implantations nationally, is extrapolated to estimate the number of women receiving implants for augmentation and reconstruction in the United States. The ASPRS (and AACS) data are not validated, however, and suffer from the problems of incomplete or inaccurate reporting inherent in surveys, especially of self-reported events. Some industry sources have suggested that ASPRS data have been overestimates, perhaps because members that respond to the survey tend to be among the more active surgeons (McGhan Medical Corp., personal communication, August 26, 1998). Others have suggested that busy plastic surgeons may have tended to overestimate the numbers of procedures they do (C. L. Puckett, Vice President, ASPRS, personal communication, September 2, 1998). The AACS surveys a different group of medical specialists with practices limited to cosmetic procedures, including general surgeons, dermatologists, facial plastic and reconstructive surgeons, some plastic surgeons, family practitioners, and obstetricians or gynecologists (Atwood et al., 1994). These specialists perform about 30% of augmentations with breast implants in the United States. The smaller sample drawn from this group is also extrapolated to a national figure, in this case for augmentation only. The AACS augmentation estimates are slightly lower than those of ASPRS (e.g., 76,407 versus 87,704 in 1996). The committee used the higher ASPRS values and larger sample in making its calculation of the numbers of women in the United States with breast implants.

Not captured in any ASPRS or AACS survey is the number of women who obtain breast implants outside the United States. Some of the implantations reported are also likely to be reimplantations that might inappropriately be counted twice in estimates of the total cohort of women with breast implants. Bright et al. (1993) found that 13% of women with breast implants in the National Health Interview Survey had replacement implants. Surveys that identify and contact women should not be affected, and the review of procedures by Terry et al. (1995) included a correction factor for procedures per woman, which may have accounted for replacements, although precise details were not provided in their report. In addition, mortality has undoubtedly affected the number of women who had implants in the 1960s (admittedly a small group) even the youngest of whom will now be 60 years of age or more.

The committee estimated that between 356,000 and 417,000 underwent breast reconstruction with implants after mastectomy for cancer. This estimate assumes that 30% of the 1 million to 1.27 million woman with implants in 1988 (300,000–381,000) had implants for reconstruction after mastectomy, to which is added the ASPRS reported number of reconstructions using implants since then—about 175,000—making a total of 475,000–556,000. No more than 75% of postmastectomy reconstruction occurs after cancer surgery. The other reconstructions follow mastectomies for other reasons, mostly prophylaxis or fibrocystic disease. Thus, the postcancer reconstruction total is approximately 356,000–417,000 women. Although the pre-1988 mortality of augmented and reconstructed women does not affect the 1988 surveys that identified living women, it may not be completely accounted for in the adjusted procedure-based data of Terry et al. (1995). Mortality in women with breast implants for augmentation is not known to be higher than in the general population, but for women implanted after mastectomy for cancer, the mortality cited by Gabriel et al. (1997) and Georgiade et al. (1985) is probably close to 30% after 10–15 years. This is slightly better than NCI's Surveillance, Epidemiology and End Results (SEER) registry statistics, probably because breast cancer patients with poorer prognosis are less likely to receive implants (Gabriel et al., 1997; Georgiade et al., 1985). The committee assumed a loss of 25%– 30% by death during 1989–97 of women who had implants for reconstruction in 1988 and those added each year since, a combined cohort with postimplant durations ranging from less than a year to several decades. This mortality rate would have resulted in a minimum of 89,000 and a maximum of 125,000 deaths over the nine years in the combined cohort. The committee felt that assumptions regarding over- or underestimations bearing on a final estimate would be rather speculative. Nevertheless, given the prevailing view that ASPRS data might be overstated, the possibility of some double-counted replacement implants, the mortality in augmented women between 1988 and 1997, and the deaths expected among cancer patients undergoing reconstruction, it seemed reasonable to adjust the final estimate downward by 150,000.

The committee judges there to have been 1 million to 1.27 million U.S. women with silicone breast implants in 1988. The National Health Interview Survey estimate was considered an outlier, and the other estimates clustered around 1 million in the late 1980s with the 1.27 million women reported by Terry et al. (1995) as an upper limit. To this was added the total of annual estimates from ASPRS survey results for 1989–1997, counting augmentations and reconstructions with implants. Explants reported from 1992 on were subtracted (replacements after explantation are included in the reported implant figures). Non-survey year implant figures were assumed to be midpoints between bracketing survey years. Non-survey year explant figures were assumed to number 12,000 in 1989 and 1990 and to be at the midpoint between 1990 and 1992 for 1991, and the same in 1997 as 1996. The implant totals from 1989 through 1997 respectively were accordingly 130,000, 130,000, 101,000, 53,000, 59,000, 65,000, 87,000, 108,000, and 146,000 (total for the period—879,000), and the explants were 12,000, 12,000, 19,000, 26,000, 32,000, 38,000, 26,000, 14,000, and 14,000 respectively (total for the period—193,000). The total cohort of U.S. women with breast implants at the end of 1997 was therefore 1.686

million to 1.956 million before adjustment (1 million or 1.27 million plus 879,000 and minus 193,000). This range of about 1.7 million to 1.95 million is adjusted downward and rounded to give a current estimate of 1.5 million to 1.8 million U.S. women with breast implants as of the end of 1997. This estimate could be projected forward each year using ASPRS or AACS survey numbers as they become available. To reach an estimate of U.S. women ever receiving breast implants, explantations (not replaced), deaths, and non-U.S. implantation should be added to the 1997 estimate. The committee did not perform this analysis in detail, but this estimate of ever-implanted women is likely to approximate 2 million women or more.

The ASPRS data also show that 90%–95% of implants currently placed are saline filled, mostly textured and primarily (65% in augmentation, almost all in reconstruction) in the submuscular position. Saline implants are used in 96% of augmentations, and saline implants and expanders are used in 86% of reconstructions. However, as noted in Chapter 3, the overwhelming majority of implants placed before the early 1990s were gel filled. Therefore, these implants, primarily single-lumen gel, standard double-lumen, and polyurethane coated, make up the majority of implants in place today. Some plastic surgeons report that the demand for gel-filled implants is increasing, although at the moment their use in the United States is limited by regulatory policies (V. L. Young, personal communication, October 16, 1998). Collis and colleagues report that in the United Kingdom the "vast majority" of augmentation involve gel-filled, textured implants in the submammary position (Collis et al., 1998). There is also a trend to more reconstructions after mastectomy and more reconstructions using tissue flaps (often without alloplastic implants). Forty-two percent of reconstructions are now done at the time of mastectomy (ASPRS, 1997). Discussion of this subject is continued later in Chapter 5.

SUMMARY

The IOM Committee on the Safety of Silicone Breast Implants was constituted to respond to a congressionally mandated request for the study of the safety of silicone breast implants from the Department of Health and Human Services. The English language, peer-reviewed, scientific literature supplemented with some data from industry and other technical reports comprised the primary information base for the description of the background, context and prevalence of silicone breast implantation and for the subsequent chapters of this report. An enormous amount of material generated from U.S. breast implant litigation, primarily the multidistrict litigation, was also available, including videotapes, compact disks, legal records, briefs, and scientific citations. Although this type of information was reviewed, it is generally not cited in this report. It is clear that adversarial legal proceedings do not generate the kind of scientific inquiry and discussion that the IOM committee process does. On the other hand, information from legal discovery and arguments can identify directions for inquiry, useful literature, and data. This information has contributed to the completeness and accuracy of this report. The statements of women with breast implants and of scientists, physicians, and others who appeared before the committee (see Appendix A and B), although often anecdotal and not peer reviewed, were helpful too. A number of important issues emerged from the committee's reviews of available information. These issues are the ones that make up the committee's charge and they are the scientific and medical questions that are suggested or explicit in the reports concerning associations between silicone breast implants and human health conditions that have appeared in increasing numbers in the world's medical and scientific literature. In Chapters 2 through 12 the committee addresses the issues as closely and conclusively as possible under the headings of silicone chemistry, implant catalogue, silicone toxicology, reoperations and local and perioperative complications, silicone immunology, antinuclear antibodies, connective tissue or rheumatic disease, cancer, neurological disease, effects on breast feeding and on children, and screening and diagnostic mammography. Descriptions of the IOM scientific workshop and public meeting and comments on other recent policy-relevant reports appear in the appendix materials.

2

Silicone Chemistry

SILICA, SILICON, AND SILICONE

Silica is the most common substance on earth. It is a constituent of most rocks. Beach sand is almost pure crystalline silica, as is quartz, which in its purest form is a clear or rosy-colored gemstone, found in geodes, or, if less pure, may be found as amethyst, agate, flint, or "petrified wood." The molecular formula of silica is SiO_2, silicon dioxide. Silicon dioxide is a three-dimensional network of silicon (Si) atoms linked by oxygen (O) atoms in a 2:1 ratio; each silicon atom is linked to four oxygen atoms, and each oxygen to two silicon atoms.

A crystalline substance is one whose atoms form a regular pattern over large distances. This regularity is usually measured by the diffraction of x-rays. The constructive and destructive interference of x-ray waveforms causes the x-ray beam to be redirected into a reproducible pattern that can be detected by photographic film. The characteristics of this pattern allow calculation of the precise atomic spacing. This regularity is also a key to the hardness and strength of most crystalline substances.

Although human exposure to crystalline silica is extensive and generally to no ill effect, tissue (especially lung) exposure to particulate silica or silica dust has well defined toxic, inflammatory outcomes (American Thoracic Society, 1997). Silica is also found in less toxic, amorphous forms (Warheit et al., 1995). Amorphous materials, in which the atoms are not found in regular arrays even though the atomic ratios are the same, do not give crystalline patterns. Amorphous forms of silica include a vitreous form like the glass used in higher-wattage halogen lamps, (e.g., automobile headlamps). Window and bottle glasses are diluted, low-melting forms of silica. Sodium and calcium oxides are used as diluents in sodalime window and bottle glass. Silica aerogel, silica smoke, fumed silica, and precipitated silica are names for amorphous silica powders that are important constituents of medical rubber-like goods, including breast implants. In fact, amorphous silica is used in almost all silicone elastomers, as well as in special-purpose isoprene (natural rubber) elastomers. Less often used is diatomaceous earth, the silica skeletal residue of diatoms, which are microscopic sea creatures (Heaney et al., 1994; Iler, 1979a,b, 1981). Some forms of amorphous silica have been approved by the Food and Drug Administration (FDA) (D. Benz, FDA, personal communication, 1998) for use in pharmaceuticals and food; they are widely distributed in foods and foodstuff manufacture (Villota and Hawkes, 1986).

Silicon is a semimetallic element, located just below carbon in the periodic table, that is not found in nature in its elemental form. It is perhaps best known as the shiny semiconducting metalloid used to make computer chips. Silicon can be made by heating silica with carbon (coke or charcoal), typically in an electric arc furnace. At high enough temperatures, the elements silicon, carbon, and oxygen can exchange places, and the driving force of the reaction is the loss of gaseous carbon dioxide (CO_2) leaving silicon and any excess carbon behind. The impure reaction product can be used to make silicones (see below) but requires extensive purification before it can be fabricated into computer chips. Although silicon is in a high-energy, unstable state with respect to its oxide, silica does not form spontaneously in air on its surface, as rust does on iron or aluminum oxide on aluminum. Like gold or platinum, silicon retains its shiny metallic appearance and electrical properties. However, silicon can burn in air to give a thick, white smoke of amorphous silica (LeVier et al., 1993).

Silicone refers to a large family of organic silicon polymer products with a main chain of alternating silicon and oxygen atoms. Typically, each silicon in the chain carries two methyl groups (CH_3–, which can also be written as Me–, where C = carbon and H = hydrogen), and the material is called poly(dimethylsiloxane) (PDMS):

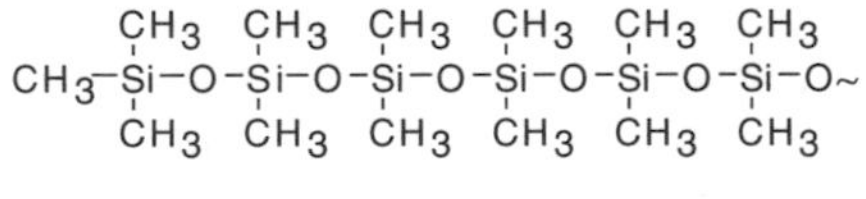

$$
\begin{array}{ccccccccccccc}
 & CH_3 & & CH_3 & & CH_3 & & CH_3 & & CH_3 & & CH_3 & \\
 & | & & | & & | & & | & & | & & | & \\
CH_3- & Si & -O- & Si & -O- & Si & -O- & Si & -O- & Si & -O- & Si & -O\sim \\
 & | & & | & & | & & | & & | & & | & \\
 & CH_3 & & CH_3 & & CH_3 & & CH_3 & & CH_3 & & CH_3 &
\end{array}
$$

The tilde (~) at the chain end implies that the sequence is repeated, typically with hundreds to thousands of silicon–oxygen links. As the number

TABLE 2-1 Viscosity of Silicone Compounds

Number of Dimethyl-Siloxane Units, DP (degree of polymerization)	Viscosity, centistrokes (cS)	Comparative Viscosity*	Reference
2	0.65		L
3	1.04	Water	L
9	3.94		L
14.5	4.5		O
22.6	6.64		O
30	9.44	Baby oil	O
40.3	12.01		O
86	26.77		O
163	52.18		O
250	82.81		O
269	100	Olive oil	L
330	138.69	Light motor oil	O
591	335.3	Heavy motor oil	O
818	968.59	Glycerol	O
960	10,000	Honey	L
1,400	1,000,000	PDMS rubber gum	L
2,600	10,000,000	Hot asphalt	L

NOTE: O = Orrah et al. (1988); L = Lee et al. (1970). *Brookfield Engineering (1999).

of units increases from two to hundreds or thousands, the compounds formed have very different properties: for example, hexamethyldisiloxane has a viscosity (0.65 centistoke [cS]) less than water (1.0 cS) and is absorbed from the gastrointestinal tract, whereas compounds with 3,000 units are relatively inert biologically and are solids having viscosities of millions of centistokes (see Chapter 4 and Table 2-1).

CHEMISTRY OF SILICONES

Silicone is made by the reaction of dimethyldichlorosilane (Me_2SiCl_2) with water to give PDMS and hydrochloric acid (HCl):

$$Me_2SiCl_2 + H_2O \longrightarrow HCl + HO(\underset{Me}{\overset{Me}{|}}SiO)_nH$$

Chlorosilane **Hydrolysate**

The $Me_2Si(OH)_2$ first formed polymerizes spontaneously to silicone hydrolysate $HOMe_2SiO(Me_2SiO)_nMe_2SiOH$, where n can vary from 0 to 50, depending on reaction conditions. Cyclic compounds are also formed in greater or lesser amounts depending on conditions.

Chlorosilanes

Me_2SiCl_2 is made from impure silicon in the "direct process." Silicon powder is heated in a stirred or fluidized bed with gaseous methyl chloride (which, in turn, is made from wood alcohol and hydrochloric acid) to produce a mixture of chlorosilanes.

$$\underset{\textbf{Methyl chloride}}{\text{Si (metal)} + CH_3Cl} \xrightarrow[\text{Cu}]{} \underset{\textbf{Chlorosilane mixture}}{MeSiCl_3 + Me_2SiCl_2 + Me_3SiCl + SiCl_4}$$

The mixture can be separated into its components by distillation of the liquid chlorosilanes. This provides sufficient purity for many applications. Me_2SiCl_2 is hydrolyzed to PDMS, which is known as crude hydrolysate at this stage (see above). Me_3SiCl is hydrolyzed to $Me_3SiOSiMe_3$, and $MeSiCl_3$ hydrolyzes to $MeSiO_3/_2$, called "T-gel," a cross-linked hard material that seems closer to sand than to silicone rubber. The 3/2 in the formula refers to the three oxygens each shared with two silicon atoms. The ratio, of 1.5 oxygen atoms per silicon atom, implies that three bonds are formed to other silicon atoms, since silicon is always tetravalent. Thus, a three-dimensional network, similar to the silica network, results, but the material is usually softer because of the valences occupied by methyl groups.

$SiCl_4$ hydrolyzes to a hydrated silica also known as silicic acid (a polymerized form of $Si(OH)_4$), which forms the drying agent silica gel when oven dried. It is a glassy, amorphous structure that has shrunk with the loss of water to give a porous, spongy structure. $SiCl_4$ is also hydrolyzed as a gaseous stream with steam. A high temperature flame of this tetrachlorosilane reacting with steam gives a white amorphous silica smoke or aerogel, which is gathered to provide the very finely divided filler used in silicone rubber.

FUNCTIONALITY AND NOMENCLATURE

Another shorthand polymer nomenclature is useful as well. $Me_3SiOSiMe_3$ is also known as M_2 in a popular shorthand that denotes $Me_3SiO_{1/2}$ as M, a *monofunctional* polymer component or "chainstopper" because it regulates polymer chain length. The 1/2 subscript indicates that only one-half of the oxygen belongs in the group, since it is shared by two silicons. In practical terms, the M (or monofunctionality) means that silicon binds to only one oxygen, and the form of the whole molecule can be deduced from this and the following information. The D in D_4 or in MD_2M refers to the *difunctional* dimethylsiloxane unit Me_2SiO, the polymer building block that can add to itself to form enormously long chains known as high polymers. PDMS is made up almost entirely of D units. Since D means that silicon binds to two oxygens (i.e., is difunctional), the silicon at one end of the polymer chain must bind to the oxygen at the other end to form a circular (cyclic) molecule (as in D_4) unless the last silicon has three methyl groups attached and is, therefore, a chainstopper, giving a chain such as MD_nM (where n can be any number). The T in T-gel refers to the *trifunctional* $MeSiO_3/_2$ which, when present as an impurity, leads to branching of polymer chains. However, its overall effect on molecular weight can be controlled to some extent by the addition of more M units, since chainstopping one of the oxygen–silicon units makes MT which is equivalent to D. The so-called Q units are *quadrifunctional* and result from hydrolysis of silicon tetrachloride ($SiCl_4$). Q can be modified with M units since M_2Q is equivalent to D because two of the oxygen–silicon units are chainstopped. The various mixtures of M, D, T, and Q control molecular weight, branching, and molecular shape and are used to formulate various types of silicone resins (varnishes, fiberglass bonding solids, pressure-sensitive adhesives, and even the release paper for protecting adhesive tapes). The symbol L is also sometimes used to denote D units in *linear* polymers, with D_n reserved for cyclics (see below). Thus, L_6 would be a linear hexamer (the same as MD_4M) with no indication of the chemical groups at the ends of the chain. The formation of cyclic, branched, or linear compounds and the substitution of other groups for methyl will change the physical and biological properties of silicone molecules, often to a very great extent (LeVier et al., 1993).

High Polymers

Pure D polymer units, without M, T, or Q, give the highest molecular weight unbranched polymers and thus are most useful for elastomer manufacture. Crude hydrolysate was once used for elastomers by polymerization with acid.

$$\underset{\textbf{Hydrolysate}}{HO(\overset{\overset{Me}{|}}{\underset{\underset{Me}{|}}{Si}}O)_nH} \xrightarrow[\text{acid}]{} \underset{\textbf{PDMS}}{HO(\overset{\overset{Me}{|}}{\underset{\underset{Me}{|}}{Si}}O)_mH} + H_2O \qquad (n = 1\text{–}50)$$

The catalyst used was usually sulfuric acid, removed from the high molecular weight PDMS by washing with water. Alternatively, acid ion-exchange resin or acid clay was used. The resin or clay could be removed by filtration in low-viscosity products or by neutralization. The limitation of polymers made from hydrolysate was the variable concentration of M, T, and Q groups, leading to uncertain properties since varying amounts of these groups caused more or less cross-linking, branching and chain length which affected molecular weight and physical properties of the final silicone product.

Methyl Tetramer (D_4)

The solution to this problem was the development of cyclic silicones, usually tetramers, as intermediates that could be highly purified. Tetramer is distilled from a kettle containing hydrolysate and a basic catalyst such as potassium hydroxide. The base forms the potassium silanolate ion via the removal of water. The silanolate ion is a powerful "rearrangement" catalyst, causing siloxane molecular bonds to exchange parts with each other. Some cyclics, mostly tetramer, are formed in a random fashion and can be distilled off. Removal of cyclics upsets the equilibrium, so more cyclics are generated, and the process continues until all of the polymer is converted to volatile cyclics. The tetramer can then be fractionally distilled to a very high degree of purity, eliminating the interfering M, T, and Q units. One of the most sensitive measures of purity is the molecular weight of a polymer made under controlled conditions. Industrial-grade tetramer can be polymerized to a molecular weight greater than several million Daltons. For even higher purity, a technique called zone refining has been used to form polymers of more than 40,000,000 Daltons (Martellock, 1966).

The D_4 tetramer is an eight-membered ring of alternating silicon and oxygen atoms with eight methyl groups attached, two per silicon (octamethylcyclotetrasiloxane):

```
Me2       Me2
  \       /
  Si—O—Si            (rearrangement)
  /      \
 O        O      <—————————————————————>      High polymer
  \      /
  Si—O—Si                 KOH
  /      \
Me2       Me2
```

$D_4 = (Me_2SiO)_4$ PDMS

The polymerization of this cyclic tetramer is somewhat different from the condensation reaction that leads to hydrolysate and higher polymers by splitting off water molecules from pairs of silanol groups. The tetramer D_4 has no silanol groups, but polymerizes by a process known as ring-opening polymerization. It is essentially the same process that led to generation of tetramer, except the equilibrium now favors high polymer, yielding about 86% high polymer with 14% mixed cyclics (Brown and Slusarczuk, 1965; Carmichael and Winger, 1965).

MD_2M, a short chain of four silicon atoms alternating with three oxygen atoms and fully substituted with methyl groups, is the chainstopper of choice in industry because it matches the reactivity of D_4. The two are heated together in the presence of a trace of basic or acidic catalyst to yield a linear polymer whose molecular weight, which controls the viscosity, is regulated by the small amounts of MD_2M. This polymerization is called equilibration because it leads to an equilibrium mixture of linear and cyclic silicones, about 14% cyclics. The latter are mostly removed by steam or vacuum distillation after the catalyst is removed. The molecular weight of crude hydrolysate is controlled by the chainstopping effect of dimethylsilanol ($-SiMe_2OH$) groups, but these are unstable since further polymerization is possible under some conditions. The silanol (–SiOH) groups can condense, losing water and increasing chain length. Conversely, siloxane (–SiOSi–) groups can, in theory, revert in the presence of water to give pairs of silanol groups, thereby decreasing chain length. Both reactions can occur under mild acidic or basic conditions. However, the reversion reaction is inhibited by the lack of solubility of water in PDMS, i.e., the physical inaccessibility of water to siloxane, so for practical purposes it does not present a problem (Martellock, 1966).

USES OF SILICONES

PDMS polymers are useful for hundreds of applications (Silicones Environmental Health and Safely Council, 1994). Low molecular weight oils (fluids) are used as (1) lubricating oils (Slipicone), (2) lubricants for syringe needles and barrels, (3) substances to improve the "hand" of fabrics and give them water repellency, (4) skin cream modifiers in cosmetics, (5) antifoam agents in the food and chemical industry, and (6) cures for stomach gas (Simethicone in Gas-X). Higher molecular weight, more viscous oils are widely used as high-temperature hydraulic and brake fluids. A list of silicone containing medical devices includes hydrocephalus shunts, foldable intraocular lenses, soft tissue implants for congenital and cancer reconstructive surgery, cardiac pacing and defibrillation devices, implantable infusion pumps, elastomeric toe and finger joints, incontinence and impotence devices, infusion ports, larynx implants, tissue expanders, and many shunts and catheters (Compton, 1997).

Silicone oil (fluid) has a very low surface energy, which causes it to spread on higher-energy surfaces and to make these surfaces water repellent. Silicone resins, highly cross-linked with T or Q units to give the required hardness, also have this effect and are used to coat plastic eyeglass lenses, or glass bottles with a very thin film to increase scratch and break resistance and aid in emptying aqueous contents. Similar resins are used as release agents in commercial bakeware. Silicone rubber films are used to coat rough-service light bulbs to increase break resistance and to capture shattered fragments. There are actually thousands of silicone products that impinge upon all aspects of modern life (Silicones Environmental Health and Safety Council, 1994).

Silicone Elastomers

$$[Me(CH_2{=}CH)SiO]_4 + (Me_2SiO)_4 \longrightarrow (MeViSiO)m\text{—}co\text{—}Me_2SiO)n$$

Me Vi tetramer **Me tetramer** **Me Vi copolymer polymethyl vinyl siloxane (PMVS)**

$$(MeViSiO)m\text{—}co\text{—}Me_2SiO)n + H(Me_2SiO)oSiHMe_2 \xrightarrow{Pt}$$

PMVS (excess vinyl) **Hydrogen-stopped PDMS**

$$\begin{array}{l}\sim O\text{-}SiMe_2\text{-}O \qquad\qquad\qquad\qquad\qquad\qquad\qquad\qquad O\text{-}SiMe_2\text{-}O\sim \\ \quad Me\text{-}Si\text{-}CH_2\text{-}CH_2 \qquad\qquad\qquad CH_2\text{-}CH_2\text{-}Si\text{-}Me \\ \sim O\text{-}SiMe_2\text{-}O \qquad SiOMe_2(Me_2SiO)pSiMe_2 \qquad O\text{-}SiMe_2\text{-}O\sim\end{array}$$

Three broad categories of silicone are used in implant manufacture: (1) platinum-cured (gel or LSR [liquid silicone rubber]); (2) RTV (room-temperature vulcanized) rubber; and (3) gum-based peroxide-cured (heat-cured) rubber. All require a final oven bake to attain optimal purity, stability, and physical properties (Lynch, 1978). The simplest of these gels is the platinum-cured gel that expanded most early implants. The original embodiment was developed for a plastic surgeon, Thomas D. Cronin, by Dow Corning. It consisted of a slightly vinyl substituted PDMS fluid that was cross-linked with a hydrogen-containing PDMS fluid in a platinum-catalyzed reaction. This means that a few silicon atoms in the chain had a vinyl (Vi) instead of a methyl substituent. The vinyl group was susceptible to bonding with a receptive hydride group on a neighboring siloxane polymer chain, creating a cross-link. This curing reaction is known as hydrosilation. It forms a very lightly cross-linked unfilled elastomer that gives the desired softness and compliance. In chemical terms, each silicon hydride group (the "hydrogen-stopped PDMS" below) adds across a vinyl double bond (CH_2=CH–in the MeVi tetramer below), thereby converting the vinyl group to an ethylene (–CH_2–CH_2–) bridge linking two polymer molecules together. Since a few of the polymer molecules had more than two reactive groups per molecule, the reaction results in a cross-linked system with no new soluble or leachable components.

Silicon Addition Cure Chemistry

The Cronin gel probably had a vinyl level less than 0.1 mole %, which was reacted with insufficient silicon hydride so that the hydrogen would be completely used up and not cause problems with hydrogen gas evolution at a later time. Therefore, the final gel had an even lower level of excess vinyl, and the cross-link density was controlled by the concentration of hydride groups added. See Table 2-2 for the composition of several versions of the Dow Corning gel.

Certain silicone fluids, chainstopped with alkyltriacetoxysilane and thickened with amorphous silica filler, cure to RTV silicone rubbers when exposed to moist air. The triacetoxy groups are hydrolyzed by the moisture and produce T groups at the chain ends, which react with each other to form cross-links and thus a rubbery structure. The hydrolysis also produces acetic acid, which catalyzes the cross-linking and accounts for the vinegary smell of this material. A tin soap such as stannous oleate or octoate is usually used as a catalyst to speed the cure of water-cured, condensation-type silicone adhesives. The filler used to confer strength is amorphous silica. It is usually treated to control its surface reactivity because the latter might impinge on the shelf life of the product. RTVs are used as adhesives and sealants in assembling the implants. Table 2-3 gives details of the composition of Dow Corning RTV.

The filler treatment involves silica aerogel filler. This filler, whose manufacture is outlined, is amorphous silica with a surface high in silanol groups. In a nonpolar environment such as silicone gum, these silanols tend to bond between filler particles, causing aggregation. Although the primary particle size is ca. 5–7 nm (LeVier et al., 1993), this aggregation can form long chains and/or agglomerates of filler particles. The agglomerated filler acts as a second cross-linking mechanism, leading to a large increase in the stiffness of an uncured gum or the hardness of a cured elastomer, clearly an unwanted outcome (Boonstra et al., 1975). Two methods have been developed to control this—process aids and filler treatment.

Process aids are typically very low molecular weight silanol-terminated silicone fluids that are added to the gum or filler mixture. The

TABLE 2-2 Dow Corning Silicone Implant Gel, Platinum Cure

No.	Chemical Name	Function	X3-0885 MDF 0193, Cronin Firm (%)	Q7-2159, Soft November 1975-September 1976 (%)	Q7-2159, Soft September 1976-July 1979 (%)	Q7-2159, Soft July 1979-January 1992 (%)	Q7-2151, Firmer Late Gel (%)
Q1-0043	Me_2-*co*-MeVi	Reactive polymer	88.48	19.77	19.77	19.77	88.18
DC-360	1,000-cS PDMS	Diluent		79.1	79.1	79.1	8.45
DC-330	PDMS with $MeSiO_{3/2}$ branching	Diluent	8.49				
Q1-0049	H-terminated PDMS	Cross-linker	3.00	1.12	1.12	1.12	3.33
Platinum II	$(Me_2ViSi)_2O$:Pt	Catalyst	0.029		0.0112	0.011	
MDF-0069	Cyclo$(MeViSiO)_4$:Pt	Catalyst		0.0126			0.045

TABLE 2-3 Silicone Adhesive to Seal Injections Sites, RTV Cure

No.	Chemical Name	Function	Q7-2198 (%)
DC-200	Hexamethyldisiloxane)	Solvent	40.31
DS Polymer	HO-terminated PDMS	Reactive polymer	48
R-972	Me_3Si-treated aerogel	Treated silica	8.23
ETS-900	Methyltriacetoxysilane and	Cross-linker	1.72
	ethyltriacetoxysilane, 1:1	Cross-linker	1.72
Sn oleate	Tin oleate	Catalyst	0.038

silanols in the process aid interact with those on the filler surface to give a stable coating and thus prevent filler agglomeration. This is also called in situ filler treatment. The coating molecules are held in place by a phenomenon known as hydrogen bonding, a moderately strong association of two oxygen atoms (of the silanol OH groups) held together by a shared hydrogen atom. Filler treatments similarly passivate the filler surface silanols. They may also rely on hydrogen bonding, (i.e., treatment of filler with D_4 vapor in a kettle). However, it is preferable and more reliable to bond M groups directly to silanol groups on the filler surface. Hexamethyldisilazane is a reagent that can bring this about. The resulting treated fillers can then be mixed more easily into elastomer compounds and yield stable products. Dow Corning has disclosed the use of hexamethydisilazane as an in situ filler treatment where it is added to the polymer along with the untreated filler. About 60% of the silanol groups react, but the resulting coverage is complete by an "umbrella effect" because the remaining silanols are not free to interact.

High-molecular-weight, viscous silicone gums filled with amorphous silica (Cab-O-Sil or Aerosil) are mixed with process aids and with peroxides such as 2,4-dichlorobenzoyl peroxide and cured under heat and pressure in metal molds. The molds help to protect the elastomer from cure inhibition by oxygen in the air, as well as to control thickness and shape (Lynch, 1978). Typically, all three types of silicone elastomers are heated or "postcured" in circulating air ovens when necessary to improve purity and stability. All three types of elastomeric materials have been used to produce silicone breast implants, joint implants, surgical drains, pacemaker covers, indwelling catheters, and the like (Batich and DePalma, 1992; Batich et al., 1996; Clarson and Semlyen, 1993; Kennan and Lane, personal communication, 1998).

SILICONE BREAST IMPLANTS

The chemistry of silicone elastomer and gel in a silicone breast implant described here is based substantially on disclosures by Dow Corning Corporation and is therefore only an example of one version of this technology. Details of implants of other manufacturers may be substantially similar but are proprietary, although similar processes have been described by NuSil chemists (Compton, 1997). Additional details of Dow Corning and other implants are discussed in Chapter 3 of this report (Lane and Burns, 1998; T. H. Lane and J. J. Kennan, personal communications, 1998; T. H. Lane et al., personal communication, 1998). The earliest Dow Corning shells were made of high molecular weight polymer (gum) filled with amorphous silica and a process aid designed to passivate the filler surface. They were mixed with 2,4-dichlorobenzoyl peroxide and cured in a heated mold. Two shell faces, front and back, were produced and then glued together to make a seamed shell. This heat-cured elastomer system was used only in the early Dow Corning implant shells designed for Dr. Cronin and in patches for sealing them; Table 2-4 lists the details. The uncured gel mixture was injected though a hole and cured in place with added heat. The hole was sealed with a patch or sealant, and the final product was thoroughly oven baked to remove all traces of volatile reactants and reaction products, especially 2,4-dichlorobenzoic acid, which may be toxic (a residue of 20 parts per million remained; T. H. Lane et al., personal communication, 1998). The gel used was the previously described platinum curing material, designed to be as soft as possible, with barely enough strength to maintain its shape (see Table 2-2). This gel was responsible for the tactile feel of the implant, roughly approximating the feel of human adipose tissue. The shell helped the gel to maintain its shape.

Both the shell and the gel were modified for a softer feel in the 1970s (see Chapter 3). The shell could be made thinner and of more uniform thickness by using platinum-cured liquid silicone rubber (LSR) and a dip-coating process similar to the process used to form surgical gloves. In the dip-coating process, the shell thickness is controlled by the viscosity and draining rate of the LSR mixture and therefore by its dilution with solvent

TABLE 2-4 Cronin Seamed Shell Elastomer, Peroxide Cure

No.		Function	MDF-0372 (%)	MDF-0070 (%)	MDF-0009 Patches (%)
SGM-11	Vi-terminated Me_2-*co*-MeVi siloxane	Reactive	65.5	66.81	64.3
MS-75D	Silica aerogel	Filler	26.85	24.05	26.36
PA Fluid	HO-terminated PDMS	Process aid	6.55	7.18	6.47
$(Cl_2BzCOO)_2$	Bis(2,4-dichlorobenzoyl) peroxide	Cross-linker	1.1	1.96	2.92

(Table 2-5). The shell was formed in one piece using a breast-shaped mandrel. The LSR was diluted to 15% solids with trichloroethylene (TCE) solvent, dipped and drained, dried, heat-set and peeled off. The large hole on the back left by the mandrel shaft was covered with an elastomer patch material (Table 2-6). This elastomer also had an amorphous silica filler whose silanol surface reactivity had been masked with M groups, probably by reaction with hexamethyldisilazane, $Me_3SiNHSiMe_3$, the reactive nitrogen analogue of M_2. The liquid gel precursor was also modified by the addition of 80% by volume of low molecular weight (1,000 cS, 25,000 Daltons) nonreactive PDMS fluid to swell the gel and make it even softer when cured (Table 2-2). This effect is analogous to the swelling of a sponge in water. Added low molecular weight silicone fluid is not chemically attached to breast implant gel. The network gel, 20% of the material mass, is a single giant molecule that is swollen by low molecular weight fluid, which compromises 80% of the mass, that can move or be extracted like water in a sponge.

BARRIER-LAYER IMPLANTS

The movement or diffusion of silicone gel fluid was addressed by Dow Corning with a fluorosilicone elastomer barrier-layer shell. Other manufacturers have used different technologies. A copolymer of trifluoropropylmethylsiloxane ($F_3PrMeSiO$) and methylvinylsiloxane was mixed with a solvent, a silica aerogel filler (in situ treated with a process aid), an alkynol cure inhibitor, MeHSiO, and platinum complex catalyst (see Table 2-5). This was dip coated at 2.5% solids to form a very thin interior layer. A second layer approximating the earlier single shell layer was then added for strength. The shell was finished as before. The function and performance of this and other barrier layers are discussed in Chapter 3.

The toxicology of silicone and silicone breast implants is also discussed there and in Chapter 4, and the biological and physical properties of some other silicone compounds are noted. As in any large chemical family, some organic silicone compounds are very toxic, some have biological activity, and some are relatively inert and do not have significant biological activity (LeVier et al., 1995).

TABLE 2-5 Implant Sealing Patch Rubber, Platinum Cure

No.	Chemical Name	Function	MDF-0081 STD (%)	Q7-2046 HP (%)	Q7-2222 HP (%)	Q7-2424 HP (%)
SGM-11	Vi-terminated Me_2-*co*-MeVi siloxane	Reactive polymer	65.00			
SGM-26	Vi-terminated PDMS	Reactive polymer		50.58	50.56	63.36
SGM-33	HO-terminated Me_2-*co*-MeVi siloxane	Reactive polymer		12.64	12.64	7.04
MS-75D	Silica aerogel	Filler	26.60			
R-972	Me_3SiO-treated aerogel	Filler		35.62	35.75	28.56
PA Fluid	HO-terminated PDMS	Process aid	6.50			
XR-63570	Me_2-*co*-MeH siloxane	Cross-linker	1.15	0.93	0.93	0.79
MeBu	Methylbutynol	Cure retarder	0.074			
ETCH	1-Ethynyl-1-cyclohexanol	Cure retarder		0.16	0.13	0.10
MDF-0069	Cyclo$(MeViSiO)_4$:Pt	Catalyst	0.64			
Platinum II	$(Me_2ViSi)_2O$:Pt	Catalyst		0.13	0.13	0.13

TABLE 2-6 Seamless Dip-Coated Shell Elastomer, Platinum Cure

No.	Chemical Name	Function	MDF-0077, O and I, STD (%)	Q7-2423, II and MSI, HP (%)	Q7-2551, FluoroSil Barrier (%)
TCE	1,1,1-Trichloroethane	Solvent	84.81	88.86	48.73
Acetone	Acetone	Solvent			48.73
SGM-11	Vi-terminated Me_2Vi-*co*-MeVi siloxane	Reactive copolymer	9.36		
SGM-35	Vi-terminated Me_2Vi-*co*-MeVi siloxane	Reactive copolymer		0.78	
SGM-24	Vi-terminated Me_2Vi-*co*-MeVi siloxane	Reactive copolymer			0.035
SGM-26	Vi-terminated PDMS	Reactive copolymer		7.03	
SGM-900	MeVi-*co*-F_3PrMe siloxane	Reactive copolymer			1.9
MS-75D	Silica aerogel	Filler			0.42
R-972	Me3Si-treated aerogel	Filler	5.6	3.16	
PA Fluid	HO-terminated PDMS	Process aid			0.15
ZnSt	Zinc stearate	Release agent	0.037	0.02	
XR-63570	Me_2-*co*-MeH siloxane	Cross-linker	0.09	0.11	
1107	MeH siloxane	Cross-linker			0.031
MeBu	Methylbutynol	Cure retarder	0.04		
ETCH	1-Ethynyl-1-cyclohexanol	Cure retarder		0.01	0.005
MDF-0069	Cyclo$(MeViSiO)_4$:Pt complex	Catalyst	0.09		
Platinum II	$(Me_2ViSi)_2$ in O:Pt complex	Catalyst		0.014	0.008

3

Implant Catalogue

GENERAL CONSIDERATIONS

There is no such thing as a "standard" breast implant. Silicone breast implants since 1962 have in common the presence of silicone in the shell with or without silicone in the contents of the shell. There are, however, a substantial number of characteristics that differentiate the more than 240 U.S.-made breast implants and expanders (Middleton, 1997). Many of these features are of slight consequence, but at least some of them have, or are reported to have, important influences on the biologic responses to, and complications of, implantation. Consideration should be given to the potential contributions of these influences as well as to the basic influence of silicone generically or of a specific silicone compound when assessing the consequences of breast implantation.

Unfortunately, the medical literature describing clinical experience with local and systemic complications of implants has often not specified the make and model of implants or their important characteristics. This has been improving, especially when reporting prospective trials (e.g., Burkhardt et al., 1986; Burkhardt and Demas, 1994; Burkhardt and Eades, 1995; Coleman et al., 1991; Hakelius and Ohlsen, 1992; Weinzweig et al., 1998). Many reports have been retrospective, however, and routinely women are unable to identify their implants. Medical records may be incomplete in this respect, or authors may not have appreciated how different implants can be and the value of taking the time to characterize implant populations by type, model, and manufacturer. Some implants were custom made for individual plastic surgeons or were made in small numbers by even the major manufacturers. Breast implants in the United States have come from one of more than ten companies, most of which no longer exist and many of which changed names and ownership over the years. Implants also were made in less usual types such as triple-lumen, gel–saline single lumen, reverse double lumen, or gel–gel double lumen. Little attention has been paid to reporting these minor product lines, and each one is likely to constitute a small number in any reported series. In many of these instances, implant records, descriptions, and specifications may not exist or may be only partially complete from the most detailed clinical source or the manufacturers themselves (Middleton, 1998a).

Not all of the implant variations noted here will have important clinical implications, but some have the potential to, are hypothesized to, or have been reported to cause local or systemic health effects or complications that are relevant to the safety of silicone breast implants. Potential associations (e.g., shell thickness and rupture, shell texturing or coating and contracture, gel or saline fill and systemic effects, gel consistency and tissue penetration, gel composition and toxic response) are noted in the relevant chapters of this report. This chapter describes the kinds of implants as far as possible, and gives important product names and dates of market entry and exit to help identify the implants that are, or might be, involved in studies reported in the medical literature and to help understand the implications of these studies. More complete knowledge of the specific characteristics of implants in use at various times might provide some guidance in interpreting clinical reports. Such information would be useful prospectively. The committee concluded that as complete information as possible about the device itself would be helpful to an understanding of the safety of silicone breast implants.

There are a number of examples in the plastic surgery literature in which an appreciation of the implants being used could enhance an understanding of the medical and scientific implications of a particular report. Relatively thick shells in early-1970s implants may have retarded the outward diffusion of high-dose intraimplant SoluMedrol and explained the reported lack of steroid complications reported by Perrin (1976) as noted later (Cohen, 1978a; Perrin, 1978). Measurements of peri-implant, capsular tissue silicon or silicone levels vary independently of implant age and capsule pharmacological reactivity but might be related to shell (or gel) characteristics (Baker et al., 1982; Evans and Baldwin, 1996; Peters et al., 1995a; Teuber et al., 1995a). One report showed a "poor but positive" correlation of silicon levels with the age of a group of implants that presumably all had low-bleed shells (McConnell et al., 1997).

High frequencies of saline implant deflation have to be interpreted in the light of implant types (Grossman, 1973; Worton et al., 1980). Early

Simaplast, Klein-type, implants were fragile and had a 76% prevalence of leakage or deflation (Williams, 1972). Early HTV (high-temperature vulcanized) models from a number of manufacturers frequently deflated (Mladick, 1993). The Jenny, Heyer-Schulte models had a reported thickness of at least 0.016 inch, or 0.40 mm, that made them sturdy (Jenny, 1994; Schmidt, 1980). Modern RTV (room temperature vulcanized) models are reported to deflate infrequently (Gutowski et al., 1997; Mladick, 1993; and see discussion in Peters, 1997).

The high prevalence of shell rupture in one gel implant was said to reflect the unique process of dipping the gel into elastomer rather than filling a preformed elastomer rubber casing used with this particular model (Meme ^{ME}, Aesthetech). Later models were said to correct this problem (Meme^{MP}) and were certainly no longer made in this way (Middleton, 1998b; Middleton and McNamara, 1995). Early Ashley-type polyurethane-coated prostheses were also prone to rupture along the seam until this was modified (Cohney and Mitchell, 1997). Prevalence of rupture differing by brand of implant has been reported by Feng (IOM Scientific Workshop, 1998), and Peters and Francel have reported major differences in rupture for silicone gel implants of different vintages, up to 95% at 12 years' implantation with thin shelled, 1972–mid 1980s-implants (Francel et al., 1998; Peters et al., 1996). Others have also reported frequent rupture for these thinner-shelled implants, although the numbers could also reflect the effects of wear on long-duration implants and the biases inherent in patient groups that are identified because they present with problems that lead to explantation (De Camara et al., 1993; Harris et al., 1993; Malata et al., 1994a; Rolland et al., 1989a).

Separate descriptions of women with saline and gel implants in patient populations with systemic signs and symptoms (Cuéllar et al., 1995a; Dobke et al., 1995) might direct further inquiry, although some report similar autoantibodies in both saline and gel implant patients and atypical disease symptoms in saline implant patients (Byron et al., 1984; Martin et al., 1993; Miller et al., 1998; Vargas, 1979). Calcification has been associated with a particular make of implant, although it can occur around any implant (Peters et al., 1998; Rolland et al., 1989b). Implant rupture after closed compression capsulotomies is reported to depend on implant vintage (Lemperle and Exner, 1993). Other examples could be cited, but it is clear that complications such as capsular contracture, rupture, and silicone migration may vary with implants from different manufacturers based on factors that are not precisely identified, including different shells, different gel consistency and diffusion characteristics, different gel chemical composition and siloxane molecular weights, different shapes, and so forth (Ksander and Vistnes, 1985).

IMPLANT TYPES

Implants come in a great range of sizes, generally from 80 to 800 cubic centimeters (cc) or milliliters in volume, although 1,000-cc implants or expanders have been used on occasion (R.A. Ersek, personal communication, 1998; Hester and Bostwick, 1990). The diameter, or largest dimension, of breast implants ranges from 7.5 to 16.8 cm and the projection, or profile, from 1.5 to 7.5 cm. These dimensions make breast implants dramatically larger foreign bodies in both surface area and volume than most other alloplastic implants, especially when placed bilaterally (Gold, 1983; Hester and Bostwick, 1990; Middleton, 1998a). Various shapes such as round, oval, teardrop, or contoured have been available.

There are a number of major construction types of implants. Single-lumen implants have a single silicone elastomer shell traditionally filled with silicone gel. The gel is composed of cross-linked silicone permeated by silicone fluid (as described in Chapter 2). The chemical composition and weight-average molecular weight of the gel differs from manufacturer to manufacturer and from time to time (Dorne et al., 1995). As measured by extraction studies, the fluid may comprise 30–80% (Council on Scientific Affairs, 1993). Changes in fluid content affect the consistency and feel of the implant. Saline (at salt concentrations similar to those of body fluids) is used to fill shells. Rarely, other materials such as dextran, polyvinyl-pyrrolidone, or recently, soybean oil have also been used.

Some of these implants (valved) may be inflatable, so that their volume can be changed during implantation. Expanders are specifically designed to be inflated incrementally postsurgically. This creates an enlarging tissue pocket either to accommodate a replacement implant after a period of tissue adjustment or, less frequently, to accommodate the expander permanently. Expanders are used most often in reconstruction. Expansion actually leads to the formation of new tissue after operative excision of tissues for cancer or other conditions. This usually entails epidermal thickening, proliferation of blood vessels, and some dermal thinning with thick collagen bundles and myofibroblasts and muscle cell degenerative changes and loss in both the experimental and clinical situation (Argenta, 1984a, b; Argenta et al., 1985a; Austad et al., 1982; Gur et al., 1998; Johanson et al., 1993; Kim et al., 1993; Leighton et al., 1988; Pasyk et al., 1982; Rowsell et al., 1986).

Since the early 1980s, designs have been available with detachable reservoirs to allow the expander to be left as a permanent placement (Becker, 1984, 1986a; Gibney, 1989). About 14% of reconstruction implants were estimated to be permanent expanders (Zones, 1992). According to American Society of Plastic and Reconstructive Surgeons' (ASPRS, 1997) data, 31.66% of breast reconstructions involve the use of some kind of an expander. Expanders can be replaced with various permanent implants. Some surgeons report advantages to augmentation patients in the use of permanent gel–saline or saline expanders with the inflation ports left in place (Berrino et al., 1998a). Inflatable implants usually are saline filled, but rarely they contain gel with provision for changing size by the addition of saline to the gel-filled lumen. Expanders contain saline in a single lumen or sometimes an expandable saline lumen inside a gel lumen. Some expanders are directionally expandable through shell modification or piggyback-bonded separate expanders (Hester and Bostwick, 1990).

Historically, single-lumen, gel-filled implants (that include polyurethane-coated implants) have been the most commonly used, approximating 60–80% of devices implanted (Middleton, 1997; Zones, 1992). However, since the 1992 FDA moratorium on gel-filled implants, single-lumen saline implants, that historically comprised 5% of implants (Gabriel et al., 1994; Zones, 1992), have almost completely replaced gel implants (see Chapter 1). Saline as the filler for implants was originally considered, but discarded by Cronin in the early 1960s, presumably because gel implants "remained normally expanded even when torn" (Cronin and Gerow, 1963) and "it seemed unlikely that leakage could be avoided for life" (Cronin, 1983a). Saline-filled implants were reported in France in 1965 (Arion, 1965) and in the United States in 1969 (Tabari, 1969—initially filled with dextran 6%). Saline implants were made earlier (1965) in New York City according to some observers (R.A. Ersek, personal communication, June 10, 1998). Their lesser popularity has been ascribed to a number of factors. These include: high deflation rates (since corrected) and leaky valves (Capozzi, 1986; Lantieri et al., 1997; Peters, 1997); a weight said to be up to 8% heavier than a comparable-volume gel implant (Barney, 1974); a fluid wave ("slosh effect") with sounds that can be heard by the patient (Asplund, 1984); and thin consistency and wrinkling that is visible through the skin and/or palpable (Gylbert et al., 1990a; Melmed, 1998; Slavin and Goldwyn, 1995). These undesirable features are alleviated to a large extent by the more tissue-like consistency of gel and its lower tendency to shift with different patient positions. Placement of the saline implant deep to the muscles of the chest and slight overfilling also minimize some of these problems (Nicolle, 1996). They must also be balanced against the problems of gel, such as gel fluid diffusion through the shell into the tissues; axillary adenopathy secondary to silicone; release of gel on implant rupture, which can be removed only incompletely by surgery and includes the possibility of gel migration and granuloma formation; higher incidences of contracture; and greater radiopacity of gel.

Standard double-lumen implants have two shells either connected or patched together or floating freely one in the other. The inner lumen is gel filled and the outer saline filled. In the case of reverse double lumen (implant expander), there is an inner saline and an outer gel-filled lumen. The idea here was that the thicker gel would minimize wrinkling, which led to leaks, while at the same time the expandable inner lumen would allow for some volume adjustment and potentially intraluminal medication (Colon, 1982). Double-gel or reverse adjustable double-lumen (gel–gel with provision to add saline to the inner gel) implants were rarely made (see company data below). The gel part of the standard double-lumen implant provides the cosmetic and other advantages of gel, and the saline part provides an inflatable or expander option and a reservoir for adrenal steroid, which, although not an FDA approved use, has been reported to minimize capsular contracture (Lemperle and Exner, 1993; Spear et al., 1991; and others, as noted in Chapter 5 of this report).

Aside from the expander and reservoir possibilities, the outer saline lumen was also supposed to form, in theory at least, an additional barrier against gel fluid diffusion or gel leakage or rupture and resulting silicone tissue residuals and granulomas (von Frey et al., 1992). This feature by itself was often ineffective (Melmed, 1998); in fact, no data could be found to support such a function. Yu et al. (1996) measured quantities of gel fluid diffusing from an explanted double-lumen implant that were consistent with amounts measured from implants of various kinds and were about twice as much as from a single-lumen gel implant explanted from the other breast of the same patient. Additional data from this group showed silicone gel fluid diffusion from double-lumen implants in greater amounts than from either barriered or unbarriered gel implants (Marrota et al., 1996a). Cocke and Sampson demonstrated silicone fluid droplets in cells of capsules of double-lumen breast implants biopsied four months after implantation by transmission electron microscopy and electron dispersion x-ray analysis (Cocke and Sampson, 1987).

The outer lumen of a double-lumen implant was designed to be punctured and deflated as a corrective to capsular contracture (Hartley, 1976), but this kind of implant did not appear to decrease the incidence of contractures (De Blecourt et al., 1989; Vasquez et al., 1987). The volume of the gel or saline outer lumen has been less than the volume of the inner lumen, varying roughly from 10 to 40% of the inner-lumen volume (Hester and Bostwick, 1990). At one time, standard double-lumen implants comprised about 12–15% of breast implants (Middleton, 1997; Zones, 1992); but since the 1992 FDA moratorium, they have given way to single lumen-saline implants and have been implanted 1% or less of the time (ASPRS, 1996). Triple-lumen implants, also seldom used, have three shells, the inner and middle filled with gel and the outer with saline.

Implants of gel alone (with no shell) were used, mostly, but not always outside the United States (Freeman, 1972, 1977). However, two gel implants without shells, the Cavon implant (CUI International) and an

Aesthetech implant are reported to have been made and sold in the United States (Middleton, 1998a). Some surgeons used small amounts of gel to fill in around implants (Middleton, 1998b), injected gel directly (Boo-Chai, 1969) or injected fluid with a catalyst to create RTV silicone gel within the breast (Conway and Goulian, 1963). Though unapproved, silicone fluid alone was formerly injected into breasts for augmentation in the United States (Ellenbogen and Rubin, 1975; Kagan, 1963; Vinnik, 1976a; see also Chapter 1 of this report).

IMPLANT SHELL CHARACTERISTICS

Implant shells are made of silicone rubber, that is, elastomer with a filler. They vary in the composition and characteristics of the elastomer (e.g., approximately 21–27% amorphous silica filler in the elastomer for the shell and in shell patches, and 16.5% in barrier coats according to Dow Corning). Specifications of other manufacturers may vary. Amorphous silica is different in its physicochemical properties and in its biologic effects from crystalline silica, which is reported not to be present in measurable amounts in implant shells or gels (see Chapter 2; see also IARC, 1997; Iler, 1981). Shell thickness also varies, ranging from 0.13 to 0.75 mm, or 0.005 to 0.030 inch. Some shells have been even thicker, and areas of some implant shells lie outside this range (J. Curtis, Dow Corning, personal communication, February 17, 1998; P. Klein, Dow Corning, personal communication, August 10, 1998; Z.F.Twardochleb, McGhan Medical, personal communication, July 7, 1998). Most shells have had smooth elastomer rubber, but increasingly, some are textured with different surface features or shell projections of varying coarseness, depending on the manufacturer.

Shell Polyurethane Coating

Texturing was a reaction to the success in reducing capsular contracture of the original 1- or 2-mm-thick poly(ester)urethane foam-textured coating of a regular silicone gel-filled implant (Ashley, 1970, 1972). The foam was produced from the polymerization of polydiethylene glycol adipate with a 4:1 mixture of 2,4- and 2,6-toluene diisocyanate and was secured by an RTV silicone adhesive primarily to single-lumen gel implants. Occasionally standard double-lumen, saline, and gel–saline implants were coated with polyurethane foam. The foam had 80–100 open pores of 200–500-mm in diameter per linear inch (Batich et al., 1989; Mishra, in FDA, 1990). About 1.35 g of foam covered an average implant (Szycher and Siciliano, 1991a).

The polyurethane coating of implants was popular. An estimated

110,000 women, or about 10% cumulatively (FDA, 1995) or 18.8% in a given year (e.g., 1990; Zones, 1992) had implants with polyurethane coating because it secured the implant and clearly reduced early contracture (Capozzi, 1991; Capozzi and Pennisi, 1981; Hester et al., 1988). The coating may not have amounted to more than a mostly temporary and no more effective form of texturing than that described below (Brand, 1984; Burkhardt and Eades, 1995; McCurdy, 1990). However, there are suggestions that polyurethane specifically inhibited fibroblasts, had some specific effects on immune cells (Bradley et al., 1994a), and either specifically or because of fragmentation into many small particles (see below and Goodman et al., 1988) was particularly effective in causing an acute and continuing chronic inflammatory response that postponed the mature fibrotic phase and accounted for delayed capsule formation (Brand, 1988; Devor et al., 1993; Sank et al., 1993; Smahel, 1978a; Whalen, 1988) with significantly less contracture than texturing of the silicone shell alone (Handel et al., 1995).

A number of reports established the success of polyurethane-coated implants in reducing the frequency of contractures in either the submammary or submuscular position in the first few years after implantation (Cohney et al., 1992; Handel et al., 1991a; Herman, 1984; Hester et al., 1988; Hoffman, 1989; Melmed, 1988; Pennisi, 1985, 1990; Wells, 1988), but it is difficult to be sure whether the long-term contracture result after disintegration of the coating was better than with other implants. For example, significant contractures occurred late in Cohney's large, long-term study (Cohney et al., 1992). An occasional synovial lining (see below) around a polyurethane implant was reported, which may also have influenced capsule formation, although that report described implants of a young age (2.5 years) (Raso and Greene, 1995). A tendency to seroma and the occurrence of late pain have also been reported (Jabaley and Das, 1986; Wilkinson, 1985). The cellular characteristics of any implant capsule most likely depend on a number of factors, some of which are as yet unknown (Hardt et al., 1994).

Polyurethane foam was said to undergo partial chemical degradation under physiologic conditions, releasing compounds that are, or could become, carcinogens in animals but are not known human carcinogens (i.e., 2, 4-toluenediamine [2, 4-TDA] or precursors) (Benoit, 1993; Chan et al., 1991a,b; Luu et al., 1994; NTP, 1978); however, these are reportedly released in very small amounts that would not present an unacceptable risk (Expert Panel, 1991; FDA, 1991b, 1995). Other evidence suggests that chemical degradation, although possible (Dillon and Hughes, 1992), may have been minimal (Amin et al., 1993; Hester et al., 1997; Szycher et al., 1991; Szycher and Siciliano, 1991a). Furthermore, epidemiological human and experimental animal evidence does not support an association between cancer and polyurethane (Brand, 1988; Cohney et al., 1992; Devor et al., 1993; Hagmar et al., 1993; Lemen and Wolfe, 1993; Sorahan and Pope 1993).

On the other hand, Sepai et al. (1995) reported levels of 2, 4-TDA in drainage from the implant operative site and, over a two-year period, in the plasma (> 4 ng/ml) of women with polyurethane-coated breast implants that were higher than had been considered previously in assessing cancer risks from these implants suggesting that the exposures and risks might be problematic. These risks had been estimated by the FDA at between 5 in 10,000,000 and 111 in 1,000,000 lifetime cancers in women with polyeurethane implants depending on the currently available data or a worst case 100% degradation to 2-4-TDA, respectively. The risk of 5 in 10,000,000 was considered reasonable by others (Expert Panel, 1991).

Given the relatively small number of women with polyurethane implants still in place, the natural breast cancer incidence in women, and the lack of evidence for polyurethane carcinogenesis, which implies at most a small effect, if any, of polyurethane in causing human cancer, it is unlikely that any study of patients with existing implants will be able to provide sufficient evidence of an association between these implants and cancer. At present, evidence is lacking to conclude that there is an association between polyurethane-coated implants and cancer, and the weight of existing evidence suggests that there is no such association. Since the implantation of polyurethane-coated breast implants within the United States is unlikely, these conflicting studies may never be reconciled.

In the human breast, the 1.5- to 2-mm foam coating separated from the implant surface and disintegrated physically as well as chemically beginning almost immediately and progressing over a few years; what remained was a mostly smooth implant with a capsule containing polyurethane fragments (Guidoin et al., 1991a,b; Hester et al., 1988; Shapiro, 1989; Slade and Peterson, 1982; Smahel, 1978a,b; Szycher et al., 1991) although there has not been complete agreement on this point (Szycher and Siciliano, 1991b). The same disintegration into scattered polyurethane fragments and migrating fibers has been observed in experimental female mice within 47 weeks (Devor et al., 1993), and half-lives for biodegradation of about 21 months or 2–3 years have been calculated, respectively, from human 2,4-TDA excretion data and explanted implants (Hester et al., 1997; Sinclair et al., 1993).

Although some studies reported that the adherent capsule was more resistant to infection (Merritt et al., 1979; Whalen, 1988), others reported major problems with eliminating infections in capsules because disintegrated foam acted as multiple foreign bodies and was often very difficult to remove (Berrino et al., 1990; Bruck, 1990; Guidoin et al., 1991a; Hardt et al., 1994; Hester, 1988; Melmed, 1988; Okunski and Chowdary, 1987;

Umansky and Wilkinson, 1985; Wilkinson, 1985). In addition to problems in removing foam fragments, the polyurethane implant itself was difficult to explant (Bruck, 1990; Cohney and Mitchell, 1997). There is insufficient evidence that infection was more frequent in these implants (Handel et al., 1991a; Hester et al., 1988; Melmed, 1988, Pennisi, 1990). The coated shell was also notably more radiopaque on mammography than an uncoated shell (Young et al., 1991a) and may have interfered with magnetic resonance imaging for rupture (Ahn et al., 1993). Domestic polyurethane foam-coated implants were discontinued in 1991.

Implant Shell Texturing

The form of texturing of silicone elastomer implant shells varied considerably by manufacturer. For example, Dow Corning Silastic MSI (Micro Structured Implant) had regular pillars 750 mm high, 250 mm in diameter, and 500 mm apart. McGhan Biocell uses an open pore network, 3.1 pores/mm^2, average size 289 mm, height 500–800 mm. Mentor Siltex has surface irregularities 65–150 mm high and 60–275 mm wide. Bioplasty MISTI consisted of pores 20–800 mm wide (Barone et al., 1992; Dow Corning, 1991, p. 20021; Jenkins et al., 1996; Maxwell and Hammond, 1993). Most of the originally smooth major construction types were sold with texturing, beginning in the mid-1980s, to minimize capsular contracture (Hakelius and Ohlsen, 1997; Hammerstad et al., 1996; Maxwell and Hammond, 1993; Pollock, 1993).

Texturing was assumed to work to reduce capsular contracture in ways similar to polyurethane; that is, tissue grew into the interstices of projections or pores, prolonging chronic inflammation, disorienting collagen fibrils, and weakening their contractile forces (Barone et al., 1992; Whalen, 1988). Some descriptions of textured gel- or saline-filled implant capsules also note the formation of peri-implant synovial tissue, that is, a joint lining-like tissue reaction that, along with a more cellular capsule, is said to check excessive contracture (Raso and Greene, 1997). The synovial cells around the implant, which appear on monoclonal antibody characterization to be the same as joint synovium, are reported to be more common around textured implants (Bleiweiss and Copeland, 1995; Copeland et al., 1994; Luke et al., 1997; Wickman et al., 1993). They are of monocyte or macrophage origin. There is suggestive evidence that some have phagocytic and transport functions that may have the capacity to transmit particulates such as silicone microdroplets or elastomer fragments (or, experimentally, colloidal carbon) outside the capsule to local lymph nodes and that others have a secretory function that may contribute to fluid surrounding the implant (Emery et al., 1994). Synovial lining has also been reported around smooth gel and saline implants (Burmester et al.,

1983; Chase et al., 1994a; del Rosario et al., 1995; Hameed et al., 1995; Luke et al., 1997; Raso et al., 1994a,b, 1995a,b).

Some studies have concluded that this synovial lining is a reaction to friction in a surgical cavity (i.e., a bursa) and is indistinguishable from the synovial lining of joints and normal bursae (Copeland et al., 1994; Emery et al., 1994). Recent analysis proposes that synovium is a transitional phase, inversely related to implant age and unrelated to other factors such as implant surface, placement, and capsule or gel fluid diffusion through the shell (Chase et al., 1996; Ko et al., 1996). Wyatt et al. (1998) recently reported 93 capsules from a variety of smooth and textured implants examined primarily during capsulectomy for contracture. The smooth implants had been in place for an average of 104 months, the textured for 67.7 months. Synovial cellular reaction decreased significantly with time around both smooth and textured implants (p = .003 and .051, respectively). Possibly synovium, beginning in bursae formed in response to friction from movement common to all breast implants, may mature over time to a fibrous tissue sheath with increasing predominance of fibroblastoid cells that were originally in the minority (Raso et al., 1994a). Other studies have concluded that synovium is a fundamental biological phenomenon in tissue spaces exposed to friction, which is seen in about 25% of implant capsules but is not particular to such sites (Schnitt, 1995). Still other reports put the percentage of synovial villous hyperplasia considerably higher (63%) in early textured implant capsules (Wyatt et al., 1998). Texturing may also cause more peri-implant fluid, in part at least due to the secretion of proteoglycans by synovial secretory cells, although some fluid around implants in general is fairly common. In a study of explants from symptomatic women, intracapsular fluid (0.2–20 ml) was found around 15% of implants, was not related to infection or any particular symptoms, but was more frequent around textured implants (Ahn et al., 1995a). Texturing is reported by some to be variably more (e.g., polyurethane, Biocell) or less effective in providing tissue fixation of implants (Maxwell and Hammond, 1993). Different patterns and depths of surface texturing seems to make a difference in cellular behavior and probably in clinical results. (For further discussion, see Chapter 5.)

Barrier Shells

In more recent times, many gel-filled implant models have had shells constructed to lessen the diffusion of silicone fluid compounds into the tissues. Either these models add one or two shell layers of diphenyl or other modified siloxanes, or they interpose a layer of fluorosilicone between the shell and the gel contents. In the case of Dow Corning, this fluorosilicone layer is reported to have limited silicone fluid "bleed" (or diffusion, as measured by various in vitro techniques designed to promote flow) to an estimated 96 mg per year per 300-ml implant, compared to 487 mg per year per implant in older models (T. Lane, Dow Corning, personal communication, April 28, 1998). Other, independent measurements of various implant models (Yu et al., 1996) put silicone gel fluid diffusion at about 300 mg per year, with considerable variation depending on implant age and manufacturer. Figures of 60–100 mg per year for pre-barrier and 5–10 mg per year for barrier implants are quoted frequently in the literature (Independent Advisory Committee on Silicone Gel-Filled Breast Implants, 1992), but these are probably just early Dow Corning estimates. Other early measurements varied between 15 and 45 mg at 12 weeks, depending on implant make (Bergman and van der Ende, 1979). In an accelerated bleed test (300°F, forced-air furnace) by Battelle, the Dow Corning Silastic II accumulated 14 mg of silicone gel fluid diffusing out through the shell at eight weeks. Implants of other manufacturers accumulated between 300 and 400 mg (Morey and North, 1986). Diffusion through the shell depends on the maintenance of a concentration gradient by the removal of fluid from the outside surface and through the capsule. Since the capsule appears to present a barrier to silicone movement, these estimates of the amount of fluid diffusion may be high, because they do not reproduce this feature (Beekman et al., 1997a; Yu et al., 1996).

In implants with a gel fluid number molecular weight of 13,840 g/mol, gel fluid diffusion averaged a number molecular weight of 11,630 g/mol (less than 0.05% low molecular weight cyclic siloxanes, D_4–D_6) or 6,194 g/mol (less than 0.4% low molecular weight cyclics, molecular weight of $D_4 = 296$) depending on the absence or presence, respectively, of a barrier coat (IOM Scientific Workshop, 1998). A minority percentage of higher molecular weight siloxanes, up to 400,000, was also reported in diffusate from implants without barrier coats, possibly from uncross-linked shell silicones (Varaprath, 1991, 1992). A silicone gel implant is said to contain about 855 parts per million (ppm) of D_4, or about 256 mg in an average-size (300-cc) gel implant (T.H. Lane and J.J. Kennan, personal communication, 1998). Using different methods, others have reported 1 mg per day of low molecular weight cyclic diffusion into surrounding hydrophilic media in vitro (Lykissa et al., 1997; E.D. Lykissa, personal communication, July 29, 1998). This figure seems high given the measurements cited above for total diffusion and the percentage of these compounds in the gel fluid. Presumably if this were to continue, the entire amount of D_4 in an implant would diffuse out in a year, which seems unlikely.

The fluorosilicone layer, which is a thin (about 10-µm) barrier coat on the interior surface of the implant shell, slowed diffusion because it had a solubility parameter quite different from that of the gel fluid. This was unfavorable to higher molecular weight silicones so diffusion was composed of relatively more low molecular weight silicone compounds, as noted above (Van Dyke, 1994; Van Dyke and Fowler, 1994). It also was not as strong as the usual elastomer rubber and typically added to shell thickness, although only slightly (about 4%). Reports of capsular and blood silicon levels in patients with implants from many different manufacturers have not substantially changed over time when shells of varying barrier effectiveness were used. In addition, several authors have reported that fluorosilicone barrier shells lose their effectiveness after two or three years, presumably due to fracture of this weaker elastomer (Baker et al., 1984; McConnell et al., 1997; Peters et al., 1995a,b, 1996; Yu et al., 1996).

Other Characteristics of Implant Shells and Gels

Rare shells, like the early polyurethane Ashley implant, had inverted Y-shaped internal dividers, presumably designed to control the shape of the gel and implant, keeping the gel from sagging to the dependent and central part of the implant. This feature was continued in the Optimam polyurethane implant until 1991. Patches in almost endless variety have been made of elastomer rubber, elastomer–Dacron, or Dacron alone [poly-(ethylene terephthalate)-based cloth]. Seal patches were used to seal holes and slits left in shells during manufacturing and to reinforce and seal the shell entries of valves or valve tubes used for filling inflatables and expanders. Fixation patches were designed in a vast array of sizes, shapes, and locations to be infiltrated by tissue and thereby keep the implant from sliding around within the breast. Fixation patches were found, or could be ordered, on almost all major implant types. Expanders meant to be replaced by permanent implants were rarely made with these patches. By the 1980s, however, fixation patches had fallen out or favor. They were felt to contribute to scarring around the implant (Williams, 1972), to a higher incidence of peri-implant calcification (Luke et al., 1997; Rolland et al., 1989b) and possibly to an increased likelihood of rupture (De Camara and Sheridan, 1993; Malata et al., 1994a). Patches as seals are still needed for manufacturing of modern seamless implants.

A variety of access ports and valves accessible through the skin have been available for inflatables and expanders, both at the implant and at a distance. Some of these remain with the implant. Some are removed after the final size of the implant has been achieved. Some valves have been reported to be quite insecure or to leak, which is said to contribute to implant deflation or microbial contamination of the saline in an implant. Middleton (1997, 1998a) listed six types of implants or expanders with valves and characterized and extensively described the various kinds of valves and patches.

The silicone gel-filled implant has undergone a number of changes over time. Its physical qualities have been altered, making it firmer or softer and more or less elastic. These changes and the addition of barrier layers and other shell changes may result in some different molecular species in gel fluid diffusion, although the fluid itself, at least in the case of Dow Corning, is said to have remained the same since 1975. Various catalysts have also been used as the manufacturing process has changed over time. Traces of these remain in the gel and could in theory diffuse through the shell. These include 1,3-diethenyl-1,1,3,3-tetramethyl-disiloxane–platinum complexes and methylvinylcyclosiloxane–platinum complexes, among others. These substances, bis-(2,4-dichlorobenzoyl) peroxide, and tin compounds such as stannous octoate or oleate or dibutyltin dilaurate (see Chapter 4 section on tin) were used in the elastomer or seal patch adhesive or RTV saline implant shells. The platinum compounds (said to be in the zero oxidative state) are generally reported to comprise 0.9 ppm of the gels and about 8–10 ppm of the shell and patch (J. Kennan, Dow Corning, personal communication, April 28, 1998; also NuSil, Compton, 1997) although this may vary with different gels or shells. The average Silastic I 305-cc implant contained 281 μg of platinum, 74% (207 μg) of which was in the gel presumably as a colloidal, elemental platinum residual (J. Curtis, Dow Corning, personal communication, April 28, 1998; Lewis et al., 1997). The conventional implant size of around 300 ml is based on company representations and actual experience with a 1,317-implant series averaging 284 cc (Middleton, 1998b) though lower averages have been reported (e.g., 247 cc, Fiala et al., 1993). Older model Silastic 0 implants contained more platinum—about 480 μg (Dow Corning IOM Scientific Workshop, 1998). Another investigator reported 4.5 μg/g platinum in gel from a Dow Corning implant, or about 1.3 mg per average implant, a higher value with questionable biological significance (El-Jammal and Templeton, 1995).[1] Analytical measurement of curing agents, solvents, and catalysts (process aids; see Chapter 2) by 48-hour dichloromethane and 24-hour 70°C saline extraction gave values of 20 ppm or less for these substances from extractions except for butylcarbitol acetate (up to 703 ppm). These substances are present at very low levels (T. Lane and J. Kennan, Dow Corning, personal communication, April 28, 1998)[2] and seem unlikely to contribute significantly to tissue levels by diffusion through the shell.

---

[1]Since the value of 207 μg is the actual amount of platinum added to about 300 g of gel, according to Dow Corning, the higher measured value is confusing.

[2]Acetone, butylcarbitol acetate, 2,4,-dichlorobenzoic acid, ethanol, 1-ethynyl-1-cyclohexanol, 2-methyl-3-butyn-2-ol, 1,1,1-trichlorethane, xylene, platinum, tin, and zinc were the substances measured.

Since silicone elastomers and gels may be irradiated under clinical conditions in patients with breast cancer, their stability and effect on the radiation beam when subjected to the doses delivered to such patients are important considerations. Although tests of a full range of elastomers and gels of various manufacturers have not been reported, the relatively small differences in silicones of various breast implants probably have minimal, if any, effect on stability or transmission characteristics. Tests of Surgitek, McGhan, and Dow Corning products have been reported. These reports and more generic reviews indicate that silicone gel breast implants should have no more clinically significant effect on radiation therapy than an equivalent amount of breast tissue or saline. Their physical characteristics and silicones themselves should remain relatively stable at dose levels up to 7,500 rads, although some discoloration of the gels and loss of compliance has been reported after irradiation (Klein and Kuske, 1993; Krishnan and Krishnan, 1986; Krishnan et al., 1983, 1993; Kuske et al., 1991; Landfield, 1983; McGinley et al., 1980; Shedbalkar et al., 1980). The radiation stability of silicone, partcularly platinum cured and phenyl methyl, is considered good (Radiation Sterilization Working Group, 1996). The cosmetic results are not adversely affected in irradiated, implant-augmented breasts when radiation is administered with careful attention to technique, according to most investigators, although there are some reports of greater frequency of capsular contracture. Contractures are more frequent and results are in general less good in immediate postmastectomy reconstruction using implants and in implantation in previously irradiated breast tissue (Barreau-Pouhaer et al., 1992; Chu et al., 1992; der Hagopian et al., 1981; Dickson and Sharpe, 1987; Evans et al., 1995; Forman et al., 1998; Halpern et al., 1990; Handel et al., 1991b; Jacobson et al., 1986; Kraemer et al., 1996; Krishnan et al., 1993; Kuske et al., 1991; Lafreniere and Ketcham, 1987; Mark et al., 1996; Rosato and Dowden, 1994; Ryu et al., 1990; Spear and Maxwell, 1995; Stabile et al., 1980; Thomas et al., 1993; Victor et al., 1998; von Smitten and Sundell, 1992), although radiation does not appear to affect contracture frequency or severity in experimental animals with implants (Caffee et al., 1988; Whalen et al., 1994). As noted elsewhere in this report (see Chapter 12), silicone gel- and saline-filled implants interfere with the visualization of the entire breast on x-ray film mammography. Relative radiolucencies of various fillers for implants were reviewed by Young et al. (1993a), and silicone gel interfered with visualization the most, followed by progressively more radiolucency with saline, bio-oncotic gel, and peanut oil fillers.

In view of the many manufacturers, major construction types, varying and changing shell elastomer rubber, gel, and surface characteristics, barrier layers, and other less meaningful differences, it is easy to appreciate why there were hundreds of types of implants. In fact, if dimensions, shape, and patch and valve characteristics are added to the variables, Middleton has estimated that as many as 8,300 different implants might have been available. Some of these can be identified by implant surface markings, which are sometimes radiopaque, or by other characteristics that are unique to a particular implant and identifiable either on explantation or by techniques such as film or MRI mammography. Identification can be useful in assessing the way implants might behave and has of course been useful in litigation (Middleton, 1997, 1998a). Presumably, gel, saline, or other filler, smooth or textured surface, barrier layer or standard elastomer shell, elastomer shell thickness, physical or chemical characteristics, other physical and chemical gel and gel fluid characteristics and compositions, and the presence and concentration of nonsilicone substances (e.g., catalysts or other substances remaining in the implant from the manufacturing process), would represent a minimum list of features that might have biomedical and health implications, either local or possibly systemic. Information on the product characteristics introduced over time by various manufacturers and distributors could help in analyzing these associations. This information, often considered in the nature of trade secrets, is not available in any detail. Even the information in this chapter was not easy to assemble and has not previously been assembled in this way.

IMPLANTS FROM DOW CORNING

Dow Corning Corporation made the first silicone gel breast implants for Dr. Thomas D. Cronin (Cronin and Gerow, 1963) in 1962. This model reflected the ideas of Cronin, who had been considering ways to improve implants through the 1950s, and of his resident Dr. Frank Gerow, in consultation with Mr. Silas Braley of the Dow Corning Center for Aid to Medical Research. After a year of development, the first implant was placed in March 1962 (Cronin, 1983a). Dow Corning continued to make these implants through 1963 in a form similar to, or the same as, that distributed in 1964, the company's first full commercial year. By the early 1970s the Dow Corning Cronin Dacron patched implant had achieved a stunning popularity of 88% of all implantations according to one survey (Williams, 1972).

Dow Corning gel used in the early Cronin and Silastic implants and officially from 1964 to 1969 and 1969 to 1975 respectively, was thick and firm. Information on these and later gels, elastomers, adhesives, and patches can be found in Chapter 2. In general, catalyst mixtures contained 0.9% platinum complexes or about 0.2% platinum (J. Kennan, personal communication, April 28, 1998), and the swelling fluid that was added to the gel was changed to (and remained) 1,000 centistoke (cS) DC-360 fluid in 1975 (T.H. Lane and J.J. Kennan, Dow Corning, personal communication, August 28, 1998). Also in 1975, the gel in the Silastic I model was changed so as to be softer and more compliant. This gel was used in the Silastic I, Silastic II (1981–1992), and textured models, Silastic MSI (1990–1992). Double-lumen models, first introduced in 1979, lagged in changing from Silastic I to II or adding MSI, but used the same responsive gel. Less compliant gel was partly reintroduced with shell changes in 1978 (522 and 529 series implants only) and 1981 (PO17 teardrop series implants only).

From 1964 to 1967, Dow Corning silicone elastomer rubber shells were thick and seamed. They were less thick and seamless from 1968 to 1973 (Cronin and Greenberg, 1970). As noted, chemical details can be found in Chapter 2 of this report. These two shells were, respectively, about 0.030 inch (0.75 mm) and 0.010 inch (0.25 mm) thick. The latter shell was made thinner and softer from 1973 to 1978 and was 0.005 inch (0.13 mm) thick on average. These dimensions presumably were described by Weiner et al. (1974) and may explain the differences in rupture rates reported by Peters and others, noted earlier. From 1979 to 1992 a high-performance elastomer shell was produced by dip coating. This shell, first used (1979–1981) only for saline inflatables, measured approximately 0.011 or 0.012 inch (0.28–0.30 mm) on average, depending on implant size, except when used in the textured MSI implants, where it was 0.020 inch, or 0.50 mm, thick. The fumed silica or silica aerogel content of these elastomers varied from about 24 to 37%.

In 1981, a 0.010-mm fluorosilicone barrier layer was added to the interior walls of implant shells filled with silicone gel. The barrier coat consisted of much the same components as the high-performance elastomer but used methylvinyl-*co*-trifluoropropylsiloxane instead of vinyl-terminated poly(dimethylsiloxane) (PDMS). As noted earlier, this barrier layer was to limit silicone fluid diffusion through the shell by changing shell solubility characteristics. It also was not as strong as usual elastomer rubber and so it could not spare elastomer thickness. Thus, the fluorosilicone layer added to the shell thickness. This barrier was said to be more effective than others (Morey and North, 1986) and was also said to be quite different from other barrier technologies and more effective at higher (nonphysiologic) temperatures (Caffee, 1992a).

After 1968, all shells were seamless. Seamless shells were prepared by dipping a form (mandrel) into an elastomer dispersion. After removal from the mandrel, the hole where the support arm held the mandrel was patched with a silicone elastomer material. Next, silicone gel was injected into the shell. For the responsive gel-filled product, the small perforation left after injection of the gel was sealed with a drop of silicone adhesive containing methyltriacetoxysilane and ethyltriacetoxysilane as cross-link-ers and stannous oleate as a catalyst. This adhesive was not used to bond fixation patches; a different form of elastomer was used for that purpose.

HEYER-SCHULTE–MENTOR IMPLANTS

In 1968, Heyer-Schulte Corporation became the first U.S. manufacturer of saline-filled breast implants. These implants had a shell thickness of 0.016 inch or 0.40 mm. The company was acquired by American Hospital Supply in 1974 and, after name changes, by Mentor in 1984. In 1968, Heyer-Schulte manufactured a polyurethane-coated silicone gel prosthesis with an internal Y-shaped baffle called the "Natural Y" prosthesis, which had previously been marketed by Poly Plastics Silicone Products (Ashley, 1970, 1972) pursuant to a 1968 patent by the plastic surgeon W. Pangman. Between 1971 and 1984, Heyer-Schulte introduced various additional models of single-lumen gel, inflatable saline, and double-lumen implants. These were mostly smooth surfaced. However, a polyurethane-coated adjustable gel–saline model was introduced briefly in 1973 (described by Jobe, 1978), and the Capozzi model polyurethane implant, which had no foam on its upper part in an effort to avoid fixation of the top of the implant and vertical wrinkling (see Chapter 5), was also available in the 1970s (Jobe, 1978). Data on shell thickness and gel characteristics were not made available by the company. Dorne reported weight-average gel molecular weights of 83,500 from a model 2000 (supposedly mid-1970s) implant, considerably higher than modern Silastic II gels (about 55,000). Slight differences in nuclear magnetic resonance (NMR) were detectable among gels from different manufacturers (Dorne et al., 1995); this was probably related to the firmer early versus the more compliant later gel.

Saline implant shell changes from HTV platinum catalyzed to RTV tin catalyzed toward the end of this period are noted to have produced dramatic improvements in abrasion resistance and durability (Gutowski et al., 1997; Mladick, 1993). Improvements in valves are also cited (see comments in Cocke, 1994; Gutowski et al., 1997; Lantieri et al., 1997; Mladick, 1993; and Peters, 1997, concerning the improved series 1600 and the problematic, leaky series 1800). Becker (1984) reported the development of his Mentor permanent expander at about this time and subsequently described an attached microreservoir that could be buried subcutaneously for long periods (Becker, 1986a).

Mentor continued the gel double-lumen and inflatable saline implant lines on acquisition of the company in 1984. In 1985, Mentor introduced a smooth reverse double lumen implant with gel outside and saline inside (the Becker implant, popular to this day as Siltex for reconstruction; Becker, 1987a, 1988) and saline expanders (in 1982, Radovan reported he had been using a Heyer-Schulte expander presumably for some time). In 1987 and 1989 the Siltex (textured) lines of implants were introduced, including the Siltex single-lumen gel, and then the Siltex (Becker) textured reverse double-lumen inflatable and textured saline inflatable implants. Clinically, the Siltex saline implant had a noticeably thicker shell than the smooth model. Women were said to prefer the smooth model, despite its higher frequency of contracture, to the often palpable and visible Siltex model (Burkhardt and Demas, 1994). Barrier shells were introduced on gel-filled models, presumably in the late 1970s. McGhan licensed barrier technology to Mentor in 1990 (Z.F. Twardochleb, personal communication, December 14, 1998).

In 1992, new (post-FDA moratorium) models of Siltex expander–implants and contoured saline implants with various valves were introduced. The elastomer from these models was used for immune adjuvant studies reported in 1996 (Hill et al., 1996). Presumably, it was improved over earlier elastomers, but specifics are not available from the company. Like those of other manufacturers, the Heyer-Schulte and Mentor lines offer various patch and valve designs. Gel suppliers for these companies were General Electric from 1970 to 1976, Dow Corning from 1976 to 1992, and Applied Silicone from 1988 to the present.

POLYURETHANE HISTORY AND MEDICAL ENGINEERING CORPORATION (SURGITEK) IMPLANTS

The polyurethane Natural Y line was continued by Heyer-Schulte through 1978. It was then manufactured by Cox-Uphoff International until 1981. In that year, the Aesthetech Corporation was formed and began manufacturing the device. It was known as the Optimam from 1982 to 1991. The Meme^{ME} was introduced as a polyurethane-coated, single-lumen gel implant without the Y septum from 1982 to 1985. The Vogue model with a Y septum was also made from 1982 to 1985 and replaced by the Meme^{MP} (Moderate Profile) without the Y septum from 1985 to 1991. The Replicon polyurethane implant without septum was made from 1984 to 1991. These lines were acquired by Cooper Laboratories until December 1988, when the Aesthetech Corporation was merged into the Medical Engineering Corporation (MEC), which continued to manufacture the Meme, Replicon, and Optimam implants until sales were suspended in 1991. Elastomer shell thickness reported for Meme was 0.003 inch, or 0.075 mm; for Replicon, 0.009 inch, or 0.23 mm; and for Meme^{MP,} 0.009 inch or 0.23 mm (dates provided by Mentor Corp.; Tobin and Middleton, 1987). These dimensions probably accounted for the changes in rupture rates of these different models noted earlier. The Microthane polyurethane foam used for Aesthetech and MEC (Surgitek) implants was fabricated from polyester foam supplied by Scotfoam (SIF 100 ppi Z M). The polyurethane was reported to have been made from an ethylene adipate triol with a molecular weight of 3,000 and toluene diisocyanate (20% 2,4- and 5% 2,6-toluenediisocyanate by weight). The molecular interface was composed mainly of polyester linkages and very few urethane linkages and was reported to yield very little TDA on enzymatic attack (Delclos et al., 1996; Szycher and Siciliano, 1991a).

The Medical Engineering Corporation (Surgitek) began distributing implants in 1971, originally various lines of gel-filled single-lumen implants, to which were added inflatable saline implants and expanders in 1974, double-lumen implants in 1977, and single-lumen gel–saline implants in 1978 (original Perras Papillon and later models). More compliant shells and gels were introduced in 1972. An unusual gel inflatable was made in 1973 (Dahl et al., 1974). The corporation was acquired in 1982 by Bristol Myers Squibb, which added high-profile models in 1982 and SCL (Strong shell, Cohesive gel, Low bleed) gel implants in 1986. The Natural Y polyurethane line was acquired by Bristol Myers Squibb in 1988. The polyurethane models were the only non-smooth-shelled models.

The first shells in 1971 were made of a General Electric (GE) Company copolymer of silicone and Lexan polycarbonate. Because of its stiffness, this was replaced by a GE silicone elastomer in 1973. From 1971 to 1976 the gel was GE 6193 MEC 122. From 1976 on, the shells were Dow Corning elastomer (Q7-2245, Q7-4735, and Q7-4750 at various times with various models, and Dow Corning 2213 on polyurethane models in 1981–1988), with an interior McGhan NuSil phenylsiloxane barrier on the SCL models. After 1976 the gels were supplied by Dow Corning and were similar to those used in its implants (Dow Corning Q7-2167/68). Peters reported that the low-bleed feature (SCL) introduced in 1986 did not seem to provide lasting protection, at least as determined by capsular and blood silicon levels (Peters et al., 1996). The company stopped distributing breast implants in 1991.

INAMED–MCGHAN MEDICAL AND CUI IMPLANTS

McGhan Medical Corporation began marketing breast implants in 1974. The company was merged with Minnesota Mining and Manufacturing Company in 1980 and subsequently acquired by First American in 1985. The company is now wholly owned by Inamed Corporation. Its implants have been sold in the United States and worldwide under the McGhan brand name. In 1975 the product line included smooth, single-lumen saline implants and expanders, single-lumen gel implants and combination gel–saline implants, and the first double-lumen implants (Hartley, 1976). Except for the single-lumen gel implants, all of these models had been updated by 1981. Individually customized inflatable implants for reconstruction after radical mastectomy were reported (Birnbaum and Olsen, 1978). Reverse double-lumen implants and expanders were added in 1987, including a double-gel model (with gel in both lumens) in 1991 and a triple-lumen model (with saline in the outer lumen and two gel lumens) in 1979. New shells were introduced periodically: a "silica free" (the exact meaning of this term is not clear) low-bleed, outer layer (Natrashiel) in 1977; a similar low-bleed shell (Natrashiel II) and a double-layer, increased-strength, decreased-bleed shell (UHP, Ultra High Performance) in 1978, and a low-bleed model containing two high-performance elastomer layers with a dimethyldiphenylsiloxane barrier layer (Intrashiel) in 1979. Gel-filled, textured and smooth models using this technology remain available.

A textured (Biocell) shell was announced in 1987 (as described earlier, Maxwell and Falcone, 1992; Maxwell and Hammond, 1993). The Intrashiel shell was the subject of an experimental study in rabbits reported in the medical literature and appeared to control silicone gel fluid diffusion from implants (Rudolph and Abraham, 1980). New shells were used on all models (except triple lumen) by 1979. In 1994, after the FDA moratorium, additional saline models were introduced. The company now sells Intrashiel, Biocell and smooth single-lumen gel, and smooth and Biocell saline models with diaphragm valves. The company's protocol for evaluation leading up to an application for premarket approval includes also a standard double lumen and a triple lumen with a gel cone within the combination gel–saline design. The company's saline tissue expander with a MagnaSite injection site, introduced in 1984, continues on the market in smooth and Biospan textured form; smooth and textured tissue expanders without the MagnaSite injection site are also available. Because the expander with the MagnaSite injection site has a magnetic locator, MRI is contraindicated in patients with these devices.

Some details of the specifications of shells and gels are considered proprietary by the company. However, measurements may be available from other sources (e.g., Intrashiel shell thickness measured 0.005–0.014 inch, 0.13–0.35 mm, in 1985; Morey and North, 1986), and other details were disclosed for this report by the company in a redacted report of confidential business information (gel implants only) that had been provided to the Independent Review Group (IRG, 1998). Shells were reported in 1994 to consist of multiple layers of modified PDMS incorporating vinyl substituents and/or modified PDMS incorporating phenyl or trifluoropropyl and vinyl substituents, the phenyl- (style 40) and trifluoropropyl- (style 246) modified silicones being the barrier layers. Treated amorphous silica is included in the shell formulation. Platinum catalysts are used, and solvents in which the shell components are dispersed during manufacture include trichloroethane or xylene (removed after dip casting). Also, in 1994 it was reported that the basic cure for the shell and silicone gel involves the reaction of a linear PDMS containing vinyl substituents with a linear, PDMS-containing silicon–hydrogen bonds catalyzed by classical platinum catalysts. Patch and injection port materials are cured using a peroxide catalyst that decomposes with the heat of the vulcanization step. The gel contains only PDMS polymers, a significant proportion of which are not bound but are entangled in the cross-linked polymer network. Approximately 2–8% of the shell and 50% of the gel by weight are extractable by hexane, slightly more by dichloromethane. Hexane extracts of shell and gel contain low concentrations of cyclic PDMS (about 520 μg/g, D_3–D_6, of which 38–99 μg/g is D_4 in gel and shell respectively, i.e., somewhat less than the Dow Corning extracts [0.05%] noted earlier) and linear PDMS along with trace amounts of solvents. Preliminary data suggest that the barrier shells reduce gel fluid diffusion by at least an order of magnitude compared with a McGhan nonbarrier shell (Eschbach and Schulz, 1994—redacted).

Silicone gel suppliers to McGhan Medical were General Electric 1975–1976, Dow Corning 1976, McGhan 1977–1984, McGhan Nusil 1984–1992, and thereafter NuSil Technology. Although undoubtedly a generic (see Dow Corning above) rather than a specific silicone gel property, a NuSil gel was reported to have adjuvant and other immune properties (Naim et al., 1993, 1995a,b). This and another gel from McGhan implants and one Dow Corning gel were later compared for strength of adjuvancy by a similar test procedure, which presumably does not reflect what happens in women with implants. Gels with greater emulsifying ability proved stronger adjuvants. This is an indication of the different characteristics of gels that can have biological implications, although it is not clear what relationship it bears to the in vivo situation in women with implants and thus what, if any, clinical significance this particular effect might have (Naim et al., 1997; see also Chapter 6 of this report).

Cox Uphoff International (CUI) began marketing implants in 1976, introducing smooth single-lumen gel (1976–1991), double-lumen (1977–1991), reverse double-lumen (1982–1993), triple-lumen (1983–1988), gel–saline adjustable (1987–1991), various tissue expanders including a permanent gel/saline model (Gibney, 1989) (1976–present), smooth dimethyl saline (1977–1991) and RTV smooth (1991–1994) and RTV textured (Microcell) (1992–1994) saline models. In 1980 and 1981, the Cavon silicone implant was made by Cox Uphoff (and later, in 1981–1985, by Aesthetech). By 1984, a DRIE (diffusion rate inhibiting envelope) low-bleed shell was introduced. Silicone gel suppliers to Cox Uphoff were Dow Corning (1976–1983), International Silicone (1981–1984), McGhan NuSil (1987–1991), Admiral Materials (1985–1989), Polymer Technologies

(1989–1990), and Applied Silicone (1990). The company was acquired by Inamed Corporation in 1989. Details on specifications of gels and shells are considered proprietary by Inamed.

BIOPLASTY AND OTHER MANUFACTURERS

After acquiring Roger Klein Mammatech in 1987 (R.A. Ersek, personal communication, March 19, 1998), R.A. Ersek, a plastic surgeon, began the Bioplasty line in 1988. The line originally consisted of MISTI (Molecular Impact Surface Textured Implant) textured single-lumen gel and double-lumen models, which were developed in 1987 and introduced in 1988. MISTI GOLD textured single-lumen polyvinylpyrrolidone (PVP, known as bio-oncotic gel) implants were introduced in late 1990 under FDA 510k provisions, followed by single-lumen PVP and saline MISTI GOLD and MISTI GOLD II textured PVP and saline prefilled and inflatable implants in 1991. Gel suppliers were Dow Corning (1987–1988), Admiral Materials (1987–1988), and Applied Silicone (1988–1992). The PVP used was low molecular weight (average molecular weight = 13,700; Beisang and Geise, 1991). Higher molecular weight PVP was used in more than 500,000 cases during World War II as a plasma expander (Bischoff, 1972). PVP was said to have much greater lubricating properties for the silicone shell, thereby decreasing friction and fold flaws; to diffuse rapidly from tissues; and to be quickly eliminated by the kidney, thus eliminating residuals or granulomas after implant rupture. These implants also had textured shells to reduce contractures and were reported to be radiolucent enough not to block mammographic visualization (Ersek and Salisbury, 1997; Ersek et al., 1993), although they were less radiolucent than triglyceride (peanut oil) filler and tended to degrade when subjected to irradiation (Klein and Kuske, 1993). Bioplasty entered bankruptcy in 1992, and its assets were purchased by NovaMed in Germany, which plans to reintroduce the slightly thicker polyvinylpyrrolidone lines to the U.S. market as Nova Gold (R.A. Ersek, personal communication, April 6, 1998). At present, NovaMed has begun domestic operations as a small company in Minnesota with plans to begin sales with saline implants first. The company has a marketing alliance with McGhan Medical Corporation (Z.F. Twardochleb, McGhan Medical Corporation, personal communication, 1999).

A number of foreign manufacturers distributed implants in the United States. The first saline implants and inflatables by Simaplast (France) were distributed as Roger Klein Mammatech (1968–1978, although some say earlier—[1965]; R.A. Ersek, personal communication, June 10, 1998). Smooth single-lumen gel, saline inflatable, double-lumen, and some polyurethane-coated implants were introduced in 1987 by Laboratoires Sebbin

(Unimed, Omega label). Koken (Japan), also known as Porex, presumably distributed gel implants with very fluid, compliant gel in the 1980s. Other companies include Unimed (Germany), PMT (Progress Mankind Technology, Germany—Integra label), Polytech (Germany, associated with Brazilian Silimed—Opticon, Mesmo, Vogue labels), Nagor (Britain), Eurosilicone (France, acquired by Polytech), and Silicone Medicale Paris (France) (Middleton, 1998a). Currently some foreign manufacturers continue to have small minority positions marketing saline implants under 510(k) provisions in the U.S. breast implant market—Hutchinson International, Inc., representing Biosil, a British company, Poly Implant Protheses, S.A. (PIP), a French company and Silimed, a Brazilian company. Little information is available about their products in the medical or other literature, and neither Biosil nor PIP responded to requests for information for this report (E. March, Medical Devices, personal communication, July 22, 1998).

CONCLUSION

The universe of implants is large, and the variation among them is substantial. In women being studied, it is often difficult to know what implants might be in place and what their characteristics might be. Companies apparently made implants for a number of plastic surgeons and often introduced designs conceived (and patented) by individual surgeons, presumably without further testing. The business was competitive, and companies introduced changes such as softer gels; barrier low-bleed (low-diffusion) shells; greater or lesser shell thickness and durability to reduce rupture and leaking and/or to enhance softness; texturing to reduce contracture; and various sizes, contours, shapes, and multiple lumens in the search for better aesthetics. These changes were introduced at somewhat different times and usually affected some but not all of a company's products. It was not possible to locate much in the way of clinical pretesting of these changes, some of which had unintended consequences. In fairness, it should be noted that testing was not required by the FDA until recently. In general, early implants were thick shelled and contained firm gel. More compliant gels were introduced between 1972 and 1975 by various companies, although the gels were primarily General Electric (departed the medical marketplace in 1976) and Dow Corning. Thinner elastomer rubber shells entered the market from 1972 to 1977, depending on the manufacturer. Various high-performance shells were marketed between 1978 and 1986. It is not clear what chemical changes made these shells high performance, although the performance referred to was greater resistance to tearing. Barrier coating, low silicone gel fluid diffusion features were added on various lines between about 1977 and

1986, and texturing was added in 1987 and 1988 (except for polyurethane coating, which was available from around 1970). The dates indicating market entry of significant new general characteristics could be helpful in considering clinical reports that do not describe implant types and specifications.

It is tempting to assume, as informal comments from some company officials and some comparative analyses imply, that implants of companies using Dow Corning or General Electric silicone gel and elastomer rubbers were made with chemical compounds and characteristics that were quite similar (Thompson et al., 1979). Clearly, gels changed over time and differed somewhat among different manufacturers who entered and left the market at various times. Thus, women were undoubtedly exposed to varying concentrations of the different molecular types and molecular weights or viscosities of silicone, but there were also surely many similarities among products from the same or very few basic manufacturers. This is the assumption that appears to underlie one recent analysis of soft-tissue responses to "approximately fourteen" precursor components of breast implants (Picha and Goldstein, 1991). With respect to elastomers, they were identified only 45% of the time in the series of up to 50 reports reviewed by Foliart (1997).

In general, it can be concluded that there have been at least three "eras" (referred to as generations by others, as noted later in this report) and a number of lesser variations in breast implant manufacture. In the first era, dominated by Dow Corning, there were thick-shell, thick-gel, patched, smooth-surfaced implants with low rupture rates, high contracture, and probably moderate to high gel fluid diffusion rates; in the second era, thin-shell, compliant gel, smooth-surfaced gel and HTV saline implants with high rupture and deflation rates, high contracture, and high gel fluid diffusion rates; and in the third era, stronger-shell, barrier-layer, compliant gel, textured gel- and saline-filled and stronger RTV saline implants with as-yet incomplete data, but presumably lower rupture and deflation rates (although not enough time has elapsed to predict this with confidence), lower gel diffusion rates, and lower contracture rates. This latter era may continue to the present or may have given way to a fourth era with changes resulting from the FDA moratorium on gel implants, the predominance of saline implants from the two remaining manufacturers, and the requirements for study protocols. In any event, differences in local and perioperative complications caused by these implants from different eras clearly have implications for the safety of silicone breast implants as described further in Chapter 5. It seems reasonable to conclude that both the physical and the chemical characteristics of implants should be spelled out clearly in product changes, introductions, and investigations because they may influence patient reactions and patient health. Moreover, as noted in Chapter 5, it would be desirable to accumulate information on the safety, complications, and health effects of a stable group of implants and not make changes until the safety, complications, and health implications of these changes are known.

4

Silicone Toxicology

SCOPE AND CRITERIA FOR THE TOXICOLOGY REVIEW

This chapter reviews studies of the toxicology of silicone compounds carried out over the past 50 years. It does not review immunological studies, except occasionally when immune system toxicology is part of a report covering other toxicology. Otherwise, immunological studies are discussed in Chapter 6. Silicone compounds include a great many chemical entities; a recent compilation lists toxicological data on 56 different siloxanes (Silicones Environmental Health and Safety Council, 1995). This chapter identifies silicone compounds as they are listed in individual reports, but it is organized by route of exposure not by type of compound. Silicone fluids, gels, and elastomers are covered since they are components of silicone breast implants.

Although the most relevant exposures are reviewed, that is, tissue injections and subcutaneous implants, the committee, unlike other recent reviews (Kerkvliet, 1998) also decided to include other (nonimplantation) exposure routes, such as dermal, oral, and inhalation, since data from such studies may provide some insights into systemic silicone toxicology. The committee included citations on the toxicology of silica in the reference list of this report, because there has been considerable mention of silica as a component of breast implant elastomers. However, the toxicology of silica is not reviewed here because the committee found no valid scientific evidence for the presence of or exposure to silica in tissues of women with breast implants. Some compounds not found in breast implants (and identified as such) are included briefly, sometimes to complete a survey of silicone species and other times because they have been mentioned in the current debate on the toxic effects of implants. It is important to note that toxicology studies often report silicone dose levels substantially in excess of any doses that could be achieved on a relative weight basis in women with silicone breast implants.

Earlier in this report, the committee emphasizes the relevance of published, peer-reviewed scientific reports and assigns secondary importance to technical reports from industry. In this chapter, however, studies done in-house by industry or by commercial testing laboratories have been analyzed. Such reports are often reviewed first in-house, then by the sponsor and panels of outside experts, and eventually by a regulatory agency, which also looks at original data. The conflict of interest inherent in experimentation by an organization with an economic interest in the outcome is recognized. Nevertheless, the committee found many of industry's technical studies informative, useful, and consistent with sound science. The studies cited here consisted of about 50 individual articles from the open scientific literature between 1948 and 1999 and about the same number of industry technical reports. Reviews available to the committee summarized data from some reports not reviewed by or not available to the committee. For example, the Silicones Environmental Health and Safety Council (1995) examined may reports on various organic silicon compounds that are not found in breast implants and reviewed some reports not accessible to the committee. This review was useful in presenting an overall picture of the generally low toxicity of silicones and identifying particular compounds that had toxicity. The report of the Independent Review Group (IRG, 1998) (and earlier versions of the Medical Devices Agency's work), and the report of the National Science Panel (Kerkvliet, 1998) which are described in Appendix C looked at essentially the same body of toxicology information as the committee. The IRG report included proprietary data not available to the committee, and as noted, the committee examined routes of exposure and listed silica references neither of which are included in the IRG or National Science Panel reports. Since the IRG, which had some proprietary data, concluded that silicones were bland substances with little toxicity, such data seem unlikely to have changed the committee's findings in any substantial way. Also, the committee believes that the inclusion of dermal, oral and inhalation toxicology studies in this report provided additional security in conclusions about the biological and toxicological behavior of relevant silicones.

Kerkvliet lists three major reasons why toxicology studies are helpful in assessing the safety of a drug or consumer product such as silicone breast implants. (1) Toxicology studies in animals may identify a hazard—that is, whether a given product can cause adverse health effects. (2) Studies may also clarify dose responses—that is, how much of an entity is necessary to produce effects. (3) Studies may provide mechanistic information—that is, how and under what circumstances an agent produces effects (Kerkvliet, 1998). Such studies, reviewed here, will not "fulfill the manufacturers' responsibility to demonstrate the safety of . . . implants" as Kessler urged in 1992 (Angell, 1995), since unanticipated events cannot be predicted or complete safety proven. Accumulating qualitative and quantitative data on the general toxicity of silicones, however, allow a reasonable degree of confidence that silicone compounds in breast implants are not hazardous.

BRIEF HISTORY OF SILICONE TOXICOLOGY

The principles of safety evaluation have not changed much over the past 50 years. However, analytical tools, the ability to measure chemicals in the body, and the science of molecular biology, which allows association of complex changes in a few cells or molecules with various disease states, have advanced considerably. These advances affect evaluations of the toxicology of silicones over time and are reflected in more recent studies.

One of the first (if not the first) systematic evaluations of the toxicology of commercial silicones was conducted during World War II at the Dow Chemical Company. Silicone intermediates (chlorosilanes and ethoxysilanes) and selected commercial silicones were tested in rats, rabbits, and guinea pigs. The chlorosilanes and some ethoxysilanes were found to be highly corrosive; they represented significant industrial handling hazards. Methyl- and mixed methyl- and phenylpolysiloxanes, on the other hand, had very low toxicity. For practical purposes, they were divided into three groups: fluids, compounds, and resins. Five methylpolysiloxane and two methylphenylpolysiloxane fluids were tested (hexamethyldisiloxane, 0.35 centistoke [cS]; dodecamethylpentasiloxane, 2 cS; DC 200 fluid, 50 cS; DC 550 fluid, 550 cS; DC 702 fluid, 35 cS; DC 200 fluid, 350 cS; and DC 200 fluid, 12,500 cS). None of these killed rats or guinea pigs when given orally at doses up to 30 ml/kg. Some of the fluids had laxative effects not unlike mineral oil. DC 200 fluid (50 cS) "seemed literally to flow through the animals." The fluid with the lowest viscosity (hexamethyldisiloxane, 0.65 cS) did not have a laxative effect, but produced some mild inebriation and subsequent central nervous system depression. This suggests that there might be some absorption of this compound from the gastrointestinal tract. Repeated administration of DC 200 oil (350 cS) by stomach tube, up to dose levels of 20 g/kg, did not produce gross signs of toxicity such as reduced weight gain, changes in organ weight, or organ pathology.

Intraperitoneal injection was well tolerated, except for hexamethyldisiloxane, which produced extensive adhesions within the peritoneal cavity. This compound also produced inflammation and necrosis at the sites of subcutaneous and intradermal injections and proved lethal on repeated intraperitoneal injections. Other silicone fluids in the peritoneal cavity elicited only reactions "typical . . . of an irritating foreign body" with nodules containing the fluid in the omentum and visceral peritoneum. Eye irritation was transitory and no skin irritation was observed with these fluids (Rowe et al., 1948).

Shortly after the report by Rowe et al., Kern et al. (1949) reported their results from feeding rats 0.05%–0.2% silicone-containing diets (a polydimethylsiloxane [PDMS], G.E. Dri-Film, No. 9977) and injecting silicone suspensions at unknown (but probably low) doses, intraperitoneally and intravenously in mice, and intra- and subcutaneously and in the muscles of rabbits. Hematological and gross and microscopic pathology examinations after 13 weeks were all normal, and the animals had no loss in body weight or other signs of toxicity (Kern et al., 1949).

Two silicone compounds (DC 4 Ignition sealing compound and DC Antifoam A) were examined. Both agents caused transient conjunctival irritation, but no corneal damage when introduced directly into the eyes. No skin irritation was seen. Feeding of Antifoam A at concentrations up to 1% to rats did not produce any untoward effects. In a six-month feeding study in dogs, Antifoam A also exhibited no toxicity (Child et al., 1951). Three types of silicone resins (DC 2102, a methylpolysiloxane, DC 993, a methylphenylpolysiloxane; and DC Pan Glaze, which was similar to DC 993) were evaluated. Acute oral administration of up to 3 g/kg in guinea pigs was not toxic (higher doses could not be administered), and intraperitoneal injection in rats or dermal application in rabbits produced no signs of irritation. Rats fed Pan Glaze at concentrations up to 3% for 50 days gained weight normally, and on microscopic examination, their organs did not show any signs of toxicity (Rowe et al., 1948, 1950).

The studies described by Rowe et al. (1948) reflect state-of-the-art toxicity testing at that time. They were done in a respected laboratory by competent toxicologists. The untoward effects observed with some compounds did not alarm toxicologists. These effects were found only after exposure to high doses of the test agent. According to an old classification, substances with a probable human lethal dose in excess of 15 g/kg were considered practically nontoxic (Casarett, 1975). These investigators commented that "for the past few years, an attempt has been made to keep pace with the rapid development of these products so that toxicological information would be available upon which the health hazards of these materials could be evaluated." Only a few selected samples from each class of compounds were studied, but the experimental toxicology of silicone compounds did not yield data that suggested a need for fundamental, mechanistically oriented experimentation.

When these and some other early studies were reviewed in 1950, silicone fluids with a viscosity of 350 cS were described as having exceedingly low toxicity. Some animal toxicity tests, such as oral and subcutaneous administration and eye irritation, were even performed on one of the authors of this study (Barondes et al., 1950). By then-current standards of toxicology, silicone fluids had to be considered harmless, devoid of any obvious acute toxic potential, and thus presumably safe.

THE CURRENT DATABASE

A recent review of silicone toxicology summarized a substantial database (Silicones Environmental Health and Safety Council, 1995). This document does not list any references which makes it impossible to determine whether the data were published or to discover when the studies were done. It is not possible, therefore, to evaluate adherence to modern good laboratory practice regulations, protocols, and procedural requirements. Carcinogenesis studies done before the mid-1970s had different protocols and procedural requirements than later studies and, by today's standards, must be considered less reliable. This may apply to other test systems as well. The Silicones Council review analyzed a total of 629 studies (see Table 4-1), more than half of them done with PDMS linears (Chemical Abstracts Service [CAS] No. 63148-62-9). Compounds that are of concern because a large number of people are exposed to them and because they are found in breast implants, that is, D_4 and D_5 (where D_4 and D_5 represent cyclic tetramer and pentamer, respectively), comprise 17% of studies. There are few chronic lifetime or carcinogenesis studies (less than 3%) and immunological studies (less than 5%). Acute and subacute toxicity and irritation studies are in the majority (57%). Some of the Silicones Council studies summarized briefly in this current database may also be reviewed subsequently in other parts of this chapter. As noted, this material presents an overall picture of silicone toxicity based on a general review of many data sources covering a wide variety of compounds. Specific studies on breast implant compounds are relied on by the committee for conclusions relevant to the safety of silicone breast implants, however.

RESULTS OF STUDIES IN FOUR MAIN GROUPS

Group I

A: Dimethylsiloxanes

A total of 123 reports on cyclic polydimethlsiloxanes (D_3, D_4, D_5, and D_6) were reviewed. These compounds are volatile and potentially of concern in manufacturing; however, they also are used in consumer products, such as hair sprays, and are found in breast implants, although in very low amounts (see Chapter 3). They are practically nontoxic on ingestion, dermal application, or inhalation, although they are mildly irritating when placed directly on the skin or in the eyes. Subacute gavage studies showed that these compounds had no untoward effect other than a reversible increase in liver weight due to increases in both cell number and cell size at doses ranging up to 2,000 mg/kg. Skin application did not cause toxicity; however, some D_5 penetrates the skin. No signs of toxicity were observed in subacute and chronic inhalation studies, except the development of hepatomegaly in some animal species, which was reversible on cessation of exposure. No evidence for carcinogenicity was found. Bacterial and mammalian mutagenicity studies were generally negative. Developmental and reproductive studies failed to show teratogenic effects or effects on fertility, except when exposure conditions were high enough to cause maternal toxicity in a rabbit study with D_4. Immunotoxicity was studied following intraperitoneal, intramuscular, subcutaneous, and dermal exposure. D_4 had a substantial adjuvant effect for humoral but not cell-mediated immune reactions when injected subcutaneously. Pharmacokinetic studies showed that these compounds are absorbed following oral administration or inhalation, but that skin penetration is very poor. Most of the compounds were excreted in the urine following intravenous administration.

B: Linear Dimethylsiloxanes

Fifty one reports on L_2, L_3, and L_4 (where L = linear polymer) were reviewed. Linear polymers of this size are unlikely to be found in breast implants (Kala et al., 1998; reference not found in the original but added for this report, see Chapter 2). Systemic toxicity after oral, dermal, or inhalation exposure is low. However, linear siloxanes appear to have significant potential for dermal irritation in animals and humans. An in vitro study with human cells suggested that the materials are biocompatible. Evidence for modulation of immune function was obtained in some tests, although the biological significance of these findings was questioned.

TABLE 4-1 Summary of Toxicity Studies

CAS No.	Group	Acute	Subacute or Subchronic	Chronic	Irritation
541-05-9 D_3	IA	3	3	2	
556-67-2 D_4[a]	IA	8	15		11
541-02-6 D_5	1A	9	12		12
541-02-6	1A	1			1
540-97-6 D_6	1A	2	1		
Mixture[a]					
107-46-0	1B	21	6		
107-51-7	1B	1			
141-62-8	1B	1	2	2	
Mixture					
141-63-9	1C		2		3
677-62-90-7	1C	1			
69430-24-6	1C	1			
68037-74-1	1C	1	1		
70131-67-8[a]	1C	11	1	3	
63148-62-9[a]	1C	52	45	9	88
2554-06-5	II	2			
546-56-5	II	1			
2374-14-3	II	9	6		
68037-59-2	III	2			
67762-94-1	III				1
680-83-14-7	III	3			
Mixture					
999-97-3	IV	11			
2627-95-4	IV	8	1		
Others					
Total[b]		149	95	16	116

[a]Denotes human data are available. [b]Sum of all studies: 629.

C: Polydimethylsiloxanes

A total of 516 reports on L_5, L_6, L_7, L_9, L_{13}, L_{16}, D_7, D_8, D_9, D_{15}, D_x (cyclosiloxanes, dimethyl(cyclopolydimethylsiloxanes), DMPS (dimethylmonomethylpolysiloxanes, dimethylpolysiloxanes), DMSS (dimethylsilicones and siloxanes, reaction products with silica), SSHS (siloxanes and silicones, dimethyl hydroxy-terminated), PDMS, and L_x (linears) were reviewed. The database on the toxicity of these compounds is extensive. Acute exposure by different routes showed only minimal toxicity. The compounds have minimal potential for skin irritation. Subchronic studies involving oral administration of the agents did not reveal any systemic toxicity. On prolonged dermal application, sometimes under occlusion,

Developmental, Reproductive	Pharmaco-kinetic	Immunological	Cytotoxicity, Mutagenicity	Bio-compatibility
			3	
5	12	3	9	
	2	1	6	1
	1			
	1	1	3	
	1		8	3
		2		1
		1		2
	1			
	2	1	1	1
2			5	1
66	19	19	41	5
1			1	
			3	
			7	
		1		2
1				
			2	
			1	
		1		
			3	
75	39	30	93	16

some edema and scarring are observed, but no systemic toxicity. Implants of these materials under the skin usually produce granulomatous inflammatory changes and fibrosis. Subcutaneous implantation of PDMS gels in rats produced local sarcomas, such as are commonly seen in rats implanted with inert foreign bodies (solid-state carcinogenesis). An oral carcinogenicity study failed to produce any positive data. Multiple tests found a lack of genotoxicity. Tests for reproductive toxicity following oral or dermal exposure failed to show any clearly positive results. On occasion a small increase in fetal abnormalities was found, although the agents are not considered teratogenic.

In 29 of 35 studies, no effects on the male gonads were found. The summary document, without providing references however, mentions that some PDMS fluids given by gavage at 3.3 ml/kg for six days were associated with reduced seminal vesicle weights, whereas others, given for up to 20 days at similar doses, had no such effects. Spermatogenic depression was found in two of ten rabbits treated with 2 ml/kg PDMS for 20 days. Dermal application of 2 ml/kg for 28 days decreased testicular weight. In the case of one PDMS fluid (not characterized), a no-observable-adverse-effect level (NOAEL) of 50 mg/kg per day for a 28-day exposure was established. All of these dose levels are orders of magnitude greater that could be achieved in women with breast implants on a milliliter- or milligram-per-kilogram body weight basis. No immunotoxic potential was identified, although in some studies, adjuvant activity was noted with an increase in humoral but not cell-mediated immunity. The results were not seen with any consistency, and studies were often of poor quality. The absence of virtually any toxicity following acute exposure by oral and dermal routes was confirmed in human volunteers.

Group II—Non-Dimethyl Siloxanes

Thirty reports were reviewed. The acute oral LD_{50} (mean lethal dose) of these compounds is influenced by solvent effects. Reproductive studies indicated some adverse effects on the male reproductive tract. In addition, the agents produced severe ulceration and necrosis of rabbit skin during the 21-day treatment. Significant histopathological changes in rabbit liver and kidney were seen after four days' treatment at 3.3 mg/kg. No genotoxicity was observed. Agents in Group II are polymer precursors, and no exposure is anticipated outside manufacturing sites. The committee found no evidence that these compounds are in breast implants.

Group III—Other Siloxane Polymers and Copolymers, DHPS, DMMVS (siloxanes and silicones, dimethyl, methylvinyl), and DMDS (siloxanes and silicones, diphenyl)

Ten reports were reviewed. The studied compounds are reactive, and they cross-link easily. Use of the toxicity of starting materials is not appropriate in judging the toxicity of cured cross-link products. There appears to be limited industrial exposure and no exposure of the general public. Acute toxicity, irritation, and sensitization are minimal. These compounds are not known to occur in silicone breast implants.

Group IV—Other Materials

Forty-four reports were reviewed. Toxicity following oral exposure is low, and for inhalation a one-hour LC_{50} (50% lethal concentration) between 23 and 111 mg/ml was measured. The lowest-observable-adverse-effect level (LOAEL) for lung hemorrhage was 5.6 mg/l. Tetramethyldivinyldisiloxane was severely irritating to the skin under occlusive conditions. No evidence for genotoxicity or immunotoxicity was reported. These compounds are not known to occur in silicone breast implants.

TOXICOLOGY OF SUBCUTANEOUSLY IMPLANTED OR INJECTED SILICONES

Acute and Subchronic Studies with Silicone Fluids and Gels

Early toxicological experiments were designed to evaluate the effects of silicone liquids and solids implanted under the skin of experimental animals. Such experiments mimic silicone breast implants in many ways, although there are some important differences. Silicone breast implants are more complex. They may have varied surfaces, including coating with polyurethane. They may also contain many different chemical species, including potentially toxic compounds such as platinum. On the other hand, in many of these studies, actual gel and elastomer components of breast implants were tested.

In one early study, medical series 360 Dow Corning PDMS fluid, 350 cS, was injected in massive (up to 540 ml over 27 weeks) doses subcutaneously in rats and guinea pigs. There was very little or no local inflammation. The injected fluid became encapsulated by thin, transparent connective tissue in multiloculated cysts. No systemic toxicity was observed. However, it was not clear whether the material was eventually absorbed, redistributed within the body of the animals, or excreted (Ballantyne et al., 1965). To further elucidate this point, mice were injected subcutaneously or intraperitoneally with 1 ml of Dow Corning 360 silicone fluid, 350 cS, followed by intravenous carbon particles to induce reticuloendothelial blockade. Silicone was found in macrophages in regional lymph nodes in all animals and in macrophages in the adrenal in some intraperitoneally injected animals. Unlike the previous high-dose experiment, all other organs were normal (Ben-Hur et al., 1967). A high-dose exposure in man, multiple massive subcutaneous injections of silicone (1 liter at a time), eventually led to diffuse tissue distribution of the material in various organs (primarily the lungs) of this patient who succumbed to adult respiratory distress syndrome (Coulaud et al., 1983).

In mice as in rats, subcutaneous injection of 5 ml of Dow Corning 360 medical fluids did not produce any untoward effects (Andrews, 1966). The same author reported the case of an 18-year-old woman injected subcutaneously twice with 20 ml of 360 fluid. In examining a blood smear, neutrophils and mononuclear cells containing clear vacuoles were seen, which presumably contained silicone. The smear, however, was taken from an incised injection site where leukocytes had direct access to a silicone deposit, and this finding could not be confirmed by Hawthorne et al. (1970), who examined white cells from rats with high silicone exposures (see below). Nedelman (1968) injected various room temperature vulcanized (RTV) medical-grade Silastics mixed with Dow Corning 360 fluid and stannous octoate catalyst subcutaneously in the back of hamsters and supraperiostally in the jaw and palate of rabbits in doses of 0.5–2.0 ml and followed them for one week to three months. He reported that the Silastic was well tolerated and elicited only a mild connective tissue response. In another study in mice, Rees et al. (1967) observed a redistribution of silicone fluid within the body when injected in 1-ml amounts intraperitoneally or in larger amounts subcutaneously (6 ml in a single dose, 1 ml in repeated doses). Deaths occurred when the mice received more than 7 ml of PDMS by subcutaneous injection, an amount corresponding to about 280 ml/kg or about 14 liters in an average woman. Macrophages, presumably containing silicone, accumulated in multiple organs, including adrenal, lymph nodes, liver, kidney, spleen, ovaries, pancreas, and others (Rees et al., 1967). Whether the wider distribution of silicone injected at high doses results from access to, and distribution by, the circulatory system is unknown. The study by Rees et al. prompted Autian (1975a) to warn against the injection of silicone fluid in humans. He was also influenced by the local complications of silicone injection in women, which were well known by that time. Ashley et al. (1971) briefly reported injecting Dow Corning MDX 40411 in amounts ranging from 1 to 500 ml into mice, rats, guinea pigs, rabbits, and monkeys, with the formation of thin capsules, very little tissue reaction, and no systemic effects. This 350-cS fluid was also injected in small (4 ml) amounts into patients for cosmetic effect without complications. Very few data were reported, and the follow-up of the patients was three months on average (Ashley et al., 1971). Cutler et al. (1974) observed no ill effects on mice of PDMS fluid similar to Antifoam A mixed with 6% amorphous silica injected subcutaneously (0.2 ml) or fed at 0.25 and 2.5% from weaning for 76 weeks. Distribution to liver, spleen, kidneys, and perirenal fat was not detected.

In a more recent study, Dow Corning silicone 360 fluid and gel (1 ml per mouse), and elastomer and polyurethane (0.6-cm-diameter disks) were placed subcutaneously in B6C3 Fl mice (Bradley et al., 1994a,b). Animals were examined first over a 10-day period, then for 180 days. Silicone implantation did not affect any of the selected toxicological endpoints, including survival, weight gain, body and organ weights, hematology, serum chemistry, and bone marrow cytology. No effects on humoral immunity or cell-mediated immunity were found, and host resistance in two bacterial models was not altered.

Although, on occasion, widespread tissue distribution with potentially toxic or even fatal outcomes is seen when very large doses of silicone fluid are deposited subcutaneously or intraperitoneally (1 liter or more in humans, 7 ml in mice), quite substantial amounts are usually well tolerated. A subcutaneous injection in rodents (and most other animal species) is not directly comparable to a subcutaneous injection in humans however, because in most animals a large potential space is provided between mobile skin and underlying muscular fascia that can accommodate a substantial amount of fluid. In humans, silicone, if injected in large amounts, may be forced into the circulation and thus to distant organs, as suggested in the cases mentioned earlier (Andrews, 1966; Coulaud et al., 1983).

Silicones are present in medical devices and instruments (e.g., coatings for tubing and syringes). This has prompted some investigators to inject silicones intravenously, intraperitoneally, or even into the subdural space of the lumbar spinal cord. Intravenous or intracardiac injection of 2 ml of PDMS in dogs did not produce any changes in clotting time, hemoglobin concentration, or plasma surface tension. No changes in electrocardiograms or electroencephalograms were noted (Fitzgerald and Malette, 1961). These authors cited others who had injected larger doses intra-arterially or intravenously causing embolisms in various organs. Intraperitoneal injections of Dow Corning MD 44011, a silicone fluid that was actually injected in women for breast augmentation (see Chapter 1), at doses up to 62 ml in 60 rats were tolerated without any apparent adverse effects for up to one year (Hawthorne et al., 1970). Intraperitoneal injections of up to 3 ml of PDMS in mice resulted in a reduction of cell size in abdominal and pericardial fat tissue. In addition, in many abdominal organs such as adrenal, liver, kidney, spleen, pancreas, ovary, and lymph nodes, focal silicone-containing macrophage infiltrates were seen (Rees et al., 1967). Migrating silicone could produce granulomas on the surface of organs (Brody and Frey, 1968). In the course of investigating adjuvant effects, Lake and Radonovich (1975) reported that intraperitoneally injected low molecular weight silicones (L_3, L_4, D_4, L_5) caused a transient (48 hour) increase in interferon production and a reduction in colloidal carbon clearance by macrophages of the reticuloendothelial system in mice. Higher molecular weight silicones did not have these effects.

PDMS lubricant used in disposable syringes was injected into the lumbar subdural space in rabbits (0.3 ml) and monkeys (0.5 ml) and into the cisterna magna of rats (0.1 ml). No signs of neurotoxicity or histopathological alterations attributable to the silicone injections were observed. All of the radiolabeled silicone injected intracisternally remained in the brain, spinal cord, and vertebral column (Hine et al., 1969). Chantelau et al. (1986) calculated that 0.15–0.25 mg silicone lubricant might be lost from an insulin syringe with each use, or about 200 mg per year, assuming multiple injections per day for diabetes. Others have reported lower estimates of 30–40 μg from an insulin syringe with each use, or up to 30 mg in a year (Collier and Dawson, 1985). An average lifetime human dose would be at most several grams of silicone if the higher estimate was used; Hine's doses in experimental animals, therefore, equal or exceed lifetime human doses on a milligram-per-kilogram body weight basis. In another study, direct injection of silicone gel into peripheral nerve did not result in findings of toxicity of silicone to nerve tissue (Sanger et al., 1992).

Short-Term Studies with Solid Implants

Solid silicone implants also were generally well tolerated by experimental animals. Dogs, examined up to one year after implantation of sponges subcutaneously, intraperiostally, or placed directly onto bone, tolerated the implantation well, and the material was not invaded by bone or periosteum (Marzoni et al., 1959). Actual breast implant materials, such as Dow Corning Q7-2245 elastomer, in a biological safety screen consisting of tissue cell culture, systemic toxicity, rabbit intracutaneous and pyrogen tests, guinea pig sensitization, and rabbit 90-day implants, elicited no local or systemic responses (Munten et al., 1985), nor did Q7-2167/68 gel in a similar screen (Malczewski, 1985a). Subcutaneous implantation of medical-grade polysulfone-based silicone elastomer in rabbits was not carcinogenic up to 18 months. This study was of insufficient duration to be conclusive, however (Lilla and Vistnes, 1976).

In another implant study, nine different Silastic materials were implanted subcutaneously, intramuscularly, and intraperitoneally into 20 young adult purebred beagle dogs for six months to two years. The materials provoked a minimal foreign body reaction and the formation of a fibrous capsule but no general adverse effects (Dow Corning Corporation, 1970). Two years is, nevertheless, a short time compared to a life expectancy in beagles of 12–15 years. Thus, this study does not allow conclusions on such long-term effects as carcinogenesis.

James et al. (1997) recently evaluated one-week and two-month local cellular responses to PDMS, compared with the responses produced by impermeable cellulose acetate Millipore filters. Expression of leukocyte antigens for helper–inducer, T-suppressor–cytotoxic, and macrophage leukocyte antigens, proliferating cell nuclear antigen, and in situ labeling of DNA strand breaks as indicators of DNA damage and apoptosis were measured. The response to silicone did not differ from the response to impermeable cellulose acetate filters. On the other hand, porous cellulose filters, known not to produce local sarcomas, produced more intense inflammatory responses but minimal fibrosis. Within the fibrotic capsule surrounding the tumorigenic implants, cell proliferation and apoptosis were increased and associated with DNA breaks. The authors pointed out that persistent DNA damage and elevated cell proliferation are usually associated with genomic instability and malignant transformation. Similar studies might thus be carried out on human tissue surrounding silicone implants. Van Kooten et al. (1998) in the course of evaluating human fibroblast proliferative responses to smooth and variously textured Dow Corning Medical Grade Silastic found no influence of toxic leachables that might have been released from the silicone samples using 3-(4,5-dimethylthiazole-2-yl)-2,5-diphenyl tetrazolium bromide (MTT) conversion testing of cellular biochemical activity.

Long-Term (Carcinogenicity) Studies

From the moment silicone compounds became available for implants in humans, long-term effects were of particular concern. It was recognized that subcutaneous implantation of silicone compounds in rodents would produce local tumors at the implantation site. Solid-state carcinogenesis had been discovered in the 1940s and was a well-known phenomenon in plastics toxicology. In addition, the possibility was entertained that implants might release agents capable of producing tumors at distant sites. In a study of carcinogenesis in which animals were observed for up to two years, silicone rubber implanted intraperitoneally did not produce any tumors, but subcutaneous implants caused local sarcomas (Hueper, 1961). An RTV silicone elastomer with a stanous octoate catalyst was also implanted under the skin, intraperitoneally, and subdurally in the brain. No implant-related tumors were found during an observation period of up to 22 months (Agnew et al., 1962). A review of the entire literature on solid-state carcinogenesis induced by silicone compounds was published in 1967. In rats, but not mice, local sarcomas developed at the sites of silicone rubber implants (a 29–40% incidence following placement of single implants). Silicone gel or fluid produced only one sarcoma in 30 rats and no tumors in mice. The authors also pointed out that many of the reported experiments were not lifetime and therefore of too short duration to evaluate carcinogenicity properly (Bryson and Bischoff, 1967).

In 1972, Bischoff again reviewed silicone toxicity and carcinogenicity. Despite problems with the referencing of this review that interfere with discovery of the original data, the summarized data show a significant trend for tumor development in female, but not male, rats following intraperitoneal injection of silicone fluid. Subcutaneous administration of silicone fluid produced no tumors in rats, but an increased incidence of mesenchymal tumors was observed at the injection site in mice. No such tumors were found with controls (it is not clear how controls were injected). Bischoff (1972) concluded that silicone fluid had a low-grade carcinogenic potential in rodents. In the absence of the original data, it is difficult to evaluate this conclusion. However solid silicone compounds, implanted subcutaneously, clearly produce local tumors of mesenchymal origin at the site of implantation in rats. Silicone shares this property with numerous other agents.

The salient features of solid-state carcinogenesis have been reviewed (Autian, 1975a). The phenomenon is seen in rodents, mainly rats. Implantation of an inert material (e.g., acrylic, cellulose, Teflon, glass, bakelite, silicone, polystyrene, polyurethane, polyethylene) under the skin elicits, after a latent period, the local growth of a mesenchymal malignant tumor. To have such an effect, the implant must have a minimum size. Smooth implants are more effective than rough or perforated disks. Initially, the foreign body will be surrounded by granulomatous tissue that eventually forms a thin capsule. If the foreign body is removed within the first six months after implantation, no tumors develop. Removal of the test material later may or may not be followed by tumor development, but if the tissue pocket is removed, regardless of timing, no tumor will develop. The same amount of material introduced in powdered form under the skin does not produce tumors.

Later studies of the carcinogenicity of silicone implants, gels or solids, confirmed their ability to produce local sarcomas in rodents. In rats, silicone implants produced significantly fewer tumors at the implant site than did polyvinyl chlorides or polyhydroxyethyl methacrylate (Maekawa et al., 1984). Silicone amputation stump implants were placed in dogs, and the animals were observed up to 10 years (Swanson et al., 1984). While there was a benign foreign body giant-cell reaction to local silicone, no silicone particles or giant-cell responses were observed in distant organs, and the implants were well tolerated.

Surgitek breast implant components, silicone gel-SCL, silicone gel-Meme, silicone elastomer SCL, and standard elastomer coated with type A adhesive and polyurethane foam were examined in a two-year rat study with negative (Millipore filters, 0.65-μm pore size) and positive (Millipore filters, 0.025-μm pore size) controls. Test materials were implanted subcutaneously in the back at four different sites, and the animals were observed for up to 104 weeks. Survival was comparable for the negative control group and the polyurethane foam group, but significantly decreased in all other groups. However, body weight gains were similar in all groups. Subcutaneous tissue masses at sites of implantation were found in all groups. Tumor incidence ranged from 3% (polyurethane foam) to

53% (positive controls), and the two silicone gels had incidences of 27 and 19%, respectively. Most tumors were malignant, but rarely metastasized, and all were of mesenchymal origin. There was no evidence of systemic toxicity during the conduct of this study. At both interim and final sacrifice, there were no changes in organ weight, clinical chemistry, or hematology that could be attributed to an effect of the test agents. Age-associated inflammatory, degenerative, or neoplastic changes were seen on pathological examination, but the groups did not differ significantly. It was concluded that implantation of silicone gel-SCL or silicone gel-Meme at a higher dose than usual in humans did not produce any signs of systemic toxicity in female rats (Lemen and Wolfe, 1993).

Most recently, a lifetime implant study with Dow Corning Q7-2159A silicone gel, used in breast implants, tested whether a silicone implant would produce tumors at other than the implant site. A group of animals with subcutaneous polyethylene disk implants was also examined. The study, begun in 1990, involved a total of 700 female rats. Seven groups were formed: a control group, three groups receiving silicone gel implants (total surface areas 6.6, 18.0, and 48.8 cm^2), and three groups receiving polyethylene disks (total surface areas 0.79, 3.1, and 12.6 cm^2). The animals were observed for 104 weeks. Data for survival, body weight gain and food consumption, incidence of neoplastic and nonneoplastic lesions, organ weights, hematology, urinalysis, and clinical chemistry were all analyzed with appropriate statistical methods, designed to show dose-responses, trends, and significance of differences in lesions among treated and control groups (Klykken, 1998). The design, execution, data analysis, and quality control procedures used in this study represent today's state of the art in the conduct of carcinogenesis bioassays. Survival was somewhat shorter in animals that had silicone gel- or polyethylene-induced sarcomas at the implantation sites. In non-tumor-bearing animals, life span was not reduced. Incidence of local tumors increased with implant surface area and was higher in the polyethylene-treated animals. Silicone gel did not produce tumors at a site distant from the implantation site. Similarly, there were no observations of systemic toxic effects in silicone gel-implanted animals.

There was weak statistical evidence of decreased incidence of mammary gland malignant and benign epithelial tumors following gel exposure and of thyroid c-cell carcinomas and adenomas in animals treated with the largest polyethylene disks, compared to controls. In all animals, including the ones with implant site sarcomas, a reduced tumor incidence was also found for brain, mammary gland, pituitary, and all sites combined. Others have suggested that silicone gel implants might be associated with a lower incidence of malignancy in experimental systems. Dreyfuss et al. (1987) noted that a group of 60 rats with experimental silicone gel-filled implants experienced fewer mammary cancers caused by injection of *N*-methyl-*N*-nitrosourea 14 days after implantation than were seen in 60 rat control groups or groups with gel, elastomer, or polyurethane implanted as component sheets rather than fabricated into implants. This was the only positive finding in a group of negatives involving exposure to different silicones and different timing of injections (Dreyfuss et al., 1987). In another study, tumor size was diminished in the presence of tissue expanders in rats injected with mammary cancer cells compared to control and sham-operated rats. In still another study, rats with silicone implants in three locations, including beneath the mammary gland, developed fewer tumors after *N*-methyl-*N*-nitrosourea injection compared to sham controls, and mice with implants developed fewer spontaneous carcinomas compared to mice with implants of free gel or silicone sheets or sham operations (Ramasastry et al., 1991; Su et al., 1995). These studies and the epidemiological evidence of lower relative risks of breast cancer in implanted women (cited in Chapter 9) are suggestive, but they are not adequate to provide conclusive evidence for a decreased cancer risk in women with silicone breast implants.

Reproductive Toxicity Following Implantation with Silicones

Most women who receive silicone breast implants are of childbearing age. For this reason, reproductive, developmental, and teratologic effects of exposure to silicones and the effect of silicone implantation on breast feeding are particularly relevant. Many of the human data on exposure and responses to silicone are reviewed in Chapter 11. The reproductive toxicity and teratogenesis of some silicones relevant to those found in breast implants have been addressed directly in a few experimental animal studies.

Dow Corning 360 medical-grade fluid, 350 cS, and two other PDMS fluids were administered in comparatively high doses (20, 200, or 12,000 mg/kg) to male and female rats, mice, and rabbits. Basic guidelines issued by the Food and Drug Administration (FDA) for reproductive toxicity testing were followed. General reproductive performance (exposure of males and females before and during gestation), embryogenesis (exposure of pregnant females during the critical period of gestation), and postnatal performance were evaluated. Altogether, several hundred rats, rabbits, mice, and their offspring were examined, and no adverse teratologic, reproductive, or mutagenic effects were observed (Kennedy et al., 1976).

PDMS fluid, 350 cS, at dose levels of 5, 10, and 20 g/kg body weight was injected over ten days in one group of pregnant rats and all at once in another group of rats one week before mating. The sole effect observed was a significant postimplantation loss in the 5- and 10-g/kg PDMS dose groups of predosed animals. This effect prompted use of the predosing regimen and dose levels of 1, 10, and 20 g/kg PDMS in a definitive assay with 0.85% saline controls. The 20-g/kg dose level was selected to approximate the exposure of a 50-kg woman to sudden and complete rupture of two 500-g silicone gel breast implants. In this final test, no clinical signs of toxicity were evident in the mothers. No effects were found in the fetuses, and no postimplantation loss was observed. Under the conditions tested, the compound had no teratogenic effect (Bates et al., 1985, 1991).

In a later study, Surgitek silicone gel-SCL, silicone gel-Meme, and polyurethane were implanted under the skin of rabbits at six different locations, 17 rabbits per group. Doses were calculated to represent up to three times the expected human exposure for the gels and up to ten times for the polyurethane. After six weeks the rabbits were mated and then killed on gestation day 29. There were no effects of the treatment on implantation efficiency, pregnancy rates, fetal viability, postimplantation loss, or fetal weights. In animals exposed to polyurethane, some fetal malformations were observed, but the incidence per litter was not significantly different from controls. These findings were considered incidental. Materials implanted under the skin did not appear to produce either maternal toxicity or fetal abnormalities (Lemen, 1991).

More recently, silicone gel Q7-2159A and elastomer Q7-2423/Q7-2551 were evaluated for reproductive toxicity and teratogenesis in rats and rabbits. Altogether, the studies examined three different dose levels for the gel (3, 10, and 30 ml/kg) and two different disk sizes for the elastomer. In the reproductive toxicity studies, 30 male and 30 female rats were used per group, and in the teratology study, 25 pregnant rabbits were used in each group. Test articles were implanted in male rats 61 days, and in female rats 47 days, before mating and in female rabbits 42 days prior to insemination. Implantation of the gel or of the elastomer disks and their continuous presence before or during pregnancy and lactation did not cause observable effects in parents or neonates and had no discernible teratogenic effects. These two studies reflect the current state of the art in reproductive toxicity and teratogenesis testing (Siddiqui et al., 1994a,b). Finally, a two-year gel implant study of Dow Corning Q7-2159A and Dow Corning MDF-0193 in rats has been reviewed (Ruhr, 1991). This report examines the data for evidence that silicone implantation leads to changes in the male or female endocrine system. Fifty male and female rats were implanted with the test materials, and no changes in the endocrine system were found during what amounted to a lifetime study.

Distribution and Migration of Subcutaneously Implanted Material

The fate of subcutaneously implanted silicone has been directly addressed in a few studies. A total of eight male rats received a single subcutaneous injection of PDMS fluid labeled with carbon-14 (^{14}C). More than 94% of the radioactivity remained at the site of injection, and very small percentages (around 0.1%) were detected in expired air, urine, and feces. Less than 0.02% was eventually found to have migrated to different tissues, presumably via the lymphatics (LeBeau and Gorzinski, 1972). The movement of subcutaneously implanted, radiolabeled PDMS gel Q7-2159A was followed over a 20-week period (Isquith et al., 1991). Male and female CD-1 mice received a middorsal 0.5-ml implant of gel synthesized by equilibrating [^{14}C]octamethylcyclotetrasiloxane with dodecamethylpentasiloxane under acidic conditions. Over a period of 20 weeks, only 0.006% in males and 0.009% in females was found to be mobile. A very small amount of radiolabeled silicone was excreted, in large part during the first week postimplantation. What remained in the body beyond the injection site was found primarily in lymph nodes draining the implantation site. The injection sites were collected, but not analyzed. This precludes calculation of the usual mass balance (silicones not specifically measured elsewhere were assumed to have remained in the injection depot), but generally, silicone concentrations (calculated from radioactivity) in different tissues and organs were micrograms per gram of tissue, orders of magnitude lower than the amount injected (500 mg). In a report from the FDA, Young (1991) reanalyzed data from a 1966 Dow Corning study of the movement of [^{14}C]poly(dimethylsiloxane) injected subcutaneously in mice and followed over 90 days. A small fraction of the injected radioactivity appeared in the urine and feces with a half-life of 2 days initially and 56 days for redistributed radioactivity, but 99.97% of the silicone was stable (Young, 1991). These studies appear to show that very little of a gel implant leaves the site of deposition.

Raposo do Amaral et al. (1993) injected rats with 2 ml of silicone gel at two different sites. The animals were killed at intervals of 3, 7, 15, 30, 60, 180, 240, 420, and 450 days. The authors did not detect any silicone gel in lung, heart, spleen, liver, stomach, or gonads, although they could see it in the local tissues surrounding the capsule formed around the injected gel. No silicone was found in the regional lymph nodes draining the implant. However, these tissues were examined for silicone by light microscopy, which is an insensitive detection method. The reaction of local lymph nodes to injected silicone gel (1.5 ml injected subcutaneously into male Wistar rats), was measured with rigorous quantitative morphometric techniques at intervals up to 365 days (Tiziani et al., 1995). There was no evidence of lymph node hyperplasia, giant cells, or silicone droplets.

There was no morphometric difference in lymph nodes from gel-injected or saline-injected animals, and it was concluded that the silicone gel had not migrated. Swanson et al. (1984, 1985) evaluated a patient at autopsy after 12 years' exposure to silicone elastomer joint implants and also evaluated three dogs with elastomer implants after 10 years' exposure. Silicone elastomer particles were found locally around the implants, but a complete organ and reticuloendothelial system review revealed no particles at distant sites and only a few silicone particles in an axillary node of the autopsied patient (Swanson et al., 1984, 1985). Silicone rubber fragments placed in the peritoneal cavities of rats were found in the spleens of these animals, associated with a giant-cell reaction after four days (Guo et al., 1994). Barrett et al. (1991) found silicone particles locally and in regional nodes (when examined) of patients with penile implants. Examinations for particles in more distant sites were not undertaken. These examples are typical of reports of local and some regional node presence of silicone elastomer particles from various kinds of implants, which generally provoke some giant-cell, but no systemic, reaction (Barrett et al., 1991). Inflammatory reactions are limited to joints exposed experimentally to particulate silicone elastomer in rabbits by injection (or in humans from joint implants); unexposed joints are not inflamed (Worsing et al., 1982). More distant migration of small (median diameter, 73 μm) silicone particles to lung and lymph nodes and, less frequently, to kidney and brain was observed in seven female dogs injected with a silicone–polyvinylpyrrolidinone paste. There was no tissue reaction around the particles (Henly et al., 1995). Tiziani et al. (1995) concluded from this sort of evidence that regional node reactions were more likely to particulate elastomers than to silicone gel implanted in their drainage areas.

In a recent study, mice received subcutaneous injections of 250 mg of breast implant distillate, a low molecular weight siloxane mixture containing D_3, D_4, D_5, D_6, L_5, and L_6 (Kala et al., 1998). These materials are released by gel fluid diffusion from breast implants in very low concentrations (see Chapter 3). Animal tissues were analyzed at 3, 6, 9, and 52 weeks by gas chromatography–mass spectroscopy. Commercially available D_4, D_5, and D_6 were used as standards. The distribution of individual cyclosiloxanes in brain, heart, liver, kidney, lung, lymph nodes, ovaries, uterus, spleen, and skeletal muscle was measured. Concentrations for the individual cyclosiloxanes were all in the range of less than 1 μg (brain, liver) to a maximum of 7 μg (lymph nodes, ovaries) per gram of tissue. When calculated as total cyclosiloxanes, concentrations were highest in lymph nodes, uterus, and ovaries after six weeks, in the range of 1 to 14 μg/g of tissue. The authors reported that they could detect silicone in all organs examined up to one year later. Linear siloxanes were found at 4 to 5 μg/g of brain and up to 8 μg/g of lung. Large variations in the concentrations of the siloxanes between individual animals were noted. This study shows that in mice a small percentage of low molecular weight siloxanes injected in the suprascapular area can migrate in microgram amounts to different tissues. The experiment gives data on tissue concentrations only.

A mass balance study—that is an analysis of the amount of siloxanes injected, distributed, and excreted—was not carried out in this experiment. Such an analysis, usually a part of tissue distribution studies of chemicals as noted earlier, would have provided information on how much silicone was dislocated from the injection site, retained, or lost from the animal. The data on the total siloxane concentrations in different organs allow others to estimate a mass balance, however. Average organ concentrations were 7 µg/g wet tissue weight at most. If uniform distribution is assumed for a 25-g mouse, this provides for a total of 175 µg siloxane distributed from the injection site, or about 0.07% of the administered dose (250 mg). By allowing for the fact that the migratory part of the gel (a low molecular weight siloxane fluid distillate), not the gel itself, was injected, these results are consistent with those of Isquith discussed earlier. Kala et al. (1998) reported similar weight gains at one year in control and experimental mice, suggesting that in this study, a large (10 g/kg) dose of low molecular weight linear and cyclic siloxanes appears to have been well tolerated. In a subsequent study, this group injected even larger doses of a distillate containing D_3–D_6 intraperitoneally in mice and observed inflammatory changes in liver and lung. The LD_{50} for distillate was about 28 g/kg body weight, and for D_4 alone 6–7 g/kg body weight (Lieberman et al., 1999). It is not clear what relevance these studies have for women with silicone breast implants, since test article doses were given that were orders of magnitude greater than possible from breast implants, and LD_{50}s in these ranges have historically been considered indicative of lack of toxicity (Casarett, 1975; Marshall et al., 1981). It was also not clear to the committee why a distillate, instead of an extract or simply reference compounds, was used, since the possibility that some of these compounds were created during distillation once again raises the question of relevance for women with silicone breast implants.

GENERAL TOXICOLOGY OF SILICONE COMPOUNDS, INCLUDING LOW MOLECULAR WEIGHT CYCLIC AND LINEAR POLY(DIMETHYLSILOXANES)

Exposure to silicone compounds is widespread. A comparatively small number of people in industry may experience high exposures by dermal or inhalation routes. A large population may experience low-level exposure through consumer products including food. Toxicity testing has thus had to consider these routes of exposure. The committee has reviewed some of the studies of dermal, oral, and inhalation exposure to silicone in experimental animals for this reason and also because such studies provide some insights into the systemic toxicity of silicones that may be relevant to the toxicology of silicone breast implants.

Dermal Exposure

There are few studies on direct dermal toxicity of silicones, probably because early investigators recognized that silicones had no skin irritating properties and were generally considered nontoxic (Barondes et al., 1950). Nevertheless, a study conducted in rabbits with trifluoropropylmethylcyclotrisiloxane revealed some toxicity. In the highest-dose group (400 mg/kg), 40% of the animals died, and there was significant reduction in body weight gain (Siddiqui and Hobbs, 1982). Dermal (and oral) exposure to some organopolysiloxanes, not found in breast implants, resulted in adverse effects on the reproductive systems of male and female rats, rabbits, and dogs. Dermal application for 28 days produced testicular or seminal vesicle atrophy in rabbits (Bennett et al., 1972; Hayden and Barlow, 1972). Maternal weight loss, increased resorption, and decreased viability of young were observed in female rabbits treated dermally with a phenyl-methylcyclosiloxane. However, the material was not considered teratogenic. Application of the same silicone fluids to human skin did not lead to an increase in silicone blood or urine concentration (Hobbs et al., 1972; Palazzolo et al., 1972). Although some interest in these compounds has been expressed by women with implants or by other investigators, there is no evidence that they are found in silicone breast implants.

Oral Exposure

Oral toxicity for most silicone compounds is very low. For two silicone oils (poly(*sec*-butylmethylsiloxane) and polydimethylsilicones), the LD_{50} was greater than 24 g/kg. Agents with such a high LD_{50} are generally considered nontoxic (Marshall et al., 1981). More recently, the oral toxicity of Dow Corning 200 fluid, 10 cS, a PDMS fluid, was examined in a 28-day and then a 13-week feeding study. Rats received the test material in the diet at concentrations from 1 to 10% in the 28-day study and from 0.5 to 5% in the 13-week study. Corneal opacities, identified as corneal crystals, and other corneal inflammatory changes were noted in the higher-dose groups, presumably due to direct contact with the fluid on the fur. Changes in clinical chemistry were limited to a significant decrease in mean triglycerides, and in low-density and very low density lipoproteins. A NOAEL could be set at greater than 100,000 parts per million (ppm) of the test substance, provided the corneal lesions were the result of a topical effect for the 28-day study, and at greater than 50,000 ppm for the 13-week study (Tomkins, 1995). Dow Corning 200 fluid, 350 cS, another PDMS fluid, was evaluated in a similar experiment. The same corneal lesions were noted both in the 28-day and the 13-week studies, and again were attributed to topical contact. No changes in clinical chemistry were noted. In the 13-week study, male and female rats were also given the test substance by gavage (500 and 2,500 mg/kg per day). The NOAEL for this substance could be set at greater than 50,000 ppm, again if the corneal lesions are assumed to be the result of a topical effect (Tomkins, 1995).

Some silicone fluids may be absorbed from the gastrointestinal tract. In one male monkey given ^{14}C-labeled Dow Corning 360 fluid, very little absorption occurred, and more than 90% of the radioactivity was eventually recovered in the feces (Vogel, 1972). On the other hand, in rats repeatedly given octamethylcyclotetrasiloxane (D_4) approximately 23–33% of the silicone species were detected in urine, and less than 0.3% was found in the feces (possibly resulting from contamination by urine) (Malczewski et al., 1988). Metabolites originating from exposure to D_4 are under investigation (Varaprath et al., 1997), as are studies designed to clarify whether inducers of hepatic drug-metabolizing enzymes alter its metabolism (Plotzke and Salyers, 1997). In commenting on the results of these studies at the Institute of Medicine (IOM) scientific workshop, Meeks noted that these metabolic changes were similar to those induced by common sedatives (McKim 1995, 1996a,b; see R. Meeks, IOM scientific workshop, 1998).

Some early studies examined the carcinogenicity of orally administered silicone compounds. Rowe et al. (1950) fed Dow Corning Antifoam A at a concentration of 0.3% to rats over their lifetime. Survival and growth rate were not affected. However, survival rates, in both controls and exposed animals were not very good by today's standards. No tumors were found, but the low survival rate and the use of only one dose that did not approach a maximum tolerated dose, which is required in current practice, make this negative study inconclusive (Rowe et al., 1950). Carson et al. (1966) fed Dow Corning Antifoam A and Dow Corning 360 fluid, 50 and 350 cS, at 1% of diet to rabbits and rats for 8 months and 1 year, respectively. They observed no differences in body weight, organ weight, hematological, urine, or serum chemistry tests, the microscopic examination of organs, or overall survival between control or experimental groups. Earlier, Kimura et al. (1964) had reviewed studies of methylpolysiloxane.

A silicone antifoam compound consisting of a mixture of 6% finely divided (amorphous) silicon dioxide and 94% PDMS was administered in the diet, at concentrations of 0.25 and 2.5% to male and female outbred mice, respectively (Cutler et al., 1974). This experiment was begun at weaning and terminated 76 weeks later. In the same study, some animals received a single subcutaneous injection of 0.2 ml silicone or 0.2 ml paraffin. All visibly altered tissues as well as lung, heart, stomach, small intestine, spleen. liver, and kidney from about ten male and female mice in each treatment group were examined microscopically. No treatment-related increase in nonneoplastic or neoplastic lesions was found. Cysts and some fibromas were observed at the injection site in mice injected with silicone oil or paraffin, the latter producing fibromas more frequently than the former. Although carcinogenesis was not observed at the dose levels examined, this study performed in 1974 would not fulfill today's criteria for a carcinogenesis bioassay. The study was terminated early, histopathology was incomplete, and no indication was given of how close the higher dose used was to a maximum tolerated dose.

Although the studies of polydimethylsilicone reviewed so far offer little evidence of toxicity, this is not true for all silicone compounds. A series of papers, published in the early 1970s, provides experimental evidence that certain organosiloxanes have estrogenic activity. Several agents were evaluated. The most active of them was *cis*-2,6-diphenylhexamethylcyclotetrasiloxane. This and similar chemicals caused an array of effects in the reproductive systems of male animals and on reproduction in female animals (Bennett et al., 1972; Hayden and Barlow, 1972; Hobbs et al., 1972; LeFevre et al., 1972; LeVier and Boley, 1975; LeVier and Jankowiak, 1975; LeVier et al., 1975; Nicander, 1975). Some human data are available from patients with prostate cancer. The biological half-life varied between 14 and 23 hours (Pilbrandt and Strindberg, 1975). As noted earlier in this chapter, women with breast implants and some recent investigators have expressed an interest in these compounds. However, the toxic effects of these compounds have not been observed in experimental silicone gel implant toxicological studies, and there is no evidence that they are present in silicone breast implants.

Inhalation Exposure

Because silicone compounds are present in hairspray and shampoo, adverse health effects following inhalation of these compounds have been explored. The toxicity of aerosolized D_4 was evaluated, first in a dose-setting study of four weeks' duration, then in a three-month study (Kolesar, 1995a,b). Exposures were six hours a day, five days a week at concentrations of D_4 ranging from 200 to 1,333 ppm (2.4–15.8 g/m^3, grams per cubic meter) eventually reduced in the three-month study to 12 g/m^3 (1,000 ppm). The animals were observed for clinical signs of toxicity, and food consumption was monitored. A few animals died during the first week when exposed to 15 g/m^3, necessitating reduction of the dose to 12

g/m^3. No treatment-related clinical signs were observed at the lower dose levels, but changes in hematology and clinical chemistry were seen. Enlargement of the liver and its cells was dose dependent and more pronounced in females. Changes in the respiratory tract were interpreted as adaptive responses to mild irritation. In females exposed to the highest concentration (12 g/m^3), minimal to marked vaginal mucification accompanied by moderate degrees of ovarian atrophy was noted. A separate group of animals was allowed to recover in air for one month following the exposure. Practically all of the abnormalities eventually disappeared, indicating reversibility of the effects of exposure. These exposures are considered quite high.

In a later study, Fischer 344 rats were exposed to D_4 at concentrations ranging from 7 to 540 ppm (80 mg to 6.4 g/m^3) for six hours a day, 5 days a week, for 28 days (Klykken et al., 1997). In addition to the usual endpoints measured, immune function was assessed by splenic antibody-forming assay and enzyme-linked immunosorbent assay (ELISA). The only change noted was liver enlargement, which was reversible after a two-week recovery period in male rats exposed to 540 ppm and females exposed to 20–540 ppm (0.24 to 6.4 g/m^3). No immune system changes were observed.

This protocol was repeated with D_5, except that exposures ranged from 0.4 to 3.5 g/m^3 (expressed as milligrams per liter in the original, 27–240 ppm) (Kolesar, 1995c,d). At one month, all animals survived and gained weight normally. Upon termination of the study, only slight interstitial inflammation in the lung and some liver cell enlargement were noted in the highest-dose group. In the three-month study, reduced weight gain was observed in the highest-dose group. Hematology, clinical chemistry, and urinalysis were unremarkable. Histopathological changes were observed in the lungs of animals exposed to the higher concentrations of D_5, both those killed immediately after exposure and those allowed to recover for an additional month in air. More frequent interstitial ovarian and vaginal lesions were also seen in the highest-dose group. Exposures used in all these studies were quite high, perhaps unrealistically so.

The effects of inhaled D_4 and D_5 were also evaluated in reproductive toxicity tests. Male and female rats were exposed to D_4 concentrations ranging from 70 to 700 ppm (0.83–8.3 g/m^3) for six hours a day for a minimum of 28 days or for 70 days prior to mating. Exposure continued throughout the gestation and lactation periods (except on day 21 of gestation and days 1–4 of lactation). Offspring were further exposed following weaning on day 21 until day 28. They were thus potentially exposed to the test agent while in utero, throughout suckling, via inhalation or dermal contact during lactation, and via inhalation after weaning. Maternal toxicity consisting of slight reduction in body weight gain and hepatomegaly at autopsy was observed at dose levels of 300, 500, and 700 ppm (3.5, 5.9, and 8.3 g/m^3). In the highest-dose group, there was a consistent and reproducible reduction in fetal implantation sites and a decrease in mean live litter size. In the offspring, no exposure-related signs of toxicity were observed (Stump, 1996a). No effect on litter size or pup viability and no signs of maternal toxicity were found in a study with D_5, when maternal animals were exposed to concentrations of 26 and 132 ppm (0.38–1.9 g/m^3) (Stump, 1996b).

Decamethylcyclopentasiloxane (D_5) was also evaluated in a different laboratory (Lambing, 1996). Exposures were six hours a day, seven days a week, for a total of 28 exposures, with exposure concentrations ranging from 10 to 160 ppm (0.15–2.4 g/m^3). A two-week recovery period was included in the experimental design. There were no test-related effects on survival, clinical condition, body weight gain, food consumption, clinical chemistry, and urinalysis at any exposure level. There were no adverse effects on immunoglobulin M (IgM) antibody response to a T-dependent antigen (sheep red blood cells). Changes noted were a 5% decrease in hematocrit, enlargement of the liver, and increased lung weight, all reversible upon cessation of exposure. Microscopically, increased alveolar macrophage accumulation and some interstitial inflammation in the lungs were observed. Goblet-cell hyperplasia was found in the nasal passages, which was thought to be reversible. If the histopathological changes confined to level one in the nasal passages are taken into account, the no-observed-effect-level (NOEL) would be less than 10 ppm. A NOAEL for systemic toxicity (liver weight increase) was identified at 75 ppm (1.1 g/m^3) and for immunosuppression at 160 ppm (Lambing, 1996).

Presumably because some systemic effects such as liver enlargement were observed during inhalation of D_4, a series of pharmacokinetic studies has been initiated. Rats were exposed by nose-only inhalation technique to D_4 labeled with ^{14}C. Concentrations used ranged from 7.5 to 716 ppm (90 mg to 8.5 g/m^3). The animals were killed immediately after exposure and at selected intervals thereafter up to 168 hours. The animals retained approximately 5.5% of the total radioactivity delivered. Radioactivity was found in all tissues and reached maximum levels between zero and three hours after exposures, except in fat, which seemed to serve as a depot for radioactivity. Half-times of retention for combined radioactivity ranged from 68 hours in plasma to 273 hours in various tissues. Radioactivity was mostly excreted by breathing and excretion was most rapid within the first 12 hours. An initial rapid decline followed by a longer terminal elimination phase was also observed in a study where rats were exposed for 14 days, first to unlabeled, and for 1 day to labeled, D_4 vapor

(Ferdinandi and Beattie, 1996a,b, 1997). Exposures in these inhalation studies reached very high levels.

Studies have been performed to examine the implications of liver enlargement (McKim, 1995, 1996a,b). Male and female rats were exposed for four weeks to D_4 at airborne concentrations of 70 and 700 ppm. Animals were killed from 3 to 28 days after exposure and after 7 and 14 days of recovery. In females, liver size increased early during exposure. At the end of the study, liver weights were approximately 110% of controls in females and 117% in males. However, following cessation of exposure, there was a rapid decrease in liver weight. Some liver enzymes and proteins were increased. It was concluded that D_4 acted like a "phenobarbital-type" inducer in rat liver. Essentially similar observations were made in studies with inhaled and oral D_5 (McKim, 1997). A metabolic study in rats showed that 75 to 80% of intravenously administerd ^{14}C labeled D_4 appeared in urine as dimethylsilicone diol, methylsiliconetriol and five other minor metabolites within 72 hours (Varaprath et al., 1997).

Because D_4 is found in personal care products such as hairsprays, shampoos, and deodorants and, together with D_5, has been found in indoor atmospheres, a potentially large number of people are exposed daily (Shields et al., 1996). Very small amounts of these compounds are found in breast implants (see Chapter 3), constituting exposures substantially lower than those possible from other, ubiquitous sources. Recent studies have examined the effects of inhaled D_4 on humans. At a concentration of 10 ppm, a one-hour inhalation did not alter human lung function. Deposition of D_4 was calculated to be around 12%. Measurement of plasma concentrations showed a rapid nonlinear blood clearance. Immune function was evaluated by several parameters, such as measurement of serum acute-phase reactants, interleukin-6 (IL-6) levels, establishment of lymphocyte subsets, blast transformation in isolated peripheral mononuclear cells, natural killer (NK) cell cytotoxicity, and in vitro production of cytokines. No signs of an immunotoxic or systemic inflammatory response were found (Looney et al., 1998; Utell et al., 1998).

The authors pointed out that their studies did not preclude possible immunological effects with exposures of longer durations or at higher concentrations. Since the route of exposure was via inhalation, the negative findings should not be relied on when assessing the immunological effects of implanted silicones in humans. Nevertheless, the low order of toxicity observed when D_4 is absorbed and distributed systemically after administration by inhalation or oral routes, tends to support the observations of lack of D_4 toxicology after systemic exposure by implant or injection. The committee did not find data that would allow comparisons between possible systemic exposure to D_4 from common consumer products to large numbers of the general pupulation and estimated exposures from silicone gel-filled breast implants.

In Vitro Assays

Few in vitro studies on silicone materials have been published in the open literature. The LC_{50} of D_4, decamethyltetrasiloxane (L_4), and tetramethyltetravinylcyclotetrasiloxane (D'_4) on B-cell lymphoma, plasmacytoma, and macrophage cell lines ranged from 30 to 50 micromolar (8.6–14.4 mg/l, D_4). At lower concentrations, there were biochemical signs of cytotoxicity. Exposed macrophages produced more IL-6 than did untreated cells (Felix et al., 1998). On the other hand, WI-38 human fibroblast, mouse fibroblast, and Chinese hamster ovary cells, when grown in contact with silicone gel used in breast implants, were not adversely affected, even when exposed up to 12 days. Flow cytometry, a sensitive analytical technique, did not reveal any changes in cell-cycle characteristics (Cocke et al., 1987).

Results from in vitro mutagenicity assays are not conclusively negative, although they are suggestively so. Poly-*sec*-butylsilicate ester (Silicate Cluster 102, Olin Corp.) and PDMS (SF-96, G.E. Corp.) were negative in the Ames test (TA-1535, TA-100, TA-1538, and TA-98), with and without metabolic activation (Marshall et al., 1981). In 1988, it was reported that 12 silicone compounds all tested negative for genotoxicity in salmonella (Ames test), Saccharomyces cerevisiae, and Escherichia coli test systems. Hexamethyldisiloxane (L_2) and D_4 at one dose and several other compounds, among them methyltriethoxysiloxane, produced sister chromatid exchange, although often no dose-response relationship was found, and the results were considered inconsistent. Chromosome aberrations were also found with some of the compounds (Isquith et al., 1988). In an evaluation of the mutagenicity of Dow Corning 7-9172 Part A (used to make gel) with several tester strains, with and without metabolic activation systems, no positive responses were found (Isquith, 1992). Six siloxanes were recently examined for mutagenic activity in rat fibroblasts (Felix et al., 1998). Only one compound, tetravinyltetramethylcyclotetrasiloxane was found to give a weak positive response. The study was prompted by the observation that silicones could produce plasmacytomas in highly sensitive mouse strains. Since only one compound was found to be mutagenic, it was concluded that possible nonmutagenic mechanisms might also be responsible for plasmacytoma development.

PLATINUM

The potential toxicity of several platinum compounds has received some attention because they have been used as catalysts in the manufacture of silicone gels and solids. Platinum is present in small amounts in implants (see Chapter 3, in which the amount of platinum and the question of its form are discussed). Reports that this platinum is in the form of platinate (Lykissa et al., 1997) are unconfirmed (Lewis and Lewis, 1989; Lewis et al., 1997). Inhalation of platinum compounds is recognized as a problem in the smelting and refining industry. Platinum can produce chemical pneumonitis (Furst and Rading, 1998). Inhalation of complex salts of platinum, but not elemental platinum, can cause progressive allergic and asthmatic reactions. Skin contact with platinum, particularly its chlorides, which are powerful skin sensitizers, can cause contact dermatitis (American Conference of Governmental Industrial Hygienists, 1998). Cisplatin, an agent used in cancer chemotherapy, is highly toxic to the gastrointestinal tract, kidney, bone marrow, and peripheral nervous system. This compound does not occur in silicone breast implants, however.

Early toxicity tests, conducted on a minimum number of animals, showed little if any signs of toxicity for two platinum compounds, Dow Corning Platinum Nos. 1 and 2 (Groh, 1973). Acute oral toxicity was greater than 6.8 g/kg, and upon instillation of the liquids into the eyes of rabbits, only a slight and transient irritation was noted. Moderate to marked skin alterations were seen after repeated application of the undiluted substances. Edema and hyperemia were mentioned, but without any quantitative scores. Studies with Dow Corning X-2-7018 gave essentially similar results (Groh, 1972). The platinum catalysts, when compounded into an elastomer, were nontoxic to human embryonic lung cells in tissue culture. However, in liquid form, the catalysts were toxic, although this effect was abolished for Platinum No. 2 by heating. This seems to indicate that compounding might eliminate toxicity by inactivating reactive sites (Jackson, 1972). The oral toxicity of TX-82-4020-02 (H_2PtCl_6 reacted with tetramethyldivinyldisiloxane and then diluted with Dow Corning SFD-119 fluid) was greater than 20 g/kg, and no signs of toxicity were observed during a two-week observation period or upon autopsy of rats (de Vries and Siddiqui, 1982).

BALB/c female mice received injections of ammonium hexachloroplatinate in the left footpad. Comparison of the weight of left popliteal lymph nodes with nodes collected from the right hind leg showed that five, six, and seven days later, the weight of the lymph nodes was increased. This was taken as evidence that platinum in its multi-valent state has immunogenic potential (Galbraith et al., 1993). The skin sensitizing potential of Platinum Nos. 2 and 4 was recently examined in a study with guinea pigs (Findlay and Krueger, 1996a,b). On day 1 of the test, the guinea pigs received six intradermal injections of Dow Corning 2-0707 Intermediate (Platinum No. 4) or Dow Corning 3-8015 (Platinum No. 2) intradermally into the skin of the back over the shoulder region. Negative (phosphate-buffered saline) and positive (1-chloro-2,4-nitrobenzene) controls were similarly injected. On days 7 and 8, the same agents were reapplied, this time topically and under occlusion. A first challenge was applied on day 22 and a second challenge on day 29; 24 and 48 hours after the challenge doses, the skin was examined and scored for signs of irritation with a quantitative procedure (Draize scale). For this experiment, both agents were found to be moderate skin sensitizers in guinea pigs although previous studies were said to be inconsistent with this result (Lane et al., 1998). Available data provide little evidence that the platinum catalysts would have a particular systemic toxicity. They may have sensitizing potential, but it is not clear whether this is a function of the platinum itself or of the entire molecule.

Harbut and Churchill (1999) reported a small case series of eight women with the onset of asthma at varying intervals after placement of silicone breast implants. These authors speculated that the respiratory signs and symptoms were the result of exposure to hexachloroplatinate in their implants. No evidence for this was reported. Conclusions regarding platinum toxicity in women with breast implants should await evaluations that positively relate platinum to the symptomatology; these might include some or all of elevated serum platinum levels, positive skin prick tests for platinate, positive radioallergosorbent (RAST) or other tests for platinum-specific antibodies, remission of allergic symptoms or reduction of serum platinum levels or skin prick or other allergic tests on explantation in women with no other known exposures to platinum (Biagini et al., 1985; Rosner and Merget, 1990). Absent these tests, diagnoses of platinum toxicity in women with implants are speculative only. Since allergies and asthma are extremely common in the general population, they should be common in women with breast implants, yet epidemiological studies do not report this. These complaints are not prominent in lists of problems with breast implant patients (see Appendix B of this report), and one cohort study of 222 women with breast implants and 80 control women without implants found breathing difficulties to be significantly less frequent ($p < 0.05$) in the women with silicone breast implants (K.E. Wells et al., 1994). It should also be kept in mind that platinum exposure from vehicle exhaust catalysts is increasing and is reflected in serum levels but not in any known health condition (Farago et al., 1998). The committee could not find any such positive platinum-specific evaluations in women with breast implants and thus finds that evidence is lacking for an association between platinum in silicone breast implants and local or systemic health effects in women who have these implants. If the platinum in breast implants is in zero valence form in the final cured state in excess vinyl as reported by Stein et al. (1999), and if it is in microgram quantities as is usually added to gel (Lane et al., 1998), as the current evidence suggests, then a biologically plausible rationale for platinum related health problems in women with silicone breast implants does not presently exist. Many silicone-containing implants other than breast implants (listed in Chapter 2) are found at high frequency in the general population and presumably contain platinum also; the committee is not aware of any evidence that platinum toxicity is present in these persons.

TIN

The committee reviewed information bearing on the possible effect of tin on the safety of silicone breast implants. Stannous octoate, stannous oleate or dibutyltin dilaurate catalysts are generally involved in formulation of only part of an implant, e.g., the adhesive sealant in the case of Dow Corning and McGhan Medical or the RTV elastomer shells of saline implants in the case of Mentor and McGhan Medical Corporations. HTV gel-filled shells are platinum catalyzed (B. Purkait, personal communication, Mentor Corporation, May 1999; Eschbach and Schulz, 1994). Tin has been added at low concentrations (e.g., 0.038% stannous oleate to formulate adhesives [about 1.4 μg of tin per Dow Corning implant] or targeted at 70–80 parts per million tin from dibutyltin dilaurate in the case of Mentor saline implant shells and about the same in the case of McGhan shells). Tin has been analyzed at non detectable to 0.73 ppm in saline or dichloromethane extracts of Dow Corning implant silicone gel (J. M. Curtis, Dow Corning, personal communication, May 11, 1999, Lane et al., 1998) or non detectable by inductively coupled plasma atomic emission spectroscopy and cold vapor atomic absorption spectroscopy in saline, ethanol, methylene chloride or hexane extracts in the case of Mentor implant shells (B. Purkait, Mentor Corporation, personal communication, May 1999), or measured within a range of 15 to 100 parts per million in saline shells and non detectable in saline extracts of shell elastomer by inductively coupled plasma atomic emission spectroscopy (R. Duhamel, McGhan Medical Corporation, personal communication, 1999). Normal tissue concentrations of tin can be higher than the levels in implants (0.25-130 ppm, Clayton and Clayton, 1994). Total tin in an average implant[1],

[1]This depends on saline shell weights which are quite variable, ranging it is said, from a lower limit of 5 g (B. Purhait, Mentor Corporation, personal communication, 1999) to 10 to 30 g (J.M. Curtis, Dow Corning Corporation, personal communication, 1999) to a maximum upper limit as high as 100 g (with a lower average value; R. Duhamel, McGhan Medical Corporation, personal communication, 1999). Also, these weights are dependent on implant model and whether the shell is smooth or textured.

therefore, could vary from 1 or 2 μg to 10 mg as an upper limit in Dow Corning, Mentor or McGhan implants.

The toxicology of inorganic and organic tin was reviewed extensively for the U.S. Public Health Service (Agency for Toxic Substances and Disease Registry, 1992) and a few studies of particular tin soap catalysts are available from industry. Human data for organotins are sparse to nonexistent as are experimental animal data on parenteral exposures. The human permissible industrial exposure limit for organotin of 0.1 mg/m^3 calculates to a maximum exposure of 14.3 mg/kg per day (American Council of Governmental Industrial Hygienists, 1998). In general, animal data indicate oral toxic levels at more than 10 mg (for the most toxic), although absorption of oral doses is poor, and on inhalation no observable adverse effect levels (NOAELs) over 1 mg/m^3. RTV elastomer with stannous octoate was implanted under the skin, intraperitoneally and subdurally in rats. Although no toxic or carcinogenic effects were observed over 22 months, this early study was not designed to examine tin toxicity (Agnew et al., 1962). Other similar implant studies of stannous octoate catalyzed elastomers were also negative but were not designed to evaluate tin (Nedelman, 1968). Likewise, Dow Corning elastomers with 1, 3 and 5% stannous octoate were implanted subcutaneously and intramuscularly in rabbits for 10 or 30 days, and no clear dose response was observed, only the usual foreign body reaction. In another Dow Corning study, the oral LD_{50} was 3.4g/kg (R. Meeks, Dow Corning, personal communication, 1999). Studies of dibutyltin dilaurate found LD_{50} levels ranging from 85 mg/kg intraperitoneally to between 175 and 1240 mg/kg body weight orally. In general, these substances were not carcinogenic (Agency for Toxic Substances and Disease Registry, 1992; American Conference of Governmental Industrial Hygienists, 1998; Clayton and Clayton, 1994; Hazardous Substances Data Bank; Mellon Institute of Industrial Research, 1994; National Cancer Institute). These data suggest that toxic effects of even the most toxic (triorganotins—which have not been found in breast implants) tin compounds are seen at doses above those possible from breast implants even in the most unlikely event of complete release of all the tin into the breast. Moreover, the tin in breast implants appears to be of relatively low toxicity among organic tin compounds, and given the difficulty in extracting it, as noted above, and the durability of silicone elastomer, as noted elsewhere in this report, unlikely to be significantly available to surrounding tissues. The committee concluded that there is currently no evidence for toxic effects of retained tin catalysts at the very low exposures likely from silicone breast implants.

CONCLUSIONS

Historically, silicone toxicology has tended to focus on short-term, acute and subacute studies and has suffered from a proportionate dearth of chronic, lifetime, and immunologic studies, as noted earlier in this chapter. Presumably, this reflects early conclusions that silicones were inert. Some silicones have clear biological effects. None can be said to be inert, if this implies an absence of tissue reaction, but the term has perhaps been a used as a proxy to indicate that the toxicity of many silicones is of such low order that they comprise a useful class of biomaterials for medical implants.

Older silicone toxicology studies have deficiencies by current standards, but the body of toxicological information is substantial and improving. More chronic studies are being done, although modern regulatory requirements will undoubtedly generate a closer identification of silicones (and other substances) in implants and more specific toxicological studies of appropriate duration. Nevertheless, no significant toxicity has been uncovered by studies of individual compounds found in breast implants. Toxicology studies have examined carcinogenic, reproductive, mutagenic, teratologic, immunotoxic, and local and general toxic and organ effects by exposure routes that are varied and range to very high dose levels. Even challenges by doses that are many orders of magnitude higher than could be achieved on a relative-weight basis in women with silicone breast implants are reassuring. Toxic effects that have been found occur at very high, even extreme, exposure levels (e.g., D_4, D_5). The fact that some organic silicon compounds may have, as one would expect with any large family of chemical compounds, biologic or toxicologic effects is not relevant to women with breast implants since these compounds are not found in breast implants, as noted here and in Chapter 2.

Studies using whole fluids, gels, elastomers, or experimental implant models injected or implanted in ways that are directly relevant to the human experience with implants are also reassuring. These studies show that depots of gel, whether free or in implants, remain almost entirely where injected or implanted. Even low molecular weight cyclic and linear silicone fluids appear to have low mobility. Half-lives of low molecular weight silicones in body fluids and tissues have been measured infrequently, but known values appear to be on the order of 1 to 10 days. In general, there do not appear to be long-term systemic toxic effects from silicone gel implants or from unsuspected compounds in these gels or elastomers detected by these animal experiments.

Some have speculated that platinum found in silicone gel and elastomer may be responsible for allergic disease in women with silicone breast implants. Very little platinum, microgram quantities, is present in implants, most investigators believe it to be in the zero valence state, and it likely diffuses through the shell at least over a considerable period of time. Evidence for resulting systemic disease at such exposures is lacking. Toxicological studies of tin compounds used in silicone breast implants are scarce, and generally not of parenterally administered tin. The data on organotins indicate that tin catalysts are among the less toxic, and they have not been extractable from implants shells by saline and some organic solvents. Based on the data available, the committee concluded that evidence is also lacking for tin toxicity at the very low amounts present in saline implants and at the virtually absent levels in gel filled implants.

5

Reoperations and Specific Local and Perioperative Complications

INTRODUCTION

This chapter addresses the frequency of local and perioperative complications associated with breast implants. Later chapters of this report deal with long-term safety, particularly in terms of cancer and connective tissue disease. Local and perioperative complications are important outcomes in their own right, and to the extent that they lead to significant further medical interventions or impair the achievement of expected and desirable results, they are also relevant to implant safety. Five-year reoperative or secondary surgery rates or average number of implants placed per breast or per woman provide approximations of the sum of these complications. They are important to safety because, even though breast surgery is of low systemic morbidity, every operation and the attendant anesthesia carry risk. Many of the same complications that occur when implants are placed may occur when they are removed, revised, or replaced, e.g., infection, hematoma or seroma, pneumothorax, tissue necrosis (Rohrich et al., 1998a). Furthermore, other interventions such as closed capsulotomies, extra manipulations for mammographic screening or diagnosis, and medical care for rash, pain, infection and the like are often not included in reoperation and multiple replacement data and can be contributors to, or comorbidities with, the need for surgery. These other interventions can be very frequent; for example, as many as 192 closed capsulotomies in 140 patients (254 implants) have been reported (Brandt et al., 1984). Patient satisfaction, or the lack of it, is another indicator that can generate further interventions, as noted in Chapter 1. It should be kept in mind with respect to the following discussion that implants, surgical experience, surgical techniques, and perhaps other factors have evolved since the studies reported here were undertaken, so current experience may differ. This argues for careful prospective studies as the committee concludes at the end of this section.

This chapter addresses the following topics because they have significant effects on implant safety: reoperation or secondary procedures as indicators of overall frequency of local and perioperative complications; aggregate complications in breast reconstruction; aggregate complications in breast augmentation; rupture and deflation; factors contributing to loss of implant shell integrity; detection of gel implant rupture; strength and durability of implant shells; frequency of implant rupture and deflation; description of implant fibrous tissue capsules and contractures; capsular, local breast, and distant tissue exposures to silicone and their complications; frequency of saline implant capsular contracture; barrier implants and contractures; effect of implant surface and contracture; effect of local adrenal steroids and contracture; presence of bacteria around implants, antimicrobial treatment and contracture or other complications; hematomas, their frequency and relationship to contractures; the effect of implant placement on contracture; and other relevant complications including pain.

Many other local and perioperative complications in addition to those noted above require explantation or other secondary surgical or medical interventions. A reasonably complete list (see Table 5-1) would include fibrous contracture of the implant capsule; gel implant rupture (with or without migration of silicone gel outside the capsule) or saline implant deflation; filler port or implant valve malfunction; shell folds or wrinkling; infection of the surgical wound; infection around or within the implant; infection associated with toxic shock syndrome; hemorrhage and hematoma; seroma; swelling of the breast; various skin rashes and other skin manifestations such as localized morphea; epidermal proliferative reactions (Spiers et al., 1994); middermal elastolysis; edema; blistering; cysts (Copeland et al., 1993); ulceration; necrosis of the skin, nipple or mastectomy or reconstruction flap; exudation of silicone through the skin or from the nipple (Erdmann et al., 1992; Leibman et al., 1992; McKinney et al., 1987); implant extrusion, misplacement, or displacement; silicone granuloma; axillary adenopathy; sensory loss and paresthesia; pain; abnormal lactation (Hartley and Schatten, 1971; Mason, 1991) and/or galactocele (DeLoach et al., 1994; Johnson and Hanson, 1996); thoracic skeletal asymmetries (Dickson and Sharpe, 1987; Peters and McEwan, 1993); pneumothorax (Brandt et al., 1984); and calcification. "Bleed" or diffusion of small quantities of mostly lower molecular weight linear (and cyclic) silicone gel fluid compounds through the silicone elastomer shell (and to a

TABLE 5-1 Reported Local and Perioperative Complications

Implant fibrous capsular contracture	Skin rashes
Gel implant rupture (intra- and extracapsular)	Skin blistering, cysts, and necrosis
Gel migration	Swelling of the breast
Silicone granuloma	Nipple or flap necrosis
Axillary adenopathy	Implant extrusion
Silicone exudation through skin or nipple	Implant misplacement
Saline implant deflation	Implant shifting or displacement
Implant filler port or valve leakage	Acute and chronic breast and chest wall pain
Operative wound infection	Loss or change in sensation of the breast or nipple
Peri-implant infection	Chest wall skeletal changes
Intra-implant infection	Pneumothorax
Infection with toxic shock syndrome	Peri-implant calcification
Hemorrhage at the operative site	Lactation and galactocele
Peri-implant hematoma or seroma	

lesser extent outside the fibrous capsule) is also reported as a complication, but gel fluid diffusion is intrinsic to the design and physical characteristics of gel-containing implants (see Chapter 3 of this report).

Many of these complications have been cited in the approximately 100,000 adverse event reports to the Food and Drug Administration (FDA) summarized by Brown et al. (1998). This chapter does not rely on that reporting system, however. The FDA system is sensitive to national publicity and includes voluntary reports, which frequently consist of undocumented assertions (Brown et al., 1998), and is therefore subject to distortions of the frequency and nature of implant adverse effects.

OVERALL FREQUENCY OF LOCAL COMPLICATIONS

Several studies with representative cohorts of 583 to 7,008 women address the frequency of secondary interventions in saline- and gel-filled implants for both augmentation and reconstruction (Gabriel et al., 1997; McGhan Medical Corporation, 1998; Mentor Corporation, (1992). Gabriel et al. (1997) reported that 178 (23.8%) of all 749 Olmstead County women of the usual age distribution, noted in Chapter 1, who were implanted at the Mayo Clinic (95% with gel-filled implants) had clinical indications requiring reoperation ranging from explantation to drainage of a hematoma over an average 7.8-year follow-up after implantation. This amounted to 18.8% of the 1,454 breasts implanted. Multiple complications occurred in 61% of these. Although the incidence of complications requiring surgery after augmentation or reconstruction did not differ at two months, by the end of the fifth year when 83% of all first complications had occurred, the percentage of patients with complications after reconstruction (30–34%) was almost threefold that after augmentation (12%). Only surgical complications were analyzed, and some that may be important, such as silent ruptures, may have been missed. The frequency of complications reported in this study is consistent with the frequencies reported in other studies cited later, especially given the long average follow-up in this series.

The McGhan AR90 preliminary report (McGhan Medical Corporation, 1998) describes the 583 women of the usual age distribution who agreed to participate in this study and received McGhan 1990s, mostly textured, single- and multilumen gel-filled implants, 549 for augmentation and 34 for reconstruction, with a five-year follow-up. In this cohort, 23% of augmented women and 42.4% of reconstructed women required secondary surgery ranging from explantation to evacuation of hematoma or seroma, to correction of implant placement or contracture, to biopsy during the five-year study period. These are underestimates because implant rupture was diagnosed by physician evaluation; and therefore a number of silent ruptures were likely missed. Explantation is overestimated since about one-third (or roughly 6 and 14% of augmentation and reconstruction secondary surgeries, respectively) were at patient request because of safety concerns prevalent during the entry period (1990–1992) of this study not because of clinical indication.

The McGhan large simple trial (LST) (McGhan Medical Corporation, undated) was a one-year prospective observational study of all 2,855 women of the usual age distribution who agreed to participate in this study and received McGhan 1990s, predominantly textured, room temperature vulcanized (RTV) saline-filled implants, 81.1% for augmentation. Women entered this trial in 1995 and 1996. The cumulative results after a year for four complications (infection, deflation, explant, and severe [Baker Class III or IV] capsular contracture) were 18.9 and 35.9% of women following augmentation and reconstruction (includes revisions), respectively. These figures are more reflective of actual clinical conditions since saline implant deflations are likely to be observed, and women are much less likely to have requested explantation of saline implants on nonclinical grounds. While secondary surgical frequencies were not identified as such, they are likely quite similar although probably slightly higher than the cumulative percentage for the four complications, since these complications are highly predictive of surgical intervention. Additional complications in this cohort will occur in the one- to five-year interval. Comparison of these results with overall complications of the previously cited AR90, long follow-up gel-filled implants is inappropriate.

Women receiving Mentor gel-filled implants (and some receiving expanders) were enrolled in the company's adjunct study. At the three-year follow-up, there were 3,559 women with reconstructions and 3,449 women with augmentation, almost all with low-bleed, gel-filled implants. The overall frequency of infection was 2.8–4.3% in reconstructions and 1.3% in augmentations. The overall Class III–IV contracture prevalence was 12–13% in reconstructions and 11% in augmentations. The overall frequency of rupture was 1.3–1.7% in reconstructions and 0.7% in augmentations—but these ruptures were determined by physical examination only (Purkait, Mentor Corporation., IOM Scientific Workshop, 1998).

In addition to these studies, Gutowski et al. (1997) reported the outcomes of 504 patients with 995 predominantly Heyer-Schulte–Mentor saline implants in an 11-center retrospective cohort study. These patients represented the 41.5% of those identified by the plastic surgery centers that were successfully interviewed, but it is not clear how patients were identified or what proportions of the total number of women with implants at the centers were identified. This uncontrolled accession of patients raises significant concerns about the interpretation of any results. Implants were placed almost entirely (93.8%) for augmentation, evenly divided between submuscular and submammary positioning in 1980–1989, and were followed for an average of six years. Of these women, 20.8% underwent secondary surgery, primarily for replacement, removal, or capsulotomy. The complications of infection (0.2%), hematoma (1.6%), and seroma (0.1%) were infrequent. Deflation occurred in 55 implants (5.5%) and 51 women (10.1%). Deflation (and rupture) frequency differed by implant model. Only about 4.2% of the predominant late model RTV implants deflated. These probably represent minimum figures (Gutowski et al., 1997).

Fiala et al., (1993) reported the results of a survey of 106 women representing 62.9% of a cohort of 167 women who could be located from the original 304 women who had undergone breast augmentation from 1973–1991. Their implants were primarily smooth silicone gel (70.8%) but also included some polyurethane-coated (27.1%) and a few textured implants. In this survey, 73.9% of women reported being "highly satisfied," 19.8% of women underwent secondary surgery, and the complications were mostly contractures. Contractures occurred more often as time progressed and significantly more in submammary than submuscular implants. There were fewer contractures, though not statistically significantly, around the polyurethane compared to the smooth implants (Fiala et al., 1993). Edworthy et al. (1998), surveying the experience of a population of 1,112 unselected women with silicone gel-filled implants, found that 214 women (19.25%) had undergone secondary surgical procedures and 38.5% of breasts implanted (average of frequencies reported for left and right breasts) had Class III–IV contractures. The odds of a woman needing more than one implant per breast over time are high, and placement of as many as 16 implants per woman has been reported (Roberts et al., 1997). In one small cohort of 52 mostly (67%) augmented women who agreed to participate in the study, out of 138 consecutive women with breast implant problems, the average was 3.19 gel implants per woman over an average of 11.9 years (Wells et al., 1995). In another small cohort (N = 60) of consecutive women undergoing immediate reconstruction with expanders, 2.78 operations were required on average for each woman, 0.78 for complications and 2.00 for original expander insertion and the following permanent implant replacement (Slavin and Colen, 1990). Shanklin and Smalley (1998a) reported 3.45 implants per women in a small experience (N = 130) with patients self-selected for problems and a 49.3% frequency of procedures in addition to implant replacement including 15.4% closed capsulotomies. Although the data were reported in a way that made it difficult to aggregate them, each woman appeared to have undergone 1.8 to 1.9 operations, many of which were on the normal breast for correction of asymmetry in the series of 109 women with delayed postmastectomy reconstructions reported by Houpt et al. (1988). Worseg et al. (1995) reported 83 secondary operations in a cohort of 77 women implanted with inflatable (saline or dextran) Heyer-Schulte–Mentor implants with a mean follow-up of nine years. There was an average of 1.08 secondary operations per woman, predominantly for deflation (23.9%) or severe contracture (37.6%). Similarly, Middleton (1998b) reported a series of 1,251 women seen since 1992 at the University of California at San Diego with a diverse array of implants who were referred for magnetic resonance scans because of suspected implant problems. He found that 15.35, 30.56 and 45.19% of these women required replacement implants within five years following augmentation, cancer mastectomy, and prophylactic mastectomy, respectively. This population, which was referred for problems, averaged 1.54 implants per breast (Middleton, 1998b).

These studies covered different follow-up periods, different kinds of implants, and different indications for implantation. Some were surveys, some record reviews, and some prospective observational trials. Each group was of unknown relation to the total group from which it was selected with respect to the events being studied. The results, therefore, cannot be compared scientifically. Although a quantative estimate is not possible, it appears that a significant number of women can expect additional procedures in the first five years after implantation. Women with implants for reconstruction and with gel-filled implants appear more likely to be at the upper end of the range of frequency.

Breast Reconstruction After Mastectomy

Perioperative and local complications are significant medical and patient events. Some complications are procedure related, that is, they would occur independent of the presence of an implant, and some are implant dependent and may vary with the characteristics of the implant, as noted in Chapter 3. This is particularly clear in reports that compare perioperative complications in reconstructions after mastectomy with matched mastectomy patients without reconstruction, in a sense "operative controls." O'Brien et al. (1993) in a short follow-up study, reported a similar complication frequency of 28% (*N* = 82) in 289 mastectomized women who were not reconstructed, compared with 31% (*N* = 35) in 113 women who were reconstructed, primarily with subpectoral expanders, after mastectomy. Most perioperative complications were the same, but seromas requiring one or more aspirations were present in 19% (*N* = 55) of those without reconstruction and only 3% (*N* = 3) of those with reconstruction. Implant-related problems occurred in 14% (*N* = 16) of the reconstructed women, including eight who required explantation (O'Brien et al., 1993). Vinton et al. (1990) in a study primarily about immediate, surgical complications, reported a similar total complication rate of 48% in 305 women undergoing modified radical mastectomy without reconstruction and 37% in 90 women with mastectomy and immediate reconstruction, primarily with expanders. Again, seromas were more frequent in the nonreconstructed group (30% versus 13%), and the reconstructed group had a 6% prosthesis complication rate with 4% requiring explantation (Vinton et al., 1990).

With respect to total short-term complications in reconstruction, these reports suggest that the implant may prevent seromas. Other complications such as infection, hematoma, and epidermolysis or skin necrosis occur with about equal frequency in women undergoing mastectomy who have implants and those who do not. The frequencies of early complications in implanted and nonimplanted women after mastectomy are roughly equal in these reports, but implant related complications are underestimated because of the short follow-up. Comparisons such as these are not possible in augmented patients because there can be no operative controls. In reconstruction after mastectomy, surgery is a precondition and the avoidable risk is only the implant-dependent fraction; in augmentation, surgery is not a precondition, and the risks of silicone implants may not be as separable from the operative risks. Implant technology designed to minimize risk is important in both instances.

Similar results are reported from case series of implant patients. Noone et al. (1985) reported on 85 women undergoing immediate reconstruction after mastectomy with saline and double-lumen implants with short follow-up and the usual complications of skin necrosis (15%), seroma or hematoma (12%), extrusion (4%), infection (2%), and severe contracture (11%)—or 44% overall—15% of which (contracture, extrusion) were clearly implant dependent. In addition, secondary surgery later was required for open capsulotomy and explantation in 14.4%. Francel et al. (1993) reported 57% revision surgeries with permanent saline implants or expanders in immediate reconstruction after mastectomy and 30% in delayed reconstruction, with minor complication frequencies of 8.1 and 14% respectively, and implantation failures of 3.5% in both groups. Eberlein et al. (1993) reported 19 (27%) secondary surgical procedures (replacement or capsulotomy) and 8% prosthetic loss in 71 women with submuscular double-lumen implants after mastectomy, and Bailey et al. (1989) reported 18% implant loss in 165 women reconstructed with submuscular expanders or gel implants. Crespo et al. (1994) reported 115 consecutive implant reconstructions at the time of mastectomy using McGhan double-lumen smooth implants. Secondary surgery was performed in 20% of these women, and there were 5% infections, 8% explantations, 11% seroma or hematomas and 3% tissue flap necroses (Crespo et al., 1994).

Gylbert et al. (1990a) reported breast reconstruction in 65 women with randomly selected gel or saline implants followed for an average of six years: 6 of 37 (16%) patients with saline implants required replacements because of deflations, and three other operations were needed for misplacement, severe contracture and extrusion (8%). This study was primarily of contracture and is reviewed again later in this chapter. Using expanders and gel implants for immediate and delayed reconstruction, Slavin and Colen (1990) had an overall complication rate of 60% (among them, 15% seromas, 13.3% skin necrosis, 8.8% extrusion, 6.7% infection) in 60 consecutive immediate reconstructions involving expanders. Kroll and Baldwin (1992) had 23% "failures" (poor aesthetics or failure to complete reconstruction) at 22 months' follow-up in 87 women reconstructed immediately with expanders, followed by permanent replacement with polyurethane or other gel-filled implants.

Schlenker et al. (1978) studied 89 women with immediate or delayed reconstruction after simple mastectomy for fibrocystic disease over 6 months to 12 years. They removed implants in 28% of these patients for infection, extrusion or necrosis. Using primarily the Mentor 1600 inflatable saline implant, Schuster and Lavine (1988) reported 98 women undergoing immediate submuscular reconstruction after subcutaneous prophylactic mastectomy over a nine-year period. Eighteen patients suffered tissue loss, and there were three extrusions, among a number of less troublesome complications (Schuster and Lavine, 1988). In a study of wound complications in implant or expander immediate breast reconstructions in 112 women, Furey et al. (1994) observed complications in 25 patients (22.3%) and removed 8 implants; other complications were not reported. Camilleri et al. (1996) reported 111 consecutive women reconstructed using the Becker (reverse double-lumen, gel outside) permanent expander with an average follow-up of only one year. Complications more typical of expanders, such as wound dehiscence (8%) and filling port failure (6%), occurred in addition to contracture (9%), expander infection and removal (5%), skin flap necrosis and expander exposure (5%), and other sequelae such as pain on expansion (20%). Despite these complications, 89% of women expressed satisfaction to the plastic surgeon on follow-up (Camilleri et al., 1996).

Gibney (1987) using CUI or Heyer-Schulte expanders for reconstruction in 65 women with three to seven years of patient follow-up, reported 5.8% of breasts with contractures, 2.5% with infections, and 4.5% with deflations, resulting in loss of the implant in 4.6%. Mandrekas et al. (1995) compared 19 women with immediate to 25 women with delayed reconstruction using subpectoral smooth tissue expanders after cancer mastectomy. The longest follow-up was seven years, but most complications were assessed by one year. These included one seroma, one infection, one skin necrosis, one valve deflation, ten Class II–IV contractures and two malpositions—16 complications in 15 (34%) women, more frequent in delayed reconstruction. There were no rheumatic complaints (Mandrekas et al., 1995). Mahdi et al. (1998) carried out a prospective trial using the McGhan reverse double-lumen expander in 16 immediate and 4 delayed subpectoral reconstructions followed for an average of 10.1 months. There were seven reoperations for correction of placement, one hematoma, and two filler port problems. Follow-up was insufficient to evaluate rupture or contracture (Mahdi et al., 1998).

Spear et al. (1991) reported 76 women with 89 double-lumen implants for immediate reconstruction, randomized to 16 mg methylprednisolone in the outer saline lumen or to controls. Except for a lower frequency of contracture in the steroid group, the two groups were comparable three years after implantation. There were a total of 38 operative revisions, 2 significant infections, 3 extrusions, 16 fluid collections, 6 instances of skin necrosis and 26 Class II–IV contractures. Spear and Majidian (1998) subsequently reported 171 immediate postcancer mastectomy reconstructions with textured McGhan expanders in 142 women. Expanders were mostly replaced by textured saline implants, and follow-up after completion of reconstruction averaged 19 months. There were 14 (8.1%) skin necroses, 2 (1%) hematomas, 6 (3.5%) infections, 8 expanders and 11 implants (6.4%) requiring replacement and 5 (3%) significant capsular contractures. Equal or better results using textured expanders were reported by Fisher et al. (1991; see also Maxwell and Falcone, 1992; Russel et al., 1990; Beasley,

1992 who reported infrequent loss of expanders and rare contractures). In a review of a large experience with saline expanders (currently the most widely used technology for reconstruction according to the 1997 American Society of Plastic and Reconstructive Surgeons [ASPRS] survey), Woods and Mangan (1992) implied that results at the low end of reported complications could be achieved through experience and care.

As earlier, these studies include a number of variables. However, based on these reports, it appears that women, historically, could expect early (postoperative) complications, up to 30%–40% after reconstruction with implants, because reconstruction typically involves a significant surgical procedure to begin with (i.e., mastectomy for breast cancer). In addition to the surgical complications from mastectomy and implantation, there are the usual complications that depend on the presence of the implant.

Breast Augmentation

Using Mentor implants for submammary augmentation, with a follow-up of four or more years for 87%, Capozzi (1986) reported 3.4% of breasts with contractures, 3.4% with deflations at intervals from nine months to seven years, and 100% satisfaction in 100 women between 1976 and 1985. Cocke (1994), using Heyer-Schulte–Mentor saline implants in 75 women for augmentation, mostly submammary, followed for 1.5 to 13 years, reported 29% (N = 22) secondary surgeries and 52% (N = 39) complications (23 contractures requiring treatment). McKinney and Tresley (1983) reported a series of 58 women using Heyer-Schulte saline implants in the submammary position, with a number of complications including deflation (N = 9), infection (N = 4), capsules (N = 14), and hematomas (N = 9). In a letter report, Bell reported 10 deflations on average at 32 months of the same implant model in a series of 193 women (Bell, 1983).

Others have reported very infrequent failures. Mladick (1993) summarized results from his experience with saline augmentation over 17 years in 1,327 women with 9.1% secondary surgery. Most of these implants were modern RTV saline inflatables, but high termperature vulcanized (HTV) saline implants had been used earlier. Although the average follow-up was short, only 28 months, as is often the case, the deflations of the older implant models were 37.7% compared to the 1.33% for the more recent model, and complications were infrequent, mainly contractures in 1.1% of breasts, and no infections (Mladick, 1993). Frequent deflations (5–8%) were reported with the early saline models by others (Grossman, 1973; Regnault et al., 1972). Lavine (1993) reported placing 2,018 saline implants, with 4.2% of patients needing revisions, 1.1% Class III–IV contractures, and 2.3% deflations of all implants, but only 0.56% deflations of recent model Heyer-Schulte inflatables. The follow-up of these implants ranged from 6 months to 13 years (Lavine, 1993). These reports also include a number of different variables, but they generally find a lower complication frequency, more consistent with the overall reoperation frequencies cited earlier, which were based mostly on results of women with implants for augmentation.

SPECIFIC COMPLICATIONS

The important events for the safety of breast implantation are those that require significant interventions and seriously detract from the desired cosmetic objective. These include gel implant rupture (especially extracapsular) or saline implant deflation, severe contracture, infection, significant hematoma, severe and continuing pain, granuloma and axillary adenopathy, and implant displacement and extrusion. These are events that may require surgical revision, extensive medical or surgical attention or explantation, or leave the patient with deformity and discomfort. The occurrence of individual local and perioperative complications varies enormously among reports. Differences in complication frequency result from multiple factors: (1) individual unexplained variability in biological reaction to the device (e.g., fibrous capsular contractures); (2) differences in women's ages, physical conditions, habits, comorbidities and indications for implantation; (3) differences in types of implants and their physical and chemical characteristics, as described below and in Chapter 3; (4) differences in the design, adequacy, and reporting of clinical and basic research that may distort the true biological and medical picture; and (5) variable techniques and skills of surgeons and other medical personnel (e.g., operative techniques and skill and/or coincident medical interventions such as antibiotics, antiseptics, closed capsulotomies, steroids, treatment for cancer, and others).

In the discussions that follow, evidence for the contributions of these factors to a particular complication or the frequency of complications is reviewed. In some instances, a role is likely but speculative. In other instances, there are data to support objective statements, at least of limited or suggestive evidence of an association. Although a great deal has been learned, much more work on biologic variation is needed to fully understand the influences of this factor. As noted earlier, there are differences in the frequency of complications in women who receive implants for augmentation and for reconstructions and in those with immediate and delayed reconstructions. Although age may not influence most complications, the amount of body tissue and fat available for implant coverage, habits such as smoking or alcohol abuse (which could affect tissue viability), and significant medical illness (diabetes) are reported to make a difference (Cohen et al., 1992). Implant types and characteristics are important in a number of ways, as noted here and Chapter 3. Deficiencies in design and reporting of research may result in confusing or even misleading or incorrect information concerning complications. These problems are mentioned elsewhere in this report. Differences in surgical skill or technique may also play an important role. It seems intuitively reasonable that this should be so, given the great variation in reported results, which often appears to have no other obvious explanation. Although few studies explore these factors, techniques, and skills, some reports claim that they are critical in explaining frequencies of hematoma, infection, contracture, or other complications that differ greatly from the average values cited in the medical literature (e.g., Freeman, 1967; Mladick, 1993). The roles of some of the specific medical interventions are detailed further below.

In addition, several major operative approaches to implant placement are described in the medical literature (Salomon and Barton, 1997). The operative incision can be made in the axillary fold (and the implant placed under direct vision or endoscopically), in the circum- or periareolar position, or in the inframammary fold. The implant can be placed subcutaneously, under the mammary gland on the chest muscles (submammary, subglandular), or under the chest muscles (submuscular, subpectoral), depending on the status of the breast and a number of other factors including surgeon–patient preferences. The axillary incision is generally not visible unless the arm is raised; the inframammary incision lies under the breast and is covered by normal clothing. Circum- or periareolar incisions are usually around the inferior pole of the nipple-areolar complex from 9 o'clock to 3 o'clock. Some of these approaches may give better operative exposure for control of bleeding or may allow greater ease of insertion of bulky implants. They may also make operative scars, which can be unsightly in 2 to 5% of patients, less visible (Baker, 1992). Some concern has been expressed also that periareoloar incisions may be more likely to interfere with subsequent lactation and breast feeding (see Chapter 11). The periareolar approach may interrupt some lactiferous ducts, but inferior pedicle mammaplasty interrupts ducts substantially, and many women are said to breast-feed successfully after this procedure. Some have speculated that any interference with breast feeding may be due to compression by the implant. In any event, no conclusive evidence was found that these different surgical approaches have significant influences on complications related to the safety of breast implants.

Implant Rupture and Deflation

All silicone gel implants are subject to the bleed or diffusion of gel fluid composed of relatively low molecular weight linear and cyclic silicone compounds through the implant silicone elastomer shell. The compounds range in molecular weight from 5,200 to 400,000 but are primarily less than 25,000 or 10,000 in implants without or with barrier shells. The higher molecular weight compounds may be from uncross-linked shell silicones (Varaprath, 1991, 1992). The large, highly cross-linked poly-(dimethlysiloxane) (PDMS) molecule of the gel cannot diffuse through the shell, and gel does not appear outside the implant unless there is a physical passage caused by a breach in the integrity of the shell. Diffusion is potentially important if silicone fluid or other substances inside the implant are toxic, if low molecular weight compounds can permeate the capsule and get into the circulation or into local lymph nodes with adverse effects, or if the fluid contributes to local reactions such as capsule formation, infection, or local effects that have systemic consequences. As the implant ages, silicone penetrates intact capsules and appears in breast tissue outside the capsule more often. This does not necessarily relate to frank ruptures or result in granulomas or adenopathy, however (Beekman et al., 1997a). These questions are taken up elsewhere in this report.

Factors Contributing to Loss of Shell Integrity

Silicone gel fluid is regularly found on and outside the shells of gel-filled implants. Implant rupture, a loss of integrity of the implant shell of varying severity, is diagnosed only when silicone gel itself is present outside the implant. This may occur, at one end of the spectrum of severity, through tiny flaws or pinholes in the shell, such as these caused by inadvertent needle sticks during suturing at implantation (Goldwyn, 1969), open capsulotomy, or other surgery, or through injection, needle biopsy or aspiration of seromas and hematomas. Wrinkles or folds are observed in 15–67% of measurable gel or saline implant shells by methods such as palpation, mammography, or observation at explantation (Frankel et al., 1995; Ganott et al., 1992; Gylbert et al., 1990a; Rolland, 1989a). Explant cases may not be representative and are probably high-end estimates. Tears can occur because a shell distorted by folds abrades itself through the continuous motion of the breast and implant on the chest wall or through muscular contraction over a submuscular implant (Schmidt, 1980). Such abraded areas can be detected by scanning electron microscopy (Young et al., 1996a). Older implants and those with tight capsules have been noted to have significant distortion, folding, and often calcification which suggests ample opportunity for wear (De Camara et al., 1993). Some of these defects may not be visible to the eye, but they have been characterized by scanning electron microscopy that can define small fold flaws and suture needle holes (Brandon et al., 1997a,b).

The breast may be subjected to considerable compressive force during squeezing maneuvers to break fibrous capsules in closed capsulotomies (Gruber and Friedman, 1978) and when greater-than-necessary compression is used during routine film mammography or mammography modified for better visualization of breasts with implants (Eklund et al., 1988). Both of these maneuvers have been associated in some reports with implant rupture or deflation and rarely with other complications such as infection, gel migration, silicone granulomas and exudation of gel from the skin and nipple, or conversion of intra- to extracapsular rupture. During mammography, this is very unusual and rarely, if ever, has been proved conclusively and should not discourage mammographic screening for breast cancer (Addington and Mallin, 1978; Andersen et al., 1989; Apesos and Pope, 1985; Argenta, 1983; Bassett and Brenner, 1992; Beraka, 1995; Brandt et al., 1984; Cocke, 1978; Cohen et al., 1997; De Camara et al., 1993; Edmond and Versaci, 1980; Eisenberg and Bartels, 1977; Eklund, 1990; Feliberti et al., 1977, Goin, 1978; Gruber and Jones, 1981; Hawes, 1990; Huang et al., 1978; Hueston and Hare, 1979; Laughlin et al., 1977; Pay and Kenealy, 1997; Pickford and Webster, 1994; Renfrew et al., 1992; Robinson et al., 1995; Scott et al., 1988; Wilflingseder et al., 1983; Williams, 1991; Zide, 1981).

Recurrence of contracture after either open or closed capsulotomy is substantial when patients are followed long enough and has been reported to range from 23 to 89% (Baker et al., 1976; Brandt et al., 1984; Burkhardt et al., 1981; Hetter, 1979; Hipps et al., 1978; Little and Baker; 1980; Moufarrege et al., 1987; Vecchione, 1977). Complications after closed capsulotomy are reported to reach 10%–12%. and primarily involve distortion, displacement, rupture (with migration of gel), infection, and bleeding. Rarely, severe persistent pain and extrusion, among other complications, may also occur (Gruber and Jones, 1981; Laughlin et al., 1977; Nelson, 1980a). Such data support those who question the wisdom of this procedure. In a follow-up to his survey of closed procedures, Nelson (1981) reported a complication prevalence in 5,579 open capsulotomies of 6.24%, primarily hematoma, displacement, and infection.

Open (operative) or closed capsulotomies have significant safety implications because they have historically been performed, often repeatedly, on women with contracture of the implant fibrous capsule. These procedures may be performed in a third to almost all cases, depending on surgeons' and women's tolerance of this complication and confidence in the effectiveness of the procedure (see above references and those in the discussion of contractures). Peters et al. (1997) reported that in their series of 100 consecutive explants, 36% had had at least one closed and 54% at least one open capsulotomy. Baker (1975) commented that he performed open capsulotomies in all Class IV and 50% of Class III contractures and had 40% recurrences. He performed closed capsulotomies in cases with any firmness, repeated without limitation, and had 31% recurrences (Baker, 1975). Moufarrege et al. (1987) reported doing multiple closed and open capsulotomies on 82% (134 out of 164) of women with contractures, 28% of their series of 482 women who received silicone gel implants between 1973 and 1978. They noted that 18% of women with contractures were satisfied despite contracture and declined further intervention. Recurrences after closed capsulotomies occurred in 67% on the first attempt, 80% after the second attempt, and 90% after a third attempt. Similarly, recurrences after open capsulotomies occurred in 54% after one, 56% after two, and 71% after three attempts in the same breast. More than three attempts to relieve contracture by capsulotomy were fruitless (Moufarrege et al., 1987). In view of women's tolerance for contracture without seeking medical attention, the subjective nature of contracture assessment by surgeons, the loss to follow-up of women with implants, and the varying periods of follow-up for a problem that continues to accumulate over time (all noted elsewhere in this chapter), reports of the frequency of contracture recurrence after capsulotomy are probably underestimates.

Gruber et al. (1981) wrote that they performed open capsulotomies in 72–100% of breasts with Class III and Class IV contractures. Nelson's (1980a) survey of closed capsulotomies found 30,001 of these procedures in 114,617 augmentations. Capsular contracture-related procedures made up 27.5% of secondary procedures in augmentation and 14.3% in reconstruction in the McGhan (1998) AR90 study. Other sources of trauma, ranging from gunshot wounds to automobile accidents to tight hugs, may also burst the shell (Cohen et al., 1997; De Camara et al., 1993; Dellon et al., 1980; Wise, 1994a,b). Some shells are broken or abraded during insertion. Some shells that are diagnosed as ruptured are actually broken on explantation (Slavin and Goldwyn, 1995).

At the most severe end of the spectrum of loss of integrity, the implant shell can become completely disrupted and float in a pool of silicone gel and fluid. In other instances, only small quantities of gel may escape through small holes such as those described earlier. If the fibrous capsule surrounding the ruptured implant is intact, it can contain the silicone in more or less the same shape and to the same effect as the implant shell. This occurs in what is called an intracapsular rupture. Such a rupture is often asymptomatic, without cosmetic effect and imperceptible on physical or radiological examination. If the fibrous capsule is weakened and bulges, a ruptured (or intact) implant can adopt, or conform to, this new shape. If the capsule has lost its integrity at some point, varying amounts of silicone gel can escape the capsule entirely. This gel can either reincapsulate close by in the breast tissue (Argenta, 1983; Mason and Apisarnthanarax, 1981) or migrate along tissue planes to other parts of the body, usually the axilla and chest or upper abdominal wall (Ahn and

Shaw, 1994; Goin, 1978; Hueston and Hare, 1979). Occasionally, gel migrates to even more distant sites, including inside the thoracic cage, down the arm, or into the groin. Rarely, this causes damage to structures such as neurovascular bundles, the formation of granulomas and cysts, and/or the breakdown of overlying tissues (Capozzi et al., 1978; Edmond and Versaci, 1980; Foster et al., 1983; Hirmand et al., 1994; Kao et al., 1997; Masson et al., 1982; Persellin et al., 1992; Sanger et al., 1992; Teuber et al., 1995b, 1999; Walsh et al., 1989). Extracapsular rupture can be present with implants that are completely ruptured and collapsed, or it can be associated with implants that are ruptured but not collapsed (Middleton, IOM Scientific Workshop, 1998).

Rupture of saline implants is referred to as deflation. Because saline, unlike silicone, is a physiologic solution and is rapidly absorbed in tissue, it does not remain or accumulate where deposited. The collapse and loss of aesthetics of the implant generally occur over one to two days (Rheingold et al., 1994) but can be quite gradual with small perforations or valve leaks. These leaks may cause deflations (as few as two to three drops over 12 hours in vitro), which may become apparent slowly over as long a period two years and are observed as partial deflations (Dickson and Sharpe, 1987; Nordström, 1988; Peters, 1997; Rapaport et al., 1997). Deflation, even partial, usually should not pose a diagnostic problem except in multilumen implants where the deflation of a small outer saline-filled lumen may, as was the designer's original intent, escape notice. According to Rees et al. (1973b) water (but not salt) may pass through the silicone elastomer shell in response to an osmotic gradient despite the insolubility of silicone in water, but usually there is no reason for disequilibration because at physiologic salt concentrations the osmotic pressure is the same on both sides of the shell. If the shell and valves remain intact, only small increases or decreases in volume over time are reported (Cederna, 1996). For unknown reasons, larger volume changes have been reported to develop over the years in rare cases (Botti et al., 1994; Robinson and Benos, 1997). Volume changes in intact saline implants might reflect correction of an osmotic imbalance due to variation in human body fluid and saline filler osmolality by movement of water into the implant lumen (Frisch, 1997, 1998). In vitro experiments found that volume changes pursuant to osmotic gradients occurred slowly, over six months to a year. Subjecting the implant to pressure, which might occur especially in the submuscular position or with severe contracture, accelerated the movement of fluid out of implants. This might explain some in vivo changes (Rubin, 1983), or in some cases with inflatable implants the valve leakage could be so slight that it was not apparent and partial deflation was mistakenly ascribed instead to movement of fluid through the shell (possibly what happened in Cederna, 1996, and other studies).

Needle sticks at implant placement surgery are a significant cause of early deflation although, as noted, this may not be apparent for several months. In one study, about 1% of implants sold were returned because of perioperative deflation. Small needle holes were discovered in about 7% of these (Rapaport et al., 1997). Small holes were found in 75% of saline implants involved in one series of deflations (Rheingold et al., 1994). Abrasion and compression cause deflation of saline implants in ways similar to their effect on gel implants. However, saline implants lack the solidity and supportiveness of the gel interior and the lubrication of silicone fluid on the shell surface. They are therefore more prone to wrinkling, fold flaws, surface abrasion, and consequent deflation. Fold flaws have been associated with underfilling of saline implants, which causes wrinkling, especially of the upper part of the implant. These fold flaws have been cited as an important cause of deflation (Gylbert et al., 1990a; Lantieri et al., 1997; Worton et al., 1980). Even with overfilling or attention to proper filling of newer implants, however, a smooth saline implant or a non-adherent textured implant may still sag toward the bottom of a large tissue pocket in the breast, producing some collapse and vertical, so-called traction wrinkling of the superior part (Tebbetts, 1996). As described earlier, these implant problems are common, and submammary or subcutaneous placement of saline implants often allows these wrinkles to become easily visible through the skin. Skin wrinkling over a wrinkled implant can be quite pronounced and require corrective interventions. It has been reported with a frequency of 3.3–5% in subglandular, smooth saline implants for augmentation (Cocke, 1994; McKinney and Tresley, 1983; Mladick, 1993). In reconstructed patients, skin wrinkling with smooth saline implants has been reported to occur in as many as 26% of cases (Gylbert et al., 1990a). In two additional studies, skin wrinkling occurred with 14% of saline compared to 3% of gel smooth implants or 7.3% of saline compared to 2.1% of gel textured implants (Asplund, 1984; Handel et al., 1995).

The valves and valve–shell interfaces of saline implants and expanders can also leak or become incompetent under increased pressure in the implant. Some have reported average pressures of 4.5 mm of mercury (Hg) in implants in soft breasts and 11.5 mm Hg in hard breasts and pressures of as much as 320 mm Hg during closed capsulotomies (Jenny, 1980). In other instances, such pressures are known to reach levels on the order of 93 mm Hg or 126 cm of water [H_2O] or more, which is substantially greater than historic test standards (Caffee, 1993a; described in FDA, 1992b). Peters (1997) also demonstrated in vitro that valves that appear competent may leak saline slowly under pressure.

Detection of Rupture of Gel-Filled Implants

As noted above, intracapsular rupture of gel implants can go unrecognized. There may be no patient complaints and no physical diagnostic findings. The sensitivity of commonly used imaging technologies, such as film mammography, is reported to be around 50%, and some report a sensitivity as low as 15–20% (Ahn et al., 1994a; Bassett and Brenner, 1992; Robinson et al., 1995; Samuels et al., 1995), although there are some who claim it is much higher (Cohen et al., 1997; also see Chapter 12). Ultrasound may detect more ruptures. Magnetic resonance imaging is generally reported to have a sensitivity of around 90% in experienced hands, but this technology is currently too costly and time-consuming for routine screening. Physical diagnosis of extracapsular rupture, when the shape or feel of the gel mass has changed, is much easier, although occasionally such changes can escape detection (Edmond and Versaci, 1980). The changed contour of the gel is also observed on film mammography, although contour irregularities may be secondary to accommodation of an unruptured implant to, or herniation through, a capsulotomy defect. Presence of gel is reported outside the capsule in about 12–26% of ruptures (Ahn et al., 1994a; Berg, et al. 1995; Frankel et al., 1995; Gorczyca et al., 1994a; Middleton, 1998b). It has been as high as 35% in selected series (Andersen et al., 1989). These figures generally refer to more fragile second generation implants and come from case series of patients who present because of problems and, therefore, may overstate complications. There are also reports of series of 19 or 30 instances in which there has been implant rupture without any extracapsular movement of gel (Beekman et al., 1997a; Malata et al., 1994a) or a low proportion of extracapsular movement, e.g., 5.7% of ruptured implants (Peters et al., 1997). Extracapsular rupture is also more easily detected on ultrasound and MRI.

The diagnosis of rupture of a gel implant is important because the release of silicone gel and fluid into the tissues may result in local complications. An intracapsular rupture may become extracapsular, and both are generally, but not always (Hardt, IOM Scientific Workshop, 1998), agreed to be an indication for explantation (Young., 1998). Moreover, rupture should be anticipated at some point since implants have a finite life span, although what this might be with current models is not certain. Careful explantation and direct visual examination are the standard for diagnosis of silicone gel-filled implant rupture, both unsuspected or silent, and for confirmation of rupture. Explantation allows only a retrospective or confirmatory diagnosis. It is not a prospective means of resolving the question of presence or timing of rupture in an individual patient.

Capsulectomy along with explantation is recommended if the implant is ruptured (Rohrich et al., 1998b; Young, 1998). Although Thomson (1973) reported that capsules left at explantation were reabsorbed, this is not necessarily the case. Retained capsules can interfere with adequate compression for mammography, can confuse mammographic diagnosis of breast cancer if calcifications are present (Hardt et al., 1995a; Peters et al., 1995d) and may lead to further complications necessitating additional surgery (Copeland, 1996; Hardt et al., 1995a; Hayes et al., 1993; Peters et al., 1995d; Rockwell et al., 1998; Stewart et al., 1992).

Implant Shell Strength

A number of additional factors could contribute to implant rupture. As discussed earlier, some shells were thicker and stronger than others. Different implants had valve or valve attachments that were more or less secure. Manufacturers developed elastomers with various performance characteristics, that also affected implant integrity. The manufacturing process itself has been cited as a possible contributor to deflation by Rubin (1983) who noted changes by scanning electron microscopy such as accentuation of defects in the surfaces of saline implants subjected to 3/4-pound tension.

Although not universally agreed upon, it appears that the elastomer shell is relatively stable in vivo once the effects of gel fluid permeation, that can decrease the tensile strength of shells not protected by barriers to gel fluid diffusion by around 30%, are taken into consideration (FDA, 1992a, p. 75). The shell appears to maintain strength, rupture resistance, and bulk material stability as determined by measurements of mechanical and chemical properties and cross-link density over many years of implantation. In Silastic II explants, elongation values were greater than those recommended by the American Society for Testing and Materials (ASTM) for 12 years (ASTM, 1983a; Brandon et al., 1998a,b). Analyses of elastomer by nuclear magnetic resonance (NMR) have reported or suggested some chemical changes, but the quantitative effects of these on shell strength were not assessed (Pfleiderer et al., 1995; Picard et al., 1997). A number of reports have cited decreases of modest proportions in silicone elastomer strength characteristics either in materials testing or in non-breast implants in mid-length, one-to-two year studies (Langley and Swanson, 1976; Leininger et al., 1964; Roggendorf, 1976; Swanson and Lebeau, 1974). Some more marked decreases were found in one long-term study of pacemaker leads (Dolezel et al., 1989), but a shorter-term in vitro investigation of the material found physicochemical and strength properties were maintained (Kennan et al., 1997).

The resistance to rupture and deflation observed in some studies is quite good, but there is a considerable experience that describes rupture and deflation prevalence as increasing, sometimes markedly, with time after implantation. This increased prevalence may relate to repeated stressing, folding, and abrading of an implant, especially with tight capsules and incidental trauma of various kinds (Cohen et al., 1997; De Camara et al., 1993; Gutowski et al., 1997; Malata et al., 1994a; Peters et al., 1994a, 1996; Phillips et al., 1996; Young et al., 1996a, 1998). Shell strength and rupture resistance can be measured by tensile strength, elongation, tear resistance, and modulus, which are measurements (and standards) of the ability of an elastomer to stretch and withstand measured stresses and tearing forces. Greenwald et al. (1996) measured the shell tensile strength (resistance to stress and strain) and modulus of 25 smooth gel implants explanted after 2 to 18 years and found consistently less strength over time in older implants with considerable scatter of results. As the authors point out however, the explants were not compared to control devices, and the makes and models were not described; the implants were those removed by one of the authors from consecutive women between 1991 and 1994 (Greenwald et al., 1996). Phillips et al. (1996) also tested a series of 29 explants, 4 months to 20 years of age, and found considerable variation. They concluded that shell strength diminished with age, although they also noted considerable differences over time among implants of various types and manufacturers. They tested an unused Silastic II breast implant to validate their methods, but otherwise had no controls. Van Rappard et al. (1988) testing implants of the same make, noted a decrease in bursting strength with implant age. Marrota et al. (1998) compared explants with unused implants made by the same manufacturer; unfortunately, implant types were not specified in this short report, but explants in general had 25% less strength.

Addressing these problems, Wolf et al. (1996, 1997) and Brandon et al. (1997a,d, 1998a–f, 1999) described measurements of a large series of explanted and unused (some same lot) control gel implants of ages up to 28 years, manufactured primarily by Dow Corning, both as is and after gel fluid extraction. They also reported that gel fluid permeation in vivo decreases various parameters of shell strength. In the aggregate, physical properties of shells weaken but are not dramatically changed by length of implantation when measured after extraction of gel fluid, nor does scanning electron microscopy detect significant, visible surface deterioration in regions of nonwear even after 28 years in vivo. Different types and manufacture of implants have quite different physical parameters. Shell thickness varied twofold when measurements were made in a number of different places. Most striking was the lot-to-lot variation in implants of the same type from the same manufacturer. For example, tensile strengths of Silastic I and Silastic II models from different lots varied 3.5-fold and from minimum to maximum between the two types by fivefold. Strength parameters of two 28-year-implanted Silastic0 implants' were decreased 20–40% by gel fluid permeation, but both extracted and nonextracted values fell within the range of control Silastic I (same elastomer) shells and were higher than ASTM standards (Brandon et al., 1997a–f, 1999; Wolf et al., 1996 and 1997; and see also Frisch and Langley, 1985; Swanson, 1973; Swanson and Lebeau, 1974).

Chawla and Hinberg (1996) also found that shells implanted for up to seven years maintained surface integrity, and neither they nor Ratner et al. (1994) were able to demonstrate free silica at the shell surface by any of a number of techniques. Peters (1981) tested a small number of gel and inflatable prostheses, some explanted, some unused, with a compression (burst) test and found no pattern, extreme variability among implant types, and lot-to-lot variability. Rupture occurred at pressures ranging from 0.62–10.8 pounds per square inch (psi) considerably lower than the pressures measured in various kinds of closed capsulotomy, 10–15 psi, (Gruber and Friedman, 1978) which was the objective. Different makes and models of implants clearly will have different tolerances for closed capsulotomy (Lemperle and Exner, 1993). Curtis and Hoshaw (1998) plotted Dow Corning mechanical test data against duration of implantation from approximately 5–20 years and observed no degradation with increasing in vivo duration, although there was considerable scatter of results.

These results reflect the nature of silicone chemistry and manufacture. They indicate that rupture will depend on the manufacturer, type and model and even the lot of saline and gel implants, as well as on underlying physical parameters such as designed thickness and chemical formulation. Any analyses of rupture resistance and shell strength or of rupture prevalence in cohorts of women should try to control for these confounding variables. As indicated earlier, rupture also will depend on distortion, wear, and stress in the body, untoward events, and perhaps other unknown factors.

Biomedical polymers, including silicone, may absorb or adsorb certain lipids and lipoproteins (Carmen and Mutha, 1972; Chin et al., 1971; Dong et al., 1987). One investigator has proposed that the absorption of lipids by an elastomer may weaken it over time (Caffee, 1993b). Although lipids were reported in Silastic sheet implants and in explant silicone elastomer shells at low levels, <0.2% (Pfleiderer et al., 1995; Picard et al., 1997), and at less than 1% by weight in slabs of silicone elastomer implanted in dogs for two years (Swanson and Lebeau, 1974), others have not found them (Chawla and Hinberg, 1996). In discussing this issue, Frisch claimed that lipid adsorption accounted for at best an early but stable weight increase of about 1.5–2% and very little, if any, loss of elastomer strength. The effect of lipids, if present, on shell rupture remains hypothetical; only small decreases in physical strength of the elastomer were found in the dogs of Swanson and Lebeau (1974), and Swanson (1973) observed lipids generally below 1% with no relationship to duration of implantation or fracture of the elastomer in the elastomer of finger joints that had been implanted for up to five years.

The Frequency of Rupture and Deflation

Rupture reports have been based on findings at explantation, detection by various mammographic technologies (often confirmed, at least in part, by explantation) and descriptions or surveys of results in cohorts of patients. None of these is absolutely reliable. Explant series are the standard for diagnosing rupture and for confirming rupture suspected by other means, but they undoubtedly include some ruptures that occur during implantation and explantation procedures. Further, women undergoing explantation are a special subset of the population of women with implants, and even of the population of women with ruptured implants. Mammography series may be drawn from explant series, may involve groups of women with suspected problems, or may depend on a less-than-certain diagnosis, although MRI has an excellent record. Case series reported from practitioners or facilities have the advantage that they can be (unless selected in some way) more representative of the population of women with implants, but the detection of rupture depends on patient complaint, routine screening film mammography, or physical examination, all of which are subject to considerable error and lack of sensitivity (see, for example, data on mammography sensitivity and Malata et al., 1994a, who suspected clinically only 6 of 19 ruptures seen on explantation, including 10 intracapsular ruptures with complete shell disintegrations). The accuracy of very low rupture rates reported by manufacturers based on returns, complaints, legal proceedings and other sources probably suffers from these same problems of ruptures' going undetected and unreported.

The medical literature on rupture of gel implants includes reports of prevalence ranging from 0.3 to 77% (Beekman et al., 1997b; Berg et al., 1993, 1995; Chung et al., 1996; Cohen et al., 1997; Davis et al., 1995; De Camara et al., 1993; Destouet et al., 1992; Dowden, 1993; Duffy and Woods, 1994; Gabriel et al., 1997; Gorczyca et al., 1992; Harris et al., 1993; Ko et al., 1996; Malata et al., 1994a; Middleton, 1998b; Nelson, 1981; Netscher et al., 1995a; Park et al., 1996b; Peters et al., 1996; Phillips et al., 1996; Robinson et al., 1995; Rohrich et al., 1998a; Rolland et al., 1989a; Slavin and Goldwyn, 1995; Weizer et al., 1995; Yeoh et al., 1996; Young et al., 1996a, 1998). These are reports of either the percentage of women who have one or both implants ruptured or the percentage of all the implants placed that have ruptured. Since patients may have two implants, only one of which is ruptured, rupture frequency by number of implants is usually lower. The list of references here omits some mammography series that could have been cited because they report low numbers, patients are often referred for problems and ruptures are not always confirmed by explantation (see Chapter 12). The very low value, 0.3%, was from a review of 307 women examined by ultrasound and thus subject to the level of sensitivity of this technology. Three confirmatory explantations and six confirmatory MRIs were performed in the 307 women. One explant was clearly ruptured. The other, which was discounted, was covered with sticky silicone and was probably a small leak. This implant probably should not be counted as intact. This would raise the prevalence to at least 0.6%, with another upward correction of unknown magnitude for the ruptures missed due to the lack of sensitivity of ultrasound.

Deflation does not pose the same problems in definition, or generate the same research interest or attention in the literature because its detection is not prone to the uncertainties associated with gel rupture, and release of implant contents is of little consequence beyond the loss of aesthetic effect. Because of the reliability of detection, saline deflation estimates are much firmer than those for gel-filled implants. Women do not always seek medical attention from their operating surgeon for deflation, however, so it should not be assumed that these complications are always discovered and reported. Gutowski et al. (1997) noted that women had not notified the responsible plastic surgeon of 10 of 55 deflations, and no intervention was taken for some of these; in this large survey, deflations occurred in 10.1% of women and 5.5% of implants. Lantieri et al. (1997) reported their experience with 709 implants in 407 women who responded to a questionnaire mailed to 454 women who had received saline inflatable implants in their two facilities in France and the United States between 1981 and 1995 (489 smooth Mentor and 220 textured Mentor Siltex breast implants). The indication for implantation was reconstruction, usually delayed, in 40% of breasts; augmentation in 41%; and replacement in 19%. There was no significant difference in deflation between smooth or textured implants, between submammary or submuscular placement, or by indication for implantation. The overall deflation prevalence was 6.6%, with an average follow-up of 7.1 years, and underfilling was highly significantly associated with deflation; fold flaws were observed in 81% of deflations. In this report of implants filled on average to 103.1% of design capacity, the Kaplan–Meier survival curve showed a deflation rate of less than 1% at 12 months (Lantieri et al., 1997).

Presence of deflation at the end of one year in the McGhan LST was 3.9% of patients receiving implants for augmentation and reconstruction combined (McGhan Medical Corporation). Deflations varied between 1.33 and 37.7% of implants, depending on type, in the experience of Mladick (Mladick, 1993) and similarly between 0.56 and 20% of implants in Lavine's (1993) series comparing the 1600 with the 1800 (defective valve) Heyer-Schulte–Mentor model. In the patient cohorts cited earlier in the discussion of aggregate complications, deflation usually was not the focus of the report and varied between 2.6 and 16% over different periods of follow-up for a number of different inflatable saline implants and expanders. In a discussion of explantation of gel-filled implants, Robinson (1992) noted 0.6% deflations of 1,600 mostly recently placed saline implants of unknown model and manufacture. Rheingold et al. (1994) reported a survival analysis of 67.34% at slightly less than ten years. They commented that their "study confirms the obvious: Inflatable breast implants deflate with time."

Rubin (1983) reported his own experience with saline inflatable implants. He found 29 deflations in 478 implants from three different manufacturers, or 6% over five years (not counting those [*N* = 14] noted to be defective at the time of implant surgery) and commented that he expected to see more deflations with time. In a survey of plastic surgeons with 528 responses, he found 1,181 leaking implants of 13,200 reported, or 8.95% over an unknown period of time (Rubin, 1983). Gutowski et al. (1997) reported an actuarial survival estimate at ten years of 90.2–95.2%. Some underreporting is probable since, as noted earlier, not all women seek attention from their surgeons for deflation (Rheingold et al., 1994; Gutowski et al., 1997). Other reports on saline implant and expander deflation are very variable. Some frequencies are quite high (e.g., 76%), but since they include early implants that are known to have had problems, they have little to teach about what can be expected in terms of deflation of modern saline implants and expanders (Bell, 1983; Williams, 1972; Worseg et al., 1995; Worton et al., 1980). Taking implant type and model into account and reviewing relatively recent representative case series, the committee concludes that modern first-year deflations might be of the order of 1–3% of implants and that this percentage would rise slowly with time (see Capozzi, 1986; Francel et al., 1993; Gutowski et al., 1997; Lantieri et al., 1997; McGhan (undated); Mladick, 1993; O'Brien et al., 1993; Schuster and Lavine, 1998; Vinton et al., 1990).

Estimates of gel implant rupture can start with measures from cohorts of women examined in inclusive follow-up reviews or from routine screening of populations. Gabriel et al. (1997) reported 5.7% ruptures in a 7.8-year mean follow-up of 749 women, 3.9% of 1,454 implants, based on chart review. An unknown number of ruptures undoubtedly went undetected (Gabriel et al., 1997). At 10.7 years, Harris et al. (1993) detected 22 ruptures (6.5%) in 336 gel-implanted women routinely screened by film mammography, with 42% followed up with ultrasound. In view of the low sensitivity of film particularly, but also of ultrasound mammography (Ahn et al., 1994a; see also Chapter 12), a significant number of ruptures must have escaped detection (Harris et al., 1993). In the McGhan (1998) AR90 clinical study, the five-year cumulative risk of rupture suspected by symptoms or physical examination was 4% of augmented patients (2.6% of implants in augmented women) and 9.8% of reconstruction patients (6.3% of implants in women with implants for reconstruction). Similarly, at two years, a 1990 Dow Corning observational study reported no ruptures in 69% of an original cohort of 360 augmented women returning for evaluation (Bowlin et al., 1988). The prevalence of rupture detected on physical examination in the Mentor adjunct study (1992) was 1.3% at the three-year follow-up of about 8,000 women. The low sensitivity of these detection methods (and, especially for Dow Corning, the short follow-up) inevitably means an underestimate of implant rupture (Bowlin et al., 1998; McGhan Medical Corporation, 1998; Purkait, Mentor Corp, IOM Scientific Workshop, 1998). Destouet et al. (1992), Dowden (1993), and Peters and Pugash (1993) screened consecutive routine patients by film mammography, physical examination confirmed later for a subset by explantation, and ultrasound. Ruptures were detected, respectively, in 4.6% of women at 10 years, 4.5% at an unknown interval, and in 8% at 8.5 years.

Clearly in all of these instances, detection was attempted with low-sensitivity technology and significant numbers of ruptures were missed (Destouet et al., 1992; Dowden, 1993; Peters and Pugash, 1993). The explant or selected series, on the other hand, presumably overestimates prevalence (Young et al., 1998). The survey of Nelson (1981) represents an interesting hybrid between these two study types, explant and routine follow-up or screening series. He reported rupture in 15.9% of 5,579 breasts undergoing open capsulotomy. The selection bias of this series is unknown. Of these, 57% had previously been subjected to closed capsulotomy. The duration of implantation was not reported (although it may have been a relatively few years given the usual time of onset of contracture), and the implants in question were most likely of the thin-shelled, second generation variety. Nevertheless, this represents a considerable number of ruptures identified by direct observation in a large group of women with presumably a cross section of implant models who were gathered because of only one problem and thus not subject to the more obvious bias of explant cohorts (Nelson, 1981).

Unless the increasing prevalence of implant rupture with age can be shown to correlate with specific kinds of implants having specific fragility (Peters et al., 1996), it seems reasonable that the relationship between implant age and rupture, noted earlier, reflects a real trend (Goldberg et al., 1997). Capsular contracture and implant distortion tend to continue over time, although no studies were found that provided conclusive evidence of an association between contracture and rupture or deflation (Lantieri et al., 1997). Stress and incidental trauma also accumulate over time. Shells are nonuniform in thickness and strength even within the same lot, and they can be expected to weaken after implantation due to permeation by gel fluid. They may then gradually lose strength over more prolonged times. Thus, deflation and rupture can be expected, as the data show, to continue over time.

Authors cited above reported that 96% of gel implants ruptured at or beyond 10 years (De Camara et al., 1993); up to 63% ruptured at 12 years or more (Cohen et al., 1997); 62.5% of those in situ for 10 years ruptured (Malata et al., 1994a); 71.2% ruptured at 14 years, and 95.4% ruptured at 20 years according to a survival analysis (Robinson et al., 1995); increasing failure was reported between 10 and 15 years, and 50% ruptured at about 15 years (Beekman et al., 1997b), 69–70% ruptured at 6 years or more (Peters, 1994a), 49% ruptured (includes leaking) at 10 years (Rohrich et al., 1998); and frequency of pinholes and frank ruptures increased from 8% at 0–5 years to 61% at 10 years to 73% at 20 or more years (Young et al., 1996a, 1998). Different rupture percentages have been found according to implant vintage. First-generation implants (1963–1972) had no ruptures, second-generation implants (1972 to mid-1980s) were 95% ruptured at 12 years, and third-generation implants (late 1980s to date) had only 3.5% ruptures by 1992 (Peters et al., 1996). Other investigators have reported similar findings. In fact, they found no ruptures in third-generation implants (Francel et al., 1998). On the other hand, the large series ($N = 161$) described by Yeoh et al. (1996) of 4- to 27-year-old, primarily Dow Corning gel-filled prostheses, which had 25% ruptures, did not show a correlation of implant age with rupture. The analysis by Gutowski et al. (1997) indicated 5–10% deflation at ten years for saline implants of recent vintage. A very high, in fact unacceptable, frequency of deflation is reported for older models, as noted earlier.

It is not possible to predict current rupture frequencies or rates. Rupture depends on implant type, model (and lot), and manufacturer; implant physical characteristics; silicone gel fluid permeation, which weakens implants; and the many other factors that stress, compress, and abrade implants. The reported high rupture prevalences cited above reflect experience with a great many thin-shell, compliant gel models according to the dates of explantation from these reports. Clearly it is possible to build an implant of sufficient strength to endure a long time, as the experience with first-generation 1960s thick-shell, thick-gel implants shows (Brandon et al., 1999; Peters et al., 1996). It is unknown where the balance of sturdiness, durability, and cosmetic softness versus wear and stress in the body lies, and whether implants in current use with short histories will also reach the end of their lives at 10 to 15 years as data seem to imply for older models. Silicone gel fluid permeation of the shell seems to have a deleterious effect on durability, more so at high percentages of extractable fluid. Contracture, which is more common in gel implants, may be a risk factor for rupture (Feng, IOM Scientific Workshop, 1998), although there is insufficient evidence for this (Lantieri et al., 1997). Gel-filled implants have a softer HTV shell than saline implants. These factors, and indeed some of the studies summarized in this section, suggest that rupture may be more common in current gel-filled implants than current saline-filled implants and expanders, other things being equal, although properly conducted new studies will be needed to resolve this point as suggested below. Neither the submuscular or submammary site of implantation nor the augmentation or reconstruction indications appear to be important variables for rupture.

Estimates of rupture frequency of gel-filled implants must consider the bias problems of explant series, which are likely to seriously inflate rupture rates while providing an accurate diagnosis through direct examination, against the advantages of studying a more random group of women with the associated problems of underreporting of rupture that are inherent in insensitive diagnostic tools. Experience relying more heavily on random case series or explant series that identified recent implants (see Bowlin et al., 1998; Destouet et al., 1992; Dowden, 1993; Francel et al., 1993; Gabriel et al., 1997; Harris et al., 1993; McGhan, 1998; Peters and Pugash, 1993) suggests a relatively modest number of ruptures. The size, sensitivity of detection, duration of implantation, and other problems of these studies also suggest the need for an upward adjustment or considerable caution in relying on them to predict current rupture experience.

On the other hand, the variation, selection bias, and inclusion of implants no longer in use in most explant series do not provide a good basis for an estimate of modern or future rupture frequencies. The ruptures of gel-filled implants with certain characteristics such as soft, thin shells and compliant gels with high levels of extractable gel fluid, referred to as second generation, are substantial but are not really at issue. Experience with these implants clearly implies that women who still have them will need them removed or replaced, but it cannot be used to predict modern implant rupture frequency. (The very high deflation rates of early HTV saline implants are also generally accepted.) Rupture rates or frequencies of modern implants will not be known until long-term, prospective observational studies of sufficiently large and random cohorts of women are completed, using sophisticated and reliable detection methods such as MRI by skilled and experienced investigators. The recent experience of

Brown et al. demonstrates that good agreement on ruptures defined by MRI can be achieved among experienced experts (Brown et al., 1999).

Preliminary and admittedly anecdotal reports from such experts suggest that the frequency of rupture in third-generation implants is much lower than the prevalence reported for second-generation implants (Middleton, IOM Scientific Workshop, 1998). The committee stresses that a determination of rupture (and deflation) prevalence or rate in such a way is of value, should include a determination of other complications and characteristics of implantation in a disciplined way, and should be carried out because of its implications for the safety of silicone breast implants. Such a study or studies will be valuable only for implants of the same types and with the same physical–chemical characteristics. If manufacturers change silicone implant formulations or shell thicknesses or modify gel-filled implants in other ways such as by changing gels, studies of these defined formulations would have to be carried out. Until such time, only a guess at the order of magnitude of gel-filled implant rupture can be hazarded.

Keeping in mind the results of explant series of modern implants and other recent observations as noted above, the committee is of the opinion that, with a conservative guess at upward adjustment to account for underdiagnosis, a modest number (perhaps less than 10%) of modern gel implants will have ruptured by five years and that ruptures will continue to accumulate and prevalence will increase in ensuing years. Whatever the actual rupture prevalence or incidence, the safety implications of rupture and deflation noted here include the risks of additional surgery and anesthesia when explantation or replacement of an implant (and capsulectomy) is required to remove silicone or to address the loss of aesthetics in saline- and gel-filled implants. Operative interventions to treat granulomas and significant axillary adenopathy may also be required, though infrequently. There will also be the rare complications of gel migration and tissue damage at more distant sites and whatever health conditions may follow tissue exposure to silicone gel.

Implant Capsules and Contracture

Placement of an implant in the body causes a reaction in the tissues that varies depending on size, shape (Matlaga et al., 1976), and surface texture and porosity (James et al., 1997; Salthouse, 1984; Taylor and Gibbons, 1983). Other surface physical characteristics, such as charge and energy, chemical characteristics of the implant, location of the implantation site, and animal species studied also make a difference (Bakker et al., 1988; Ksander et al., 1981). These differences affect the ability of some materials to adsorb body proteins of various kinds, to activate certain cells, to cause the production of cellular factors and cytokines that may influence cellular proliferation and other activities both locally and perhaps systemically, and to excite inflammatory reactions of varying extent, intensity, and type of cell participation. All implants, including all breast implants, provoke some form of this general foreign body tissue reaction.

The production of an enclosing capsule of fibrous scar tissue around the implant is an important component of the foreign body reaction and significantly affects the effectiveness of breast augmentation or reconstruction with implants. Contracture of this capsule, if severe, causes often painful and disfiguring squeezing and distortion of the implant (and overlying tissue). At the extreme, it is compressed into its smallest volume, a sphere, rather than the shape designed to achieve normal breast contour. The contributing causes and management of this variably occurring complication are important and incompletely resolved issues in breast surgery. It is the adverse event most frequently reported to the FDA (Brown et al., 1998).

The reaction to a foreign body is a normal part of the body's intrinsic defense mechanisms. Silicone elastomer, gel, fluid, or some other component of a breast implant might also provoke an immune response as part of the body's reaction to implantation. In this case, certain cells would recognize specific foreign molecules associated with the implant and would initiate immune cellular proliferation and the production of specific protein antibodies to these molecules, and/or proliferation of, and the specific targeting by immune cells to attack these molecules. Changes in the local tissue reaction and possible systemic effects would likely follow an adaptive immunological response in addition to a foreign body or innate response. The committee did not find scientific evidence for this, but such questions are discussed further in the following chapter.

Whatever the contributing causes, the breast implant capsule can be described by its numbers, orientation, and types of cells and cell products. Different types of breast implants will produce differing capsules. Some have speculated that damage to the breast during implant placement, which could lead to fat necrosis, mammary gland degeneration, and muscle atrophy, may also contribute to capsule thickness and contracture (Smahel, 1978b), although there is insufficient evidence to support or refute this. Of course, the healing of an operative wound is a part of the response to implantation. In elementary terms, the early response to tissue injury and to the presence of an implant consists of the migration and activation of many different cells including polymorphonuclear leukocytes (PMNs) and mononuclear cells. PMNs disappear within a few days, but monocytes, lymphocytes, and fibroblasts remain around the implant. Monocytes differentiate into macrophages, and some of these cells coalesce to become foreign body giant cells. Fibroblasts are stimulated to proliferate and produce collagen, and new capillaries develop. An array of different kinds of lymphocytes may be present (Katzin et al., 1996; Miller, IOM Scientific Workshop, 1998).

Contracted capsules, like hypertrophic burn scar, contain greater amounts of glycosaminoglycans and proportionately more chondroitin 4-sulfate, characteristics of immature scar (Vistnes et al., 1981). The types of collagen (I, III, and V) in capsules surrounding different types of implants and expanders and of different degrees of severity and age are similar to the types in breast dermis and commonly observed cutaneous scar. Contracted capsules have more collagen than soft capsules and normal dermis (Marshall et al., 1989; McCoy et al., 1984). Gradually the process and capsule become mature and take on more of the appearance of normal scar tissue with few cells around smooth implants and a thicker, more cellular, chronic inflammatory appearance with less regularly organized fibrous tissue around textured or polyurethane foam-coated implants. The fibrous tissue capsule surrounding breast implants is described in a number of reports (e.g., Copeland et al., 1994; Emery et al., 1994; Hameed et al., 1995; Kasper, 1994; Lesesne, 1997; Luke et al., 1997; Raso and Greene, 1997; Smahel, 1977; Wickman et al., 1993; Wyatt et al., 1998; Yeoh et al., 1996).

On direct visual observation, the usual implant capsule is a variably thin, grayish, glistening membrane. Microscopically, smooth-surfaced gel or saline implant capsules may have a flattened unicellular lining or a layer of pseudoepithelial cells next to the implant, overlaid with a regularly and linearly oriented dense collagen network that progresses to looser, better-vascularized connective tissue merging with the surrounding breast tissue. Synovial linings are also seen around smooth implants. Macrophages, multinucleated giant cells, T lymphocytes, fibroblasts, and occasionally other cells such as eosinophiles and plasma cells, are seen in varying numbers, although the older capsules generally have fewer cells set amid regularly oriented fibrous connective tissue.

Capsules of textured implants are likely to have a palisaded secretory and phagocytic synovial multicellular layer without a basement membrane next to the implant, overlaid by a thicker, more disoriented, cellular and vascular connective tissue layer progressing to loose connective and adipose tissue in the surrounding breast tissue. Occasionally the synovial layer, especially in capsular infolds, assumes a papillary hyperplastic appearance (Hameed et al., 1995). This villous hyperplasia has been reported around 63% of textured implants at less than five years, decreasing significantly to 7% after five years (Wyatt et al., 1998). Capsular synovium is apparently of mesenchymal origin and is believed to be a reaction to the shearing movement of the implant. The synovium secretes proteoglycans, chondroitin 4-sulfate and keratan sulfate, which may lubricate the prosthesis–capsule interface, and there has been speculation that these substances may help to diminish contracture (Lin et al., 1994; Raso and Schulte, 1996). The synovial layer may diminish over time, as noted in Chapter 3, and as reported in a long-term study with findings of statistically significant decrease in synovial lining around textured and smooth implants over time (Wyatt et al., 1998). Synovium has been described around all kinds of breast implants including smooth saline implants (McConnell et al., 1997).

Fragments of the elastomer shell are seen in capsules around saline implants (Jenny and Smahel, 1981; Vargas, 1979), particularly from textured shells, but no droplets of silicone fluid. Silicone fragments, up to 1 mm in size, are found inside giant cells and in aggregates of giant cells called granulomas mostly in textured saline implant capsules. If these are permanent implants, not expanders, synovium may be less frequent with increased cellularity (Lesesne, 1997). Silicone shards and microfragments from other kinds of (nonbreast) implants provoke similar inflammatory reactions and granulomas, as do other kinds of polymers under similar circumstances (Needelman, 1995; Peimer et al., 1986; see Chapter 4). This cellular reactivity to elastomer may be due to the microfragment form, since bulk elastomer does not seem to provoke cytotoxic responses in cell culture (Lockhorn et al., 1996). With gel-filled implants, silicone fluid is seen at various depths of the capsule or outside it as small droplets ingested by macrophages or histiocytes or in extracellular spaces (Beekman et al., 1997a; Wickham et al., 1978). Silicone gel is present in the capsules around ruptured implants. Granulomas containing silicone gel or fluid may also be present. There are no obvious differences between a capsule exposed to fluid diffusion or to gel from an implant rupture (Luke et al., 1997), but vacuolated cells (macrophages) and silicone droplets differentiate capsules around gel from those around saline-filled implants. The effects of phagocytosed silicone gel microdroplets on individual macrophages are incompletely known, but appear relatively benign in some investigations of short term reactions (Azizsoltani et al., 1995). In polyurethane capsules, vacuolated cells, more giant cells, hemorrhage and hemosiderin pigment and fragmented polyurethane are seen (Smahel, 1978a).

Myofibroblasts, which are smooth muscle-like cells derived from fibroblasts, are characterized by 6 to 8 nanometer microfilaments, indented nuclei, desmosomes, and basal lamina and are implicated in capsule contracture and generally detectable in capsules in varying numbers (Rudolph, 1983). These cells contract and relax in response to smooth-muscle stimulants and relaxants, but their role in capsular contracture is still theoretical. They may cause contraction of the capsule, which then becomes fixed as fibrous tissue is laid down (Baker et al., 1981; Ryan et al., 1974), and they disappear after the contracture is mature and fibrotic

(Lossing and Hansson, 1993; Rudolph et al., 1977, 1978). Myofibroblast quantification was attempted in experimental animal wounds. Peak levels of these cells, about 75% of fibroblasts, were reached at 2 weeks after wounding, and myofibroblasts disappeared at 12 weeks. The frequency of these cells was apparently the same in all of the experimental wounds and independent of the degree of contracture (McGrath and Hundahl, 1982; Rudolph et al., 1977). In implanted women, however, myofibroblasts are seen over much longer periods of time, are present particularly in contracting capsules (where they are said to contain greater amounts of contractile [actin] protein) and to a much lesser extent in soft capsules, and are also seen in reoperated breasts and breasts with both saline and, more frequently, gel implants. Removal of the implant (foreign body) results in disappearance of the myofibroblasts and their associated peptide growth factors (Lossing and Hansson, 1993; Rudolph et al., 1978).

Macroscopic calcification (or mineralization) has been reported in 10–33% of capsules although these reports generally describe implant series that were problematic, symptomatic, or explants (Destouet et al., 1992; Peters and Smith, 1995; Peters et al., 1998; Rolland et al., 1989a,b). Capsular calcifications involve calcium phosphates and were not associated with silicone (or talc) deposits by electron probe microanalysis in one study (Raso et al., 1999). Calcification is particularly associated with implant shells with patches and more fibrous, long-duration capsules. It can occasionally be severe, causing pressure atrophy of breast and underlying muscle tissue, and it can be seen on mammography (Benjamin and Guy, 1977; Cocke et al., 1985; Fajardo et al., 1995; Frazer and Wylie, 1995; Gumucio et al, 1989; Hayes et al., 1993; Leibman, 1994; Luke et al., 1997; Redfern et al., 1977; Reynolds et al., 1994; Rolland et al., 1989b; Schmidt, 1993; Vuursteen, 1992; Yeoh et al., 1996; Young et al., 1989). Peters et al. (1998) have emphasized that calcification is associated with all first generation implants. Calcification surrounds most of the implant but does not always affect Dacron patches. In this large study of 404 silicone gel-filled breast implants of all three generations, calcification was related to first generation implants (100%), implant duration, and implant rupture. About 50% of second generation implants in place over 16 years, or ruptured and in place over 11 years, had associated calcification. Calcium phosphate was reported as hydroxyapatite in both heterotopic bone and spherulitic aggregates of crystal in the capsule near the implant surface. Although most reports of calcification, and the data in this IOM report refer to silicone gel implants, calcification in the form of hydroxyapatite crystals is occasionally described stuck to the surface of saline implants (Peters et al., 1998; Schmidt, 1993). Talc is also present in 49–71% of capsules (Kasper and Chandler, 1994; but any role for talc is purely speculative and unlikely, as noted by Peters, 1998). Calcification of deposits of silicone injected into the breast has been reported as quite common (Inoue et al., 1983; Koide and Katayama, 1979), but in these mammography case series the silicone was very likely adulterated and calcification was more prevalent in association with paraffin injection.

During the process of formation and maturation of the capsule an array of chemical mediators, growth factors, enzymes, and various cellular factors are activated and inactivated at various times to effect the various stages and processes of the foreign body and inflammatory reactions (Anderson, 1988, 1993; Lossing and Hansson, 1993; Tang and Eaton, 1995; Ziats et al., 1988). Cellular behavior and appearance change on exposure to silicone (McCauley et al., 1990). In comparative studies, however, different polymers including silicone may have greater or lesser, but not categorically different effects on the release of these factors and on cell behavior (Anderson et al., 1995; Bonfield et al., 1989a, 1991; Cardona et al., 1992; James et al., 1997; Kao et al., 1994; Kossovsky et al., 1993; MacDonald et al., 1996; Miller et al., 1989; Miller and Anderson, 1989; Naidu et al., 1996; Petillo et al., 1994; Sevastianov and Tseytlina, 1984; Taylor and Gibbons, 1983; Wilsnack and Bernadyn, 1979). Also, when the silicone shell of a breast implant (expander) was coated with a 0.3–0.5 mm layer of pyrolytic carbon, the cellular types and proliferative activity of capsules underwent modest quantitative but not qualitative change (Bosetti et al., 1998).

An understanding of the host response to implants is important to experimental and clinical attempts to manage their undesirable and desirable aspects and to the overall safety of the implantation process. Some have argued for an adaptive immune component in silicone breast implant tissue reactions (Kossovsky, 1993). Others have tried to immunize animals to silicone gel, elastomer, or fluid using powerful adjuvants and have failed to observe a difference in the tissue reaction to subsequent silicone implants in either normal or immune deficient (nu/nu) animals (Brantley et al., 1990a,b; Klykken et al., 1991a,b,c). A study of expression of helper (CD4) T cells, suppressor (CD8) T cells, (CD11 b/c) macrophages, and indicators of proliferation, DNA damage and apoptosis revealed no difference in acute and chronic capsules around Silastic or cellulose acetate (James et al., 1997). Other, investigators however, found restriction of receptors and cell types, suggestive of an immune response in capsules compared to control breast tissue (Ladin et al., 1994). The general tissue–polymer response was recently reviewed without supporting an adaptive immune response (Laurencin and Elgendy, 1994).

Capsules vary from 0.25 to 4 mm in thickness, with an average of 1.3–1.4 mm. (Emery et al., 1994; Ersek et al., 1991; Hardt et al., 1994; Raso and Greene, 1997; Rolland et al., 1989a; Williams, 1972). They are occasionally much thicker (13 mm, Baldt et al., 1994). If grossly abnormal with heavy calcification or ossification, capsules may measure up to 2.2 cm (Peters and Pritzker, 1985; Peters et al., 1998). Contracted capsules vary in thickness. Some say they are thicker (Caffee, 1992c; Ersek et al., 1991—five to tenfold difference, Class I versus Class III–IV; Lossing and Hansson, 1993; Rudolph et al., 1978), whereas others say they are not necessarily thicker but may in fact be thinner than uncontracted capsules (Gayou, 1979; Smahel, 1977; Vistnes and Ksander, 1983; e.g., mean thickness of 17 contracted capsules 0.47 mm, of 6 normal capsules 0.52 mm (Vistnes et al., 1981). The committee found no study in which manufacturer, type, and model were held constant and the only variables were contracture severity and capsule thickness. Grossly ruptured gel implants provoked significantly thicker capsules than intact capsules in experimental animals, however (Vistnes et al., 1977), and consistent with this presumed reaction to exposure to silicone gel and gel fluid, capsules around saline implants are thinner than those around gel and textured implants. Capsules around textured implants tend to take on the imprint of the pillared surface of these shells of those implants, with a greater likelihood of fluid accumulation in cysts within the capsule or in the space around the implant (Jenny and Smahel, 1981; Malata et al., 1997; Rothfuss et al., 1992); probably due to the presence of synovial linings with secretory function. Ahn et al. (1995a) found 0.2–20 ml of fluid within capsules around 15% of breast implants of all kinds in a small group of symptomatic women.

Some investigators have reported that smooth gel-filled implant capsules tend to thicken over time (Ersek et al., 1991; Wickman et al., 1993). Capsules around nontextured implants tend to become mature and stable after 9 to 12 months, and some have emphasized that most (89–93%) contractures are observable within the first postoperative year (Little and Baker, 1980; Malata et al., 1997; Moufarrege et al., 1987; Vogt et al., 1990). However, others have reported that, clinically, contractures continue to accumulate, although at lower frequencies, through the first 24 to 36 months after implantation and taper off thereafter (Brandt et al., 1984; Ersek, 1991a; Gayou and Rudolph, 1979; Rheingold et al., 1994).

By use of presumably more sensitive and quantitative techniques (applanation tonometry; see below), slow continued subclinical contraction has been measured in the one- to five-year interval after implantation. The risk of contracture continued to increase each year for five years in the McGhan (1998) AR90 five-year observational study of gel implants following augmentation and for three years after reconstruction. Reporting on a series of 186 implants, Peters et al. (1997) observed that Class III–IV contractures continued to accumulate over time, reaching 100% around silicone gel-filled implants at 25 years. In a large, long-term study primarily of contracted capsules, Wyatt et al. (1998) noted that the presence of a dense collagenous capsular architecture increased over time around smooth implants. After five years, the parallel collagen fibers tended to become disoriented, significantly so around textured implants. Also, peptide growth factors are reported to be continuously present in capsules around breast implants and to subside only on removal of the foreign body (Lossing and Hansson, 1993). It is likely, therefore, that contracture is a progressive phenomenon that increases slowly with time (Hakelius and Ohlsen, 1997; Handel et al., 1995; Lossing and Hansson, 1993; McCraw and Maxwell, 1988; Peters et al., 1997). Also, as noted elsewhere in this report, some technologies to reduce contracture may become less effective over time (barrier layers, polyurethane), and in such cases, contractures could accumulate over longer periods (Cohney et al., 1991, 1992; Handel et al., 1995).

A foreign body reaction and the formation of a capsule are expected consequences of breast implantation. The contraction of the fibrous connective tissue of this capsule to the point of discomfort and loss of cosmetic effect is an undesirable but common complication. This complication is essentially a cosmetic problem, but it is associated with health and safety to the extent that it leads to frequent operative interventions such as open capsulotomy, explantation or replacement with both operative and anesthesia risk, as well as the risk of infection or other complications that accompany surgery. In a recent explant series, 72.5% of implant removals were performed for the indication of contracture (Beekman et al., 1997b). Certain characteristics of capsules—such as thickness, Class III or IV contracture, associated granulomas, calcifications, and infection among others also may obligate capsulectomy, which can be a significant procedure accompanying explantation or replacement, may require an hour of additional operative time, and may force difficult decisions about further plastic interventions if tissue cover is inadequate (Young, 1998). Contracture may also lead to other interventions that carry risk, such as closed capsulotomies with possible hematoma or rupture, migration of silicone gel and a need for further surgery, or it may impair the use of diagnostic technologies such as screening or diagnostic mammography for the detection of cancer and other conditions, by making it much more difficult or impossible to achieve adequate breast compression and visualization of much of the breast tissue. The foreign body reaction, formation of a fibrous capsule, and its contracture are likely no more common in breast than in other implants, but the soft tissue, cosmetic role of the breast implant means that these reactions or complications have a substantially greater effect on the safety and performance of this implant, as just discussed.

Assessment of Capsular Contracture

The foreign body reaction is intrinsic to human physiology. Contracture, however, is an excess of fibrosis that may go beyond the patient's usual biological response and occurs, at least in part, individually by breast, presumably influenced by local, poorly understood factors—one of which may be the presence of bacteria, which would be random (Burkhardt, 1988). It could also be argued that the loss of aesthetics with one hard, distorted breast is more disturbing than with two symmetrically affected breasts. Burkhardt has pointed out that contracture should be reported as the percentage of breasts, not of patients. Burkhardt's calculations show how lower contracture percentages, if due to random local factors, can give progressively more misleading impressions if reported as patient percentages. For example, 80% of breasts contracted would yield 90% of patients with contractures statistically, and percentages close to this have been observed in actual clinical practice; 30% of breasts would yield 51% of patients, and 16% of breasts would yield 30% of patients (Burkhardt, 1984). Not everyone agrees that contracture is random, however, even though contractures observed in patients in clinical practice seem to be a mixture of unilateral and bilateral, and in some reports all contractures are unilateral (Milojevic, 1983). The finding of Class III contractures on one side and Class I on the other in monozygotic twins with identical implants three years postoperatively is also interesting, although anecdotal, evidence (Poppi, 1985). Malata et al. (1997) have commented that in some instances, different implants may have been inserted and caused this variation and that, in any case, it does not seem logical that even if local factors were controlling they would not be somewhat similar in the same woman.

Repeated efforts have been made to devise scientifically rigorous clinical assessments of contractures. These include applanation tonometry to compare, over time or between breasts, the relative imprint area on a disk placed on top of the breast in the supine position (Asplund et al., 1996; Gylbert, 1989; Hakelius and Ohlsen, 1992) or, using a standard weight disc, to calculate intramammary pressure (Moore, 1979); mammometry to measure comparative softness after manual compression (Barker, 1978); calipers to measure the compressibility of the breast over time (Burkhardt et al., 1982, 1986; Gylbert and Berggren, 1989) or modified to allow force–distance calculations (Hoflehner et al., 1993); tonometers to measure the compression pressure of the breast at intervals in the clinical course (Gruber and Friedman, 1981; Hayes and McLeod, 1979; Mulder and Nicolai, 1990); a durometer to measure breast hardness (Truppman and Ellenby, 1978); and standardized pictures to be rated by observers (Asplund and Nilsson, 1984). Applanation tonometry is the most frequently used of these techniques, but none has become universally accepted.

The Baker classification has continued as the most common standard, essentially as originally proposed (Baker, 1975), although modifications have been used by some investigators (Burkhardt and Demas, 1994; Gylbert et al., 1989) or suggested by Spear and Baker (1995). This system, though not quantitative, has the advantage of describing the actual clinical factors important to cosmetic effectiveness. Although undoubtedly subject to some bias when used by the operating surgeon on his or her own patients, it has good interrater agreement when applied by experienced personnel who do not have a personal interest in the results of care or research trials. Agreement ranges upward of 83% and is even better between the two major groupings (Groups I–II versus III–IV) at the border between acceptable and unsatisfactory (Coleman et al., 1991; Gylbert et al., 1989; Malata et al., 1997). This classification rates a breast as follows: Class I—the augmented breast feels as soft as an unoperated one; Class II—the breast is less soft, and the implant can be palpated but it is not visible; Class III—the breast is more firm, the implant can be palpated easily, and it (or distortion from it) can be seen; and Class IV—the breast is firm, hard, tender, painful, and cold. Distortion is often marked. Class I and II breasts are considered clinically satisfactory. Class III and IV are not.

As noted earlier in this report and in the literature, women have shown considerable tolerance for contracture, either by not seeking medical attention for Class III or IV contractures or by pronouncing themselves satisfied with their implants when surveyed (Gylbert et al., 1989, 1990a). The history of breast augmentation with implants (see Chapter 1) began with unsatisfactory substances that were often extruded or, in the case of paraffin, led to devastating tissue reactions. The twentieth century history, however, demonstrates a continuing willingness of surgeons (and women) to experiment with a series of technologies that have progressively improved contracture rates. The original "open-pore" implants, polymer sponges such as Ivalon and others, produced 100% Class III–IV contractures (Broadbent and Woolf, 1967), and needless to say, augmentation was not in great demand at that time (see discussion of prevalence in Chapter 1). The introduction of silicone gel implants with Dacron patches in the early 1960s reportedly lowered the incidence of serious contractures to around 75% (Gylbert et al., 1989), and the elimination of patches and use of smooth single-lumen gel implants reduced contractures further to about 50% or less (51.5% in gel implants followed an average of 8.5 years, Fiala et al., 1993; see also Brandt et al., 1984; Domanskis and Owsley, 1976; Gylbert et al., 1990a; Moufarrege et al., 1987; Shapiro, 1989). From these beginnings the problem of contracture has been addressed, but not eliminated, in a number of ways. These include reducing the exposure of breast tissue to silicone fluid by using saline implants or gel implants with barrier shells, addition of steroids to the saline lumen of single or multiple-lumen implants, measures to control infection and hematoma, positioning of implants under the pectoral muscle instead of the mammary gland or breast skin, and development of polyurethane and textured implants.

As with ruptures, the reported prevalence of contracture depends on a number of factors, such as varying detection, the assembly of cases which may or may not be symptomatic or have other biasing factors, the different placements of implants, and timing of assessment and length of follow-up. Studies that attempt to examine unselected groups of women and account for these factors can give a perspective on contracture prevalence. Such studies are cited in the discussion that follows. Reports of high modern contracture prevalence probably reflect selected case series, for example, Solomon's (1994b) report of 71% Class IV contractures in 639 women with silicone gel implants at 440 days on average after placement.

Tissue Exposure to Silicone and Contracture

There are some data defining the amount and characteristics of the silicone gel fluid diffusing through the barrier and nonbarrier shells of implants from some manufacturers, but they are far from complete (see Chapter 3 and below). The total amount and definition of molecular species diffusing over specific units of time in the actual clinical situation for a given implant are not known. Qualitatively, silicone droplets are often visible in capsular tissue, however, and their presence has been said variously to correlate (Barker et al., 1978; Domanskis and Owsley, 1976; Wilflingseder et al., 1974) or not to correlate with capsular thickness and contracture (Gayou, 1979; Rudolph et al., 1978; Thuesen et al., 1995). Measurements in these studies are too subjective to constitute reliable indicators of capsular silicone content. Silicone droplets (from gel implants) or fragments (from saline or textured implants) are also seen from time to time in breast tissue capsules, both intra- and extracellularly in axillary lymph nodes (Barnard et al., 1997; Thuesen et al., 1995; Vargas, 1979), and in the dermis of the scar at the operative insertion site, probably silicone gel fluid rubbed off the implant during implantation (Raso et al., 1996). Such droplets in capsular tissue and within distended macrophages have been proven to contain silicon (Winding et al., 1988). Quantitatively (what is presumed to be), silicone has been measured in the circulating blood or serum and in capsules, breast, and other tissues, mostly by technologies that measure the presence of elemental silicon, not a specific organic form such as siloxane. Attempts have been made to correlate these measurements with the clinical findings, but they have been variable and inconclusive, as noted below.

The technologies for obtaining an accurate determination of silicone, as silicon, in blood and tissue have evolved continuously. Results have been reported in different units, and actual readings have varied enormously as different technologies have been used and increasing care to eliminate contamination of sample from ubiquitous environmental sources or loss from sample due to volatilization has been exercised (see review of Cavic-Vlasak et al., 1996; and also Peters et al., 1995c). This has made it difficult to interpret results with confidence. In fact, it is difficult to be sure in various reports that contamination has been completely avoided. Silicon intake in the diet and in water or other drinks (including silicone, Kacprzak, 1982) can be substantial and can vary widely (20–50 mg SiO_2/day, Bellia et al., 1994; reflected as daily urinary silicate excretions in this range, Berlyne et al., 1986; from 0.68 to 17.3 mg per liter of mean silicon compounds in drinking water in various U.S. cities, Morykwas et al., 1991; 9–14 mg of silicon ingested per day, Cavic-Vlasak et al., 1996). Silicone parenteral, oral, dermal or inhalation exposures are substantial and variable, with sources including lubricants in syringes (see Chantelau and Berger, 1985; Chantelau et al., 1986; Collier and Dawson, 1985), antifoams in foods, surfactants, emulsions, polishes, water repellents, textile finishes, fluid and powder treatments in skin and suntan lotions and other cosmetic products, antiperspirants, hair care products, shaving cream, anti-foams in many pharmaceutical products, and so on as is often reported in the labeling of these common consumer products (Cavic-Vlasak et al., 1996; Shields et al., 1996; Silicones Environmental Health and Safety Council, 1994).

Poly(dimethylsiloxane) is about 37.8% (Kala et al., 1997, Thomsen et al., 1990) or 38.3% (Garrido and Young, 1999) elemental silicon by weight, and the technologies that measure silicone concentrations in various tissues usually detect the element silicon in the silicone and express results as weight of silicon per milliliter of serum or fluid or per gram of tissue or tissue dry weight. These values could be converted, of course, to the approximate weight of PDMS by multiplying by 2.6. However, this should be done with care, since, although it is likely when silicone droplets are seen—it cannot be assumed that the silicon is in the form of silicone; it may be in other silicon compounds. Some of these technologies measure silicon in gross blood or tissue samples, (e.g., atomic absorption spectroscopy, gas–liquid spectroscopy, inductively [or direct] coupled plasma atomic emission spectroscopy, and mass spectroscopy). Other technologies can locate and identify silicon in microscopic sections using energy dispersive x-ray analysis or scanning electron microscopy (Winding et al., 1988). Silicone compounds can be identified by NMR, Fourier transform infrared microspectroscopy (FTIR) and laser Raman microprobe, the latter two useful in microscopy (see review of Cavic-Vlasak et al., 1996 for discussion of these and other technologies).

Normal serum silicon levels, which vary slightly from blood or plasma levels (Bercowy et al., 1994), have been determined mostly, but not always, from groups of women assembled as controls for implant studies or studies of renal disease. These analyses have been controlled with calibration curves against known standards of hexamethyldisiloxane and analysis of tissues spiked with this compound (Evans et al., 1994, 1996) or other silicon-containing standards, including bovine liver tissue standards, recovery of spiked samples, repeat assays, and the like. Average serum (unless otherwise noted) silicon levels reported include <0.2–68 (mostly <0.6) μg/ml (Bercowy et al., 1994); 0.265 μg/ml in plasma of men (Berlyne et al., 1986); 0.6 μg/ml (Dobbie and Smith, 1982a, 1986, converted from micromoles per liter, 35.6 μmole/L = 1 μg/ml); 0.17 μg/ml in plasma (Gitelman and Alderman, 1992); 0.22 μg/ml (Hosokawa and Yoshida, 1990); 0.25 μg/ml (Jackson et al., 1998); 0.03–0.209 μg/ml (Leung and Edmond, 1997); 0.02542 μg/ml, mean, and 0.02175 μg/ml, median (Macdonald et al., 1995); 0.1498 μg/ml in blood (Malata et al., 1994a); 0.01–0.25 μg/ml (Marco-Franco et al., 1991); 0.11 μg/ml in blood (Mauras et al., 1980); 0.02528 μg/ml, mean, and 0.01705 μg/ml, median in blood (Peters et al., 1995); 6.24 μg/ml in blood (Sun et al., 1996), 0.14 μg/ml (converted from micromoles per liter, Roberts and Williams; 1990), 0.27 μg/ml and 0.23 μg/ml, mean 1 week and 1 month, respectively, postpartum (Tanaka et al., 1990, converted from micromoles per liter), and 0.13 μg/ml (Teuber et al., 1995a, 1996). These values have been compared to measurements from women with silicone gel breast implants. The serum or blood values from women with breast implants have been found by some to be not significantly different from normals listed above and reported at the same time—0.1355–0.1680 μg/ml in women with intact or ruptured implants (Malata et al., 1994a), and a mean of 0.02711 μg/ml, = or median of 0.02531 μg/ml (MacDonald et al., 1995). Others report approximately double levels in women with breast implants compared to the normal levels reported (see above, e.g., mean, 0.03909 μg/ml, median 0.03345 μg/ml [Peters et al., 1995a], 16.16 μg/ml [Sun et al., 1996] and 0.28 μg/ml [Teuber et al., 1995a; 1996]). Much of this serum (or plasma) silicon in normal men and women, and presumably in women with implants, is in the form of silicic acid or magnesium or calcium silicate and is excreted as such by filtration (and in some instances tubular secretion) by the kidney (Adler and Berlyne, 1986).

Garrido et al. (1994, 1996) found blood values by NMR that were below their detection limits in normal women and several orders of magnitude higher (i.e., milligram versus microgram quantities) than those cited above in women with breast implants (31–143 millimole, total silicon) and also detected silicone breakdown products. An effort to confirm these results by NMR in implanted women was unsuccessful. If the microgram values in blood and serum cited above are correct, these levels are below the detection limit of the NMR technology used (Macdonald et al., 1995; Garrido and Young, 1999; Taylor and Kennan, 1996). If the milligram values reported by Garrido et al. are correct then gram quantities of silicone are in the circulation at any given time. If such elevated blood levels are correct, one would expect that levels of at least the same order of magnitude would be seen in body tissues that must be in some sort of equilibrium with blood and, in fact—at least for lower molecular weight silicones—are known to be in equilibrium with blood (see descriptions of D_4 and D_5 toxicology in Chapter 4). Such levels have not been reported by any technology except NMR (Garrido et al., 1994) in other human tissue than capsules around gel implants, and studies reporting these capsular levels also report levels in tissue in the few microgram range (see below). It was recently suggested that the 1994 analysis of Garrido et al. (1998) might have to be rethought (Garrido et al., 1998; MacDonald, 1999). In addition, studies have not confirmed the presence of crystalline silica (suggested as a breakdown product of silicone) in breast capsular tissue (IRG, 1998; Pasteris et al., 1999). Serum or blood levels of silicon do not correlate with whether an implant is intact or ruptured (Jackson and Dennis, 1997; Malata et al., 1994a; Peters et al., 1995a; Teuber et al., 1995a, 1996) or the duration of implantation (Jackson and Dennis, 1997; Peters et al., 1995a; Teuber et al., 1995a, 1996). The marked difference between capsular levels (or even pericapsular breast tissue levels) and blood–serum or distant tissue levels raises a question about the feasibility of movement of silicone (specifically from gel and elastomer) into the bloodstream and its dissemination from such depots with high concentration gradients. This question requires further investigation.

Almost all studies have agreed that there are baseline levels of silicon in normal breast and other tissues. Values reported range from the detection limit of 2.00 ng/g to 9.46 μg/g dry weight of heptane-extracted organosilicon in breast in a comparative autopsy case series of implanted and nonimplanted women. Some higher values in spleen and lung tissues were seen in the nonimplanted than in the implanted cadavers (95th percentile, 134.4 and 45.22 μg/g dry weight, respectively, versus 58.92 and 16.00 μg/g dry weight). The majority of implanted women in this report had at least one positive axillary node (presumably) by light microscopy for extra- or intracellular silicone (Barnard et al., 1993). Other reports include the following: 0.5–6.8 μg/g tissue in breast, liver, spleen, and subcutaneous tissue in an autopsy case series of women without implants (Evans et al., 1994); 0.25–2.4 μg/g dry (breast) tissue in women without implants (Leung and Edmond, 1997); median levels of 27 μg/g and mean levels of 60.5–64 μg/g dry (breast) tissue in an operative, breast reduction, control series, range 4–446 μg/g (McConnell et al., 1997; Schnur et al., 1996; Weinzweig et al., 1998); and 0.025–1.460 μg/g dry weight in heptane extracts of normal breast tissue (Peters et al., 1995a).

Elevated levels of silicon are reported in capsules around intact saline implants, but not in breast tissue beyond the capsule. Reports include capsule levels in saline tissue expanders of 44–1,380 μg/g tissue (Evans and Baldwin, 1996); median capsular levels of 7.7 μg/g dry (heptane extracted) weight (Peters et al., 1995a); median capsule levels of 71.5 μg/g with a mean of 140.7 μg/g and median breast tissue levels of 28.0 μg/g with a mean of 56.5 μg/g dry weight (Schnur et al., 1996). In an extension of their 1996 report, Evans and Baldwin (1997b) reported control cadaver silicon tissue levels from various organs averaging 2.2 μg/g tissue, with a median of zero and undetectable levels in >50%. Levels in the capsules of silicone elastomer port-a-catheter chemotherapy implants averaged 8.04 μg/g tissue; levels in capsules of saline implants or expanders averaged 292 μg/g tissue with a median of 110 μg/g tissue; and levels in non-breast tissue sites of women with saline and gel implants averaged 3.2 μg/g tissue, with a median of 2.7 μg/g tissue and undetectable levels in 18%, that is, not significantly different from controls. Apparently tissue silicone levels are increased even around small short-term non-breast silicone implants. (Evans and Baldwin, 1997a,b). The saline inside an implant contains on average 10–12 μg/ml silicon, and when the implant deflates this silicon is released into the capsule (presumably as silicone) and some probably reaches the surrounding breast tissue (McConnell et al., 1997). Deflated saline implant capsule and tissue levels reported include the following: capsule, range, <5–2818 μg/g dry weight (McConnell et al., 1997); capsule, median, 198 μg/g and mean 883 μg/g; and breast tissue, median and mean, 116 μg/g dry weight (Schnur et al., 1996).

Very high silicon levels are reported in capsules around silicone gel implants and intact and ruptured implant capsules: 15–9,800 μg/g of PDMS in formalin--fixed tissue (Baker et al., 1982); 75–9,000 μg/g tissue (Evans and Baldwin, 1996); average levels in capsule around silicone gel implants of 1,439 μg/g tissue, with a median of 490 μg/g tissue (Evans and Baldwin, 1997b); 29–496 μg/g dry weight in presumably intact implant capsules (Leung and Edmond, 1997); a median of 11,492 μg/g and a mean of 11,613 μg/g in intact implant capsules with a median of 85 μg/g and a mean 490 μg/g in breast tissue. Levels reported for ruptured implant capsules are: a median of 13,590 μg/g and a mean of 14,683 μg/g, with a median of 64 μg/g and a mean of 3,332 μg/g in surrounding breast tissue, and axillary lymph node levels of 11,879 μg/g dry weight (McConnell et al., 1997). Capsules of intact and ruptured implants measured 9,979 μg/g, range 371–152,000 μg/g dry (heptane extracted) weight (Peters et al., 1995a); 0.252–116.9 μg/gram dried capsule (Sun et al., 1996); a median of 8,118 μg/g and a mean of 13,685 μg/g in intact implant capsule, with a median of 73.0 μg/g and a mean of 265.3 μg/g in breast tissue, a median of 12,666 μg/g and a mean of 14,751 μg/g in ruptured implant capsule with a median of 216.0 μg/g and a mean of 2,430 μg/g dry weight in surrounding breast tissue (Schnur et al., 1996); capsules of intact, 1,400 μg/g, and ruptured or possibly ruptured implants, 5,600–6,800 μg/g tissue of heptane extracted silicone (Thomsen et al., 1990). Using NMR, levels of 0.05–9.8% silicone by weight were reported in excised capsules of gel implants (Garrido and Young, 1999). A number of reports have confirmed a two-to tenfold variability of silicon levels from location to location in capsular tissue, as well as some variation in capsules from each breast in the same woman. If silicone levels are related to contracture, the relationship appears to be unpredictable and random (Baker et al., 1982; Evans and Baldwin, 1997b; McConnell et al., 1997).

One study detected silicone degradation to silica and "high coordinated silicon complexes" inside gel implants (Pfleiderer et al., 1993a), and some reports speculate that electron microscopy or FTIR may indicate some degradation forms of silicone in tissue (Greene et al., 1995a; Hardt et al., 1994). Other investigators, however, using NMR and laser Raman microprobe have reported that the silicone inside the gel implant and in the capsular tissue is chemically the same, i.e., only PDMS (Centeno et al., 1994; Garrido and Young, 1999), and that implant gel is stable in vivo over prolonged periods (Dorne et al., 1995). The weight of current evidence does not support the detection of silica or other silicone degradation products by the reported technologies. There is no correlation between implant age and capsular silicon level in most reports (Baker et al., 1982; Barnard et al., 1997; Evans and Baldwin, 1997b; Peters et al., 1996; Schnur et al., 1997), although one analysis of intact gel implants found a significant correlation between implant age and silicon levels (McConnell et al., 1997). Also, a qualitative analysis of silicone migration through the capsule found greater migration with implant age (Beekman et al., 1997a). A few investigators have reported that there is no correlation between the integrity of the implant and silicon capsular levels (Evans and Baldwin, 1996; McConnell et al., 1997; Peters et al., 1995a). Not surprisingly, silicone is found microscopically or analytically in tissue around non-breast silicone elastomer implants (Evans and Baldwin, 1997a; Needelman, 1995; Peters et al., 1995a). A preliminary report of implanted rabbits described more silicone per gram of tissue in capsules from ruptured than from intact gel implants, and tissue silicone levels in organs of implanted animals were the same as controls except for brain and capsule in which significantly higher levels were measured (Marotta et al., 1996b).

These data define in part the exposure of women to silicone from breast implants, which appears to be primarily and usually from the implant, its capsule, and the immediately surrounding breast tissue and axillary lymph nodes. Silicon found in distant tissues apparently reflects human exposure to ubiquitous silicon or silicone from the environment, and concentrations in tissue and fluids of women with implants are not significantly higher than control values from women without implants. This does not mean that all implant silicone is accounted for. Small amounts of low molecular weight compounds from gel fluid are likely to diffuse or be transported away from their source and to be subject to lung, hepatic, or renal clearance, as some elevated blood levels (if accurate) might imply. This is consistent with animal studies using carbon-14 (^{14}C) labeled silicone. Only 33–47 µg of 500,000 µg of silicone gel (with 80% extractable 1,000 centistoke, ^{14}C-labeled PDMS fluid) implanted without a containing shell in the backs of mice left the implantation site over 20 weeks the majority of which was excreted in urine, most of the balance being found in regional nodes (FDA, 1992a, vol. I, pp 86–87, vol. II, pp 94–96, Isquith et al., 1991, see also the review of distribution and pharmacokinetics of D_4 and to some extent D_5 in Chapter 4). The substantial variation in silicon measurement levels reviewed here, however, raises a question of the reliability of some of these data, which appear to be outliers and suggests caution in extrapolating from these results. Because one cannot be sure how reliably contamination or volatilization was ruled out in reports, and therefore how accurate silicon determinations were, the committee believes that the situation calls for an effort to develop and agree on standardized technologies and normal biologic measurement values that can be used as accepted references in research and clinical medicine.

Silicone exposure, as measured by capsular silicon levels, was not found to be associated with connective tissue or autoimmune disease-like signs or symptoms (Evans et al., 1996; Evans and Baldwin, 1997b; Weinzweig et al., 1998). These data also provide a context for considering the association between implants and local complications. Evidence for a relationship of tissue silicon concentrations and changes in the breast, including capsular contracture, is insufficient. Silicon levels were correlated with microscopic changes such as foamy histiocytes and vacuoles; that is, the levels were associated with microscopic signs of silicone in the tissue, but not with inflammation, giant cells, or calcification (McConnell et al., 1997). Silicone levels were also correlated with an abundance of fibroblasts and lymphocytes, silicone droplets in the tissues, and sparseness of plasma cells (Thomsen et al., 1990). Thomsen's report stands alone in suggesting a direct relationship, measured by quantitative analytic techniques of silicone equivalents, between increasing silicone capsular tissue levels and increasing fibrosis. Using a semiquantitative technique, energy dispersive x-ray analysis (which suffers from the sampling problems of electron microscopy), Jennings et al. (1991a,b) reported that tissue silicon levels were lower in more severely contracted than in soft capsules. However, these levels were higher in capsules around gel than around saline implants and diminished rapidly with distance from the implant (Jennings et al., 1991a,b).

Other evidence for the relationship of silicone exposure to contracture depends on the lesser frequency of contracture observed with implants that deliver less silicone to the tissue, (e.g., saline and, at least initially, barrier implants). Capsules around saline implants have been reported to have less microscopically detectable silicone, as noted earlier in this chapter. Barrier implants allow diffusion of smaller quantities of silicone gel fluid through the shell in vitro, but the actual measured implant capsular tissue silicon levels between one manufacturer's barrier and nonbarrier implants did not reveal a difference (Peters et al., 1996), and one study comparing gel fluid diffusion amounts among different implants removed from patients did not find differences between barrier and nonbarrier shells (Marotta et al., 1996a). This may reflect the known individual variability of silicon tissue levels or the loss of barrier effectiveness over time as suggested in this and other reports.

Frequency of Capsular Contracture—Saline Implants Compared to Gel Implants

As noted earlier, reports of the frequency of capsular contracture suffer from many of the same problems as studies of breast implant rupture in the plastic surgery literature. Reports use different units (percentage patients, percentage breasts); some give Baker class, others do not, some use Class II–IV, others Class III–IV. In addition, there are many variables such as submammary or submuscular placement, use or nonuse of steroid, mixing of different makes of implants, variable and too short follow-up periods, and noncomparable study and control groups. In general, however, the results seem to support a lower frequency of contracture around saline implants compared to gel. The following frequencies refer to Class III–IV contractures, unless otherwise noted.

Asplund reported contractures in 55% of capsules around gel and 20% of capsules around saline implants in women with reconstructions (Asplund, 1984). Similar figures, 50% in gel and 16% in saline implants, were reported for this same group of women five years later by Gylbert (Gylbert et al., 1990b). McKinney and Tresley (1983) reported contracture frequencies of 36% around gel and 24% around saline implants in breasts of augmentation patients. Hetter (1979) reported gel implant capsular contractures of 64% and saline implant capsular contractures of 40% in women augmented in multiple surgical practices with different models of implants. Cairns and de Villiers' (1980) contracture results for augmentation were 81.1% with gel, and 8.3% with saline implants. Reiffel et al. (1983) reported "firmness" in a group of 307 women from three plastic surgery practices receiving gel and saline breast implants primarily in the 1970s. There was a statistically significant greater frequency of firmness in the whole group after augmentation with gel implants (61%) than with saline implants (23%), and the differences were similar and statistically significant in each practice taken separately. In this study follow-up was generally short, from 6.8 to 29 months. Edworthy et al. (1998) reported 36.3% Class III–IV contractures in left breasts and 40.7% in right breasts of women with gel-filled implants (*N* = 1,112) and 18.2% Class III–IV contractures in left and 22.3% in right breasts of women with saline-filled implants (*N* = 352) in a large survey series of augmentations. Their aggregate figures for contractures per patient were 56.8% of women with gel implants and 40.5% of women with saline implants.

Other substantial numbers of Class III–IV contracture of capsules around gel-filled implants have been reported: 79% at 15–21 years after submammary augmentation (Gylbert et al., 1989); 44% of gel submuscular implants (Hakelius and Ohlsen, 1997); 40% of augmented breasts with "firmness" leading to reoperation in more than a third (Domanskis and Owsley, 1976); 45% of augmented breasts with Class II–IV contractures needing capsulotomies (Brandt et al., 1984); 56% Class III–IV contractures of 60 breasts augmented with double-lumen implants in the placebo arm of an antibiotic treatment trial (Gylbert et al., 1990a), and 14.6% of 1,454 breasts requiring reoperation in 749 women (Gabriel et al., 1997). Very low rates of contracture around saline implants have been reported in two large series: 1.3% (Lavine, 1993); and 1.1% (Mladick, 1993). Also 1.9% contractures were reported in a smaller experience (Capozzi, 1986). However, in the large series of Gutowski et al. (1997), Class III–IV contracture (as graded by the patients) plus the number of patients requiring open or closed capsulotomy totaled 20.4% of patients; the prevalence of Class III–IV contracture reported by Rheingold et al. (1994) was 9.5%, and by Francel et al. (1993) in immediate and delayed reconstruction using implants or expanders was 11% and Worseg et al. (1995) reported 37.6% contracture. All of these saline implant series had adequate to good length of postoperative follow-up.

The Class III–IV contracture frequencies for mostly textured, saline implants at 12 months cumulative follow-up in the modern McGhan LST of 2,855 women were 6.2% overall, 5.5% for augmentation, 10.6% for reconstruction, and 8.8% for revision. Undoubtedly, contractures will continue to occur beyond 12 months. The figures for gel implants in the McGhan AR90 five-year clinical study were 9.3% of augmented breasts and 4.9% of reconstructed breasts. The better value for reconstructions at five years may be explained in part by the predominance of textured implants used for reconstruction (94.4%) versus augmentation (62.1%) and in part by the submuscular placement used for reconstruction (98.1%) versus augmentation (50.9% submuscular, 49.1% submammary). Historically, contracture has been found to be more frequent following reconstruction (reviewed in Environ, 1991). The 1990 Dow Corning figures at two years were 17.6% Class III–IV contracture for Silastic II, and 8.6% for Silastic MSI implants in augmentation (Bowlin et al., 1998). All of these studies have so many variables, such as different vintages and manufacturers of implants, follow-up, placement, texturing, and indications for implantation among others, that it is not possible to draw a firm conclusion about the frequencies of contracture in capsules around saline- or gel-filled implants, but the evidence suggests that women can expect more contractures around gel implants than around saline implants if these are the only variables.

Barrier Implants and Contracture

Barrier-coated shells also decrease tissue exposure to silicone by slowing the diffusion of gel fluid through the implant shell at least for some years. Animal experiments in mice, guinea pigs and rabbits showed qualitatively less silicone in tissue around "low bleed" implants and softer, less contracted capsules (Barker et al., 1981, 1985; Caffee, 1986a). Implants with a McGhan barrier to gel fluid diffusion (presumably the dimethyl diphenylsiloxane, Intrashiel, technology) were compared to standard gel-filled implants in rabbits. Silicone was observed and confirmed by scanning electron microscopy or electron dispersive x-ray analysis in significantly more (11 of 20) capsules around standard implants than in capsules (1 of 10) around barrier implants, although there was no difference in capsule firmness (Rudolph and Abraham, 1980). In a very preliminary study, Price and Barker et al. (1983) expressed the opinion that Silastic II barrier implants appeared to be lessening contracture. They were less sure about Intrashiel implants. Their findings consisted of eight "contractions" of unspecified severity in 170 (4.7%) breasts after very short follow-up. Chang et al. (1992) compared conventional implants from several manufacturers and low-bleed gel Silastic II implants in women augmented submuscularly. At more than a year of follow-up, with conventional implants the Baker scores averaged 1.65. There were 16% Class III–IV contractures. The low-bleed implants had a Baker score average of 1.07. There were no Class III–IV contractures. These were significant differences (Chang et al., 1992). Biggs et al. (1993) compared their low-bleed and conventional results at more than a year follow-up. There was no significant difference between the percents of patients with Class I soft breasts, but in submuscular cases the percent Class III–IV contractures was minimally significantly lower with low-bleed implants. In women with submammary implantation, the low-bleed implants produced significantly fewer severe contractures than the conventional smooth single-lumen gel implants.

The definite proof of a relationship between tissue silicone and contracture in humans is lacking since no study of adequate power has held all other variables constant and compared actual tissue silicon measurements to contractures. There is considerable inconsistency among various reports as noted earlier. In the reported literature, qualitative assessments of silicone droplets or a few measurements of silicon may or may not correlate with contracture severity. On the other hand, silicone fluid injected into breasts causes fibrosis and walling-off of silicone deposits, and gel implants are associated with much higher capsule and tissue silicon measurements. Saline-filled and barrier-coated implants appear to be associated with lower tissue silicone exposure and fewer and less severe contractures compared to conventional gel implants in a preponderance of the studies cited above. Fibrous capsules form around any foreign body, and contracture of these capsules is undoubtedly multifactorial, however. Until definitive studies are carried out, it seems reasonable to assume, based on current evidence, that silicone fluid and gel may contribute to contracture rate and severity and that this can be beneficially influenced by barrier technology or by substituting saline filler.

Effect of Implant Surface on Contracture

Experimental work on the effects of surface characteristics of foreign bodies and clinical experience with polyurethane foam-covered implants suggested that providing breast implants with a "rough" or textured surface might result in fewer and less severe contractures. Capsular reactions to texturing and polyurethane have been described earlier in this chapter and in Chapter 3. Some experiments in rats and rabbits failed to show an advantage of textured implants or showed some advantage only with expanders (Barone et al., 1992; Bern et al., 1992; Bucky et al., 1994; Caffee, 1990). Other studies in the same kinds of experimental animals revealed decreased capsular contractures around the textured implants which were related in some cases to the depth and spacing of the texturing; in other cases there were strikingly different prevalences (Brohim et al., 1992; Cherup et al., 1989; Clugston et al., 1994; Maxwell and Perry, 1995; Smahel et al., 1993). Texturing seems to have differing effects on capsule characteristics depending on the characteristics of the texturing. In some cases, almost no effects are noted if surface deformities are shallow (den Braber et al., 1997), but in other instances where (human) cellular activity was studied on elastomer surfaces with shallow (0.5 m) grooves of varying width and spacing, fibroblast proliferation and orientation differed as the surface changed (van Kooten et al., 1998). In one study, lower reactivity of capsular tissue to smooth muscle stimulants was also observed (Malata et al., 1993).

With few exceptions, a number of clinical trials or observational studies have supported the association of texturing with less severe capsular contracture. Asplund et al. (1996) found 3–9% Class III–IV contractures around textured implants and 10–20% around smooth-surfaced gel implants from the same manufacturer, measured by three techniques (two of which provided a statistically significant difference) in submuscular augmentation. In a study directed primarily at exploring the role of infection in contracture, texturing provided a significant enhancement of contracture control for the saline inflatable implants of one manufacturer (Burkhardt and Eades, 1995). A study designed to further explore antibacterial effects in submammary augmentation compared textured and smooth saline implants of another manufacturer and found, respectively, 2 and 40% Class III–IV contractures (Burkhardt and Demas, 1994).

A prospective controlled trial using submammary gel-filled, low-bleed implants that were identical except for texturing produced Class III–IV contractures in 58% of smooth and 8% of textured implants (Coleman et al., 1991). A five-year follow-up of these women produced essentially the same highly significant results—11%, and 59% Class III–IV contractures in the textured and smooth devices, respectively, and 31% replacements for the smooth implants (Malata et al., 1997). Using implants of yet another manufacturer, Ersek (1991b) reported double-lumen (with steroid) implant Class III–IV contractures of 34.5% for smooth submammary, 7.9% for submuscular, 2.5% for textured submammary, and 0% for textured submuscular implants. Hammarsted et al. (1996) reported that postmastectomy reconstruction patients implanted with double-lumen textured and smooth gel implants (from different manufacturers) with intraluminal steroid had, respectively, 9 and 24% Class III–IV contractures. McCurdy (1990) compared two different textured gel implants with polyurethane-coated implants and smooth double-lumen implants and found that texturing was as effective as polyurethane in eliminating contractures, whereas smooth implants produced 25% contractures.

In a study with a short follow-up of women with breast augmentation using gel implants, Pollock (1993) reported 21% of patients with Class II–IV (13%, Class III–IV) contractures around smooth, barrier shell implants and 4% with Class II–IV (2%, Class III–IV) contractures around textured implants with otherwise the same shells from the same manufacturers. These results are biased against finding a beneficial effect of texturing since the smooth implants were more often (24% versus 1%) placed in the submuscular position, which should have lessened contractures of their capsules. In a comparison study of patients with textured and smooth surfaced, but otherwise identical, gel-filled implant placed in opposite sides, the textured implant was unequivocally preferred by the women and rated better by surgeons in terms of contracture (Hakelius and Ohlsen, 1997). The Dow Corning 1990 multisite study of its smooth and textured gel implants reported half as many Class III–IV contractures around the textured as around the smooth implants (Bowlin et al., 1998). Vogt et al. (1990) reported a multicenter survey using textured double-and single-lumen implants, some with steroid or antibiotics, compared to historical controls. After 12 months the contractures around textured implants were 1.8% overall, compared to the historical controls of 25% and 22% (Little and Baker, 1980; Moufarrege et al., 1987; Vogt et al., 1990).

In a rare negative study, Handel et al. (1995) used a corrective factor for different follow-up periods and reported similar contracture frequency around various saline and gel smooth, textured and polyurethane implants from a number of manufacturers. In a second negative study, 20 consecutive patients at least two years after unilateral mastectomy were given either textured or smooth expanders, followed shortly thereafter with textured or smooth gel-filled implants. There was no difference in contracture or the thickness of capsules between the two groups, although the textured implant capsules contained many silicone fragments (Thuesen et al., 1995). In another, more impressive negative study, Tarpila et al. (1997) augmented a small group ($N = 21$) of women in the submammary position with a randomly placed textured saline implant in one breast and a smooth saline implant in the other. The implants were the same size and shape from the same manufacturer. Class III–IV contractures were 38% around the smooth and 29% around the textured prostheses, results that were not significantly different statistically (Tarpila et al., 1997).

These authors speculated that textured (and thicker) shells may reduce gel fluid diffusion from gel-filled implants which would explain the reduction in contracture around these implants. However, it would not explain how textured saline implants reduce contractures in most studies, where there is no gel or gel fluid diffusion, and also where fragments of silicone elastomer in tissue are more frequent than in smooth implants. There is no evidence for lower silicon levels in capsules around textured implants, and as noted earlier, these capsules have clearly different cellular characteristics that most probably play a role in their effect on contracture. Although studies that control all variables except texturing and have adequate numbers are not available, this evidence suggests that capsular contracture is less with textured implants than with smooth surfaced implants.

Effect of Steroids on Contracture

Local adrenal cortical steroid treatment may also play a role in contracture and in the safety of silicone breast implants. Steroids have been placed in the lumen of saline implants, in the saline lumen of double-lumen implants, or in the tissue pocket that receives an implant. It is speculated that steroid in single-lumen implants may deliver higher tissue concentrations and thus provoke more steroid complications than in double-lumen implants. In the latter the diffusion may be divided into both an outward to the tissue and an inward to the gel lumen direction. This presupposes that steroid concentrations are made equal in the unequal saline volumes of the two implant types by adjusting total dosage, and also assumes that the effects of such adjusted total dosage depend on concentration relationships. These are unproved assumptions. Exactly what happens to forms of methylprednisolone (SoluMedrol) or triamcinolone (Kenalog) placed in the lumen of saline implants could not be determined from reports found in the breast implant literature. Conflicting in vitro studies found that steroid diffusion out of the implant was very slow—a few months to years in duration—and likely varies with the physical and chemical characteristics of the implant shell. Continuing steroid diffusion probably results in exposure of surrounding capsular and breast tissue to pharmacologic concentrations of steroids over prolonged periods of time as clinical experience suggests. Berman et al. (1991) concluded that about 30% of the methylprednisolone might be in the shell at any one time depending on its thickness, or depending on the drug's chemical formulation, it might be variably subject to hydrolysis or crystallization from solution (Berman et al., 1991; Cohen, 1978a; Cucin et al., 1982; Morykwas et al., 1990; Perrin, 1976; Spitalny et al., 1981). In addition, as Gutowski et al. (1997) recently noted, steroid inside saline implants may be, in their experience, a risk factor for twofold increments in deflation rate. Manufacturers have pointed out that the interaction of this chemical with the implant shell has not been investigated adequately, and its use cannot be recommended (Gutowski et al., 1997). In addition, delivery of steroid from a breast implant is not an FDA-approved usage.

Because of the known effects of steroids on scar formation and inflammation, Peterson and Burt (1974) instilled 60 mg of triamcinolone into the pocket on one side of eight bilaterally augmented women and noticed that the treated side was consistently softer than the other over a follow-up period that ranged from a few months to a year. This study had insufficient follow-up, small numbers and unblinded assessment. Some subsequent communications reported failure of this technique (Brownstein and Owsley, 1978; Kaye, 1978; Price, 1976). For example, Biggs and Yarish (1990) reported that 14% of breasts treated with periprosthetic steroids had Class III–IV contractures and only 4% of breasts without steroids had this complication and Vasquez et al. (1987) also found that steroid-treated breasts had more, but not significantly more, contractures: 40.7% with, versus 31.7% without periprosthetic triamcinolone.

On the other hand, Hipps et al. (1978) found Class II–IV contractures in 26% of women with implants for augmentation in a series treated with 60 mg of triamcinolone in the pocket around smooth gel implants, compared with 35% contractures in the no-treatment group. Baker (1975) reported a 10% decrease in Class II–IV contracture when 20–40 mg of triamcinolone was placed in the tissue pocket. And Lemperle (1980) commented that 20 mg of triamcinolone crystals in the pocket on one side seemed to produce a softer augmented breast, but also a number of perforations due to tissue atrophy at the location of the crystals. Local instillation of triamcinolone around implants in experimental animals failed to produce a marked effect on capsules (Vistnes et al., 1978), or, in fact, any effect on capsules or intraprosthetic pressures (Moucharafieh and Wray, 1977). Reduction in contractures to 5% was noted after placing 62.5 mg of methylprednisolone in each saline prosthesis (Perrin, 1976), and recommendation of this treatment was repeated by Hartley (1976). Addition of 40 mg of triamcinolone to the lumen of saline implants produced marked thinning of the overlying tissue, inferior displacement of the implant, and ptosis of the breast with impending extrusion after a few months. These complications did not appear when 20 mg of methylprednisolone was substituted (Ellenberg, 1977). A case of late erosion of a medium-sized arterial branch with substantial hemorrhage and implant loss has also been reported after triamcinolone at 40-mg dosage (Georgiade et al., 1979).

Experimental results reported by Ksander et al. (1978) using high dose triamcinolone inside implants produced a number of extrusions and disorganized, loosely knit, thinner capsules in the steroid treatment group, although there was no measurable effect on hardness (Ksander et al., 1978). In a later study, methylprednisolone at two dose levels (0.1 and 1 mg/ml) had a significant effect on capsule histology and compressibility (Ksander, 1979). Subsequent reports of the use of 62.5 mg methylprednisolone confirmed steroid complications of severe ptosis of the breast, inferior displacement of the implant, atrophy and bluish discoloration of overlying tissue, and implant extrusion as long as two years postoperatively and the need for replacement of 70% of the implants in one series (Cohen, 1978a; Cohen and Carrico, 1980; Oneal and Argenta, 1982; Persoff, 1978). Lemperle (1980) found that using 50 mg in the outer lumen of double-lumen prostheses resulted in the need to replace the implants with single-lumen gel implants after a year, although con-tractures fell from 57 to 16% in his patients.

Carrico and Cohen (1979) reported that methylprednisolone in the tissue around the implant had no effect on contracture (control and treatment frequencies both 50%) and provoked no steroid complications. Methylprednisolone at doses greater than 20 mg within the saline implant, however, led to steroid complications in 61.5% of breasts and to 4% Class III–IV contractures, while doses of 20 mg led to steroid complications in 8.3% of breasts and 4.2% contractures. Because the same total dose may be contained in different volumes of saline used to inflate the outer lumen of the implant, concentrations of the drug may vary, and in this study, higher concentrations appeared to correlate with increasing steroid complications (Carrico and Cohen, 1979). Ellenberg and Braun (1980) reported their results with 20 mg or less methylprednisolone in double-lumen implant augmentations compared with a control group of gel implants. The control contracture rate was 67.6%. Those with 5–15 mg of methylprednisolone experienced 11.9% contractures and 2.4% steroid problems, those with 20 mg methylprednisolone experienced 9.9% contractures and 3.6% steroid problems (Ellenberg and Braun, 1980).

In a study of a large number of patients comparing single-lumen gel implants with double-lumen implants containing 12.5 mg of prednisolone, contracture frequencies were 19% in augmentations, 54% after subcutaneous mastectomy, and 64% in post mastectomy reconstructions with the gel implants without steroids. Contractures decreased to 4%, 14.9% and 24.4% in these same categories when steroid-containing double-lumen implants were used (Lemperle and Exner, 1993). In a randomized and controlled study, Spear et al. (1991) compared the Class II–IV contractures and steroid complications of smooth double-lumen implants with and without 16 mg of methylprednisolone, assigned randomly to two well-matched groups of women undergoing submuscular reconstruction, 44 breasts with steroid and 45 without, followed for a minimum of three years. Contractures were 14% in the steroid group compared to 44% in the non-steroid group, and there was no difference in complications between the two groups.

McCurdy (1990) compared textured gel implants from two manufacturers with polyurethane-coated implants and smooth double-lumen implants with and without 20 mg methylprednisolone in submammary augmentation. Although the follow-up was short in some groups, in general the Class III–IV contractures were zero and 3.9% around polyurethane-coated implants and steroid-added double-lumen implants compared to 25% with the no-treatment smooth double-lumen implants. The prevalence of local steroid complications was 17.1%, however.

Although the total dose appears to be an important variable, it is likely that the intraluminal concentration of steroid also plays a role, as suggested by the data of Carrico and Cohen (1979) and the subsequent reanalysis and discussion by Cohen and Carrico (1980). The much higher complication rate reported by McCurdy (1990) than by Spear et al. (1991) whose doses were similar (20 versus 16 mg) but whose concentrations were markedly different, (i.e., 100 mg versus 40 mg per 100 ml of saline), is also suggestive. In an inflatable saline implant, the steroid is contained in a much larger volume and thus is present at a much lower concentration. Some authors report that the total dose of 20 mg in these cases never causes a problem (Guthrie and Cucin, 1980). It is logical to assume that the higher concentration gradient associated with the more concentrated steroid would expose the tissue to a higher dosage of the drug, although probably for a shorter time. In an analysis of their data by concentration of steroid in the implant, Cohen and Carrico (1980) concluded that methylprednisolone should be administered according to concentration in the implant and not according to total dose. Based on their clinical findings, they recommended 5–10 mg/100 ml of saline as a reasonable level that would minimize, but not eliminate, steroid complications and at the same time have an effect on contractures.

This suggestive evidence for an effect of intraimplant adrenal cortical steroid in decreasing contracture has to be balanced against the occurrence of steroid complications, the possible weakening of implant shells, the availability of other modalities to reduce contracture, and the nonapproved status of this intervention. The studies cited have, in general, design problems, including small numbers, lack of controls, varying dose levels, and placement of the steroid in implants with varying shell characteristics, among others. The committee believes that, at a minimum, before this treatment can be recommended, the behavior of a particular implant as a delivery vehicle and the therapeutic results and complications of a defined dosage to tissue in properly controlled and randomized studies would have to be determined.

Role of Infection and Antimicrobial Treatment

The safety of breast implants is affected by infections in a number of ways. Surgical wound infections necessitate medical and surgical interventions. Infections of the implant or implant pocket often require extensive treatment, including removal and replacement of the implant (e.g., Rheingold et al., 1994). A small number of these infections are caused by unusual and recalcitrant microbes, including various fungi, mycobacteria, and clostridia that resist rapid resolution or resolution without implant removal. These organisms differ from the usual bacteria found in wounds or infecting implants perioperatively, such as *Staphylococcus aureus, β hemolytic streptococci,* or less virulent staphylococcal species. A diverse array of bacteria can be cultured from the surface of, or from breast tissue around, implants often with no clinical signs, such as *S. epidermidis* and related species, *Propionibacterium acnes* and related species, *S. aureus,* anaerobic diphtheroids and more rarely *Streptococcus A and B, Escherichia coli, Enterococcus, Corynebacterium, Klebsiella, Pseudomonas* and infrequently others (Ablaza and LaTrenta, 1998; Ahn et al., 1996; Brand, 1993; Clegg et al., 1983a; Coady et al., 1995; Courtiss et al., 1979; Dobke et al., 1995; Foster et al., 1978; Gylbert et al., 1990b; Hunter et al., 1996; Lee et al., 1995; Netscher et al., 1995b; Peters et al., 1997; Truppman et al., 1979; Virden et al., 1992; Williams et al., 1982; Young et al., 1995a). Some of these latter organisms, and occasionally fungi, may also be found within saline expanders and inflatable implants, where they can survive and even proliferate possibly supported by glucose that diffuses into, and has been measured within, the implant (Blais, IOM Scientific Workshop, 1998; Chen et al., 1996; Coady et al., 1995; Nordström et al., 1988; Young et al., 1997). Presumably they enter through the punctures in the inflation ports (Liang et al., 1993). These periprosthetic organisms are usually discovered on aerobic and anaerobic culture of implants, pockets and capsules. They are often not involved in clinically apparent perioperative infection problems, which for the most part are caused by *S. aureus,* hemolytic streptococci or some less virulent staphylococci, are infrequent, and occur within a month after surgery (Courtiss et al., 1979). In general, studies of infection suffer from the use of varying culture technologies, some failing to culture anaerobically or for a long enough time, some with greater or lesser vigor and thoroughness in sampling the implant surface or peri-implant tissue (Virden et al., 1992).

Local, perioperative infections are generally treated with antibiotics and resolve, although they may contribute to pain or other complications. The frequency of these infections is reported in many case series and ranges around 1–4% after augmentation and significantly higher after reconstruction (e.g., 13%, Bailey et al., 1989; 6%, Courtiss et al., 1979; 5%, Crespo et al., 1994; 7%, Eberlein et al., 1993; 5.8%, Furey et al., 1994; 2.5%, Gibney, 1987; 2%, Noone et al., 1985; 3%, O'Brien et al., 1993; 5%, Slade, 1984; 13%, Vinton et al., 1990) including one report of very high numbers of infections, 8 of 15 patients (53%), in women undergoing immediate postmastectomy reconstruction with expanders (Armstrong et al., 1989). Gabriel et al. (1997) reported a combined total of 1.1% of breasts, implanted primarily for augmentation, reoperated for infection. Brandt et al. (1984) reported 3.9% infections in gel augmented breasts. Biggs et al. (1982) reviewing an 18-year experience reported 2–7.6% of patients reoperated for removal of infected implants at various stages in the evolution of this practice (Biggs et al., 1982).

The McGhan LST found 1.1 and 6.9% of breasts with infections after saline augmentation and reconstruction, respectively, and the McGhan AR90 (1998) five-year experience of infection with gel implants was 0.7% of augmented breasts and 0% of reconstructed breasts. The Mentor adjunct study (1992) found 4.3 and 1.3% infections at the three-year follow-up of gel implantation for reconstruction and augmentation, respectively. Very infrequent infections in saline implant augmentation were reported by Gutowski et al. (1997), 0.2%; and by Mladick (1993), 0%. A frequency of infections in mostly inflatable saline implant augmentations of 1.5% was reported by Rheingold et al. (1994). A survey by Brand of 73 plastic surgeons using a diversity of implants found frequencies of infection of 0.06–0.16% for implants in augmentations and 0.3–6% for implants in reconstructions. Since a long time interval was covered and "only severe infections" were reported, considerable underreporting is probable in this survey (Brand, 1993). In a Centers for Disease Control and Prevention (CDC) survey of 2,734 plastic surgeons with a 67% response rate, wound infection after augmentation was reported in 0.64% of patients (Clegg et al., 1983b).

Some wound infections are not treated successfully with antimicrobial therapy and result in loss of the implant (Courtiss et al., 1979). Very rarely, there are very serious or lethal complications such as staphylococcal, streptococcal, or other bacterial toxic shock syndrome (Barnett et al., 1983; Bartlett et al., 1982; Brown et al., 1997a; Giesecke and Arnander, 1986; Holm and Muhlbauer, 1998; Oleson et al., 1991; Poblete et al., 1995; Tobin et al., 1987; see also Walker et al., 1997, for a case after explantation and granuloma excision). Very rarely also, an infection may occur in an otherwise well-tolerated implant many years after surgery without an apparent inciting event (Ablaza and LaTrenta, 1998).

In addition there is evidence that infection is associated with increased frequency and severity of implant capsular contracture and thus with the interventions that accompany this complication. The tissue of the breast is open to the environment through the lactiferous ducts, which are colonized extensively by normal skin flora, both aerobic and anaerobic bacteria, primarily *S. epidermidis*, *P. acnes* and anaerobic diphtheroids. As a result, bacteria can be recovered from 91.6% of female breasts, usually bilaterally (primarily coagulase-negative staphylococcal and propionibacterial species, Ransjö et al., 1985). Implants themselves, implant pockets, or capsules and nipple secretions have yielded 23.5–89% positive bacterial cultures, using various techniques (Ahn et al., 1996; Burkhardt et al., 1981; Courtiss et al., 1979; Dobke et al., 1995; Gylbert et al., 1990b; Netscher et al., 1995b; Peters et al., 1997; Thornton et al., 1988; Virden et al., 1992).

These bacteria, particularly gram positive bacteria, have been shown in vitro to be able to adhere within two minutes to, and colonize, all types of silicone breast implants (Jennings et al., 1991a,b; Sanger et al., 1989). They are often located in a bioslime film on the surface of the implant (Dougherty, 1988), where they are largely protected from antibiotic action (Evans, 1987), and they presumably contribute to infections after implant surgery. Thornton et al. (1988) found that some postoperative breast infections were associated with the same organisms that they had cultured at the time of surgery (both for implantation and for breast reduction) from deep within the breast, primarily coagulase negative staphylococci. In this series of 30 patients (19 with breast reductions), contracture was associated with positive cultures, but the numbers were too small to achieve statistical significance (Thornton et al., 1988).

In rabbits with implants contaminated with *S. epidermidis* compared to sterile controls, the contaminated capsules were Class III–IV and two to three times thicker with more dense collagen than the control Class I–II capsules (Shah et al., 1981). In a subsequent study, the effect of intraluminal cephalosporin was evaluated in this protocol, and the thickness of the capsules around contaminated, antibiotic-containing implants was significantly reduced (Shah et al., 1982). At about this time, cephalosporin (and gentamycin) had been found to diffuse from Heyer-Schulte saline implants in significant concentrations for up to six months (Burkhardt et al., 1981). Guinea pigs formed capsules more rapidly after experimental implants were dipped in staphylococcal broth cultures overnight (Kossovsky et al., 1984). Quantitative data in this report were sparse, and the effect of coating an implant with broth before placement may be an uncontrolled, confounding variable. Others have experimented with iodinated silicone implants. Implants containing povidone–iodine (Betadine) were found to inhibit bacterial growth in vitro due to the diffusion of free iodine through the shell. Saline implants placed in mouse tissue pockets contaminated with *S. aureus* had capsules 2.8 times thicker than povidone–iodine implants similarly placed or saline implants placed in sterile pockets (Birnbaum et al., 1982; Morain and Vistnes, 1977). Since iodine degrades the silicone shell, this is not a clinically useful observation (Morain, 1982).

Broadbent and Woolf (1967); Burkhardt et al. (1986); Courtiss et al., (1979); and Dobke et al. (1995) reported clinical associations of positive cultures with contracture, and Netscher et al. (1995) found a significant association of Class IV contractures with positive periprosthetic explant capsule cultures. Virden et al. (1992) performed routine and special research cultures with 55 silicone implants (38 gel- or saline-filled implants and 17 expanders) removed from 40 women. Class III–IV contracture was observed around 24 (63%) implants and 3 (18%) expanders, and cultures (mostly research not routine) were positive (primarily *S. epidermidis*) from 56% (15 of 27) of implants with contractures and only 18% (5 of 28) of implants without contracture, a statistically significant ($p < .05$) difference. Similar to the findings of Parsons, 91% of painful contractures were associated with positive cultures (Virden et al., 1992).

Burkhardt et al. (1981) originally noted a decrease in Class III–IV contractures to 3% of breasts with implant intraluminal Keflin or Garamycin in a short follow-up study, compared to a historical control rate of 37%. They subsequently conducted a prospective randomized trial using single-lumen saline inflatable implants in the submammary position that compared a control group with four groups using a variety of antibacterial treatments, including local irrigation with povidone–iodine, antibiotic foam, and intraluminal cephalothin. They demonstrated a significant improvement in Class III–IV contracture from a control value of 41% to a combined experimental group value of 19% (Burkhardt et al., 1986). In a subsequent prospective, randomized study that looked at both texturing and povidone–iodine, the antibacterial irrigation failed to have any effect on contracture (Burkhardt and Demas, 1994), and Gylbert et al. (1990b) could show no effect on contracture of preoperative infusions of antibiotics that dramatically lowered the culture positivity of the implant pocket. This latter result is consistent with the generally held conclusion that preoperative prophylactic antibiotics are of little value (Courtiss et al., 1979) and may also reflect the fact that subclinical implant infections in a slime layer around the implant are protected from antibiotic action (Virden et al., 1992). Gutowski et al. (1997), however, reported that implants containing antibiotics experienced a lower frequency of contracture and in a final prospective randomized study that compared implant texturing from another manufacturer and povidone–iodine irrigation of the implant pocket with untreated smooth implants, a significant effect of antibacterial treatment on Class III–IV contracture was observed (Burkhardt and Eades, 1995). Dobke et al. (1995) in culturing a series of 150 explanted gel and saline (19 implants, 26% culture positive) breast implants, noted that 76% (62 out of 82) of those with Class III–IV contractures, but only 28% (19 of 68) of those without contracture were culture positive, primarily with *S. epidermidis*. This difference was statistically significant ($p < .05$) (Dobke et al., 1995). According to Burkhardt, (1988) infection explains the varying occurrence of contracture, that is, its frequent appearance unilaterally as well as bilaterally in proportions that statistically appear to represent a random (infectious) event. More recently, Peters et al. (1997) reported no association of capsular culture positivity (of 42%) with severe contracture in a series of 100 women whose implants were removed.

Dowden (1994) suggested that the presence of the subclinical infections or contaminations described above may contribute to systemic signs and symptoms such as fatigue, myalgia, diarrhea, and arthralgia, among others, in implanted women. He reported seven women, five of whom had positive cultures for *S. epidermidis* or *Propionibacterium acnes*, whose symptoms resolved and whose health returned soon after explantation (Dowden, 1994). In a study that compared women with implants without general health problems to women with implants and a similar, but somewhat more extensive constellation of signs and symptoms, including arthralgia, dry mucous membranes, fever, hair loss, and cognitive problems, Dobke et al. (1995) found health problems to be associated with positive cultures. Among women with these symptoms, implants were 81% culture positive compared to 28% positivity in those without such signs and symptoms, and among women with both the three systemic signs and symptoms and Class III–IV contracture, 95% (19 of 20) of patients had culture-positive implants.

Earlier, the same group had tested the hypothesis that a painful prosthesis signified subclinical infection. Painful breast and penile prostheses were cultured at explantation and compared with cultured expanders (removed for replacement with a permanent implant) or with cultures of malfunctioning penile implants. In the aggregate 26 out of 28 (93%) painful prostheses and 4 out of 31 (13%) devices that were not painful were infected, mostly (> 90%) with S. *epidermidis*. Replacement of infected and painful devices with sterile devices while giving antibiotics resulted in pain-free devices in nine of ten instances (Parsons et al., 1993). Others evaluating culture-positive explants have not found associations with the health problems noted above, although little in the way of description is provided (Ahn et al., 1996), and the evidence for an effect of infection on symptoms remains limited.

Also, the important data of Burkhardt would be more persuasive if the comparison control groups of smooth saline implants were not at the upper ends (27–41%) of the Class III–IV contracture rates for modern saline implants, and some studies have been negative (e.g., Peters et al., 1997). The differences in contracture frequency with saline versus gel and textured versus smooth implants are not readily explained by a bacterial theory of causation. Nevertheless, the evidence for a relationship between the presence of bacteria around the implant and contracture, although not conclusive, is certainly suggestive.

Role of Hematoma

Collection of blood, hematoma, or tissue fluids, (seroma), around implants is very like overt infection in that it complicates a small number of implantations, often requires an invasive intervention, although some resolve (or drain) spontaneously, and has been suggested as a factor in contracture. Since the frequency of clinically apparent hematoma or seroma is usually much lower than that of significant contracture, this complication is, at the most, a small contributor to contracture. Hematoma was the indication for reoperation in 3.5% of the breasts in the Mayo Clinic series (Gabriel et al., 1997). In the experience of one plastic surgery clinic 5–10.3% of patients were reoperated for hematoma over an 18-year period (Biggs et al., 1982). Hematoma or seroma was not reported in the McGhan LST or AR90 observational studies. This complication probably is reported quite variably, and often it is mentioned in case series reports only in a cursory fashion, if at all. Some of these reports of hematoma or seroma frequencies and the instances of accompanying operative interventions to provide open or needle drainage have been noted earlier in this report. Plastic surgeons vary in the use of drains (which some report prevent contracture to a meaningful extent—Brandt et al., 1984; Hipps et al., 1978) and other operative precautions to prevent or manage bleeding and the collection of blood around implants. Many surgeons use drains when implanting textured-surface implants to prevent seroma formation. Also, hematomas around implants may become infected or be associated with infections (Courtiss et al., 1979).

A hematoma frequency of 2%, most requiring reoperation, was reported by Rheingold et al. (1994) and Baker et al. (1975). Additional reports include 1.4% hematoma (Biggs et al., 1990), 5.9% (Brandt et al., 1984), 4.5% with implant loss (Artz et al., 1991), 0% hematoma or seroma (Bayet et al., 1991), 6% hematoma (Capozzi, 1986), 20% "postoperative bleeding" (Gylbert et al., 1989), 1.1% hematoma (Lavine, 1993), 0.48% of hematomas (Mladick, 1993), 2.1% hematomas (Williams, 1972) and so on, for augmentation and reconstruction with both gel and saline implants. These reports are typical for hematomas that are observed within days after implantation. Rarely hematomas occur years later in association with contracture, due presumably to microfractures of the stiff fibrous capsule. These can pose significant problems requiring more extensive surgery (Cederna, 1995; Frankel et al., 1994; Marques et al., 1992). Conversely, there are those who believe that events such as trauma, which could produce hematoma, may cause late-onset contracture (Ashbell, 1980). Observations of hematoma associated with contracture are mixed. Some report the absence of an association (Asplund, 1984; Coleman et al., 1991; Hakelius and Ohlsen, 1992), but these reports involve very small numbers of hematomas and were not designed to study the issue. Others have found a significant association between hematoma and contracture in their clinical studies (up to two- or threefold greater prevalence of contracture in implants with hematoma than in those without (Handel et al., 1995; Hipps et al., 1978; Wagner et al., 1977; Watson, 1976). In a study involving baboons, with numbers too small to have any significance, implants with blood around them had thicker and harder capsules. In another larger study with rats, hematoma had no effect on either capsular thickness or intraimplant pressure, although a combination of hematoma and steroid did elevate pressures (Moucharafieh and Wray, 1977). Caffee (1986b) also found no effect of hematoma on capsular contracture in rabbits. These studies are inconclusive. The safety implications of hematoma involve primarily the few percent extra interventions required to resolve these complications, the suggested association of infection, and the limited evidence that the incidence of contracture and its accompanying problems might be somewhat higher around implants with hematomas.

The Influence of Implant Location

The placement of implants in the submuscular position, which was originally reported by Dempsey and Latham (1968) and modified to partial muscular coverage by Regnault and colleagues has a salutary influence on the incidence of contracture, decreasing it in the latter report from 30% in the submammary group to 10% in the submuscular group (Regnault, 1977; Regnault et al., 1972). This effect is reported in a number of additional studies that cite significant decreases in contracture when comparing women with submuscular implants to women with submammary implantation of different kinds of gel-filled implants. These include decreases from 11.1% to 3% of Class III–IV contractures with some standard and some low-bleed gel implants (Biggs and Yarish, 1990); 40% to 5% of patients with severe contracture (Mahler and Hauben, 1981); 83.8% to 27.1% of Class III–IV breasts with gel implants of 12 years' duration or less (Peters et al., 1997); 41% to 8% of Class III–IV contractures with gel-filled implants (Puckett et al., 1987); improvement from 30% Class I contracture to 95% Class I contracture around gel-filled implants (Scully, 1981); average self-assessed Baker score at five years of 2.9, submammary to 2.1, submuscular using gel-filled implants (Fiala et al., 1993), and 58% submammary and 9.4% submuscular gel implant contractures (Vasquez et al., 1987).

Other reports, cited earlier, describe low rates of contracture in patients with submuscular implants studied and reported for other reasons (e.g., Chang et al., 1992). A review of the literature by Puckett, cited in another report, concluded that Class III–IV contractures occurred in 43% of breasts with submammary and 6% of breasts with submuscular implants (Biggs and Yarish, 1988). Hetter (1991) repeated his 1979 survey and reported that the contracture (firmness) rate had dropped from 64% to 8% since he had changed from the submammary to the submuscular approach. In a study of saline inflatables, Cocke reported 44% noticeable firmness in submammary implants and 19% in submuscular implants (Cocke, 1994). In a review of a large experience with polyurethane-coated gel implants, 22 of 658 (3.3%) implants in the submuscular position had Class II–III contractures (only two were Class III) compared to 14 of 237 (5.9%) submammary placements with Class II contractures (Hester et al., 1988).

A few studies compared contractures after subcutaneous implantation with those after submuscular implantation of gel-filled breast implants. Two found firmness of 31–50% in submuscular and 80–100% in subcutaneous implantation (Slade, 1984; Ringberg, 1990). A third study found 0 and 7% of breasts with Class IV and Class III contractures, respectively, in submuscular (includes both pectoral and serratus coverage), and 7 and 33% of breasts with Class IV and Class III contractures, respectively, in subcutaneous implantation in delayed reconstruction followed from one to five years (Gruber et al., 1981). There appears to be sufficient evidence to conclude that submuscular rather than subglandular or subcutaneous placement of the implant is associated with a lower incidence of severe contracture. This observation should be among the several factors considered by both the patient and surgeon in deciding between submuscular and other placement of the implant.

Not everyone agrees with a policy of routine placement of implants under the muscles of the chest wall for augmentation (Ashbell, 1980; Courtiss et al., 1974), and plastic surgeons still use the submammary approach in 32% of augmentations (ASPRS, 1997) presumably because of the better aesthetics of this placement in breasts with adequate tissue cover, and possibly because submuscular implantation has been associated with more pain. Placement has relevance for the issue of safety primarily because of its effect on contracture, which lessens the need for interventions secondary to this complication. The submuscular position may also facilitate examination of the breast for cancer, since the glandular tissue lies above the implant and is all available for palpation (Little et al., 1981, see also Chapter 12). Although the submuscular operative approach is technically somewhat more demanding, the rates of rupture, deflation, infection, hematoma, and other complications do not seem to differ significantly between submuscular and submammary placement. Occasional speculation about the submuscular position, noted below, does not have convincing nonanecdotal, experimental, or clinical support in the studies cited. It cannot be concluded that submuscular implants, being further away from potentially contaminated breast glandular and ductal tissue, are less prone to infection. There is no evidence that such implants are in some way less sensitive to silicone droplets, or might benefit from the massaging action of overlying musculature. Although the theory is intuitively attractive, there are no data in the literature available to the committee to show that placement of implants with muscular cover between them and glandular tissue results in earlier diagnosis of breast cancer by palpation or mammography, or that contracture might not be less frequent but merely more difficult to detect in this position.

Other Complications and Their Relevance to Safety

At the beginning of this chapter, local and perioperative complications were discussed. Not all of these have numerically significant, or medically and clinically important, safety implications. Although some of these conditions may be mentioned in other chapters of this report, the committee finds that for its purposes here the major influences on safety have been discussed. For example, although the reference list includes about 30 citations on the effects of radiation therapy in women with breast implants, implants themselves have good stability to clinically relevant dose levels of irradiation, they do not significantly interfere with the radiation beam and radiation therapy, and evidence that radiation can increase implant capsular contracture is limited (see Chapter 3 for discussion).

One additional problem may merit some attention. Pain associated with implantation is common enough to be considered. Localized pain results in requests for implant removal (e.g., as an indication in 19.2% of explants, Beekman, 1997b, as one of the major reasons for a 13% prevalence of replacement, Bright et al., 1993) or in interventions for relieving pain associated with contracture. Some authors have reported complaints of pain in the great majority of women with implants (107 of 114 consecutive patients, Silver and Silverman, 1996), pain manifesting as a new "chest wall syndrome" in 68% of women with implants (Silver et al., 1994), or pain in 36% of women explanted (Peters et al., 1997), but these were not representative samples of the population of women with implants. Most reports of complications do not include much if any detail on pain. It was included without discussion in the list of indications for reoperation and was the indication for secondary surgery in 1.1% of the Mayo Clinic group of 749 implanted women (Gabriel et al., 1997), and reports often cite rather low frequencies.

Wallace et al. (1996), however, reviewed the subject of pain after breast surgery using a questionnaire with a 59% return rate (282 women). Although the response rate might indicate a bias toward complaints, this group reported substantial local pain after reconstruction (up to 50%) and augmentation (38%). Pain was also more common after submuscular (50%) than submammary (21%), and after saline (33%) than gel (22%), implantation. Since the pain was worse after implantations than after reduction surgery or mastectomy alone, these authors assumed it was related, at least in part, to the implants, although significant prevalence of chronic postmastectomy pain has been reported in other surveys [12.7–17.4% of patients at various times up to a year postoperative in Kroner et al. (1992), 20% of patients in Stevens et al. (1995)]. Others have reported that pain often recedes after explantation (Peters et al., 1997). Of the augmented and reconstructed patients with pain, 20–29% required pain control medication, though for how long is not clear. Pain is one of the indications for implant removal. Capsule formation, especially under the muscles, may result in nerve compression and pain leading to a requirement for secondary procedures. Other late pain may be due to muscular compression (Huang, 1990). Usually, pain with late onset (8% and 30% of reconstruction and augmentation patients, respectively) represents contracture pain (Wallace et al., 1996). Pain is also associated with some gel implant ruptures, up to 93% in some reports (Ahn et al., 1994b; Andersen et al., 1989), is reported in association with polyurethane implants (Jabaley and Das, 1986; Smahel, 1978a; Wilkinson, 1985), and is reported in association with positive implant bacterial cultures (Parsons et al., 1993; Virden et al., 1992) or calcification around the implant (Peters et al., 1998).

There are a number of specific reports of breast pain associated with implantation (Cuéllar and Espinoza, 1996; Huang, 1990; Jabaley and Das, 1986; Janson, 1985; Lu et al., 1993, 1994; Sichere et al., 1995). These reports describe some severe chest, subscapular and arm pain syndromes, and unusual presentations in women with implants, and they list some of the indications for explantation. However, as others have pointed out, chest pain is a common complaint, and evidence to support the association of pain with implants in some of these cases, which come from highly selected groups, is not persuasive (Kulig et al., 1996; Mogelvang, 1996). As Wallace et al. (1996) discuss, pain, like sensory change, which is of similar frequency, is not surprising given the damage to the nerves to the breast and nipple during implantation and reconstruction surgery and the routine injury to the nerves including the intercostobrachial nerve (to the arm) during mastectomy with axillary dissection (Benediktsson et al., 1997 and reviewed in Courtiss and Goldwyn, 1976); see values of 41.6% permanent nipple sensory changes (Fiala et al., 1993); and 41% change (Hetter, 1979); 18% decrease in sensation (Hetter, 1991); nerve damage and paresis (Laban and Kon, 1990; Wallace et al., 1996); and partial to complete sensory loss in the nipple of 70% and in the whole breast of 12% after augmentation, although it should be noted that this was an explant series with a high (65%) incidence of breast pain (Peters et al., 1997).

CONCLUSIONS

The frequency of local and perioperative complications has been substantial in both augmentation and reconstruction of the breast with either saline- or gel-filled silicone implants. These complications have safety implications, because they may have health consequences of their own and because they may result in further operative or medical interventions that may also have health consequences. The committee sees little justification for some of these interventions, for example, closed capsulotomies or the use of steroids.

Much information in this chapter may not apply to the present and may not provide a basis for decisions concerning future experiences because past reports of complications reflect experience with implants having physical and chemical characteristics that differ from current implants and surgical practices that differ from current practices. Although the present state of knowledge does not allow definite conclusions to be drawn about the prevalence or incidence of some complications, some of the more common complications such as rupture, deflation, and contracture may be becoming less frequent due to operative and technological improvements. Information to permit conclusions about the frequency, causes, and management of complications has to be gathered based on research on a stable population of standardized devices. Much remains to be learned about the basic biology of foreign body, silicone, and other polymer interactions with tissue, although progress has been made recently.

The committee drew conclusions about ruptures and deflations, the role of silicone in contracture, saline versus gel implants, barrier shells and shell texturing, submuscular placement of implants, the roles of infection and hematomas, the use of adrenal steroid, pain and other outcomes that can affect reoperations and local and perioperative complications. In general, however, the frequency of reoperations and local complications is sufficient to be of concern to the committee and to justify the conclusion that this is the primary safety issue with silicone breast implants, and it is certainly sufficient to require very careful and thorough provision of the kind of information contained in this chapter to women considering breast implant surgery. The committee concludes that many of these risks continue to accumulate over the lifetime of a breast implant.

6

Immunology of Silicone

Silicone breast implants are associated with significant local complications. Some have studied whether these devices are also associated with systemic morbidity. Because experimental and clinical immune reactions to silicone have been said to be involved in such an association, the committee undertook an examination of the evidence for these reported reactions. An understanding of the basic immunology is also important in assessing the biologic plausibility of some reported clinical findings and some suggested associations, such as autoimmune or connective tissue disease or novel silicone associated systemic syndromes. In this chapter, the committee reviews and discusses reports from the peer-reviewed scientific literature of both animal and human immune responses, or absence of immune responses, to silicone in various forms. Included in this discussion is a brief description of a conceptual approach to investigating the immune response to silicone. Some reports on immune effects were reviewed but are not cited in this chapter. They can be found in the reference list of this report.

IMMUNE RESPONSE TO SILICONE IN EXPERIMENTAL ANIMALS

Studying effects on the immune response in various experimental animals is an approach to investigating a substance that is often employed by basic and clinical scientists. Currently available experimental data indicate that silicone gel (or some higher molecular weight silicone oils) can act as a weak adjuvant capable of enhancing antigen-specific immune reactions. Mice or rats exposed to various antigens emulsified in silicone gel produce a greater antibody reaction than if antigen alone is given (Hill et al., 1996; Naim et al., 1995a,b, 1996, 1997a; Nicholson et al., 1996). However, silicone gel was found to have weaker adjuvant activity than a widely used reference adjuvant, complete Freund's adjuvant. Furthermore, enhancement of immune responsiveness was observed only when silicone and an antigen were injected together as an emulsion in the same site. Injection of an antigen in one site and silicone gel (implant) in a different site did not augment the immune response (Bradley et al., 1994a,b; Klykken and White, 1996). Other animal studies of components of the immune response from several groups have shown that parenteral administration of silicone gel to animals induces a time-dependent decrease in natural killer (NK) cell activity (Bradley et al., 1994a,b; Wilson and Munson, 1996). The NK-cell system is an important part of the natural immune system that is believed to contribute to the initial response to infections as well to controlling the emergence of tumors. Significant reductions in tumor control or response to infections were not observed after silicone induced reductions in NK-cell activity in these studies.

Silicone gels given alone have been reported to produce disease in two different animal models. Silicone caused an acute arthritis when injected directly into the joints of one particular strain of rats, but no arthritis occurred if the gel was injected distal to the joints. Arthritis was not observed in joints that were not injected directly, and when joints were injected, local inflammation was observed, but not distant systemic effects (Yoshino, 1994). In a second animal model, Potter and colleagues (Potter and Morrison, 1996; Potter et al., 1994) induced monoclonal immunoglobulin producing B-cell tumors (plasmacytomas) in BALB/c mice following intraperitoneal injection of silicone gel. This is not a simple, silicone-specific disease model, however. These mice appear to be genetically predisposed to develop plasmacytomas on intraperitoneal exposure to other triggering agents. It has not been suggested that this model has implications for the induction of cancer in experimental animals or in humans.

Classical adjuvant arthritis does not appear to be inducible by silicones in rats or mice (Naim et al., 1995a,b; Schaefer et al., 1997), although both silicone gel and silicone oils can replace incomplete Freund's adjuvant in inducing collagen-initiated arthritis in DA rats if the collagen is mixed with the silicone (Naim et al., 1995b). Since the adjuvant arthritis model is a well-established, intensively studied animal model for inflammatory arthritis, the failure of silicones to activate similar clinical and pathologic features in experimental animals is an important finding. Likewise, exposure of 18,000 humans to mineral oil adjuvant was not followed by excess connective tissue disease over 16–18 years of follow-up compared to 22,000 controls (Beebe et al., 1972, for a discussion of connective tissue or other systemic disease and silicone breast implants, see Chapter 8). The committee concludes there is no evidence for any human adjuvant disease, as asserted by some investigators (Miyoshi et al., 1964, 1973). For review and critique of additional animal studies, see Marcus (1996).

POSSIBLE RELATIONSHIP TO AUTOIMMUNE DISORDERS

Some investigators have suggested that current experimental animal data could support an association of silicone with immune effects in humans. Several ways in which silicone might activate an autoimmune disease in silicone breast implant recipients have been proposed and explored. First, since the major histocompatability (MHC) locus is critical to the way elements of the immune system sort out, recognize, and process foreign materials and antigens, a subset of women with implants could have a special human leukocyte antigen (HLA) that makes them particularly likely to process certain antigenic moieties in silicone gels in ways that activate T-cells to induce cell-mediated immune reactivity and initiate an inflammatory reaction. Secondly, cells of the immune system might be directly activated in patients with silicone breast implants. In other disorders, immune activation is usually indicated by obvious inflammatory cell infiltrates and damage within affected tissues or by deposition of specific antibodies within such tissues. Extremely high local concentrations of cytokines either in the serum or within local inflammatory reactions in involved tissues may also indicate immune activation. Thirdly, silicone breast implants might induce reactions to autologous or self-antigens. Such autoreactivity, if induced by breast implants, should be demonstrated by self T-cell reactivity or sensitization when T-cells are exposed to self-antigens or components of silicone gels.

In exploring whether silicone breast implants cause an autoimmune disorder in breast implant recipients, the committee concludes that it is important to determine if there is an abnormal immune response in these women that is directly caused by the implant. When this is examined, the immune function and responses in healthy women with breast implants should be compared to those of symptomatic women with implants, as well as comparing symptomatic women with breast implants to symptomatic women without silicone breast implants to determine whether a specific immune system abnormality can be identified that is associated with clinically recognizable symptoms in women with breast implants.

These determinations should be supported by addressing the following questions:

1. Is there an abnormality in natural immunity?

(A) Can any evidence be found for monocyte or non-specific T-cell activation as illustrated by accurate reproducible cytokine assays?

(B) Is there any evidence that components of silicone breast implants can act as a T-cell superantigen, or as a T-cell superantigen-like molecule that is capable of activating large numbers of T-cells with antigenic specificities, by binding shared T-cell receptor epitopes?

(C) Is there any evidence for an effect of silicone breast implants on NK-cell activity?

2. Is there an abnormality in the immune response?

(A) Do women with silicone breast implants and symptoms share a particular HLA haplotype profile?

(B) Can it be demonstrated that silicone-specific T-cells are present and have been activated in women with breast implants?

(C) Can silicone-specific B-cell reactivity be demonstrated in women with breast implants?

(D) Is it possible to demonstrate T or B cell autoreactivity in women with breast implants?

STUDIES OF THE IMMUNE RESPONSE

Cytokines Representing Products of Activated T Cells

Most of the reports that have measured cytokine levels in women with silicone breast implants and in control groups have examined serum or plasma levels which is less reliable than measuring concentrations in tissues. Most studies of cytokine levels in breast tissue are case reports. An exception is the study by Mena et al. (1995) in which soluble mediators of inflammation were measured in explanted capsular tissue from women with silicone breast implants, in skin scar tissues from women undergoing reverse augmentation mammaplasty, and in synovial tissue of patients with various forms of arthritis. Tissues were cultured for 24 hours in vitro and supernatants were examined for levels of interleukin-2 (IL-2), IL-6, tumor necrosis factor-alpha (TNFα) and prostoglandin E_2 (PGE_2). No significant difference was noted between capsular tissue and controls. In particular, cytokine production from breast tissues that had been exposed to components of silicone breast implants and from skin involved in previous surgeries was not significantly different. Moreover, no correlation was recorded between systemic symptoms and actual measured cytokine production by explanted capsular tissues. Such measurements, however, may not be meaningful compared to determinations of cytokines by quantitative polymerase chain reaction (PCR), enzyme-linked immunosorbent assay (ELISA), or immune histochemistry.

A study by Ojo-Amaize et al. (1994) examined IL-1β, which is a soluble mediator of inflammation, and IL-1 receptor antagonist, also elevated in inflammatory states, in the blood of women with breast implants with and without symptoms. Differences were found between women with silicone breast implants and healthy age-matched controls, but no valid conclusions were possible because symptomatic women with silicone breast implants were not compared to well women with implants to determine if implantation itself is associated with an increase in either IL-1β or IL-1 receptor antagonist (Ojo-Amaize et al., 1994). Other studies showed no differences between women with breast implants compared to age- and sex-matched surgical patient controls when TNFα and IL-6 as well as soluble TNF receptor were examined (Zazgornik et al., 1996). Moreover, Garland et al. (1996) examined IL-6 levels in women with breast implants and age-matched women without implants; no significant differences were recorded in IL-6. Another report by Blackburn et al. (1997) looked at IL-6, IL-8, TNFα, and soluble IL-2 receptor in women with silicone breast implants compared to healthy age-matched controls. Levels of all cytokines measured were below the range of detection of the various assays, but these investigators were able to detect elevated levels of the same cytokines in the blood of rheumatoid arthritis patients studied at the same time. Few of the experimental studies include controls or testing of biomaterials for endotoxin, which could significantly affect cytokine production (Cardona et al., 1992). In a generic discussion of tissue responses to implantation with a number of different biomaterials including silicone, Anderson noted changes in tissue cytokine concentrations as a general response to biomaterial implantation (Anderson, 1988, 1993, see Chapter 5 for more discussion of and references to cytokines). None of these studies provides sufficient evidence for immune system activation in women with silicone breast implants.

Superantigens Explaining Symptoms in Women with Silicone Breast Implants

Superantigens represent a class of molecules that bind in a non-immune fashion to T-cell receptors and activate a much larger proportion of T-cells than is stimulated by conventional T-cell reacting antigens. Ueki et al. (1994) looked at whether silicate might function as a superantigen. In this study, chrysotile (a silicate) was mixed with peripheral blood T-cells from three healthy subjects. In two of these subjects, an increase in Vβ5.3 T-cells and in the other of Vβ6.7 T-cells were recorded (Ueki et al., 1994). These numbers are too small to support any conclusions, and breast implant patients are not exposed to chrysotile. O'Hanlon et al. (1996) reported a study of 20 explanted breast implant capsule tissue samples.

PCR was employed to detect T-cell receptor V-region segments as a way of identifying preferential T-cell receptor gene expression. The T-cell receptor V segments were present in 14 samples, but many different T-cell V segments were expressed (O'Hanlon et al., 1996). These observations do not support a prominent role for T-cell superantigens in any immune response—abnormal or normal—in women with breast implants. There is, at present, insufficient evidence for superantigen activation of T-cells in patients with silicone breast implants.

Natural Killer Cell Functions

Natural killer (NK) cells can be distinguished from other cells of the immune system by the expression of several distinctive markers on their cell surfaces. Some investigators have suggested that NK-cell activity may be decreased in autoimmune diseases (Sibbitt and Bankhurst, 1985; Struyf et al., 1990), but no specific mechanisms have been elucidated to indicate how decreased NK-cell activity could favor development of autoimmune disease. Consistent with animal toxicology studies noted earlier, it appears that NK cells in humans might be affected by exposure to silicone gel, since removal of silicone breast implants was followed by an increase in NK-cell function in 50% of women studied by Campbell et al. (1994). However, among the remainder, NK-cell function decreased in 26% and remained unchanged in 24%. No data were given on the normal day-to-day variability of NK-cell function in the individuals tested. Moreover, parallel studies of control groups of women without breast implants and women with breast implants who were symptomatic or asymptomatic were not presented, which considerably weakens the study. In the data published to date, there is no clear evidence that changes in NK-cell activity have functional effects or explain the signs and symptoms that characterize women with silicone breast implants who have chronic and unremitting complaints. Moreover, previous studies have demonstrated that NK-cell activity can be altered by stress, sleep loss, and various medications including corticosteroids among otherwise healthy subjects (Irwin et al., 1994, 1996; Pedersen and Beyer, 1986; Pedersen and Ullum, 1994; Shepard et al., 1994; van Ierssel et al, 1996). Whiteside and Friberg (1998) observed that geographic location, gender, age, and even occupation of control populations can affect NK-cell activity and that low NK-cell activity is observed in chronic fatigue syndrome, which has been studied extensively without a consistent correlation with immune defects having been discovered. They noted that NK-cell assays are usually single time point assays in small cohorts and rarely performed under the stringent quality control measures necessary to ensure reproducibility (Whiteside and Friberg, 1998).

STUDIES OF THE ADAPTIVE IMMUNE RESPONSE

Role of HLA

Many studies have been undertaken during the past several decades in search of susceptibility genes that may predispose certain individuals to the development of certain diseases. Much of this work has centered on the role of the human HLA locus. The presence of a susceptibility gene does not guarantee the development of a disease, but probably indicates that the disease may be much more easily triggered than in the absence of that gene. Only a few studies have provided useful information on HLA associations with symptoms among breast implant patients. Morse et al. (1995) examined whether women with breast implants and scleroderma-like symptoms shared an HLA DQ motif with scleroderma patients without breast implants. HLA types in the scleroderma patients without implants had already been determined and found to have a diminished frequency of leucine at residue 26 of the DQβ chain. A control group of healthy individuals without implants was also included for comparison. The study examined a very restricted sort of HLA polymorphism, that is, whether subjects with breast implants and scleroderma-like symptoms also had a lower frequency of leucine at residue 26 of the DQβ chain than the control group. The finding of a decreased frequency in women with breast implants and scleroderma suggested that these women are similar to typical scleroderma patients. This study does not provide evidence for a role of silicone breast implants in scleroderma. Rather this study shows that scleroderma can occur in a particular susceptible population whether or not the subjects have breast implants (Morse et al., 1995).

A second carefully designed study by Young et al. (1995b) examined whether certain HLA class I and class II MHC molecules were present in symptomatic women with breast implants, although there is a significant error associated with serological methods of typing class II molecules. Four groups were included: group 1 consisted of 77 women with silicone breast implants and debilitating fibromyalgia-like symptoms; group 2 was composed of 37 women with breast implants, but few symptoms; group 3 contained 54 healthy women without implants; and group 4 had 31 women with fibromyalgia and no breast implants. No differences were recorded in HLA class I (A, B, or C) alleles among the four groups; groups 1 and 4 had an increased frequency of class II DR53 and DR7 suggesting that symptomatic women with breast implants share HLA DR alleles with women who develop fibromyalgia (Young et al., 1995b, 1996). There is no evidence to indicate that fibromyalgia is an autoimmune disease. Current evidence suggests that HLA haplotypes of symptomatic women with silicone breast implants resemble those of symptomatic women without breast implants.

T-Cell Activation in Women with Silicone Breast Implants

In cell-mediated immunity against a particular antigen or group of antigens, T-cell clones that recognize the antigen(s) are stimulated by, and will proliferate in the presence of, that particular antigen(s). T-cells also proliferate in the presence of various mitogens which are substances that cause polyclonal nonspecific T-cell division. Mitogens do not activate the antigen-binding sites of T-cells. To date, no specific autoantigen has been identified that will stimulate T-cells of women with silicone breast implants. Many of the studies which have sought to provide evidence for T-cell activation in woman with breast implants have focused on attempting to detect silicone-specific T-cells in such individuals, that is, T-cells that divide in the presence of silicone or silicone components.

When current reports of T-cell stimulation in women with breast implants are examined, a number of methodological difficulties emerge. These include uncertainty about the physical state of the silicon or silicone used for stimulation, the composition and validity of control populations, and the procedures used in analyzing various sets of data. A critical aspect of most of the studies of T-cell reactivity is their inability to differentiate whether silicone or components from silicone breast implants are recognized as true antigens by T-cell receptors or are functioning as T-cell mitogens.

Ojo-Amaize et al. (1994) reported an enhanced T-cell response to silicon dioxide, silicon, or silicone gel in symptomatic women with breast implants. The actual physical state of the "antigen" in the preparations studied is unclear. The silicone gel was subjected to extraction before it was used, the silicon was later said to be silicate (Ojo-Amaize et al., 1995), and silicates are normally present in the circulation. Two different sets of controls were studied—one set for silicon dioxide and another for silicon and silicone gel. Data analysis used in this report was not conventional. Any individual who responded to any of the three "antigens" employed was considered a responder. Only one patient was shown to have a positive response at all three concentrations of antigen tested (Ojo-Amaize et al., 1994). The committee could not interpret the results of this study.

A subsequent report by Smalley et al. (1995a) examined the T-cell response to silicon dioxide (silica) in symptomatic women with silicone breast implants. The symptomatic patients appeared to show higher T-cell stimulation indices than age matched controls. No control group of symptomatic women without breast implants was included, and the original data were not shown in this study. In addition silica is an immunologically non-specific stimulator of macrophages (Aalto et al., 1975; Chen et al., 1996; Davis, 1991; Mancino et al., 1983), no particulate controls were included, and there is no evidence that women are exposed to silica by silicone breast implants. The observations of Garrido et al. (1994) by nuclear magnetic resonance (NMR) and the detection of silica by polarizing microscopy, on which these authors rely as evidence for the presence of silica in women with breast implants, have been seriously challenged, as noted elsewhere in this report.

Smalley et al. (1995b) also exposed lymphocytes from women with silicone breast implants, normal controls, and women with defined connective tissue disease or fibromyalgia to three mitogens and colloidal silica. In a subsequent, expanded study, they examined responses to silica in 942 symptomatic and 34 asymptomatic women with implants and 220 normal control women. In the initial study, similar responses to mitogens were observed in control and implanted women. Stimulation indices after silica were elevated in women with implants, but not to the levels observed after mitogen stimulation. In the expanded study, 91.3% (860) of the women with silicone breast implants were deemed to have mild, moderate or markedly elevated stimulation indexes compared to controls on exposure to silica (Smalley et al., 1995b). This report also includes only brief aggregate data, and the problems previously noted obtain here as well.

Testing of the technology used in these reports by Smalley et al. by submission to their laboratory on two occasions of samples from eight women with either silicone gel, saline or double lumen implants and six women who had never had any implants (but for whom false histories of breast implantation were provided) was carried out by an independent investigator. This analysis yielded an array of results that bore no relationship to the clinical status of the patients, including positive stimulation indices, from mild to marked, in all six of the unimplanted women on first testing, and reversion to negative on repeat testing in one woman in both the implanted and the unimplanted group; the mean stimulation indices of the implanted and unimplanted group on repeat testing were moderately elevated and quite similar, 92 and 87, respectively (Young, 1996b). The findings of these studies have not been confirmed by others (in fact, as noted, serious questions have been raised), and their reproducibility and biologic plausibility are questionable.

Another report by Ellis et al. (1997b), which lacked a symptomatic control group and has not been confirmed, attempted to find autoreactive T-cells by looking at T-cell stimulation by connective tissue components as well as reactions to implant biomaterial. Twenty-six symptomatic women with breast implants were studied in parallel with 23 age-matched healthy controls without implants. Of these 26 women, 15 (58%) had undergone explantation of their implants, suggesting that this was not a random group. The women with breast implants showed increased T-cell proliferation to collagen I, collagen II, fibrin and fibronectin, but no increment in reactivity to myelin basic protein, transferrin, bovine serum albumin, tetanus, octamethylcyclotetrasiloxane (D_4), or silicone gel. Antinuclear antibodies were also present at titers of 1:40 or more in five (19%) of the implant recipients, not significantly different from the healthy controls (Ellis et al., 1997b).

A study by Ciapetti et al. (1995) compared T-cell responses to silicone gel in 22 women with breast implants to those of 10 women without implants who were an average of 15 years younger. The authors reported increased proliferation of T-cells from women with breast implants on exposure to an aqueous silicone gel extract. However, a standard stimulation index was not given; instead, stimulation in the women with implants was compared to stimulation in the control group, and the difference in stimulation between the groups was much less than twofold. For unexplained reasons, the lymphocyte stimulation of augmentation patients ($N = 6$) was significant, but the stimulation of reconstruction patients ($N = 16$) was not. These positive results appear to rest on six patients. Moreover, considering the insolubility of silicone gel in aqueous media, it is not known what compounds might be present in the extract (Ciapetti et al., 1995).

Several groups have investigated the possibility of cellular immunity to silicone. Snow and Kossovsky (1989) suggested that 3 of 29 patients with ventriculoperitoneal shunts might have delayed type hypersensitivity to silicone on the basis of tissue eosinophilia associated with the shunts. However, some of the patients in this series were infected and one of these had marked eosinophilia. Moreover, the finding of eosinophilia as a marker for delayed hypersensitivity is not conclusive. Jimenez (1994) also concluded that the requirement for revision of three shunts was caused by delayed hypersensitivity. Some non-silicone replacement shunts also required revision, and infection complicated the clinical picture here also. Nosanchuk could not demonstrate delayed hypersensitivity in guinea pigs injected with Dow Corning 360 fluid (Nosanchuk, 1968a). Kossovsky et al. (1998) also examined this question in guinea pigs. The animals were injected intraperitoneally three times per week for four weeks with either: an equal volume of Dow Corning silicone fluid and sterile guinea pig serum that was mixed for 28 days at 37°C and emulsified in complete Freund's adjuvant and tissue culture medium; or tissue culture medium alone. One week after the last injection, the animals were skin tested with: silicone-serum pellet (after centrifugation) in medium; a saline-serum pellet in medium; pure Dow Corning silicone fluid; or purified protein derivative (PPD), 250 tuberculin units. The guinea pigs had a marked reaction to PPD. They also reacted to the silicone-serum pellet, but the response to silicone alone was no different than the response to saline-serum pellet. Naïve animals that received spleen cells from experimental guinea pigs gave essentially similar results. Whether the response to the silicone-serum pellet represented a reaction to denatured serum proteins resulting from the 28 day incubation or to microbial contamination of the material is uncertain. However, the data appear to exclude a response to silicone itself. Narini et al. (1995) studied delayed hypersensitivity in sheep that were injected with McGhan implant silicone gel alone, silicone gel and complete Freund's adjuvant, saline or adjuvant controls. They concluded that there was delayed hypersensitivity to the silicone gel. However, there was a significant response to silicone in the adjuvant primed sheep, strongly suggesting that this response was not antigen-specific.

Investigators attempted to immunize animals against silicone gel and studied subsequent tissue reactions on exposure to silicone. They reported no changes in tissue cellular reactions in immunized compared to non-immunized, silicone-challenged animals, suggesting that cellular changes are implant wound, rather than silicone immune, related (Brantley et al., 1990a,b; Klykken et al., 1991a–e, see Chapter 5). In addition, lymphocytes of animals immunized with silicone gel and complete Freund's adjuvant did not respond to silicone gel challenge after four weeks or eight months, and T-cell helper suppressor ratios were unchanged (Brantley, 1995b).

A study by Katzin et al. (1996) examined T-cells from breast tissue and peripheral blood of women with breast implants. Peripheral blood of control individuals (not matched to sex or age) was studied in parallel. T-cells obtained from breast tissues showed an increased prevalence of an activation marker, HLA-DR antigen, compared to peripheral blood T-cells. A decrease in the numbers of CD4+, CD45+, and RO+ helper T-cells was noted in the implant associated T-cells as compared with the peripheral blood T-cells of these patients. Comparison of peripheral blood T-cells of patients and controls revealed only a slight decrease in CD4+, CD45+, and RO+ cells in patients. The cells of the patients with implants were sometimes stained after freezing and thawing. It was not clear whether the control cells were handled in a similar fashion. Differences in implant and peripheral blood T-cell phenotypes in the same breast implant patients do not constitute a strong indication for an in vivo adaptive immune T-cell activation or an ongoing abnormal T-cell disease process.

In general, studies addressing these issues are limited, and the technical problems associated with available studies are substantial. In view of these factors, the committee concludes that studies supporting a consistent pattern of marked T-cell activation or sensitization against autologous self-antigens or silicone in patients with silicone breast implants are inconsistent and unconvincing. At present there are no conclusive data showing that silicone or any components of breast implants represent clearly defined T-cell antigens or that any individual connective tissue component has been transformed or adapted into a T-cell autoantigen capable of perpetuating a chronic inflammatory process.

EFFECTS OF SILICONE: GRANULOMATOUS INFLAMMATORY REACTIONS

Inflammation is characterized by local vascular and tissue reactions as well as generalized systemic effects including fever, leukocytosis, and production of cytokines, as noted above. Inflammation represents the body's local reaction to tissue injury. Acute inflammation is characterized by exudation of various proteins and other substances from blood and migration of polymorphonuclear leukocytes to the site of injury. With biocompatible materials such as PDMS, this phase is not prolonged (indicating that the polymer is not providing a stimulus for continued inflammation) (Anderson, 1988). In prolonged tissue exposures, as is the case with silicone breast implants, chronic inflammation seems to be the most relevant process. Accumulations of lymphocytes and monocytes, which later differentiate into macrophages, characterize chronic granulomatous reactions. The tissue reaction to silicone implants appears to be one of granulomatous inflammation. The general histological appearance of granulomas is variable but usually shows a central region of macrophages, with or without caseation, surrounded by a zone of lymphocytes and more peripherally a zone of fibroblasts. The presence of multinucleated giant cells is a key histologic feature. Foreign body type giant cells, which are more common in silicone granulomas, have centrally arranged nuclei.

The histological appearance of foreign body reactions is not specific for any particular disease process. Silicone granulomas are typical foreign body granulomas which show multinucleated giant cells and aggregates of epithelioid macrophages, surrounded by dense lymphocytic and neutrophil cellular infiltrates. Plasma cells (known to be the cells responsible for antibody production) are frequently also present (Hill et al., 1996). The granulomatous histologic lesions induced by silicone seem to vary considerably depending on the form of silicone that actually causes them (Travis et al., 1985). Silicone elastomer, for example from joint prostheses or hemodialysis tubing, usually produces an intense foreign body giant cell reaction, most prominent in adjacent lymph nodes (Christie et al., 1989; Lazaro et al., 1990). Experimentally, the inflammatory response to particulate silicone elastomer is localized to the exposed (injected) joint, other joints are not inflamed (Worsing et al., 1982). The tissue reactivity to silicone gel or oil shows less organized granulomas with cystic spaces, presumably containing the foreign material (Hardt et al., 1995b; Peimer et al., 1986; Raso and Greene, 1997).

TISSUE RESPONSE TO SILICONE

Interactions of Silicone with Plasma Proteins

The inflammatory reaction to implanted foreign materials such as silicone is similar to other foreign body tissue reactions, as noted. This reaction includes interaction with plasma proteins, recruitment of inflammatory neutrophils and monocytes, differentiation of monocytes into macrophages, fusion of phagocytic cells to form giant cells and stimulation of fibrosis (Anderson, 1988). Hydrophobic materials such as silicone elastomer are coated with host proteins within a few hours of implantation. Even in the presence of dilute protein solutions the elastomers are at least 70% covered with host proteins within one hour (Butler et al., 1997). Thus, most inflammatory cells may never make direct contact with the "naked" biopolymer, but a wide variety of plasma proteins such as IgG, albumin, fibronectin and complement components can adsorb to silicone gels or elastomers and help recruit inflammatory cells to the site of the implant. Presumably, the inflammatory cells that enter the tissues do not respond to the foreign material itself but to a surface layer of adsorbed, partially denatured plasma proteins for which there are specific receptors on neutrophils and macrophages (Anderson et al., 1990, 1995; Bonfield et al., 1989a,b). Such responding macrophages may secrete twofold more Il-1β, Il-6 and TNFα than macrophages exposed to naked silicone (Naim et al., 1998).

Formation of Giant Cells and Effects on Fibroblasts

A foreign body giant cell reaction is typical of the tissue response to silicone elastomer, but is less commonly associated with inflammation in response to silicone gel or silicone oil. Studies by several groups of workers suggest that silicone induces IL-1, TNFα or IL-6 production by human monocytes. Moreover, there also seems to be a possibility that the biomaterials used to stimulate cytokine production could possibly themselves have been contaminated by microbial products such as endotoxin lipopolysaccharide (LPS), lipoteichoic acid or similar molecules, which may be responsible for some of the observed experimental tissue reactions. This has not been investigated adequately as yet (Anderson, 1993; Bonfield et al., 1992; Miller and Anderson, 1989; B.D. Ratner, personal communication, 1998). Silicone implants eventually become walled off by the formation in vivo of a fibrous capsule, which is a normal element of the response to a foreign body. Contracture of the capsule can become a problem in some patients with silicone breast implants, as discussed in Chapter 5. Monocytes or macrophages in contact with silicone appear to produce cytokines that stimulate fibroblast growth, but this is not necessarily an adaptive immune response (Bonfield et al., 1991; Miller and Anderson, 1989).

SPECIFIC AUTOANTIBODIES INVOLVED IN SYMPTOMATIC RESPONSES TO SILICONE BREAST IMPLANTS

Anti-Collagen Antibodies

Antinuclear antibodies and specific autoantibodies, such as anti-Ro, anti-La, anti-RNP, and anti-Sm antibodies, as well as rheumatoid factor or anti-topoisomerase antibody often associated with classical connective tissue disorders such as systemic lupus erythematosus (SLE), systemic sclerosis (SSc), Sjojren's syndrome (SS), or rheumatoid arthritis (RA), have been measured in patients with breast implants. These are discussed in Chapter 7. Several other general classes of autoantibodies have also been examined with respect to whether they might be involved either directly in pathogenesis or indirectly as disease activity indicators in patients with silicone breast implants. Anticollagen antibodies have been subjected to scrutiny by investigators who concentrated on a relatively small group of patients (Bar-Meir et al., 1995; Rowley et al., 1994; Simpson et al., 1994; Teuber et al., 1993). Anticollagen antibodies were examined in breast implant patients because the symptoms experienced by these subjects often include arthralgias, skin complaints, and musculoskeletal symptoms. Anticollagen antibodies have been measured in some patients with rheumatoid arthritis and also have been implicated in some mouse models of induced arthritis.

The initial report by Teuber et al. (1993) examined anti-collagen antibodies in 46 women with silicone breast implants (2 women with previously diagnosed connective tissue disease, 38 symptomatic women, 6 asymptomatic women) and age-matched healthy women. An ELISA reading greater than three standard deviations above the mean of the controls was considered a positive assay for anticollagen antibodies. Of the 46 women with implants, 35% had positive tests for anticollagen antibodies (26% to collagen I and 15% to collagen II) in comparison to 9% of healthy controls (Teuber et al., 1993). With the exception of antibodies to denatured collagen II, these differences were significant ($p < 0.05$). Rowley et al. (1994) reported anticollagen antibody reactivity among 70 women with silicone breast implants. Many of these subjects had been included in the previous study by Teuber et al. (1993). Anticollagen activity was observed in 41% of symptomatic women with breast implants in comparison to 29% of SLE patients, 48% of RA subjects, and 6% of controls (Rowley et al., 1994).

These studies indicate that some symptomatic women with breast implants may have antibodies reacting to collagen I and II. No overall consistent pattern of reactivity is apparent by Western blotting. No data were presented by this group on healthy women with silicone breast implants or on women with functional musculoskeletal complaints without breast implants. The relevance of these antibodies to clinical symptoms was not discussed. Similar results in similar patients were reported in abstract form by Simpson et al. (1994). No clear role for anticollagen antibodies is yet apparent in any connective tissue disease.

Antisilicone Antibodies

Whether individuals with silicone breast implants ever develop antibodies to silicone is relevant to the question of the immunogenicity or potential disease producing capacity of silicone. Investigation of this question has turned out to be rather difficult because of marked technical problems in constructing a reliable assay for antisilicone antibodies. Silicone itself is sticky and viscous and can bind non-specifically to proteins or surfaces. When a substrate that is naturally sticky and gummy is used, high levels of immunoglobulins will produce falsely high ELISA readings because they adhere to plates coated with such a sticky antigenic target.

Wolf et al. (1993) developed an assay for antisilicone antibodies using bovine serum albumin bound to polystyrene plates and then coated with hydroxylsilicone. Using this assay, these workers concluded that antisilicone antibodies were increased in women with silicone breast implants, and moreover, that the highest levels of antisilicone antibodies were found in implant recipients whose implants had ruptured. A control group of symptomatic women without breast implants was lacking, and whether the women studied were symptomatic or not was not reported.

Later Rose et al. (1996) employed the same type of assay to show that women with connective tissue diseases as well as women with silicone breast implants had elevated antisilicone reactivity. Rosenau et al. (1996) could not confirm the work of Wolf et al. and could not develop an ELISA test for antisilicone antibodies using a number of variations of silicone and other conditions. Others confirmed that proteins, including antibody proteins, bind non-specifically to silicone. They failed to uncover any evidence for antisilicone antibodies (Butler et al., 1996; Van Oss and Naim, 1996). Goldblum et al. (1992) provided an example of the difficulties in determining the presence of antisilicone antibodies. An initial report of antibody to silicone (Silastic) ventriculoperitoneal shunts was retracted when it was discovered that experimental and control sera both had similar IgG binding to silicone, the variable being differential modulation by albumen (Goldblum et al., 1995). Others were unable to find antisilicone antibodies in women with silicone breast implants using similar technology (Rohrich et al., 1996), including the technology of Rosenau et al. (1996) as applied to 200 women with silicone breast implants and 500 controls (Karlson et al., 1999).

Kossovsky et al. (1993) employed the DetectSil assay for sera binding to antigens which had been modified by silicone. In this assay microtiter plates were coated first with silicone and then with various self-antigens such as fibrinogen, collagen, and fibronectin prior to applying a dilution of test serum. Binding of sera to such plates without antigen was greater than binding to plates coated with antigens, which was consistent with the known sticky qualities of silicone. Other investigators attempting to produce antisilicone antibodies in animal models have not been able to do so (Naim and van Oss, 1992; Nosanchuk, 1968a). It currently appears that a reliable assay for antisilicone antibodies is not available, and the existence of antisilicone antibodies is unproven and biologically unlikely. The Centers for Disease Control and Prevention (CDC) have expressed skepticism about such diagnostic tests for silicone breast disease (CDC, 1996). For these reasons, the committee has concluded that evidence that silicone or silicone-modified proteins are antigenic and capable of eliciting an adaptive immune response is insufficient or flawed. The evidence suggests that specific antibodies are not produced in response to exposure to silicone.

Antipolymer Antibodies

In an attempt to develop an assay specific for a silicone breast implant associated disease, Tenenbaum et al. (1993a, 1997a), Gluck et al. (1996), and Wilson et al. (1999) have reported results with an antipolymer antibody test (APA). This assay is said to measure the binding of IgG to partially polymerized polyacrylamide immobilized on nitrocellulose strips (as described in Wilson et al., 1999). This is a non-silicon-containing compound; it is unlikely that it has any antigenic similarity to PDMS or other breast implant silicone compounds. In an early abstract report of APA testing of 97 symptomatic women with silicone breast implants, 19 asymptomatic women with implants, 23 healthy controls without implants and 15 women with classical connective tissue disease without implants, APA positivity was related to severity of illness (Tenenbaum et al., 1993a).

In an unblinded survey of 667 symptomatic women with breast implants, 54.4% (*N* = 343) APA positivity was subsequently reported. This was followed by a blinded study of a highly selected group of women with silicone breast implants (50% of a clinic group of implanted women was solicited, 70% of these declined to participate). Five groups of women were tested: 34 breast implant patients with limited symptoms and disability; 26 with mild problems; 16 with moderate symptoms; and 19 with advanced symptoms and functional disability; and 15 patients with classical connective tissue disease and implants. APA positives in these five cohorts were 3, 8, 44, 68, and 20%, respectively. Twenty-three healthy clinic personnel controls were 17% positive, and 10% of 20 classical connective tissue disease patients without implants were positive. Simultaneous testing for antinuclear antibodies was carried out. There was no relationship between the two assays (Tenenbaum et al., 1997a). The division of these implant patients into severity groups was subjective. Part of the study was unblinded, and the patient group appeared to be selected in unknown ways from a group already referred for problems. A number of methodological controls were absent (for example, albumen, other polymers). Similar criticisms of this work were made at the time the report appeared (Angell, 1997; Edlavitch, 1997; Korn, 1997; Lamm, 1997).

Gluck et al. (1996) followed up this study of silicone breast implant patients by testing 48 patients with fibromyalgia, 16 patients with osteoarthritis, and 14 patients with RA. Positive APA tests were observed in 48, 19, and 7% of these groups, respectively. Wilson et al. (1999) recently reported results similar to those of Gluck et al., but assessed patients for severity and found more positive APA tests in fibromyalgia patients with severe (61%) than mild (39%) disease. They concluded that the APA test may be a marker for severe fibromyalgia although the committee is not aware of any standards or criteria for grading the severity of fibromyalgia. An agency of the Dutch government found this test to be reproducible and plans to carry out investigations on its clinical implications (de Jong et al., 1998). The specificity and clinical significance of the APA assay remain to be defined, but it is unlikely that it detects antisilicone antibodies.

In addition, Praet et al. (1999) in an abstract reported that APA assay results from the United States and the Amsterdam Red Cross Blood Transfusion Services Central Laboratory in 24 women with silicone breast implants undergoing explantation matched completely. Five preoperative and eight postoperative samples were positive. There was no correlation with autoantibodies, signs of rheumatic disease, general health, implant type or capsular contracture. There appeared to be a higher frequency of APA positivity in women with extracapsular silicone leakage than in those without, and surgery itself appeared to result in more APA positives and higher circulating APA concentrations. The statistical significance of these results was not reported.

INDUCTION OF HYPERGAMMAGLOBULINEMIA BY SILICONE

Some evidence has been presented that silicone exposure may stimulate a polyclonal hypergammaglobulinemic state in some individuals. Ostermeyer-Shoaib et al. (1994) reported elevations but also some decreases in IgG levels. Primary data were not shown, so the significance of these findings is not clear. Elevations of IgG and IgM levels were reported by Brunner et al. (1996) in, respectively, 12.6% and 7.5% of 239 patients with silicone breast implants. The frequency of increases in IgG or IgM concentrations was similar in patients with gel-filled or saline implants. In this study, however, matched controls were not examined, and information about actual levels of absolute IgG or IgM was not reported, making exact correlation and analysis difficult.

In another series, no differences in immunoglobulin levels between women with or without breast implants were found (Bridges et al., 1993a). The well controlled analysis of blood samples from the Nurses' Health Study by Karlson et al. (1999) also found no increases in IgA, IgG or IgM levels in 50 women with implants compared to 50 healthy control women without implants. Additional studies of immunoglobulin levels with some elevations (Garland et al., 1996; Silverman et al., 1996a) are discussed in relation to multiple myeloma in Chapter 9. In summary, the data on immunoglobulin levels are inconsistent, but a controlled study of an apparently random group of women did not find elevations in women with breast implants compared to matched controls.

In this connection, several groups are currently in the process of studying whether subjects with silicone breast implants are more likely than the general public to develop multiple myeloma, a lethal malignant proliferation of monoclonal plasma cells considered to be a cancerous condition. Previous animal studies by Potter et al. (1994) have demonstrated that certain susceptible strains of mice develop intraperitoneal plasmacytomas in a high proportion of instances after exposure to silicone gel from breast implants, but this is not necessarily a model for human multiple myeloma as noted in Chapter 9. Silverman et al. (1996a) reported three cases of multiple myeloma in women with silicone breast implants. These women were found among 34 patients seen in the myeloma clinic at University of California at Los Angeles (UCLA) representing 5.9% of the clinic population. In subsequent studies of different larger cohorts of women with (N = 108) and without (N = 176) breast implants, elevated immunoglobulin levels and five instances of monoclonal gammopathy were detected. Monoclonal gammopathies disappeared in two women after removal of their implants, in a third there was no change after explantation, and two women were not retested. These preliminary reports raise the possibility that silicone implants may increase the risk of monoclonal gammopathy and/or multiple myeloma (Silverman et al., 1996a). However, since benign monoclonal gammopathy is relatively frequent in the healthy population (Kyle, 1996), and since several case series and epidemiological studies do not confirm these findings, these reports provide insufficient evidence for an association (see Chapter 8).

CONCLUSIONS

Based on the data available, the committee concludes that there is no convincing evidence to support clinically significant immunologic effects of silicone or silicone breast implants. This includes: insufficient evidence for an association of a particular HLA type in women with breast implants and health conditions; insufficient evidence for silicone as a superantigen; insufficient or flawed evidence that silicone produces immune activation of cells of the immune system, silicone antibodies, delayed type hypersensitivity to silicone, cytokines as an immune response, antigen specific immune cellular infiltrates; and insufficient evidence for autoantibodies or T-cell self antigen activation. The paucity of significant, well controlled studies examining these questions is responsible for these conclusions. The committee finds that there is conclusive evidence that some silicones have adjuvant activity, but there is no evidence that this has any clinical significance. The committee has also concluded that evidence from experimental studies of the immunology of silicone does not support, or lend biologic plausibility to, associations of silicone breast implants with immune related human health conditions.

7

Antinuclear Antibodies and Silicone Breast Implants

A number of investigators have explored the frequency and titers of antinuclear antibodies (ANAs) in women with or without signs and symptoms of illness and silicone (almost always gel-filled) breast implants. These investigators have compared findings of ANAs in women with implants to findings in control groups of women, some matched by age, some concurrent, some historical, some healthy and some with similar rheumatic-like signs and symptoms. Some investigators have reported increased frequency and increased titers of ANAs in women with implants and have speculated about the implications of this finding for autoimmune disease or other immunological reactions that might result from exposure to silicone breast implants. Other investigators have not found any difference in ANA titers between otherwise similar groups of women with or without breast implants and have concluded that there is no relationship between implants and autoantibodies. Many of these studies suffer from methodological flaws, discussed below, which call into question their results or interpretations (Bar-Meir et al., 1995; Blackburn et al., 1997; Bridges et al., 1993a, 1996; Brunner et al., 1996; Claman and Robertson, 1994, 1996; Cuéllar et al., 1995a,b; Edworthy et al., 1998; Freundlich et al., 1994; Gabriel et al., 1994; Karlson et al., 1999; Lewy and Ezrailson, 1996; Miller et al., 1998; Ostermayer-Shoaib et al., 1994; Park et al., 1998; Peters et al., 1994a, 1997; Press et al., 1992; Rowley et al., 1994; Silverman et al., 1996b; Smalley et al., 1995c; Solomon, 1994a; Tenenbaum et al., 1997a; Teuber et al., 1993; Vasey et al., 1994; Young et al., 1995b, 1996; Zazgornik et al., 1996).

TECHNICAL CONSIDERATIONS NECESSARY TO INTERPRET REPORTED ANA TITERS

An understanding of the prevalence and titers of ANAs in various subsets of the population of normal individuals, and of the effects that different technical factors may have on measurement of these antibodies, is important to the interpretation of ANA results from study populations of symptomatic and asymptomatic women with silicone breast implants. The type of tissue that is used as the substrate (antigen) in the performance of the ANA test can affect the frequency of positive tests at all titers. In the mid-1980s and early 1990s, laboratories used frozen sections of mouse or rat liver as the test substrate. More recently, human tissue culture cells, such as HEp-2 cells, have replaced animal liver (or kidney) sections. Prevalence and titers of ANAs are higher when tissue culture cells, rather than mouse liver, are used as a substrate (Fritzler et al., 1985; McCarty et al., 1984). Hollingsworth et al. (1996) reported results of comparative ANA testing of 106 healthy females and 91 healthy males. There were more positive tests at all titers when HEp-2 cells were used than when rat liver was used. Also, the prevalence was nearly twice as high in normal women as in men (Hollingsworth et al., 1996). Measurements in controls using mouse or rat liver (or other tissues) cannot be compared to values from women with breast implants using human tissue culture cells.

There are differing views on what titer and what intensity of fluorescence constitute a positive ANA test. Reports of ANA prevalence in women with breast implants have not always used the same criteria to define positivity. Furthermore, differences in the performance of the ANA test and in the results obtained are common across different laboratories. These factors make it essential that studies use the same laboratory at the same time for ANA assays of experimental and control women. Strongly positive ANA tests in women with implants who have connective tissue disease undoubtedly reflect the disease. These positive ANA tests should not be ascribed to the presence of the implants. Moreover, studies from investigators with a special interest in autoantibodies or a particular connective tissue disease may have attracted a nonrepresentative group of women with implants and with connective tissue disease.

ANTINUCLEAR ANTIBODIES IN NORMAL INDIVIDUALS

In 1997, an important analysis of ANAs in normal sera was carried out by a subcommittee of the International Union of Immunological Societies' Standardization Committee (Tan et al., 1997). The objective of this study, carried out in 15 laboratories from around the world, was specification of the range of ANA titers in normal individuals and in patients with connective tissue disease. Centers for Disease Control and Prevention (CDC) reference sera for ten specific ANAs and normal serum samples in four adult age categories were provided to the laboratories. At 1:40 dilution, 31.7% of normals had a positive ANA test; at 1:80, 13.3%; at 1:160, 5%; and at 1:320, 3.3%. Results did not differ significantly across the four age categories. This absence of increasing ANA positivity with age has been reported, though infrequently, by others (Juby et al., 1994). In addition, a group of patients with soft-tissue rheumatism was studied. At a titer of 1:40, 38.5% were positive, and 23.1% were positive at a titer of 1:80. This is the kind of group whose ANA results should be compared with those reported for symptomatic women with implants who do not have a defined connective tissue disease. In contrast, nearly all patients with systemic lupus erythematosus (SLE) were positive at greater than 1:40 dilution, with the vast majority positive at 1:320. This study also found a wide variation in results across laboratories, even when the same test antigens and the same definition of positivity were used. Presumably, this was due to a number of factors, including different reagents, different skills and training of technicians, and variation in the number and sources of control sera, among others. The authors concluded that normal individuals could be successfully (but not perfectly) differentiated from those with SLE, scleroderma, and Sjogren's syndrome. Moreover, the cutoff titer of 1:160 appeared to provide an acceptable balance between sensitivity and specificity.

Gender and age affect the prevalence of ANAs in the normal population. Women are more commonly ANA positive than men (Fritzler et al., 1985; Thomas and Robinson, 1993). Most studies have shown that the prevalence of ANAs also increases with age. Slater et al. (1996) analyzed the results of ANA testing in a consecutive sample of 1,010 patients over a ten-month period. Patients 64 years of age or older had a statistically higher prevalence of ANAs. Of interest is that 23% of patients with neurologic symptoms had a positive ANA test, as did 10% of patients with constitutional symptoms. In this study, the overall false-positive rate for ANAs was 79%, that is, 79% of positives occurred in persons without defined disease (Slater et al., 1996). The age effect is also illustrated by a study of 3,492 Australians, representing more than 90% of the population of a small town, in whom the frequency of positive ANAs was 1.5% in the 31–40 year age group, but increased progressively to 13.5% in the 71–75 year age group (Hooper et al., 1972). Additional reports of high ANA values in normal populations or, particularly, increasing values with age include those of de Vlam et al. (1993); Fritzler et al. (1985); Ruffatti et al. (1990); and Xavier et al. (1995). These reports and the report by Tan et al. noted earlier cite frequencies of positive ANA tests ranging up to 31%

depending on the age of the population and the titers that are used as criteria for positivity. Some studies have also suggested that women with breast cancer may have elevated ANAs (Klajman et al., 1983; Turnbull et al., 1978); in a Japanese population, a prevalence of 15% was reported (Imai et al., 1979).

The committee finds that ANA testing is a complex and variable technology. The performance of studies and the interpretation of results require consideration of a number of variables and confounding factors, as noted above. In addition, some studies of ANA prevalence in women with silicone breast implants suffer from inadequate reporting of the details of the test technology and criteria for a positive test; inadequate descriptions of the signs, symptoms, and presence of defined connective tissue disease in some of the test populations; biased ascertainment of women with implants; inadequate descriptions or absence of control populations; uncertainty regarding adequate blinding of those who perform the assays; and questions of proper matching of control groups, among others. The result has been studies with conflicting findings, which often have flaws suggesting that the results are questionable or, through lack of information, cannot be interpreted with confidence.

ANTINUCLEAR ANTIBODIES IN WOMEN WITH SILICONE BREAST IMPLANTS

The committee reviewed 30 studies from the scientific literature on the subject of ANAs in women with silicone breast implants. Although information in some of these was substantially lacking, and some were also extensions of previous reports, they are discussed briefly for the sake of completeness. Press et al. (1992) studied 24 women referred for rheumatic complaints who had either silicone breast implants (N = 22), silicone injections (N = 1) or both (N = 1). A defined connective tissue disease was diagnosed in 11 of the 24 patients. There also were four patients with fibromyalgia, four with chronic fatigue syndrome, four with myalgias, and one with arthralgia. An ANA titer of 1:80 or more was found in 91% of the patients with defined connective tissue disease. ANAs were present in 54% of the group with symptoms but with no connective tissue disease. This study did not include three important control groups: (1) women with implants without rheumatic complaints or a defined connective tissue disease; (2) age-matched normal women without implants; and (3) symptomatic age-matched women without implants. The presence of a defined connective tissue disease in nearly half of the women studied and of rheumatic signs, symptoms, and conditions associated with ANAs in the remainder make the data very difficult to interpret (Press et al., 1992).

Bridges et al. (1993a) found that 22% of 156 symptomatic women with implants had an ANA titer of 1:80 or more; rheumatoid factor was found in 9%. Of 95 of these patients who had joint and muscle pain, 15% had positive ANAs; 22% of 32 who had joint swelling were positive; and 45% of 29 who had a defined connective tissue disease were positive. From a review of the literature and 401 patients presented in abstracts at the 1992 American College of Rheumatology Meeting, Bridges identified 5% of mostly symptomatic patients with silicone breast implants and specific autoantibodies, such as anti-Ro and anti-La, anti-Scl-70, anti-Sm, and anti-dsDNA. Positive ANA titers were found in 25% of a sex- and age-matched control group of 174 fibromyalgia patients. In contrast, only 8% of 12 women with implants without rheumatic complaints had ANA titers of 1:80 or more (Bridges et al., 1993a). Bridges and Lorden (1993) also failed to find significant elevations of ANAs in women with breast implants and sicca syndrome. In a subsequent report, Bridges et al. described 500 consecutive women with implants referred to rheumatologists, 25 age-matched controls, 25 asymptomatic women with implants, and 100 women with fibromyalgia. These women were tested for ANAs as previously reported. It is not clear whether there was any overlap of patients in the two reports, however. Of the symptomatic women with implants, 150 of 500 (30%) were positive. Positive ANA tests were obtained from 8% of the controls; 28% of the asymptomatic women with implants, and 25% of the fibromyalgia patients. A speckled or nucleolar pattern of ANA fluorescence was more frequently, but not more significantly, found in women with implants, as were very high titers in women with implants (7%) compared to normal controls (0%). This study concluded that patients with implants and those with fibromyalgia were significantly more likely to be ANA positive than normal women without implants (Bridges et al., 1996).

Teuber et al. (1993) studied 57 consecutive patients, self-referred in 1992 because of concerns about their implants. After the exclusion of eleven women with previous exposure to bovine collagen, 46 women with implants were age matched with 45 control women from the same geographical area. Implants were in place for a mean of 13.5 years, primarily for augmentation. Many of the women with implants were symptomatic, and one patient had SLE; one primary biliary cirrhosis; one small vessel vasculitis; and two had polyarthritis with ANAs. ANAs were measured using HEp-2 cells and were considered positive at titers of 1:80 or more. Of the 57 patients, 16 (35%) had a positive ANA and 11% had titers of 1:320 or more. This study was carried out only on patients preselected for symptoms or a defined connective tissue disease, and data on the prevalence of ANAs in the 45 normal control women were not reported (Teuber et al., 1993). In 1994, the same group of investigators reported on epitope mapping of antibodies to collagen found in women with implants. This study included most of the women previously reported, except those with defined connective tissue disease. ANAs were found in 19 of 70 patients at a titer of 1:80 or more. Again, no data on controls were reported (Rowley et al., 1994).

ANA testing of 200 consecutive self-referred patients concerned about their silicone gel breast implants was reported by Peters et al. (1994a). Controls were 100 consecutive women without implants referred for a variety of plastic surgery procedures. A group of 29 patients with surgically confirmed ruptured silicone gel implants was also studied. Specific autoantibodies were studied if ANAs were positive. Testing was on HEp-2 cells, and a titer of 1:100 was considered positive. Of the 200 implant patients, 4 had a defined connective tissue disease. A positive ANA test was found in 26.5% of 200 breast implant patients, 28% of controls, and 17.2% of 29 patients with ruptured implants. Titers of ANAs did not differ among the groups. Controls in this study were from the same plastic surgery practice, all patients were examined by rheumatologists, and ANAs were similar in experimental and control groups. However, the patients were a self-referred group, and ANA positivity in the control group was higher than usual (Peters et al., 1994a). This Toronto group also reported a follow-up of 100 consecutive patients requesting explantation of their gel-filled breast implants, many of whom were presumably included in the 1994 report. The same control group of women appears to have been used. In this group of highly concerned, self-selected, more symptomatic women, four of whom had connective tissue disease and ten of whom had fibromyalgia, the prevalence of ANAs was 24%, compared to 28% in the control group, and titers did not differ between the groups. ANA results after explantation would have been of interest, although the authors report that, with one exception, their patients' clinical status remained the same or deteriorated rather than improved over more than two years of observation after removal of their implants (Peters, 1997).

Claman and Robertson (1994) studied 131 women with breast implants and 19 healthy controls. The women with implants included 38 who felt healthy, 82 who had various symptoms, and 11 who had defined connective tissue diseases. ANA assays used HEp-2 cells. Fluorescence of 1+ or greater and a titer of 1:256 or more were considered positive. No positive ANAs were found in healthy women; 18% of asymptomatic women, 26% of symptomatic women, and 64% of women with implants and a defined connective tissue disease were positive. There was no correlation between presence of a positive ANA and type of implant, indication for implantation, duration of implantation or implant rupture. The controls in this study were not age matched, and there were only 19 healthy controls to compare with 131 implanted women with an array of different health conditions (Claman and Robertson, 1994). These authors reported an extension of their work in 1996, in which they tested 37 healthy control women and compared them with 75 asymptomatic women with silicone breast implants. ANA technology was the same except that a titer of 1:80 was considered positive. In this report, 3% of controls and 27% of women with implants were positive, a significant difference between the control and experimental groups (Claman and Robertson, 1996).

Cuéllar et al. (1995a) analyzed data from 300 patients (298 women) referred with a variety of musculoskeletal and other complaints. Of these, 24 had saline implants, the rest were gel-filled, but results were not sorted by type of implant. A positive ANA was defined as fluorescence of 2+ or greater on HEp-2 cells at a titer of 1:40 or more. By these criteria, 123 of 265 patients tested (46.4%) had positive ANAs. Of these patients, 185 were diagnosed as having a defined or undifferentiated connective tissue disease, fibromyalgia, or other rheumatic-like conditions. The report does not allow assignment of ANA results to any of the poorly defined categories of patients, so the data are difficult to interpret (Cuéllar et al., 1995a).

In a follow-up, the same group reported a cohort of 813 patients (810 women), including the 300 reported earlier. This report also identified 264 women without breast implants referred for ANA testing who were approximately equally divided between those with fibromyalgia and those with soft-tissue rheumatism. These women served as a control population. It is uncertain whether or how they were matched, although the mean ages of the experimental and control groups were very close. ANA assays were done using mouse kidney or HEp-2 cells. A positive test was considered fluorescence of 2+ or greater and a titer of 1:64 or more for mouse kidney and 3+ or greater fluorescence at a titer of 1:40 or more for HEp-2 cells. Most patients, 470 (57.8%), were positive using human cells as substrate, and 244 (30%) patients were positive using mouse kidney as substrate. It is not clear how the use of these different technologies was distributed between the patient and the control groups. Positive ANAs were found in 7.6% of the control population. This report also describes a selected group of women. Very little information is available on the health conditions of these women, but presumably this population consists of a number of implant patients with various connective tissue and other rheumatic-like diseases as did the original 300-patient cohort (Cuéllar et al., 1995b). As a result, conclusions on the relationship between implants and ANAs cannot be drawn from these reports.

A group of 3,380 women with silicone breast implants, self-, physician-, or attorney-referred to two physicians for evaluation relative to injury claims, was tested by a commercial testing laboratory (Roche Biomedical Labs, Burlington, N.C.) using HEp-2 cells. The prevalence of

ANAs with titers of 1:40 or more was 22%. A historical, non-concurrent, unmatched control with ANA prevalence of 5% was used. These patients complained of fatigue (83%), joint and muscle pain (83%), chest or breast pain (81%), burning of the extremities, numbness (80%), and other symptoms. The authors also found a correlation of ANAs with duration of implantation and with serum immunoglobulin G concentrations (Lewy and Ezrailson, 1996). This study reports a highly selected group of symptomatic women with low-titer ANAs and no appropriate control group.

Bar-Meir et al. (1995) studied the prevalence of 20 different antinuclear autoantibodies in the sera of 116 women with breast implants of whom 11 were caucasian. Of these women with implants, 30 had a history of implant rupture and 29 had contractures. They were compared with 134 age- and sex-matched controls. The prevalence of 15 of 20 specific ANAs was significantly higher in the silicone breast implant group than in controls. This study has incomplete data on the race of the controls, no information about how subjects were selected, and no specificity controls. The occurrence of more than twice as many patients with anti-La as with anti-Ro antibodies is unusual (Mattioli and Reichlin, 1974; Wasicek and Reichlin, 1982). Likewise, the presence of anti-Sm and anti-Scl-70 antibodies, despite the fact that only one patient each had SLE and scleroderma, suggests that there may have been false positives. In a subsequent abstract report, these U.S. and Israeli groups compared 86 asymptomatic women with implants with these 116 women and reported increased titers of 13 antinuclear autoantibodies in 2%–13% of the asymptomatic group. They concluded that anti-La antibodies were increased in both groups (Zandman-Goddard et al., 1996).

Zazgornik et al. (1996) studied 36 nonselected women with implants (77% gel filled) and 36 age-matched controls in Vienna, Austria. A positive ANA, defined as a titer of 1:80 or more using mouse liver substrate, was found in 8% of controls and 33% of women with implants (a third of these were saline or PVP [polyvinylpyrrolidone] filled). Only one of the women with implants had clinical musculoskeletal symptoms, but 29 were breast cancer patients (versus only 2 of the controls), which may have affected the results of this small study (Zazgornik et al., 1996).

Lack of information on ANA technology, deficient controls, use of less stringent (low titer) or undefined criteria for ANA positivity, and biased selection of patients handicap the interpretation of studies by Freundlich et al. (1994); Ostermayer-Shoaib et al. (1994); Silverman et al. (1996b); Smalley (1995c); Solomon (1994a); and Vasey et al. (1994). Ostermayer-Shoaib et al. (1994) reported a prevalence of ANAs in symptomatic patients with breast implants of 36%. ANA assay methods are not described, nor is there information about the titers of these antibodies or their frequency in control sera. This cohort was apparently largely self- or attorney referred (Ostermayer-Shoaib et al., 1994). Silverman et al. (1996b) studied 3,184 consecutive symptomatic, self- and attorney-referred patients with breast implants, 40 age-matched controls, 37 asymptomatic women with breast implants, and 200 consecutive fibromyalgia patients without implants from Arizona and California. ANAs were performed using HEp-2 cells. Positives were determined at titers of 1:80 or more. The prevalence of ANAs was 35% in symptomatic women with implants, 28% in fibromyalgia patients, 3% in asymptomatic women with breast implants and 5% in healthy controls. The small number of control patients, the potential selection bias, and the absence of mean age and other demographic data are problems in this study. The study results suggest that ANAs may be more closely associated with fibromyalgia, which is also suggested by the results of Claman and Robertson and Bridges (Silverman et al., 1996b). Freundlich et al. (1994) reported 50 self- or attorney-referred women with breast implants who had medical complaints. Some of these patients had defined connective tissue disease. Positive ANAs were detected in 24% of those patients. The titer used to define a positive test was not stated (Freundlich et al., 1994).

A similar study was reported by Vasey et al. (1994) in which 50 patients with symptoms and some (ca. 20%) with definite rheumatic disease were studied. No control group was assembled. An ANA titer of 1:20 was considered positive. Of these women with implants, 13 (26%) were positive (Vasey et al., 1994). Another uncontrolled study of symptomatic women mainly attorney referred was reported by Solomon (1994a) in which 44 of 176 (25%) women with implants had an ANA titer of 1:40 or more. Smalley et al. (1995c) described the presence of ANAs in sera from 231 symptomatic women with silicone gel implants. Symptoms included fatigue, arthralgias, myalgias, joint swelling, sicca syndrome, hair loss, atypical rashes, poor memory, and other symptoms "similar to and consistent with those reported by Bridges et al. (1993a)." ANAs were assayed on HEp-2 cells and tested at an initial titer of 1:40. Positive ANAs were found in 27.7% of patients. No information was provided regarding the presence of a defined rheumatic disease in these patients or whether they were examined by a rheumatologist, and there was no concurrent control group (Smalley et al., 1995c).

Young et al. (1995b, 1996) reported ANA titers in a study of human leukocyte antigen (HLA) types in four groups of women: Group I, 77 symptomatic women (primarily myalgia or arthralgia and fatigue) with breast implants; group II, 37 asymptomatic women with implants; group III, 54 healthy female volunteers; and group IV, 31 women with fibromyalgia with implants. ANA assays were performed using HEp-2 cells. A titer of 1:40 or more was considered positive. ANA titers of 1:80 or more were found in 24% of 58 symptomatic breast implant patients tested. Only

5 of 37 asymptomatic women with implants were studied, and they were negative. Sera from 11 of 31 women with fibromyalgia were tested, and 2 (18%) were positive. There was no relationship between ANA positivity and implant rupture or capsular contracture. The authors noted that there was a patient with SLE in group I. This study is of interest primarily for HLA and other data. The ANA tests were not part of the study and were carried out at patient (or patient insurance) expense; thus, there were no control sera available for ANA testing (Young et al., 1995b, 1996).

Brunner et al. (1996) surveyed 581 women who had had breast reconstruction or augmentation with implants in Munich, Germany. Of 239 who responded, six had an ANA titer of 1:80 or more. On clinical evaluation, 33.4% of the women were found to have some rheumatic symptoms (Brunner et al., 1996). In a study reported by Blackburn et al. (1997) of a small, selected group of women with implants, 70 patients referred for complaints or concerns were examined by rheumatologists, and a series of immunologic studies was performed; 5 of 58 (8.6%) patients tested had a positive ANA titer (1:40 or more). A control group was not assembled. Clinically, 3 of the 70 patients had a defined connective tissue disease (Blackburn et al., 1997).

One-half of approximately 370 consecutive silicone breast implant recipients attending a rheumatology practice between April and September 1994 were asked to enroll in a study, as were 40 nonrecipients with defined connective tissue disease. A significant number of women (N = 259, 70%) declined to participate as did 20 of the patients with connective tissue disease without implants. A control group of 23 women was recruited. The 95 participating implant recipients who did not meet criteria for a defined connective tissue disease were classified into four groups by severity of symptoms, from limited or mild to moderate or advanced, and by functional capacity, from normal to incapacitated. More than 90% of the women with implants reported fatigue and arthralgias, however, suggesting that those who participated were a selected group. There were 34 patients with limited symptoms and normal functional capacity, 26 with mild symptoms and functional incapacity, 16 with moderate symptoms and functional incapacity, and 19 with advanced symptoms and functional incapacity. Women with ANA titers of 1:40 or more in the four groups were 18, 19, 0, and 32%, respectively. Of controls, 4 (17%) were positive, and 14 (70%) of the patients with connective tissue disease without implants were positive. Overall, 26% of implanted women (compared to 17% of controls) had positive ANA tests. This study used an experimental group that appears selected (30% participation), used a control group of non-age-matched clinic personnel, had no symptomatic control group, and did not find a statistically significant difference between the women with implants and the controls (Tenenbaum et al., 1997a).

Park et al. (1998) studied 110 women in Scotland with breast implants for augmentation, of whom none had ANA titers of 1:40 or more, compared with three positive women in a group of 128 age-matched controls attending the plastic surgery outpatient clinic. In a group of 207 women with implant reconstructions after cancer mastectomy, 5 were positive compared with 4 of 88 control women who had had mastectomy for cancer without reconstruction. In this appropriately controlled study without apparent selection bias, no increase in ANA positivity was found in the women with breast implants even though human tissue culture cells were used and a titer of only 1:40 or more was considered positive (Park et al., 1998).

A Prospective Study

A recent publication by Miller et al. describes a study carried out from 1985 to 1998 of 414 women with saline- or gel-filled implants for reconstruction or augmentation. The study was designed to monitor any changes over time in the immune status of patients with breast implants by measuring rheumatoid factor, antistreptolysin O titers, C-reactive protein, and ANAs. Only the 218 patients who had these assays performed both before and after implantation are reported. Patients were divided approximately equally between into two groups, a gel implant and a saline implant group. The mean duration of follow-up for the gel implant group was 5.77 years (range 1 to 25 years), and the mean duration of follow-up for the saline implant group was 1.99 years (range 0 to 3.64 years). Positive ANAs were found in 3.57% of the silicone gel implanted patients before, and 4.16% after, implantation. In the saline implanted group, 14.15% were positive preoperatively, and 16.98% after implantation, a difference that is not statistically significant. The other measurements also were not significantly different statistically before and after implantation. The difference in values in the silicone gel and saline implant patients may reflect a change in the method of performing the ANA test, that is, using different substrates, as noted earlier. This cannot be confirmed because the methods section of the report does not describe the method for ANA assay or the criteria for a positive test. The more recent use of HEp-2 cells, which result in higher titers, may coincide with the more recent use of saline implants, however. This study is the only one of its kind discovered by the committee. The failure to obtain before-and-after samples on almost half the patients suggests a somewhat ad hoc approach, and the lack of information on ANA testing technology is an important omission. The follow-up period, especially for the saline group, was critically short also. Nevertheless, this report provides important prospective information on antinuclear autoantibody reactions to the stimulus of gel and saline breast implants in patients with a previously defined ANA status. The study also presents an interesting reverse perspective (i.e., changes after placement of implants) from the scattered, anecdotal reports of changes, some increasing and some decreasing, in ANA test results after implant removal. The similarity of results with saline and gel implants is also notable (Miller et al., 1998).

ANA and Autoantibody Analysis in Epidemiological Cohort Studies

The medical records of all women with silicone breast implants in Olmsted County, Minnesota, were reviewed by Gabriel et al. (1994). Patients were divided into those with prophylactic mastectomy (90), those with cancer mastectomy (125), and those who had implants for augmentation (534). Almost all implants were gel filled. A positive ANA test was found in 11 of a cohort of 749 women with implants and in 27 of 1,498 healthy controls (a rate ratio of 0.86, 95% confidence interval [CI], 0.42–1.70), but titers were not reported. This is a thorough review of an unbiased cohort of women by a highly regarded epidemiologic group. However, ANA determinations were performed over a number of years, probably by differing technologies and undoubtedly by different personnel, and may not be comparable (Gabriel et al., 1994).

Edworthy et al. (1998) carried out a cohort study of women with cosmetic silicone breast implants between 1978 and 1986 identified through the procedural codes of the Alberta, Canada, Health Registry. Controls were women having other cosmetic surgery. Of the women with implants, about 22% had received only saline-filled silicone implants. Of those women who provided blood samples, 324 of 1,426 (22.7%) had a positive ANA by criteria of greater than 1+ fluorescence and a titer of 1:40 or more, compared with 162 of 649 (25.6%) of the control women. A significant fraction of the total 9,200 implantations recorded were lost because of missing addresses and refusal to participate, and this study was carried out during active litigation by claimants of silicone injury. These factors raise questions of potential selection in the experimental group. Nevertheless, this study has a large cohort of women with implants and controls without known selection bias who were evaluated clinically and for ANAs in a blinded fashion (Edworthy et al., 1998).

A further analysis of the cohort from the Nurses' Health Study reported by Sánchez-Guerrero et al. (1995a,b) and discussed in Chapter 8, was carried out by Karlson et al. (1999). In 1988, 32,826 women from the group of 121,701 female nurses enrolled in the Nurses' Health Study in 1976 provided 30 ml blood samples each. From the response to a 1992 questionnaire sent to all women in the study, 1,863 women with breast implants of all kinds placed before the date of blood collection were identified as described by Sánchez-Guerrero et al. (1995a,b). Of 288 women from this cohort of 1,863 women with breast implants who did not have connective tissue disease or cancer and who had provided a blood sample, 200 women were chosen randomly. Their average age was 53.6 years at the time of blood sample, and their clinical status was unknown.

Antinuclear antibodies, specific autoantibodies, including anti-ssDNA, anti-dsDNA, anti-Sm, anti-RNP, anti-SSA (Ro), anti-SSB (La), anti-SCL-70, rheumatoid factor, and antisilicone antibodies (according to Rosenau et al., 1996) were measured in the women with implants and compared with measurements in four age-matched control groups taken from the Nurses' Health Study cohort that had provided blood samples. These groups consisted of 200 healthy women without breast implants; 100 women with insulin dependent diabetes mellitus (presumably exposed to silicone, see discussion in Chapter 4, Chantelau et al., 1986; Collier and Dawson, 1985); 100 women with defined connective tissue disease; and 100 women with at least one documented symptom or sign of connective tissue disease. Further testing for complement (C3, C4), C-reactive protein, quantitative IgG, IgA and IgM and anti-thyroglobulin, anti-cardiolipin and anti-microsomal antibody was carried out on a random 25% of all tested women. All tests were performed by blinded laboratory personnel.

A positive ANA assay, defined as a titer equal to or greater than 1:40 using HEp-2 cells, was observed in 14% of the women with implants—6% (95% CI, 1–13%) lower than in the healthy controls (20%) and 26% (95% CI, 14–36%) lower than in the control women with connective tissue disease (39%). Positive ANA assays in the women with diabetes were not significantly different (15%), and in women with connective tissue disease signs and symptoms were higher (37%). Antibody to ssDNA was significantly higher (p = 0.02) in women with implants (41%) than in healthy women (29%), a 12% (95% CI, 3–21%) difference. All other antibodies, complement, and immunoglobulin levels were not elevated in women with implants compared to healthy control women without implants. No antisilicone antibodies were detected in any of the 700 women. Additional studies of 17 women with silicone breast implants and definite or self-reported connective tissue disease were not revealing, except that this group had significantly (p = 0.02) lower anti-ssDNA (12%) than the original 200 women with breast implants. There were no differences among women with saline, gel, polyurethane, or double-lumen implants (Karlson et al., 1999).

Antibody to ssDNA is found in normals at low prevalence and is elevated in a variety of connective tissue diseases and inflammatory or infectious conditions. The significance of this antibody in these women is unknown. Clinical data are not available, elevations were not confirmed in women with implants and self-reported or definite connective tissue disease, and (in an abstract) Simpson et al. (1994) reported no difference in anti-ssDNA between 40 symptomatic women with silicone breast implants and 40 healthy control women without implants. This study provides evidence against an association between silicone breast implants and ANAs or other autoantibodies, except ssDNA. This cohort appears to be unbiased, laboratory examinations were carried out according to carefully defined techniques with attention to quality control and in blinded fashion, and several appropriate control groups from the same large group of women were analyzed in an equally blinded and careful way at the same time (Karlson et al., 1999).

SPECIFIC ANTINUCLEAR AUTOANTIBODIES IN NORMALS AND THE PREDICTIVE VALUE OF A POSITIVE AUTOANTIBODY TEST

In 1989, a study of autoantibodies in 506 sera randomly selected from 5,000 blood samples from healthy women of childbearing age in the Negev that were drawn for a study of viral antibodies was reported. Sixty women were found to have autoantibodies against at least one of ten nuclear antigens, including anti-ssDNA, anti-dsDNA, anti-La, anti-Ro, anti-Sm, and anticardiolipin. Of these women, 57 were evaluated after five years to see whether an autoimmune disease had developed. None was found to have overt autoimmune disease although 7 of the 57 had symptoms associated with rheumatic diseases such as Raynaud's phenomenon, arthritis, or multiple abortions (Yadin et al., 1989). One study showed that ANA-positive healthy women rarely (less than 1%) develop SLE, and another found that no women with highly positive ANAs developed overt disease and only 12% had any symptoms after five years of follow-up (Aho et al., 1992; Schoenfeld and Isenberg, 1989). Anticentromere antibodies are rarely present in normal individuals (Lee et al., 1993; Rothfield, 1998, unpublished data on 898 patients), but they may be found in patients with Raynaud's phenomenon. The presence of either antitopoisomerase I or anticentromere antibodies was associated with a 163-fold increased chance of developing a connective tissue disease. Gaither et al. (1987) reported that about 17% of normal sera have elevated titers of anti-Ro by enzyme linked immunosorbent assay (ELISA).

In a study potentially relevant to the finding of ANAs in symptomatic women with breast implants, Clegg et al. (1991) using mouse liver and kidney and HEp-2 cells and titers of 1:32 or more, reported 205 patients with either isolated Raynaud's phenomenon or unexplained polyarthritis, or undifferentiated connective tissue disease and found ANA positives of 55, 57 and 59%, respectively. When seen five years later, these patients generally remained the same or, in a few cases had remitted, but about 20% had progressed to defined connective tissue disease (Williams et al., 1998), indicating that frequent elevated ANAs may suggest future health problems in some groups of patients. In general, as discussed here, ANAs are also present in normal women and in the elderly, and can be associated with a number of conditions as a laboratory finding without heralding the onset of autoimmune disease.

SPECIFIC ANTINUCLEAR ANTIBODIES AND RHEUMATOID FACTOR IN WOMEN WITH IMPLANTS

Peters et al. (1994a) studied anti-Ro, anti-La, anti-Sm, anti-Scl-70 and anti-RNP antinuclear autoantibodies using an ELISA technique, but no details of the antigens used are given. In ANA-positive women with implants, anti-Ro was positive in 33.9%, anti-La in 11.3%, anti-Scl-70 in 20.7%, anti-Sm in 9.4%, and anti-RNP in 5.6%. Comparable results in ANA-positive control women were 35.7, 3.5, 10.7, 7.3, and 3.5%, respectively. These data are most unusual in the very high prevalence of (and differences in) anti-Ro and anti-La in patients and controls and in the very high prevalence of anti-Scl-70 and anti-Sm in controls and patients without SLE or scleroderma (Peters et al., 1994a). The strengths and weakness of this study have been noted earlier.

In a study of 231 symptomatic women with silicone gel breast implants, Smalley et al. (1995c) found that 5.2% had anti-DNA antibodies using an ELISA test and 20.5% had rheumatoid factor by nephelometry. No controls were reported. The authors interpreted Western blot bands at 105 and 70 kDa (kilodaltons) as being anti-Scl-70 (antitopoisomerase-I). Other bands were interpreted as reacting with other autoantigens such as Ku and Ro. There were no supporting data in which the sera reacting with certain bands were reacted with specific autoantigens. The authors did not use standardized reference sera containing specific autoantibodies such as anti-opoisomerase I or anti-Ro as controls, which are available from the CDC.

Cuéllar et al. (1995b) reported a study of 470 ANA-positive sera in which other autoantibodies, anti-dsDNA, anti-Ro, anti-La, and anti-Scl-70, were studied. Anti-dsDNA was found in six patients by indirect immunofluorescence and in six by ELISA. Anti-Ro was found in six, anti-La in four, anti-RNP in one and anti-Scl-70 in one. Anticentromere antibodies were seen by indirect immunofluorescence on HEp-2 cells in five patients. The difficulties in evaluating this study were noted earlier. Lewy and Ezrailson (1996) found anti-dsDNA autoantibodies in 17.13% of their patients, but no details of methods used were given, and there was no control group. In the report of Bridges et al. (1996), 19 patients were positive for anti-Ro, and of these, 9 were also positive for anti-La. One patient each had anti-Ro and anti-Scl-70 antibodies. Five patients had anti-RNP antibodies, one had anti-dsDNA antibodies, and one had anti-Sm antibodies. None of the normal controls, asymptomatic breast implant patients, or fibromyalgia patients was positive. This report used controls of three types, although they were not age matched. A high ANA prevalence was reported in fibromyalgia patients, and there was no information on the presence of defined connective tissue disease in the 500 symptomatic breast implant patients. Very high, specific antinuclear autoantibody prevalences were found in the previously discussed study by Bar-Meir et al. (1994). In fact the percentage of women with breast implants and at least one autoantibody (84%) was strikingly higher than in the other reports cited here.

Gabriel et al. (1994) found a similar prevalence of rheumatoid factor in implant patients and controls (both 0.5%); no difference in prevalence of antimicrosomal antibodies was found. In their large multisite study, Silverman et al. (1996b) found 13.5% of 392 ANA positive women with implants to have anti-cardiolipin antibody. They also found low frequencies of anti-DNA (0.6%), anti-Sm (0.2%), anti-RNP (0.6%) antibodies and rheumatoid factor (3.7%). Anticentromere and antithyroid microsomal antibodies were present in 4.6 and 11.7%, respectively. Young et al. (1995b) found that 10% of their 58 symptomatic patients with implants had positive rheumatoid factor. Similar results were reported by Bridges et al. (1993a). In the study by Edworthy et al. (1998), two implant patients and seven control women were anti-Ro positive, one implant patient was anti-Ro and anti-La positive, and one control was anti-La positive. Anti-DNA antibodies were found in five implant patients and five controls; Anti-Scl-70, anti-Sm, and anti-RNP antibodies were not found. Rheumatoid factor was present in 5.5% of women with implants and 7.4% of control women (Edworthy et al., 1998). This is an important study because it reviewed a very large cohort and control group, the serologic tests were performed blinded, and clinical assessments were done by rheumatologists who also were blinded. No difference in specific autoantibodies was found between controls and silicone breast implant patients.

In the study of Karlson et al. (1999) discussed earlier, the authors compared specific autoantibodies to ssDNA, dsDNA, Sm, RNP, Ro, La, SCL-70, cardiolipin, thyroglobulin, and microsomes in 200 women with implants to the same autoantibodies in four control groups. Except for anti-ssDNA, there was no significant difference in autoantibodies between women with implants and 200 healthy controls or 100 women with diabetes. A number of autoantibodies were more prevalent in women with defined connective tissue disease or signs and symptoms of connective tissue disease, as might be expected. This study provides evidence against an association of autoantibodies and silicone breast implants (except anti-ssDNA). The study examined antibodies in a large, random cohort with identified techniques, blinded laboratory personnel and four appropriate concurrent control groups (Karlson et al., 1999). In general, the reports discussed earlier of ANAs in women with implants describe ANAs that are not reactive to defined autoantigens, and specific antinuclear autoantibodies when evaluated are not found.

CONCLUSIONS

As noted at the outset, studies of ANAs in women with silicone breast implants are subject to a number of weaknesses. Results reported have varied from positive to negative in a number of experimental groups, including women with saline or gel implants and those with connective tissue disease, an array of symptoms and disabilities, fibromyalgia, or no symptoms. No differences between saline and gel implants emerge from these studies, but results are not always reported by type of implant. A number of different control groups have been reported including historical, concurrent, asymptomatic or healthy, with fibromyalgia, with soft tissue rheumatism, with connective tissue disease, and with diabetes, and they have been assessed using different ANA technologies and criteria for positivity. Studies with no controls at all are essentially case reports. Even though some may report large numbers of women, they offer only weak evidence. Different results of testing for defined antinuclear autoantibodies have also been reported. Even theoretically well designed, prospective studies (Miller et al., 1998) have problems, such as short follow-up, failure to include significant portions of the potential experimental group, and no description of the testing technology. The fact that a positive ANA test is not a disease diagnosis should also be kept firmly in mind.

The cohort studies, however, add strength to the evidence against an association between silicone breast implants and ANAs or other autoantibodies. The committee concludes that the data in support of a finding of increased prevalence, higher titers, or different profiles of antinuclear antibodies in women with gel- or saline-filled silicone breast implants compared to control women without breast implants are insufficient or flawed. The weight of the better-quality evidence suggests the lack of an association between silicone breast implants and positive ANAs. Although there are fewer data on specific autoantibodies, they also suggest no association and are insufficient to support a finding of increased prevalence or different profiles of specific autoantibodies in women with silicone breast implants.

8
Epidemiological Studies of Connective Tissue or Rheumatic Diseases and Breast Implants

Extensive recent reviews have focused on epidemiological reports studying the possibility of an association between silicone breast implants (primarily gel filled) and defined connective tissue disease (CTD) (Independent Review Group, 1998; Tugwell, 1998). A number of meta-analyses (or smaller reviews) of these reports have also been published (Hochberg and Perlmutter, 1996; Hulka., 1998; Lamm, 1998; Lewin and Miller, 1997; Perkins et al., 1995; Stein, 1999; Wong, 1996). These reviews and meta-analyses have considered a relatively standard body of literature, although there are some differences among them as to which individual reports were included or not included. The reviews also have considered connective tissue diseases, combined and individually, including particularly systemic lupus erythematosus (SLE), rheumatoid arthritis (RA), Sjögren's syndrome (SS), systemic sclerosis or scleroderma (SSc), dermatomyositis/polymyositis (D/P) and occasionally others. Taken together, they do not support an association between connective tissue disease, combined or individually, or stated another way, an elevated relative risk for these diseases, in women with silicone breast implants.Although there are some informative abstracts and letter reports (e.g., Dugowson et al., 1992; Lacey, 1998; McLaughlin et al., 1994, 1995a; Wolfe, 1995a), with a few exceptions the committee limited its review of the epidemiology of connective tissue disease to full reports in the peer-reviewed, scientific literature, and focused on connective tissue diseases, combined and individual (primarily SSc, SLE, RA, D/P, and SS), in women with silicone breast implants of any kind. Although the committee was aware of numerous case reports of connective tissue disease in women with gel-, and a few with saline-filled, breast implants, a listing of such anecdotal evidence was not considered profitable. These case reports can be found in the references of this report. Many of them have been reviewed by Sánchez-Guerrero et al. (1994), and some deficiencies of these reports have been listed by Kurland and Homburger (1996), including: poor or absent case definition; failure to apply conventional diagnostic criteria; lack of identification of type of implant; silicone injections of questionable composition; unknown disease status prior to implant; lack of a consistent latent period; and inconsistent effects on symptoms after explantation (Kurland and Homburger, 1996).

The committee found 11 published cohort studies (Edworthy et al., 1998; Friis et al., 1997a; Gabriel et al., 1994; Giltay et al., 1994; Hennekens et al., 1996; Nyrén et al., 1998a; Park et al., 1998; Sánchez-Guerrero et al., 1995a,b; Schusterman et al., 1993; Weisman et al., 1988; and K.E. Wells et al., 1994), five case control studies (Burns et al., 1996; Englert et al., 1996; Hochberg et al., 1996; Strom et al., 1994; and Williams et al., 1997), and one cross-sectional study (Goldman et al., 1995), a total of 17 epidemiological studies of rheumatic diseases. The cohort studies were carried out in different locations in the United States and abroad: Alberta, Canada (Edworthy et al., 1998), Denmark (Friis et al., 1997a), Olmsted County, Minnesota (Gabriel et al., 1994), Amsterdam, Holland (Giltay et al., 1994), national samples in the United States (Hennekens et al., 1996 and Sánchez-Guerrero et al., 1995a,b), Sweden (Nyrén et al., 1998a), southeast Scotland (Park et al., 1998), Texas (Schusterman et al., 1993), San Diego (Weisman et al., 1988), and Florida (Wells et al., 1994). The five case-control studies were performed in Michigan (Burns et al., 1996), Sidney, Australia (Englert et al., 1996), San Diego, Baltimore–Washington, D.C., Pittsburgh (Hochberg et al., 1996), Philadelphia (Strom et al., 1994), and across the United States (Williams et al., 1997). The cross-sectional study was done in Atlanta, Georgia (Goldman et al., 1995). The principal results of these studies, that is, the risk of CTD associated with silicone breast implants, are summarized in Table 8-1.

CROSS-SECTIONAL STUDY

Goldman et al. (1995) conducted a cross-sectional study using the computerized clinic records of 4,229 women, primarily with RA, seen in a rheumatology practice between 1982 and 1992. He found 721 women with connective tissue disease (12 with implants) and 3,508 control women (138 with implants) (85% of the implants were gel filled, 4 % saline filled and 12% unknown). The adjusted odds ratio for all RA and connective tissue disease was 0.52 (95% confidence interval [CI], 0.29-0.92), even

TABLE 8-1 Studies of the Risk of Connective Tissue Disease (CTD) Associated with Silicone Breast Implants

Reference	Disease(s)	Relative Risk/Odds Ratio
Burns et al., 1996	SSc	0.95 (95% CI, 0.21-4.36
Edworthy et al., 1998	CTD	1.0 (95% CI, 0.45-2.22)
Englert et al., 1996	SSc	1.0 95% CI, 0.16-6.16)
Friis et al., 1997a	CTD	1.1 (95% CI, 0.2-3.4) cosmetic
		1.3 (95% CI, 0.5-3.6) reconstruction
Gabriel et al., 1994	CTD	1.10 (95% CI, 0.37-3.23)
Giltay et al., 1994	CTD	0.44 (no CI)*
Goldman et al., 1995	CTD	0.52 (95% CI, 0.27-0.92)
Hennekens et al., 1996	CTD	1.24 (95% CI, 1.08-1.41)
Hochberg et al., 1996	SSc	1.07 (95% CI, 0.53-2.13)
Nyrén et al., 1998a	CTD	1.10 (95% CI, 0.8-1.6)
Park et al., 1998	RA	0.42 (95% CI, 0.1-15.63)
Sánchez-Guerrero et al., 1995	CTD	0.6 (95% CI, 0.2-2.01)
Schusterman et al., 1993	CTD (rheumatic disease)	1.08 (95% CI, 0.01-17.2)
Strom et al., 1994	SLE	4.5 (90% CI, 0.2-27.3)
Weisman et al., 1988	Rheumatic symptoms	N.D.
Wells et al., 1994	Arthritis	1.16 (95% CI, 0.15-9.04)
Williams et al., 1997	CTD	0.74 (80% CI, 0.2-2.02)+

NOTE: CI = Confidence Interval; N.D. = not done; * = calculated by Perkins et al. (1995); and + = combined undifferentiated and defined CTD.

though six women who had implants after the diagnosis of RA or other CTD were included (Goldman et al., 1995). Rheumatoid arthritis and connective tissue disease overall were statistically significantly less frequently diagnosed in patients with silicone breast implants than in those without implants. It is possible that detection of breast implants was incomplete, since it depended on chart data in a practice where such information would have been an incidental finding. The prevalence of breast implants was higher than usually reported for unexplained reasons (150 out of 4,229 women, 3.5%), however.

CASE CONTROL STUDIES

Burns et al. (1996) attempted to identify all cases of SSc diagnosed in individuals from 1985 to 1991 and living in Michigan for at least 18 years. Data were collected between August 1991 and May 1993. Women with SSc were identified from hospital records, rheumatologists, and the United Scleroderma Foundation; 274 women participated in the study.

Controls were 1,184 women identified by random-digit dialing who were matched to the cases by age, race, and geographic area of the state. Medical records of cases were reviewed by rheumatologists; controls reported health information by telephone interview. The accuracy of self-reporting of breast implants was confirmed by telephoning a separate population and was found to be 94%. Subjects were not informed that the object of the study was to investigate the association of implants with scleroderma. Breast implants had been placed after mastectomy for cancer in 50% of SSc patients and 43% of controls. A separate analysis for cancer versus non-cancer patients was not done. Of SSc patients, 0.7% (two) had implants compared with 1.2% of controls. One SSc patient had had her implants for 1 year, and the other for 12 years before diagnosis of SSc, and the median duration of implants (to the time of interview) in controls was 8.8 years. The implant was silicone gel filled in both of the scleroderma cases and in 12 of 14 controls. The odds ratio, adjusted for age, race, and date of birth, was 0.95 (95% CI, 0.21-4.36) (Burns et al., 1996).

A retrospective, case control study of all cases of SSc or limited SSc in Sydney, Australia diagnosed prior to 1989 was the subject of a report by Englert and Brooks (1994) and a subsequent validated update by Englert et al. (1996). Cases were identified by death certificates, hospital records, and physicians' records. Controls were patients who had visited 29 randomly selected general practitioners in Sydney since 1990. Women were interviewed, and medical records were reviewed. In this way, 287 cases and 252 controls were identified. Three cases and three controls had silicone gel breast implants before diagnosis or prior to the selected date for controls. The self-reported implant status of patients was in 100% agreement with medical records, and the adjusted odds ratio was 1.0 (95% CI, 0.16–6.16) (Englert et al., 1996).

Hochberg et al. (1996) identified 837 cases of SSc from three university arthritis clinics, and 2,507 local controls, matched for age and race who were found by random-digit dialing. SSc patients filled out a mailed questionnaire; controls were interviewed by telephone. The response rate was 73% for patients and 59% for controls. Eleven (1.31%) of the cases reported silicone gel breast implants, a median of 11 years before diagnosis of SSc. In comparison, 31 (1.24%) of controls reported gel implants. A validation study assessed the accuracy of breast implant self-report in controls on a 5% random sample, and agreement was 96.7%. (Accuracy of breast implant self report is not always so high-89.3%, Garbers et al., 1998). An odds ratio of 1.07 (95% CI, 0.53–2.13) was calculated using multiple logistic regression models adjusted for age, race, and site. This study had a power of 80% to detect an odds ratio of 1.8 or more (Hochberg et al., 1996). Although there were differences in ascertainment between controls (telephone interview) and patients (questionnaire), and some SSc patients with silicone breast implants may have died, this study provides good evidence against an association of breast implants and scleroderma.

Strom et al. (1994) reported cases of SLE from the offices of 22 rheumatologists and the Lupus Foundation in Philadelphia seen between 1985 and 1987, who had been part of an earlier unrelated study. In 1992, the authors were able to find 76% of the patients and 77% of the controls from the prior study for telephone interviews. Of 133 lupus patients, one (0.75%) was found to have breast implants compared to no implants in the 100 controls (friends). Because no implants were found in these controls, the authors calculated an odds ratio using controls from a cancer and steroid hormone study conducted elsewhere in 1980–1982 (presumably the study used for the report of Glasser et al., 1989, see Chapter 9). Although, the odds ratio was 4.5 (90% CI, 0.2–27.3), this finding was not statistically significant (Strom et al., 1994). Shortcomings of this study include the use of an unmatched control group from an earlier period with a prevalence of breast implants of 0.17% (a lower odds ratio would usually have been expected in a study group with less than 1% implants) and the very low power to detect associations between breast implants and SLE.

Williams et al. (1997) reported experience with 323 women, 156 with defined connective tissue diseases (RA, SSc, and SLE) and 167 with undifferentiated connective tissue disease, first in an abstract and subsequently in a full report. (The abstract is cited because it contains information on the distribution of breast implants and an odds ratio not found in the full report.) In the total group, three women had breast implants, one after the onset of CTD symptoms. Of the 156 women with defined connective tissue disease, one (of 40 women with SSc) had breast implants. There was no concurrent control group. Instead a historical frequency of breast implants from the survey of Cook et al. (1993) was used, which gives a national prevalence of 0.81%. This prevalence is probably an underestimate (see Chapter 1), and calculations of odds ratios based on this "control" are probably somewhat overstated. The odds ratio, which was not significantly elevated, would be even lower if it were adjusted using a higher control prevalence. The odds ratio for both defined and CTD groups combined, counting only implants that preceded symptoms, was 0.74, (80% (sic) CI, 0.2–2.02) and was 1.15 (95% CI, 0.23–3.41), counting all (three) implants (Williams and Weisman, 1994; Williams et al., 1997). The absence of a concurrent control group is a weakness of this study, as is its modest power.

COHORT STUDIES

Schusterman et al. (1993) carried out a cohort study of postmastectomy breast cancer patients between 1986 and 1992 at the M. D. Anderson Cancer Center in Houston, Texas. Records of 250 women who had breast implants and 353 who had autogenous tissue reconstructions were reviewed. Patients were also sent questionnaires regarding medically identified and treated "rheumatic diseases." The follow-up period was only 1.9 years for women with implants and 2.5 years for the control autogenous reconstructions. One patient in each group developed a connective tissue disease. The relative risk was 1.08 (95% CI, 0.1–17.2) (Schusterman et al., 1993). This study was well controlled, was from a single center, and investigates an interesting subset of implant patients. The small number in each cohort (and low power) and the very short follow-up limit possible conclusions.

Gabriel et al. (1994) reported a retrospective, population-based cohort study carried out in Olmsted County, Minnesota (the Mayo Clinic area) of all women who had breast implants between 1964 and 1991. There were two age-matched controls for each case, and these control women had a medical examination within two years of their matched case's implantation date. Connective tissue disease was self-reported with a follow-up review of medical records. The average postoperative follow-up time was eight years. There were 749 women with implants and 1,498 controls; 5 of the 749 women with breast implants and 10 of the 1,498 controls had a connective tissue disease. The adjusted relative risk was 1.10 (95% CI, 0.37–3.23) (Gabriel et al., 1994). In this study, clinical records were reviewed, limiting information on women with breast implants to this source, but Mayo Clinic records are reputed to be excellent, and experienced individuals reviewed the charts.

Giltay et al. (1994) studied women who had silicone gel breast implants between 1978 and 1990 in a clinical practice in Amsterdam. Surveys were mailed to 287 living and traceable women with implants and to the same number of age-matched controls with other breast surgery. The response rate was 82% (N = 235) in women with implants and 73% (N = 210) in controls. The average length of follow-up was 6.5 years. Evaluation was by self-report and, for those reporting CTD symptoms, a physician contact. There was no disease-specific or general relative risk reported, but 37% of women with implants and 21% of controls reported symptoms beginning after surgery, primarily painful joints and burning eyes. In a personal communication, Perkins et al. (1995) reported two CTD cases in the women with implants and four cases in the controls, with a relative risk of 0.44 (no CI reported). Not all patients were located, and some did not answer the questionnaire. A rheumatologist reviewing survey responses assessed the likelihood of rheumatic disease as 6 and 8% in controls and cases, respectively (Giltay et al., 1994). This study was done during the height of publicity about potential problems with breast implants. About a quarter of the implant patients had reconstruction after mastectomy for cancer, but cancer patients were not included in the group of age-matched controls.

Wells et al. (1994) carried out a retrospective cohort study of patients with silicone breast implants (222) or other cosmetic surgery (80) from one plastic surgeon's office in Tampa, Florida, between 1970 and 1990. In 1990 and 1991, 826 women from the practice were mailed a questionnaire inquiring about 23 signs and symptoms that may have occurred before or after surgery. This was followed by a telephone interview. The initial response rate was only 42%, and the exclusion of ineligibles reduced the final cohort further to 302 women with implants and cosmetic surgery controls without implants. The average follow-up of implant patients was four years. Medically diagnosed connective tissue disease included Raynaud's phenomenon in one woman and seven cases of arthritis. Only 3 of 27 possible outcomes differed between the two groups. Swollen axillary glands and tender axillary glands were more common in women with implants, odds ratios 7.1 (95% CI, 1.13–44.4) and 6.9 (95% CI, 1.75–27.15), respectively, and change in skin color was more common in women with other surgery, odds ratio, 0.13 (95% CI, 0.05–0.32). The odds ratio for arthritis was 1.16 (95% CI, 0.15–9.04). No patients reported scleroderma or lupus (Wells et al., 1994). The follow-up in this study was of somewhat limited duration, and results for patients who received implants for reconstruction were not separated from those receiving implants for augmentation in the analysis.

Sánchez-Guerrero et al. (1995) carried out a study using the Nurses' Health Study Cohort to investigate the association between connective tissue disease and breast implants. The 87,501 eligible women in this cohort had responded previously to biennial mailings that included questions about physician-diagnosed defined connective tissue diseases, rheumatic conditions, and "connective tissue disease not further specified." Women identified in this way completed a subsequent survey to identify those with three or more signs or symptoms of connective tissue disease or two or more swollen joints of at least six weeks' duration (cases). Criteria for cases were met by 1,294 women. Medical records were then reviewed by two rheumatologists. A screening with less stringent criteria yielded an additional 904 cases. A total of 516 women with defined connective tissue disease were identified from record review. In all, 1,183 women were found to have implants, 75 of them in the various CTD groups. A small validation study found 99 of 100 self-reports of breast implant status to be accurate (Karlson et al., 1999). The age adjusted relative risk was not greater than one for any of the above case definitions. For defined connective tissue disease, the relative risk was 0.3 (95% CI, 0–1.9) in women with silicone gel implants and 0.6 (95% CI, 0.2–2.01) in women with any breast implant (14% of implants were saline). The data in this study came from women who reported these symptoms and connective tissue disease prior to 1990 when adverse publicity about implants began to appear. Mean follow-up between surgery and disease diagnosis was nearly ten years (Sánchez-Guerrero et al., 1995). This study involved large numbers of women, who were selected only in the sense that they were health professionals who agreed to a long-term health study, and it had significant power to rule out all but the smallest risk of connective tissue disease. Furthermore, information on other than defined connective tissue disease was collected and analyzed. These considerable strengths make this an important study that finds no relationship between connective tissue disease or rheumatic conditions and breast implants.

Questionnaires on health-related items, including breast implants and diagnoses of a number of connective tissue diseases were mailed to 1.75 million women health professionals in the United States and Puerto Rico between September 1992 and May 1995. A total of 426,774 (24%) women responded, and 395,543 women returned questionnaires usable for the purpose of this study. Of these, 2.74% reported having breast implants between 1962 and 1991. Risk estimates showed a small and not statistically significant elevation in risk for each defined connective tissue disease (RA, SLE, SS, D/P, and SSc). For "other connective tissue disease including mixed" and for "any connective tissue disease," that is, any of the defined diseases, the risk estimates were significantly elevated, 1.30 (95% CI, 1.09–1.62) and 1.24 (95% CI, 1.08–1.41), respectively (Hennekens et al., 1996). This study was conducted during the height of publicity on silicone breast implants, and the overall response rate of 24% was much lower than the 70% response rate for the Nurses' Health Study reported by Sánchez-Guerrero et al. (1995) or the 100% inclusion of the Mayo Clinic study of Gabriel et al. (1994) suggesting possible selection bias. The prevalence of implants in this study was twofold higher than that in the population at large (see Chapter 1), which suggests that women with breast implants were more likely to respond to the questionnaire than women who did not have breast implants. The evidence for disease in these women rests on their own unverified self-reports, which may not be reliable. On the other hand, the large numbers of women in this study give it power to detect small changes in risk. The upper bound (1.41) of the 95% CI for "any connective tissue disease" suggests that if there is an increased risk, it is modest.

Friis et al. (1997a) reported a retrospective cohort study of all women identified in the Danish Central Hospital Discharge Register who had been hospitalized for placement of breast implants between 1977 and 1992. The register identified 1,135 women with cosmetic implants and

1,435 with implants for reconstruction. Three control groups were identified: 7,071 women undergoing breast reduction surgery, 472 women having breast ptosis corrected, and 3,952 women with breast cancer without implant. An analysis for the presence of five defined connective tissue diseases and "other defined rheumatic conditions" was carried out. The record of each patient CTD was obtained for verification by experienced rheumatologists and for implant status. Expected numbers of each connective tissue disease were calculated by multiplying the number of person-years of follow-up in the groups by the sex-specific national hospital discharge rates for each five-year age group and the calendar period of observation. For connective tissue diseases combined, the observed–expected ratio for cosmetic breast implant patients was 1.1 (95% CI, 0.2–3.4) and for reconstruction patients, 1.3 (95% CI, 0.5–3.6). For nonclassical "muscular rheumatism," there was an excess of cases for each of the four groups—cosmetic and reconstructive implants, breast reduction, and cancer (Friis et al., 1997a). This carefully designed study involved relatively large numbers of women and considered both defined and nonclassical CTD. However, only hospitalized cases of CTD were included.

Edworthy et al. (1998) attempted to contact 16,600 women identified through the Alberta Health Registry as having a breast implant or other cosmetic surgery between 1978 and 1986. Only 20% of the women could be contacted, were willing to participate, and fulfilled the eligibility criteria. The response rate was 59% (5,822) of the approximately 9,900 contacted, of whom 46% agreed to participate. No breast cancer reconstruction patients were included. After additional exclusion of some ineligibles, the final study group consisted of 1,576 women with breast implants (1,112 gel filled) and a control group of 727 women with other cosmetic procedures, with 12 and 11 years of follow-up, respectively. All women completed a questionnaire and had a blood sample taken. Women with relevant symptoms, diagnoses, or medications were invited for an examination by a nurse clinician and a rheumatologist (who were blinded to breast implant status). Symptoms, such as cognitive problems, numbness in the extremities, muscle pain, headache, and hand pain, were significantly more common in breast implant patients. There was no difference in the incidence of specific (RA, SLE, SS, SSc) or combined connective tissue disease or signs of atypical autoimmune disease in the two groups. The relative risk for all CTD was 1.0 (95% CI, 0.5–2.2) (Edworthy et al., 1998). Only 40% of women responding to the initial contact participated in this study, but the large number of women with good follow-up gives it power to detect fairly small differences in risk. The significant differences between the control and experimental groups were limited to subjective symptoms.

Nyrén et al. (1998a) reported a retrospective cohort study using the

Swedish National Inpatient Registry linked to three Swedish population registries to assemble cohorts of 7,442 women with breast implants (68% gel or double lumen) and 3,354 matched control women with breast reduction surgery discharged from hospitals between 1972 and 1993. Women in these cohorts with a subsequent hospitalization for a defined or possible connective tissue disease were identified. Diagnoses were validated by medical record review, and average postoperative follow-up was 8.0 and 9.9 years for the implant and control groups, respectively. Defined connective tissue disease (RA, SLE, SSc, SS, and D/P) was found in 29 of the 7,442 women with implants and 14 of the 3,354 controls. Standardized observed or expected hospitalization ratios were 1.6 (95% CI, 0.95–2.5) for connective tissue diseases in women with cosmetic implants, 0.8 (95% CI, 0.4–1.4) for reconstruction patients and 1.1 for all women with implants (95% CI, 0.8–1.6) compared to 1.3 (95% CI, 0.7–2.2) for connective tissue disease in women with breast reductions. No risk elevations in any of the groups were noted for any of the five defined connective tissue diseases individually or for various other unspecified CTD or rheumatic conditions such as fibromyalgia, polymyositis and others (Nyrén et al., 1998a). This study is similar to the Danish study in possibly missing cases by including only hospitalized women, but it also has relatively large numbers, considers other rheumatic conditions as well as defined connective tissue disease, and is carefully designed.

Park et al. (1998) carried out a retrospective cohort study of all patients in two comparison groups in southeast Scotland admitted to two Scottish hospitals. Women who had silicone gel breast implants for augmentation between 1982 and 1991 were compared with a control group of outpatients in a plastic surgery department. A second group, cancer patients reconstructed with silicone gel implants during the same decade, was matched with a control group of breast cancer patients without implants. All women underwent physical and clinical laboratory examinations. The study included 317 women with implants and 216 control women with a combined average follow-up of 68 months. There was one case of RA among the women with implants and one case in the controls, yielding an odds ratio of 0.42 (95% CI, 0.01–15.63). The women with implants and the controls were also similar in prevalence of symptoms such as joint pain (odds ratio; 1.07; 95% CI, 0.42–2.74), muscle pain (odds ratio; 1.17, 95% CI, 0.36–3.88), and fatigue (odds ratio; 2.01, 95% CI, 0.74–5.56). This study had good controls for both augmentation and reconstruction patients. However, it had relatively small numbers of women and according to the authors, the lowest relative risk detectable for connective tissue disease was 3.2 for reconstruction patients and 16 for augmentation patients.

Medical records for all patients receiving silicone gel implants for breast augmentation between 1970 and 1981 in a private practice were reviewed by Weisman et al. (1988). A survey was sent to the 378 patients identified, and 125 of 199 (63%) with correct addresses responded. Of 38 women who reported health problems since surgery and were interviewed, 22 were examined. Of this group, 12 women had bursitis; 7, knee pain; 14 osteoarthritis; 3 fibromyalgia; and 2 back pain. No cases of inflammatory rheumatic or connective tissue disease were discovered (Weisman et al., 1988). This was an uncontrolled study of a small group of women.

Conclusions

As noted earlier, the committee examined a number of comprehensive reviews and meta-analyses of epidemiological reports investigating associations of combined and individual connective tissue diseases with silicone breast implantation. The committee also reviewed published reports from 17 individual epidemiologic studies, which are discussed here, and took note of additional abstracts and letters. These reports and analyses generally examined connective tissue diseases combined. Of the 17 independent reports, from 6 to 12—depending on the disease in question—looked specifically at one or more of the individual CTDs listed earlier (i.e., SSc, SS, RA, SLE and D/P). A number of these reports also provided data on "other" connective tissue diseases. In only one instance was a relative risk or odds ratio significantly elevated, however. That report, based on a large number of women, found a small association of implants with combined connective tissue diseases (Hennekens et al., 1996). However, among women who responded to the study questionnaire, the proportion reporting breast implants was more than twice the estimated national frequency of these implants, which suggests selection bias. Moreover, the evidence for disease in these women consists of unverified self-reports. Thus, this study probably overstated the risk of connective tissue disease associated with silicone breast implants. If its results are valid, they rule out large increases of risk. Excluding this report, a very substantial body of evidence, consisting of a number of independent investigations and other analyses, does not provide evidence for an association of silicone gel- or saline-filled breast implants with defined connective tissue disease. Although others (e.g., Hulka, 1998) including authors of reports themselves, have pointed out problems with individual epidemiological studies, the consistency of results among many reports is impressive. As was the case with antinuclear antibodies (ANAs), data and results were rarely segregated by gel- or saline-filled implants, so no conclusions regarding associations with connective tissue disease by breast implant type are possible [see, however, Sánchez-Guerrero et al.

(1995) data suggesting a lower relative risk with gel implants]. The committee concludes that there is insufficient evidence to support an association of silicone breast implants with defined connective tissue disease. That is, given the repeated finding of no elevated risk, the evidence supports the conclusion that there is no association, and therefore no justification for the use of resources in further epidemiological exploration of such an association.

OTHER ATYPICAL SIGNS OR SYMPTOMS

The committee reviewed the literature cited earlier in this chapter and additional studies for descriptions of unusual constellations of signs or symptoms and clinical laboratory findings that might define undifferentiated connective tissue disease or a new syndrome associated with silicone breast implants, which has been proposed by some physicians (Borenstein, 1994a, cited in Tugwell, 1998; Silverman et al., 1996c; Solomon et al., 1995). Patients with undifferentiated connective tissue disease have been defined and followed as part of a multicenter project, and the association of this condition with silicone breast implants, its natural history and outcomes, and a description of its signs and symptoms have been published (Williams et al., 1997, 1998). Early undifferentiated disease was defined as at least one of the following: Raynaud's phenomenon; isolated keratoconjunctivitis sicca; unexplained polyarthritis; or at least three signs and symptoms (e.g., rash, central nervous system symptoms, pleuritis, pericarditis), and abnormal laboratory tests, (e.g., elevated erythrocyte sedimentation rate, biologic false-positive test for syphilis). At five-year follow-up, most patients with this diagnosis continue with signs and symptoms or remit, but approximately 20% were reported to have progressed to a defined connective tissue disease, usually SLE or RA (Williams et al., 1998).

In an abstract and a full report of a case control study, Williams and colleagues (Williams and Weisman, 1994; Williams et al., 1997) reported 167 women with either undifferentiated connective tissue disease (N = 89), Raynaud's phenomenon (N = 24) or unexplained polyarthritis (N = 54). As discussed earlier, 156 women with defined connective tissue disease were also reported. One woman with silicone breast implants was found in each group (specifically one woman with SSc and one with unexplained polyarthritis). Using an historical control group and counting only cases of disease occurring after implantation, the odds ratio for the combined groups was 0.74, as noted earlier. No significant risk for defined or undifferentiated connective tissue disease in women who had received silicone breast implants was found in this study, although small numbers limited its power to detect slightly increased relative risks (Williams and Weisman, 1994; Williams et al., 1997).

A case control study reported only in an abstract (Laing et al., 1996) found three women (1.46%) with implants among 205 women with undifferentiated connective tissue disease, compared to 27 women with implants in 2,220 controls (1.21%), which resulted in an odds ratio of 2.27 (95% CI, 0.67–7.71). This study also suffers from small numbers and limited power, and because it is reported in abstract form only, methodologic details are lacking, and the results have not been peer reviewed. Another abstract describing a meta-analysis of seven epidemiological studies reported a pooled odds ratio of 1.74 for non-CTD arthralgia. The absence of any data or even a history of the studies analyzed limits interpretation of this abstract (Kayler and Goodman, 1985).

Five reports (Edworthy et al., 1998; Friis et al., 1997a; Hennekens et al., 1996; Nyrén et al., 1998a; and Sánchez-Guerrero et al., 1995) discussed earlier did not study undifferentiated connective tissue disease and breast implants specifically, but did evaluate a range of conditions besides defined CTD, including early, mixed, atypical, and ill-defined connective tissue diseases; fibromyalgia; and constellations of up to 41 signs and symptoms that occur in defined and undifferentiated CTD and in rheumatic-like conditions. Another study by MacDonald et al. (1996) reported 35 cases of chronic fatigue syndrome (one breast implant in the patient and control group each), also characterized by some of these symptoms, such as fatigue, joint pain, myalgia and muscle weakness, memory difficulties, among others. These six studies collected and analyzed data on signs and symptoms that occur in these connective tissue and rheumatic-like conditions. In none of these studies was a statistically significant association of atypical disease with silicone breast implants discovered. The committee concludes that there is insufficient evidence for an association of silicone breast implants with undifferentiated connective tissue disease, and most studies suggest that there is no association.

A list of 48 signs and symptoms that might be associated with, or caused by, silicone breast implants can be found in Tugwell (1998) and 55 signs and symptoms are listed in Appendix B in this report. There is considerable overlap between these lists. Many of these signs and symptoms are also listed in reports (often abstracts) by a number of investigators (e.g., Baker, 1996; Borenstein, 1994b; Brawer, 1996; Bridges et al., 1993a; Chow et al., 1995; Cuellar et al., 1995a; Davis et al., 1995; Freundlich et al., 1994; Lewy and Ezrailson, 1996; Love et al., 1992; Mathias et al., 1996; Mease et al., 1995; Nardella, 1995; Osborn et al., 1993; Romano et al., 1995; Solomon, 1994a,b, 1996; Vasey, 1992a,b, 1994; Weiner and Paulus, 1996; Weiner et al., 1992).

In an attempt to aggregate these signs and symptoms to define a unique syndrome, a group of physicians proposed criteria for the diagnosis of a new condition [see earlier references, e.g., Borenstein (1994a) cited in Tugwell (1998)]. If such a condition could be defined and this definition applied to a reproducible set of signs, symptoms, and clinical laboratory criteria, then epidemiological studies to explore this condition in relation to silicone breast implants could be carried out. A definite diagnosis of this disease was proposed by the reference group of physicians to require the presence of a silicone gel filled breast implant and the presence of local disease, that is, any of the following: capsular contracture, rupture, more than six weeks of chest wall pain, more than six weeks of breast pain, axillary adenopathy, entrapment neuropathy, immune skin rash or immune granulomas in the implant capsule. Objectively verifiable major and minor criteria were also proposed; these include, as major criteria, symmetrical myalgia with 4–11 tender points, chronic fatigue of six-month duration, cognitive dysfunction of six-month duration, and objective sicca complex; and as minor criteria, arthralgia, enthesopathy, subjective sicca complex, cerebellovestibular dysfunction, hair loss, Raynaud's phenomenon, photosensitive skin rash, immune-mediated skin rash, improvement of two major or one major and four minor criteria within 18 months of explantation, positive ANA titer of 1:40 or more on HEp-2 cells, elevated erythrocyte sedimentation rate, and abnormal quantitative immunoglobulin G (IgG; Borenstein, 1994a cited in Tugwell, 1998; Silverman et al., 1996c; Soloman et al., 1995).

The requirement for the presence of a silicone breast implant at some time in the patient's life to make the diagnosis of this proposed disease means it cannot be diagnosed as an independent condition that can be assessed objectively. Investigations of its relationship to breast implants would be problematic at best since the condition could not exist absent a gel implant. The requirement for an implant is more consistent with a toxic reaction to silicone gel, but this perspective is not supported by available toxicological evidence (see Chapter 4). It is also of interest that there is no requirement for a saline-filled silicone implant, although atypical signs and symptoms have occasionally been reported to be associated with these as well (Byron et al., 1984; see also earlier description of CTD and Appendix B of this report). Moreover, the required presence of local disease will be fulfilled frequently (see Chapter 5), creating a large group of women eligible for this diagnosis if they display several of the required signs and symptoms (major and minor criteria), which are semiquantitative, subjective, and common in the general population.

In assessing this proposed new disease, others have also noted that there are few objective signs and that the majority of these signs and symptoms are common in the general population or frequently seen in other defined diseases (Tugwell, 1998). Hyams (1998), in a recent review

BOX 8-1
Shared Features of Symptom-Based Conditions

1. Characteristic symptoms potentially involve multiple organ systems and not a recognizable pattern of complaints.
2. Characteristic symptoms are not consistently associated with objective physical signs or laboratory abnormalities.
3. Characteristic symptoms are similar, particularly fatigue, headache, muscle or joint pains, cognitive difficulty and sleep disturbance.
4. Characteristic symptoms are experienced frequently in adult populations.
5. Characteristic symptoms are commonly caused by varied psychiatric and medical illnesses.
6. Concurrent psychiatric disorders are frequently present.
7. Young to middle-aged women are most commonly diagnosed.
8. Similar multifactorial etiologies are suspected.

SOURCE: Hyams (1998)

of symptom-based conditions, noted that a similar constellation of signs and symptoms characterizes a number of diagnoses, such as chronic fatigue syndrome, multiple chemical sensitivities, fibromyalgia, and others, including a novel silicone-associated condition. He listed the shared features of these conditions (see Box 8-1) and, in addition to the frequency of the symptoms in the general population, reinforced the significance of the absence of a specific case definition, and the lack of established diagnostic criteria that exclude well-recognized causes of chronic somatic symptoms or distinguish various symptom-based conditions from each other. This is not to question that such patients are ill, often severely so, only to suggest that whether afflicted patients are suffering from unique scientifically defined illnesses has not been established. Others have recently stressed the prevalence of this constellation of signs and symptoms, the reliance of research on self-report data, and the uncertain boundaries of the multiple associated diagnoses (Lloyd, 1998).

Many of these criteria have also been reviewed in existing studies of women with breast implants. The reports listed earlier are also, with few exceptions, uncontrolled case series descriptions. Although some describe thousands of women, by lacking controls they are essentially case reports of a selected group and therefore constitute only weak evidence of an association of implants with the described health conditions. These case or case series reports have gathered women with implants who have complaints, many of them self- or attorney referred, or patients who are seen in practices of rheumatologists who have evaluated women with implants for injury claims; that is, they do not represent an unbiased cross section of the population of women with implants.

Other reports have assessed various symptoms and signs, including some proposed for the new disease, as part of cohort studies (e.g., Edworthy et al., 1998; Friis et al., 1997a; Gabriel et al., 1994; Giltay et al., 1994; Kim and Harris, 1998; Nyrén et al., 1998c; Park et al., 1998; Wells, 1994; and Winther et al., 1998). These studies are discussed briefly above [except for those of Kim and Harris, 1998; Nyrén et al., 1998c; and Winther et al., 1998, which focus on neurologic symptoms and are discussed in Chapter 10]. They also collected data on individual signs and symptoms. For example, in the cohort study of Giltay et al. (1994), no difference was found between the prevalence of Raynaud's phenomenon in implant (3.69%) and control (3.33%) patients. Likewise in Park et al. (1998) one patient with Raynaud's phenomenon was found among 110 women with augmentations (0.91%) and three patients among 129 controls (2.34%), and there were seven cases of Raynaud's among 207 reconstruction patients (3.38%) and five of 88 controls (5.68%). Wells et al. (1994) found one case of Raynaud's phenomenon in 222 women with implants and no cases in 80 control women. The prevalence of Raynaud's phenomenon in a population of normal adult women 53.8 years of age on average was 9.6% according to Fraenkel et al. (1999).

Edworthy et al. (1998) found hand pain in 26% of women with implants and 18% of controls (a significant difference). Gabriel et al. (1994) found swollen joints in 3.34% of women with implants and 2.60% of controls, a relative risk of 1.35 (95% CI, 0.81–2.23). Giltay et al. (1994) reported painful joints for at least three months in 19.57% of implant patients and 8.57% of controls. In the cohort study of Park et al. (1998), 11 of 110 augmentation patients (10.0%) and 12 of 128 controls (9.38%) had joint pain, as did 31 of 207 reconstruction patients (14.98%) and 13 of 88 controls (14.77%). The prevalence of arthralgia was not significantly different in the patients studied (11%) and in controls (5%) in the cohort reported by Wells et al. (1994); swollen axillary glands were more common in the patients than in controls. The cohort studies reviewed here did not find sicca complex, rash, myalgia, skin tightening, or thickening significantly more frequently in women with breast implants compared to controls.

In a study that evaluated a constellation of 23 signs and symptons, there was no difference between experimental and control groups for 20 of the 23 (Wells et al., 1994). When 1,016 women with gel implants were compared with 309 women with saline implants and 609 cosmetic surgery controls by a survey questionnaire that sought information about memory difficulty, myalgia, arthralgia, numbness and headache, among others, the frequencies in the three groups were similar (Barr et al., 1998). When 105 women with breast implants were evaluated by Abeles and

Waterman (1995), only fatigue, cognitive disorder, and arthralgia were present in 50% or more of the women. Others of the 14 "key" signs and symptoms of the proposed new disease, or those commonly attributed to patients with breast implants, were infrequent (5–25%). Women averaged only 2.3 signs and symptoms and a consistent clinical picture could not be defined (Abeles and Waterman, 1995). Similar findings were reported by Weisman et al. (1998) in a study described earlier in this report. Of 125 women with implants, 38 (30%) were found to have signs and symptoms, including fibromyalgia, osteoarthritis, bursitis, or isolated back or knee pain. No atypical disease was found (Weisman et al., 1988).

Blackburn and colleagues examining a selected group of 70 physician-referred women with silicone gel implants in place for an average of 10.2 years, found one case of postimplant SLE and one case of SS and also fibromyalgia, osteoarthitis, or soft-tissue rheumatism (Blackburn and Everson, 1997; Blackburn et al., 1997). Moreover, measurement of interleukin-6 (IL-6), IL-8, soluble intercellular adhesion molecule-1 (sICAM-1), soluble IL-2 receptor (sIL-2R), and tumor necrosis factor-alpha (TNFα) in peripheral blood of varying numbers of these women did not reveal elevations compared to ten concurrent and an unknown number of historical controls (see the discussion of cytokines in Chapter 6). In 13 of these 70 women (19%), ANAs were detected at titers of 1:40 or more. These investigators also concluded that an atypical disease could not be demonstrated in these patients (Blackburn and Everson, 1997; Blackburn et al., 1997).

Considerable variation in the prevalence of individual signs and symptoms was reported when the frequencies described in case series by Vasey et al., 1992b; Solomon et al., 1994a; Freundlich et al., 1994 and Borenstein were compared (Borenstein, 1994b). Todhunter and Farrow (1998) analyzed the overlap of signs and symptoms often, but variably, described in the multiple reports and abstracts listed and discussed above, which were also examined in some of the studies of defined connective tissue disease discussed earlier. They found these signs and symptoms covered within the endpoints examined by the epidemiological studies, and these studies did not show a statistically significant association of the signs and symptoms (or defined CTD) with breast implants. They concluded that this makes a specific atypical syndrome unlikely (Todhunter and Farrow, 1998).

CONCLUSIONS

The committee finds no convincing evidence for atypical connective tissue or rheumatic disease or a novel constellation of signs and symptoms in women with silicone breast implants. Case reports, of which there are many, do not provide evidence, although they may suggest hypotheses that can be tested, as has been possible for defined CTD. A defined and testable disease is a precondition for any type of study. Given the frequency of local complications in women with silicone breast implants and the frequency and subjective nature of the symptoms that have been proposed by some to characterize a hypothetical novel disease, a large group of women would meet the criteria for this disease if such a definition were accepted. The diagnosis would ultimately depend on conditions such as fatigue, cognitive dysfunction, arthralgia, and the like which are nonspecific and common. A new disease would then be created by the discovery of an implant and its common local complications in women who had signs and symptoms prevalent in the general population or in fibromyalgia, chronic fatigue syndrome, multiple chemical sensitivities, or other less well-defined conditions. As noted earlier, silicone toxicity is conceptually more straightforward, although it is not supported by the toxicologic data reviewed in Chapter 4.

The evidence for an atypical disease or a novel syndrome is insufficient or flawed. It consists of selected case series, few of which describe a consistent and reproducible syndrome. The controlled epidemiological studies cited provide stronger, contrary evidence. In view of the paucity, weakness, and conflicting nature of the evidence, the committee concludes that there is no rigorous, convincing scientific support for atypical connective tissue or any new disease in women that is associated with silicone breast implants. In fact, epidemiological evidence suggests there is no novel syndrome.

9

Silicone Breast Implants and Cancer

Induction or promotion of malignancies of the breast or other organs by silicone implants has been the subject of studies and comprehensive reviews with negative findings. Individual case reports have raised questions regarding the carcinogenicity of silicone breast implants. These questions include whether there has been an increase in primary or recurrent carcinoma of the breast associated with silicone breast implants, whether there has been an increase in breast malignancies other than primary carcinoma of the breast associated with implants, and whether there has been an increase in non-breast malignancies in women with implants, for example, solid tumors (carcinomas) of other organs, sarcoma, lymphoma, or myeloma.

The carcinogenicity of silicone or silicone implants is reviewed in Chapter 4. Although silicone formulated into implants of the proper size, shape, and surface characteristics can induce solid-state carcinogenesis in the susceptible rodent species associated with this phenomenon, it is not a specific response to silicone. Solid-state carcinogenesis occurs in rodents with exposure to a wide array of other substances. There is no convincing evidence that it is a human risk (Brand and Brand, 1980; Morgan and Elcock, 1995). Other well-designed and implemented experimental studies of the carcinogenicity of silicones reviewed earlier were negative.

A small series of case reports of breast malignancy associated with silicone injections is reviewed in Chapter 1. This series consists of relatively few reports, and as noted elsewhere, although case reports can be a basis for formulating hypotheses, they do not constitute evidence for an association. Harris surveyed 184 surgeons performing breast implantation with a variety of pre-silicone (pre-1962) breast implants. No cases of breast malignancy were reported in 16,660 implants (Harris, 1961). Similar results were obtained by Snyderman and Lizardo (1960); only 4 of 500 plastic surgeons surveyed reported malignancies in women with pre-silicone implants. DeCholnoky's (1970) survey of 265 surgeons covered 10,941 patients; about one-third of these women had "open pore," pre-silicone breast implants, and no cancers were found. Instances of cancer associated with silicone breast implants have also been the subject of a number of case reports (e.g., Benavent, 1973; Bingham et al., 1988; Bowers and Radlauer, 1969; Cammarata et al., 1984; Dalinka et al., 1969; Frantz and Herbst, 1975; Gottlieb et al., 1984; Hausner et al., 1978; Heywang et al., 1985; Holt and Spear, 1984; Hoopes et al., 1967; Lafreniere and Ketcham, 1987; Mendez-Fernandez et al., 1980; Paletta et al., 1992; Perras and Papillon, 1973; Shousha et al., 1994; Silverstein et al., 1990a–c; Stewart et al., 1992; Travis et al., 1984).

The committee has estimated that 70% of breast implantation is for the purpose of augmentation, that is, not performed after mastectomy for cancer; in the United States in 1997 there were 1.5 million to 1.8 million women with implants, or about 1 million to 1.3 million women with implants for augmentation. Given the incidence of breast cancer in the general population, tens of thousands of cases of breast cancer would be expected to occur over time in a cohort of this size. In fact, breast cancer is reported in association with implants in the epidemiological studies cited below or in examinations of the effectiveness of mammography (see Cahan et al., 1995, and other studies in Chapter 12) as an expected event.

In 1997, Brinton and Brown reviewed many studies relating to the carcinogenicity of silicone breast implants and concluded that these studies found no association of breast implants with breast carcinoma, although they noted that some potential outcomes, such as non-breast malignancies and breast sarcomas, or factors such as life-style, latencies, and others were not adequately addressed. Lamm (1998) also reviewed some of the epidemiological studies and, in a meta-analysis of four cohort studies, reported a standardized incidence ratio for breast cancer that was significantly less than one (0.70; 95% CI, 0.55–0.87), suggesting that breast implants were associated with a decreased risk of this disease.

A number of epidemiological studies, both cohort and case control, of the potential associations between breast (or other) cancers and silicone breast implants provide good evidence that these implants do not result in a higher frequency of breast cancer. Summary data from these studies are listed in Table 9-1. Two small case control studies (Malone et al., 1992) of two age groups of breast cancer patients with odds ratios less than one

TABLE 9-1 Studies of Silicone Breast Implants and Cancer

Reference	No. of Patients (cancer or implant)	SIR, OR (adjusted)
Berkel et al., 1992	11,676 (implant)	0.48 (no CI)
Brinton et al., 1996	2,174 (cancer)	0.6 (95% CI, 0.4–1.0)
Bryant and Brasher, 1995	10,835 (implant)	0.76 (95% CI, 0.6–1.0)
Deapen et al., 1997	3,182 (implant)	0.63 (95% CI, 0.4–0.9)
Friis et al., 1997b	1,135 (implant)	1.0 (95% CI, 0.4–2.0)
Glasser et al., 1989	4,742 (cancer)	1.0 (95% CI, 0.3–3.3)
Kern et al., 1997	680 (implant)	0.67 (95% CI, .02–2.17)
McLaughlin et al., 1998	3,473 (implant)	0.7 (95% CI, 0.4–1.1)
Park et al., 1998	186 (implant)	No cancers observed

NOTE: CI = confidence interval; OR = odds ratio; SIR = standardized incidence ratio.

are not included here, because they were reported only by letter with little detail.

Berkel et al. (1992) reported the association of breast augmentation with breast cancer for all women in Alberta, Canada, who had implants between 1973 and 1986. The expected number of cancers was estimated from data from the Alberta Cancer Registry. The implant cohort was compared to a cohort of all women in Alberta who developed breast cancer ($N = 13,557$). The average follow-up of the implant cohort was 10.2 years, and the average length of time from breast augmentation to the diagnosis of breast cancer was 7.5 years. The standard incidence ratio was 0.476, significantly lower than expected ($p < 0.01$) (Berkel et al., 1992).

Bryant et al. (1994) reported some problems with the study methods of Berkel et al. that tended to introduce a bias resulting in an underestimate of the standardized incidence ratio. In a subsequent report, this group reanalyzed the original data, and a number of new standardized incidence ratios were reported (0.76, 0.81, 0.85, 0.68), depending on induction periods of 0, 1, 5, and 10 years, respectively; these ratios did not differ significantly from each other, nor was the incidence of breast cancer shown to be significantly higher or lower than in the general population (Bryant and Brasher, 1995).

Brinton et al. (1996) reported a population-based case control study of 2,174 cases of breast cancer and 2,009 age- and geographically matched controls. The odds ratio for augmentation in breast cancer patients, 0.6 (95% confidence interval [CI], 0.4–1.0), after adjustment for a number of factors, including age, race, body size, and family history of breast cancer, among others, suggested a lower association of breast implants with breast cancer.

In a series of studies, Deapen and colleagues described the association with breast cancer in a cohort of breast implant patients in the Los Angeles area over a 14-year period (Deapen et al., 1986, 1997; Deapen and Brody, 1992, 1995). The 1997 study reports 3,182 women collected from private practices in Los Angeles who had breast implants (74% gel filled) between 1953 and 1980 (91% since 1970). Data on breast cancer were obtained from the Los Angeles County Cancer Surveillance Program through 1991. The average follow-up was 14.4 years (range 0.04–20 years), and the median interval from implant to diagnosis of breast cancer was 10.3 years. The standardized incidence ratio (SIR) was 0.63 (95% CI, 0.428–0.895), indicating a significant decrease in breast cancer in the women with breast implants (Deapen et al., 1997).

Using the Danish Hospital Discharge Registry, 1,135 women with cosmetic breast implantation were identified with an average age of 31 years and an average follow-up of 8.4 years (Friis et al., 1997b). There was no increase in the standardized incidence ratio for all cancers ($N = 27$) or for breast cancer ($N = 8$): SIR = 1.1 (95% CI, 0.7–1.6) and 1.0 (95% CI, 0.4–2.0) respectively. No cases of multiple myeloma were observed in the implant patient cohort (0.1 case expected). These data update the preliminary report of McLaughlin et al. (1994).

Glasser et al. (1989) reported 4,742 breast cancer patients 20–54 years of age diagnosed between 1980 and 1982 and 4,754 controls who were part of a large U.S. case control study of cancer and steroid hormone use. The mean interval from implantation to diagnosis or interview was six to seven years. The adjusted odds ratio for breast augmentation was 1.0 (95% CI, 0.3–3.3) (Glasser et al., 1989).

Kern et al. (1997) studied 680 cases of breast implantation in women with no prior history of cancer using the Uniform Hospital Discharge Data Set from 34 Connecticut hospitals during 1980–1993. The Connecticut Cancer Registry was used to verify cancer cases. Women with implants were compared to 1,022 control women undergoing tubal ligations, a less-than-ideal control group in several respects. Mean follow-up of the women with implants was 4.6 years and of the control group 5.4 years. The implant group had relative risks for breast cancer and nonbreast cancers of 0.67 (95% CI, 0.2–2.17) and 0.21 (95% CI, 0.07–0.60), respectively. No cases of multiple myeloma or sarcoma were observed (Kern et al., 1997).

McLaughlin et al. (1994, 1995a, 1998) briefly reported on cohort studies from Denmark and Sweden. The Danish study, first reported by letter (McLaughlin et al., 1994), found standardized incidence ratios less than one for breast cancer and for all cancers; the results were reported in more detail by Friis et al. (1997b), as reviewed earlier. The Swedish study was mentioned first in a letter (McLaughlin et al., 1995a) and then expanded and reported in a brief communication (McLaughlin et al., 1998). This communication described a study that consisted of 3,473 women undergoing breast augmentation mostly after 1976 with an average age at implantation of 30 years and an average follow-up of 10.3 years. The standardized incidence ratios (based on Swedish national cancer rates) for all cancers ($N = 74$) and for breast cancer ($N = 18$) were 1.1 (95% CI, 0.8–1.3) and 0.7 (95% CI, 0.4–1.1), respectively. A small increase in lung cancer (SIR = 2.7; 95% CI, 1.1–5.6), no significant excess of lymphoproliferative malignancy, and one case of multiple myeloma (expected cases not reported, but presumably somewhat less than one) were observed (McLaughlin et al., 1998).

Park et al. (1998) analyzed data from two groups of women from southeast Scotland who had implant surgery for augmentation or reconstruction at two Scottish hospitals. These groups are analyzed for antinuclear antibodies and connective tissue diseases. The group receiving silicone gel implants for augmentation consisted of 186 women. Although only 110 were seen on follow-up for the study, data on breast cancer were available for all 186, and no breast cancers occurred.

These epidemiological studies of breast cancer and silicone breast implants are strikingly consistent in showing no association. Some of the studies have very small numbers (and therefore low power), some have control groups that may not be exactly comparable (e.g., tubal ligations), and others have follow-up intervals after implantation that may be short in relation to reasonably expected latency periods between exposure and the onset of malignancy. The committee concludes, however, that there are sufficient studies with consistent and convincing findings of no association between breast cancer and implants.

Several of the epidemiological studies reviewed here also collected data on all cancers, or non-breast cancers, and found no associations with breast implants (e.g., Friis et al., 1997b; Kern et al., 1997; McLaughlin et al., 1994 and 1995a). The Deapen and Brody (1992, 1995) reports also contained information on all cancers; in 3,112 implant patients, 45 cancers (versus 50 expected) were found, and a standardized incidence ratio of 0.90 (95% CI, 0.66–1.20) was calculated. Vulvar and lung cancers were increased. No cases of multiple myeloma were observed versus 0.6 expected (Deapen and Brody, 1992, 1995). Although these data are not conclusive, they are generally negative; occasional increases in a particular cancer are not consistent and are likely due to chance or confounding factors. The committee concludes, therefore, that there is limited evidence that silicone breast implants are not associated with non-breast cancers.

A number of investigators have studied recurrence of cancer or death due to breast cancer in patients with silicone implants for breast reconstruction after mastectomy. Birdsell et al. (1993) found that survival in implanted and nonimplanted patients was similar. Breast cancer recurrence in 306 reconstruction patients (207 with submuscular implants) followed for a mean of 6.4 years was similar to that reported in the scientific literature (Noone et al., 1994a). Johnson et al. (1989) reported that their experience with recurrence of or death from breast cancer in 118 mastectomy patients after reconstruction with implants was similar to their experience with mastectomy patients without implants. Similar results with implant patients and recurrences were also reported briefly and then in a large series comparing relapse-free intervals in women with and without reconstruction with implants after mastectomy for cancer by Georgiade et al. (1982, 1985). Petit et al. (1994) compared 146 women with silicone gel implants for reconstruction to 146 matched cancer mastectomy patients without implants who had 9- and 12-year follow-ups, respectively, and reported a relative risk for local recurrence of 0.5 (95% CI, 0.3–1.1) and of death from breast cancer of 0.5 (95% CI, 0.3–1.0). Park et al. (1998) studied 289 postmastectomy implant reconstruction patients (176 matched to mastectomy controls without implants) and reported a relative risk of recurrence and death (all cases) of 0.83 (95% CI, 0.48–1.45) and 0.51 (95% CI, 0.23–1.11), respectively. These data present a consistent picture that implants do not increase breast cancer recurrence rates or decrease survival rates in patients after reconstruction with implants.

BREAST SARCOMAS AND OTHER TUMORS

Because silicone solid-state carcinogenesis results in sarcomas in susceptible rodents, the prevalence of breast sarcomas in women has been explored. It is difficult to assess whether there has been an increase in tumors of the breast other than primary carcinomas because malignancies other than primary carcinomas are rare, have not had uniform classification over the years, and probably have not been reported consistently in tumor registries (Callery et al., 1985). Tumors of stromal or fibrous origin arising in the capsule of a breast implant in humans would, presumably, be analogous to those caused in solid-state carcinogenesis in rodents. Such tumors with fibrous, myeloid, and fatty tissue patterns do occur in the breast but are rare, constituting 0.5–1% of primary breast malignancies (Tang et al., 1979). These malignant tumors with the potential to metastasize have been grouped under the term "stromal sarcomas." At present, there is no evidence that breast sarcomas have increased in frequency or are occurring unusually in women with silicone breast implants. Only two reports were found in a review by Lorentzen (1988) for the Public Health Service: Kobayashi et al. (1988); (a stromal sarcoma) and Morgenstern et al. (1985); (a pseudosarcomatous carcinoma—felt by a departmental scientist to be an undifferentiated sarcoma), both after silicone injections. Sarcomas were not found in the epidemiological studies reviewed earlier of all, or non-breast, malignancies occurring in women with implants. Deapen et al. (1997) found no sarcomas in their own study and reported a review (personal communication of M. F. Brennan) of sarcomas occurring at Memorial Sloan-Kettering Cancer Center of which 0.5% were in the breast but none in women with implants (Deapen et al., 1997). The National Cancer Institute's Surveillance, Epidemiology and End Results (SEER) data have been reviewed for changes in the incidence of breast sarcoma from 1973 to 1986 (extended to 1990 by Engel et al., 1995) that might have occurred consequent to the increasing prevalence of breast implantation during that time. May and Stroup (1991) found no increase, and Engel and Lamm (1992) also found no increase on reanalysis of the data to allow for a ten-year latency between exposure to silicone and appearance of sarcoma. Breast sarcoma was and remained extremely rare, 0.12–0.13 case per 100,000 woman-years (Engel and Lamm, 1992; Engel et al., 1995; Lamm and Engel, 1989; May and Stroup, 1991). This evidence consistently fails to support an increase in breast sarcoma associated with silicone breast implants, although analysis of the national data would not be expected to detect small increases in breast sarcoma because of the rarity of that condition.

Another rare fibrous tumor that can infiltrate extensively into surrounding structures but does not metastasize is classified by the term "desmoid." Rosen and Ernsberger (1989) reported their experience with 22 cases of breast desmoids. One of these cases was associated with saline implants that had been in place for several years. Four other cases of desmoids in association with breast implants have been reported (Dale and Wardlaw, 1995; Jewett and Mead, 1979; Schiller et al., 1995; Schuh and Radford, 1994). Dale and Wardlow (1995) reviewed the literature and found less than 75 other cases of desmoids reported in women without breast implants. The relation of these tumors to previous trauma, scars from previous surgery, fibroadenomas and fibrocystic disease was noted. Desmoids occur rarely; there is no evidence of an increase in frequency, and they are apparently associated with fibrosis, which occurs in the breast in conditions other than implantation. It is possible that a desmoid could occur very rarely in association with the fibrotic response that forms the capsule around a breast implant, but there is no evidence to conclude that this occurs with increased frequency in the presence of silicone breast implants.

Several case reports and review articles indicate that the incidence of primary breast lymphoma is 0.05–0.53% of primary breast malignancies (Petrek, 1987a,b) In recent years there have been a few case reports of lymphoma developing in breasts in relation to silicone implants (Benjamin et al., 1982; Cook et al., 1995; Duvic et al., 1995; Krech, 1997). These lymphomas were of several varieties including follicular cutaneous T-cell (mycosis fungoides and Sézary syndrome) and neoplastic T-cell lymphoma. Proximity to the implants and foreign-body reaction with giant cells were noted. Significant increases in lymphomas were not found in several epidemiological studies (Friis et al., 1997b; Kern et al., 1997; McLaughlin et al., 1998). The committee also noted two reports of squamous cell carcinoma arising in the capsule of a breast implant (Kitchen et al., 1994; Paletta et al., 1992).These case reports are few in number and do not constitute evidence for an association of these malignancies with breast implants.

The question of a relationship between exposure to silicone and subsequent development of monoclonal gammopathy of undetermined significance (MGUS) or multiple myeloma in humans was raised by Salmon and Kyle (1994) in commenting on the induction of plasmacytomas after intraperitoneal injection of silicone gel in genetically susceptible strains of mice (Potter et al., 1994). This question is also discussed in Chapter 6 of this report. Salmon and Kyle emphasized, as does this report, that experimental plasmacytomas can be induced only under special conditions in genetically susceptible mice, that they differ from multiple myeloma, and that agents other than silicone can induce this response in susceptible mice.

Garland et al. (1996) reported five Florida women diagnosed with immunoglobulin G myeloma from 1990 to 1993 after 2–12 years' exposure to silicone gel implants. Three of these women were 45 years of age or less. Garland concluded that these three cases of multiple myeloma in women with implants were several times the number expected in the State of Florida (Garland et al., 1996). Tricot et al. (1996) reviewed 114 women with multiple myeloma seen from 1992 to 1995; 9 (7.9%) of these women had silicone breast implants. Silverman et al. (1996a) reported three women with silicone breast implants and multiple myeloma; 2 were from a small series of 34 multiple myeloma clinic patients. Although these reports raise the question of an association, as uncontrolled case reports they cannot support a conclusion.

Garland et al. (1996) also studied immunoglobulin levels in a small sample of referred sera from women with silicone breast implants and found 30% of these women to have elevated levels. Silverman et al. (1996a) reviewed immunoglobulin levels in 630 symptomatic women with silicone breast implants of 14 years' mean duration and found elevated immunoglobulins in 23%. In neither of these studies was the frequency of other conditions that might be associated with increased blood levels of immunoglobulins fully assessed in the patients with elevated values. Five women with MGUS were found; two of these women (of four contacted) reverted to normal immunoglobulin levels after removal of their silicone gel implants. Other studies that tested immunoglobulin levels in women with implants—some finding an increase, and others not—have been discussed in Chapter 6. Also, a large study, which was part of a major epidemiological cohort study of connective tissue disease and rheumatic symptoms in women with breast implants, did not find elevated immunoglobulin levels in women with implants compared to healthy controls without implants (Karlson et al., 1999).

Epidemiological studies reported by Deapen and Brody (1992, 1995), Friis et al. (1997b), Kern et al. (1997), and McLaughlin et al. (1998), discussed earlier, have not observed significant (or any) numbers of myeloma cases in women with breast implants. The committee concludes that evidence for an association between silicone breast implants and multiple myeloma or MGUS is insufficient.

CONCLUSIONS

There is a consistent, substantial, long-term base of scientific evidence bearing on the experimental carcinogenicity and clinical breast or other cancer experience with silicone and silicone breast implants. Based on its review of this evidence, the committee concludes that the available evidence does not support an association of silicone or silicone breast implants with experimental carcinogenesis (other than rodent solid-state carcinogenesis), primary or recurrent breast cancer, breast sarcoma or other solid tumors, lymphoma, or myeloma. If anything, evidence (though limited) suggests a lower risk of breast cancer in women with silicone breast implants.

10

Neurologic Disease and Its Association with Silicone Breast Implants

EPIDEMIOLOGIC STUDIES

Two recent epidemiological studies, carried out in Denmark and Sweden, used national hospital discharge registry databases to identify women with breast implants and compared them to age-matched women who had undergone breast reduction surgery. Nyrén et al. (1998c) studied three large cohorts in Sweden—3,502 women with cosmetic breast implants, 3,931 women with implants for reconstruction, and 3,351 women who had undergone breast reduction surgery. On review of a 2,500-woman sample from the cosmetic implant group, 24% were found to have saline implants. A ten-year follow-up of these women was performed through cross-linkage within hospital discharge registers. Neurologic diagnoses examined included multiple sclerosis, neuritis of the optic nerve, amyotrophic lateral sclerosis, diseases of the nerve roots and plexus, mononeuritis of the upper extremity (median, ulnar, and radial nerves), mononeuritis of the lower extremity, Guillain-Barré syndrome, and Meniere's disease. Charts of all women with neurologic diagnoses were reviewed. Overall the relative risk for any of the neurologic diseases was 0.8 (95% confidence interval [CI], 0.5–1.4). Following removal of prevalent (preexisting) and misclassified cases identified through chart review, there was a significant deficit (relative risk, 0.5; 95% CI, 0.2–0.9) of multiple sclerosis and a marginally significant deficit of mononeuritis of the upper limb (relative risk, 0.5; 95% CI 0.2–1.0) in implant patients (Nyrén et al., 1998c).

The Danish study followed 1,135 women with breast implants and 7,071 women in the comparison breast reduction group. The same neurologic diseases were examined, with the addition of myasthenia gravis, other demyelinating central nervous system neuropathies, and motor neuropathy. Cases were not verified. No increased relative risk for defined neurologic disease in the implant group relative to the comparison group was found. The relative risk in the implant group was 1.7 (95% CI, 0.9–2.9), but a similar excess of neurologic disease was found in the breast reduction control group. The relative risks for several individual neurologic conditions were not significantly elevated, and on chart review, 38% of the cases (5 of 13) of neurologic disease were discovered to have had their onset before breast implantation (Winther et al., 1998).

Another recent publication addressed the issue of sensorineural hearing loss (Meniere's disease) associated with silicone breast implants. A group of 119 of 184 women with Meniere's disease or progressive hearing loss and 100 age-matched controls responded to questionnaires (64.7% response rate) and provided serum samples to measure the presence of the 68 kiloDalton (kDa) protein found in some forms of autoimmune hearing loss. There was no significant association of silicone breast implants with Meniere's disease or progressive hearing loss (odds ratio, 1.42). The presence of the 68-kDa protein was not significantly associated with the presence of silicone breast implants (Kim and Harris, 1998). The committee has concluded that these well-designed epidemiological studies provide limited evidence for the lack of association between breast implants and neurologic disease.

CASE SERIES AND REPORTS

Pathological findings in nerve and muscle biopsies from 55 women with breast implants were reported in an abstract by Vogel and Edmondson (1996). Biopsies were examined by light and electron microscopy and by teasing the nerve fibers. Pathology was observed in 6 of 55 biopsies, including 3 with axonal neuropathy, 1 with granulomatous neuritis and myositis, 1 with chronic inflammatory demyelinating polyneuropathy (CIDP), and 1 with Charcot-Marie-Tooth disease. The authors concluded that only conventional neuromuscular disease was found in these women (Vogel and Edmondson, 1996).

Additional pathological and toxicological reports are reviewed in Chapter 4. Hine et al. (1969) did not find evidence for neurotoxicity on injection of silicone syringe lubricant into the lumbar subdural space and cisterna magna of rabbits, monkeys, and rats. Silicone was implanted subdurally in the brain of rats with no observable effect (Agnew et al., 1962). No direct evidence of silicone gel toxicity to peripheral nerves was observed when gel was injected directly into or around the sciatic nerve of rats, although an inflammatory response followed by fibrosis was seen (Sanger et al., 1992).

Also silicon concentrations were somewhat elevated in brains of rabbits exposed to gel implants that had been cut open, but not in rabbits with intact gel or saline implants. No pathological changes were observed in the brains of these rabbits (Marotta et al., 1996b). These results are reported briefly with no individual data and are unconfirmed. No accumulation of silicon in sural nerves of women with breast implants were found by Evans et al. (1996), and toxicological studies of silicone distribution after injection subcutaneously of gel distillate in mice showed, if anything, lower brain concentrations of cyclic compounds and moderate concentrations of linears (Kala et al., 1998; see Chapter 4).

In response to inquiries to the American Academy of Neurology (AAN) regarding scientific reports that associated neurological disease with silicone breast implants, the AAN Practice Committee performed an extensive search of the scientific literature from 1975 on (Ferguson, 1997). This search discovered 14 reports focusing on a variety of painful syndromes, for example, involvement of the brachial plexus by a ruptured silicone breast implant (Collins et al., 1995). A Call for Comments in the AAN newsletter produced some anecdotal responses, a published abstract (Rountree et al., 1995), several published papers and unpublished manuscripts from Ostermeyer-Shoaib and colleagues, and an article from Rosenberg (1996) that reviewed medical records of 131 patients that had been examined by Ostermeyer-Shoaib et al. (Rosenberg, 1996).

The published abstract by Rountree (1995) reported 330 women who were injury claimants and 248 controls. Antinuclear antibody (ANA) frequency was no different for women with silicone breast implants and controls. The prevalence of antibodies to ganglioside M1 (anti-GM1) was 3.3% in patients with ruptured implants, not significantly different from 5.4% in patients with intact implants. Age-adjusted prevalence was 19.1% in patients with ruptured implants compared to 7.1% in patients with intact implants, a difference that was still not statistically significant. It was proposed that rupture increases with age and this increases the risk of anti-GM1 antibodies. Two reports by Ostermeyer-Shoaib and colleagues (Ostermeyer-Shoaib and Patten, 1996a; Ostermeyer-Shoaib et al., 1994), discussed below, were critically reviewed in the report of the Practice Committee (Ferguson, 1997). Problems identified included the following: (1) both papers are case series whose findings have not been replicated by other groups; (2) clinical presentation, symptoms, and physical findings were not associated with laboratory data for the individual neurological diagnoses; and (3) as reported by Rosenberg (1996), a review of the medical records from 131 of these patients found little data to support the neurological diagnoses. The Practice Committee concluded that existing studies do not support any association or causal relationship between silicone breast implants and neurologic disorders.

Ostermeyer-Shoaib and colleagues published numerous abstracts describing self- or attorney-referred women with silicone breast implants and neurological syndromes (Ostermeyer-Shoaib and Patten, 1993a,b,c; Ostermeyer-Shoaib et al., 1992). Results from the first 100 consecutive referrals from 1985 to July 1992 of women with silicone breast implants who developed symptoms after implantation were reported in 1994 (Ostermeyer-Shoaib et al., 1994). This group of 100 women had increased to 1,500 by December 1993. Subjects were studied by history, physical and neurological examination, and a plastic surgery consultation. All subjects had 20 to 30 symptoms. The most common were weakness (95%); fatigue, myalgia morning stiffness, joint pain, and memory problems (81%); sicca complex (71%); shortness of breath (63%); and joint swelling (58%). History and physical examination provided diagnoses of polyneuropathy in 83, multiple sclerosis-like syndrome in 10 (with peripheral neuropathy present in eight of these), motor neuron disease in 5, and myasthenia gravis in 2 patients. The criteria used to establish these diagnoses were not reported. Symptoms and physical signs were tabulated only in the aggregate and therefore could not be linked to a diagnosis. Magnetic resonance imaging (MRI) of the brain in 84 patients demonstrated multiple white matter lesions in 19 women, but the distribution of these lesions was not specified. Thirteen women had multiple small ischemic lesions; this type of lesion is frequently considered part of normal aging. Assay of 28 spinal fluid samples revealed oligoclonal bands in 13, but the number of bands was not specified. Axonal neuropathy was diagnosed by electromyography in 4 patients, and 53 had an abnormal sural nerve biopsy with significant loss of myelinated fibers. It is surprising for the electrodiagnostic findings to reveal so few abnormalities in the presence of significant pathology in the large myelinated fibers. Randomly elevated autoantibodies, such as ANA, rheumatoid factor, anti-GM1, anti-MAG (myelin-associated glycoprotein) and antisulfatide, were measured. The committee can find no pattern of results or of clinical or laboratory evidence that would allow an assessment of the accuracy of any of the diagnoses.

In a second publication, Ostermeyer-Shoaib and Patten (1996a) summarized findings in 26 patients with silicone breast implants that they believed had a systemic disease involving the central nervous system. A referring neurologist had made the diagnosis of atypical multiple sclerosis with physical findings of optic neuritis, hyperreflexia, spastic paraparesis, stocking-glove sensory loss, nystagmus, and ataxia. MRI had demonstrated white matter lesions in 21 of these women. Visual evoked responses were prolonged in 14 of 23. Lumbar puncture found oligoclonal bands in 18 of 23, and electromyography was abnormal in 9 of 19, including 4 with carpal tunnel syndrome, 3 with myopathic units, and 1 with denervation (Ostermeyer-Shoaib and Patten, 1996a). Despite these varied electrodiagnositc findings, all 15 sural nerve biopsies were abnormal. The committee notes that these results do not fit any known pathology, are clinically inconsistent, and have not been reported by any other group.

Rosenberg (1996) reviewed the medical records of 131 patients examined by Ostermeyer-Shoaib and Patten. He found all patients had non-neurologic symptoms that included fatigue (82%), numbness or paresthesias in the upper extremities (50%), headache (47%), numbness or paresthesias in the lower extremities (41%), back pain (37%), gait disturbance (35%), neck pain (35%), dizziness (34%), blurred vision (18%), and diplopia (8%). Neurological examination was normal in 66% or revealed abnormalities that were rated as mild or subjective. The most common finding, varying sensory abnormalities, was present in 23%. Muscle weakness was present in 18% in a variable distribution. Reflexes, abnormal in 8%, were increased in all but one patient who had absent ankle jerks. Both mental status and cranial nerve abnormalities were found in 3%. Gait disturbance was present in 2 patients, although 46 had complained of this. Twenty-one antibodies were tabulated and found to have a prevalence similar to that in the general population. Rosenberg noted one case of multifocal motor neuropathy with an elevated titer of anti-GM1, a condition described in the neurological literature. Decreased perfusion by brain SPECT, reported in 67%, showed no consistent pattern. Electrodiagnostic testing was abnormal in 12 of 48 women, but these were primarily entrapment syndromes or root compression. Electrodiagnostic findings of axonopathy and myopathy in three women were not supported by clinical findings. Diagnostic imprecision and preconceptions were exemplified by the use of the term "silicone encephalopathy," which was applied whenever any cognitive complaint existed, even with normal mental status testing. White matter lesions found by MRI were scattered nonspecifically (27%), or the few lesions present were not in a periventricular distribution as found in multiple sclerosis. The diagnosis of chronic inflammatory demyelinating poyneuropathy (CIDP) in 23% did not meet the clinical, electrophysiological, or neuropathological criteria for this condition. Rosenberg found support for some specific diagnoses in the 131 patients: depression (16), fibromyalgia (9), radiculopathy (7), anxiety disorder (4), multiple sclerosis (4), other psychiatric disorders (3), multifocal motor neuropathy (1), dermatomyositis (1), and carpal tunnel syndrome (1). However this review of medical records did not uncover any causal link between silicone breast implants and neurological disease (Rosenberg, 1996).

A neuroimmunologic evaluation of 200 symptomatic patients with breast implants and 100 symptomatic patients with chronic fatigue tabulates only laboratory data and provides an extensive methodological description. Antibodies to myelin basic protein, myelin associated glycoprotein (MAG), asialoganglioside GM1, and sulfatide were measured, and lymphocyte subsets were defined. The absence of demographic or clinical information limits any meaning that might be assigned to these laboratory data (Vojdani, 1995a). An abstract by Shanklin and Smalley (1996a) reports their examination of sural nerve biopsies from women with silicone breast implants using polarizing microscopy. These authors reported detection of quartzite silica scattered throughout the nerve at the outer surface of the myelin and speculated on how silicone might be transformed to silica in the body (Shanklin and Smalley, 1996a). However, there is no credible evidence that silicone is degraded to crystalline silica under physiologic conditions. There is also no credible evidence that crystalline silica originates from breast implants or is found near implants (see Chapter 5 of this report). Furthermore, polarizing microscopy is not a reliable technology for detection of crystalline silica (IRG, 1998; see Young, IOM Scientific Workshop), and examination of sural nerves in cadavers of women with silicone breast implants did not reveal elevated silicon concentrations (Evans et al., 1996).

CONCLUSIONS

The available studies suggesting neurologic disease, with the exception of obvious local problems due to the physical presence of silicone gel which can compress nerves following implant rupture and migration of the gel, have defects that limit any conclusions to be drawn from them. Furthermore, basic toxicological and animal experimental studies do not find pathology that would support a causation of human neurologic disease by silicone breast implants. Two epidemiological studies suggest that there is no elevated relative risk for neurological disease in large cohorts of women with silicone breast implants. The committee finds that the evidence for a general neurologic disease or syndrome caused by, or associated with, silicone breast implants is insufficient or flawed.

11

Effects on Pregnancy, Lactation, and Children

It has been suggested that children born to, and breast-fed by, mothers with silicone breast implants might be adversely affected by transmammary or transplacental delivery of silicone during either breast feeding or pregnancy. Silicone might be available for transmission since periprosthetic breast tissue, regional lymph nodes, and possibly more distant sites in such women are exposed to silicone fluid by gel fluid diffusion, to silicone gel in cases of implant rupture, and to silicone elastomer from implant shells. Mothers with breast implants might also have problems with breast feeding due to the effects of implant surgery, the implant itself, or fear of lactation insufficiency and transmission of complications to their infants. The committee has reviewed the effects of breast implants, especially silicone gel breast implants, during pregnancy and lactation.

EFFECTS OF SILICONE BREAST IMPLANTS DURING PREGNANCY

The ability of silicone to pass the placental barrier depends on factors such as the size of the silicone molecule. The concentration gradient of silicone in the maternal and fetal circulation is also important. This gradient in turn is dependent on other factors, including the amount of silicone in the maternal–fetal circulation, the protein-binding ability of silicone, and the uterine blood flow. Whether silicone crosses the placenta has not been evaluated in women, but there is little evidence of any elevation of blood or serum silicon or silicone concentrations in women with silicone breast implants, and elevations reported in two studies have been modest and have not been confirmed by subsequent studies (see below and Chapter 5 of this report).

The committee is not aware of any studies of reproductive or teratologic effects of silicone in humans. However, reproductive and fetal developmental effects of polydimethylsiloxane (PDMS) fluid have been evaluated in rats and rabbits, and mutagenic potential was evaluated in mice. Teratologic and mutagenic effects were not observed at the dose levels and in the species employed (Kennedy et al., 1976). Subcutaneously implanted silicone elastomer and silicone gel at several dose levels did not induce maternal or developmental toxicity before or during pregnancy and lactation, did not have adverse effects on parents or neonates, and did not impair reproductive performance in either male or female rats or pregnant female rabbits (Siddiqui et al., 1994a,b). These and other relevant studies are reviewed in Chapter 4. Evidence from these studies for toxic effects of silicone during or after pregnancy is lacking.

EFFECTS DURING LACTATION

Effect on Breast Milk

Many drugs and chemicals that appear in the maternal circulation may be detected in breast milk (Berlin, 1989). Characteristics that affect a compound's ability to traverse the mammary gland epithelium, appear in human breast milk, and become available to a nursing infant include its degree of ionization, molecular weight, lipid solubility, and protein-binding capacity. Except in the rare event of direct rupture of a deposit of silicone into a milk duct (Leibman et al., 1992; Shermis et al., 1990), to be transferred to breast milk, silicone must diffuse or be transported across a number of cell membranes. The evidence reviewed in Chapter 4 does not support diffusion or transport of silicone gel across membranes that presumably would exclude substances of high molecular weight. The evidence does suggest limited mobility of lower molecular weight linear or cyclic species, but these compounds are present in very low concentrations in breast implants, do not appear to be highly mobile in experimental distribution studies, and are subject to the body's clearance mechanisms.

Some proteins from maternal or external sources have been found in milk—for example, cows' milk proteins and maternal immunoglobulin G (IgG)—and these proteins can be found in the serum of breast-feeding infants. Transport of these proteins probably occurs through clefts between mammary alveolar cells (Berlin, 1989). Most other proteins do not cross from maternal circulation into breast milk. Ions, such as sodium and iron, do not cross well either, except for those such as lithium, with low atomic weights.

The determination of silicon or silicone in human body fluids by current technologies is discussed in Chapter 5. Reported blood and tissue measurements are reviewed there, as are the problems in attaining accurate and reproducible results and the varied sources of silicon and silicone that either contribute to dietary intake and affect biological concentrations or constitute environmental contaminants in analytical measurements. In addition, Chapter 5 notes that analyses of tissue and body fluid samples usually measure concentrations of the element silicon and do not differentiate between inorganic and organic (silicone) silicon-containing compounds.

Although, as noted earlier, silicone could enter breast milk through direct extension from deposits in breast issue, there is no evidence that this is other than a rare event, and it has not been reported in breastfeeding women with implants. Measurement of silicon or silicone concentrations in breast milk of women with implants might provide some insights into whether silicone reaches breast milk by other means. Jordan and Blum (1996) reported silicon measurements from a U.S. laboratory in 69 breast milk samples by inductively coupled plasma atomic emission spectrometry. The implant status of women providing these samples was not mentioned, but all showed a silicon concentration of less than the detection limit, 0.05 μg/ml. Tanaka et al. (1990) reported breast milk silicon concentrations in healthy postpartum Japanese women without implants averaging 0.171 μg/ml and serum concentrations of 0.27 μg/ml. These higher results may be due to an increased intake of silicon in the high-fiber, high-silicon diet of the Japanese population; they may also reflect the known, ubiquitous analytical problems caused by contamination with environmental silicon (Semple et al., 1998). In a Dow Corning laboratory, no difference was found between breast milk samples (1.2 parts per million [ppm]), control samples (2.1–3.9 ppm), and water blank (0.4–3.1 ppm) samples. These outlier results undoubtedly reflect analytical difficulties as the authors note (Curtis et al., 1991).

In a study of breast milk from women with silicone breast implants compared to controls, no significant difference was found. Breast milk was tested for silicon concentrations in 10 women with silicone gel breast implants (0.063.7 ± 0.041 μg/ml) compared to 20 women without breast implants (0.061 ± 0.035 μg/ml) measured by graphite furnace atomic absorption spectrophotometry (Lugowski et al., 1996; and personal communication, 1998). In a later report, Lugowski et al. (1998) compared breast milk and blood silicon concentrations in 14 and 15 blood and milk samples, respectively, from women with silicone gel implants and 23 and

29 blood and milk samples, respectively, from women without implants. Mean blood concentrations were 0.0743 and 0.1038 μg/ml, and mean milk concentrations were 0.0587 and 0.0511 μg/ml in women with implants and control women, respectively. There were no significant differences in blood or milk silicon concentrations between these two groups (Lugowski et al., 1998). In yet another report from the same laboratory comparing 15 lactating women with silicone breast implants to 34 lactating control women, mean silicon concentrations in breast milk were 0.0555 ± 0.035 and 0.0511 ± 0.031 μg/ml, respectively, and in blood were 0.0793 ± 0.087 and 0.10376 ± 0.112 μg/ml, respectively. The mean silicon concentration measured in store-bought cows' milk was 0.7089 μg/ml and that for 26 brands of commercially available infant formula was 4.4025 μg/ml (Semple et al., 1998). These last three studies taken together suggest that lactating women with silicone breast implants are similar to control women without implants with respect to the concentrations of silicon in their breast milk and blood. Silicon concentrations in cows' milk exceed concentrations in human breast milk by a factor of ten and are even higher in infant formula. Five different samples of cows' milk yielded silicon concentrations ranging from 0.667 to 0.778 μg/ml. Even higher concentrations of silicon were measured in 26 brands of infant formula (0.796–13.796 μg/ml). The high values for silicon in cows' milk and infant formula found by Semple et al. (1998) do not necessarily imply a high silicone content, however. There are likely multiple sources of both silicon and silicone in processed and manufactured foods, which may be related to silicon in cows' feed, silicone antifoaming agents, or packaging techniques involving silicone, among other factors. The results from this laboratory appear to represent accurate values since collection of samples was scrupulously controlled to avoid contamination and samples were prepared in a class 100 "ultraclean" laboratory.

Although only modest numbers of women were enrolled in these studies, breast milk from women with silicone implants appears to have a relatively low concentration of silicon, especially when environmental forms of silicone and silicon are accounted for. Breast milk concentrations may reflect blood silicon concentrations and, as noted earlier, may therefore be in large part inorganic, although as noted earlier, women in industrialized countries have ample exposure to silicone in a number of ways (Adler and Berlyne, 1986). Semple et al. (1998) have also demonstrated that two alternatives to breast milk, cows' milk and infant formula, contain considerably more silicon than breast milk. Infants may have significant exposure to silicone in infant formulas, cows' milk, bottle nipples, and infant pacifiers. Silicone, as a component of Simethicone-containing proprietary drops, is also considered safe and effective as a treatment for colic or gastrointestinal hypermotility in infants and children. One such product (Mylicon) contains 67 mg of PDMS/ml (Berlin, 1994). The committee concludes that there is convincing evidence that infants breast-fed by mothers with silicone gel breast implants receive no higher silicon intakes from breast milk than infants breast-fed by mothers without breast implants. Infants receiving cows' milk or commercial infant formula feedings are likely to have significantly higher silicon intakes than breast-fed infants. Evidence that any likely exposure to silicon or silicone has effects on infant health is lacking. The proportion, if any, of silicone in measurements of silicon in the samples discussed remains to be investigated. The oral toxicity of methylated siloxanes is very low, however, and these siloxanes are generally recognized as safe (for oral exposure) by the Food and Drug Administration (FDA) when used as indirect food additives as reviewed in Chapter 4 of this report (D. Benz, FDA, personal communication, 1998).

Breast Implants and Problems with Breast Feeding

Under the influence of rising concentrations of estrogen, progesterone, and prolactin during pregnancy, the breast increases in water, fat, and electrolyte content. The overall increase in breast volume is approximately 0.75 pound per breast. This increase in size may cause breast discomfort in women who have implants, especially those with capsular contractures, i.e., beyond the discomfort normally experienced by pregnant women (Lawrence, 1989; Riordan and Auerbach, 1993).

The prevalence of breast-feeding problems in the general population is not well defined, but both maternal and infant factors account for the cessation of breast feeding or for lactation insufficiency. Although insufficient milk supply is the major reason reported by mothers for early termination of breast feeding in both developed and developing nations (Gussler and Briesemeister, 1980), other maternal factors may contribute to insufficient milk supply such as sore nipples, let-down reflex inhibition, engorgement, blocked milk ducts, infection and return to work. Infant problems also are related to insufficient supply of breast milk, for example, poor weight gain (Hill and Schatten, 1991; Melnikow and Bedinghaus, 1994).

Few studies have evaluated women with silicone breast implants during pregnancy. In the survey by de Cholnoky (1970) of 265 plastic surgeons and 10,941 breast augmentation procedures (including 149 silicone injections and 6,304 silicone gel, Cronin-type implants), plastic surgeons reported that women tolerated implants without significant complaints during pregnancy and nursed babies adequately. Whidden (1986), in a report of 2,228 women who had breast augmentation procedures with either silicone gel- or saline-filled implants, noted that problems with breast feeding were not encountered. The value of these reports is limited since no information is provided on the number of women who breast-fed their infants, the duration of breast feeding, any problems they might have had, or how women were evaluated for lactation sufficiency. In the epidemiological study of children of women with silicone breast implants in Denmark discussed below, there was incomplete information on breast feeding (Kjoller et al., 1998).

Three studies have focused on the effects of augmentation mammaplasty on lactation sufficiency. Neifert et al. (1990) studied 319 first-time mothers who breast-fed healthy, full-term infants. Although the relative risk of lactation insufficiency was threefold greater for women with a history of breast surgery (95% confidence interval [CI], 1.65–5.9), only 5 of the 22 surgeries were for breast augmentation with implants. Surgery with a periareolar incision was almost five times more likely to be associated with insufficient milk compared to no surgery. Breast incisions in other locations were not associated with lactation insufficiency (Neifert et al., 1990). Hurst reported retrospectively on 42 mothers with breast implants for augmentation and 42 mothers without implants matched for age, delivery type, breast-feeding experience, and other factors, who were selected from 5,066 mother–infant records from a Texas hospital. Both groups of mothers received the same intensive lactation support and counseling from a hospital-based lactation program. The frequency of lactation insufficiency was significantly increased in women with implants (27 out of 42, 64%) compared to women without implants (3 out of 42, 7%). Periareolar incision was most associated with breast-feeding insufficiency, although the frequency of lactation insufficiency in augmentation by the submammary or axillary approach was statistically significantly increased compared with women without implants. No data were available on the type of implants (Hurst, 1996).

In a survey of 292 women with saline-filled breast implants, 46 women reported subsequent pregnancies and 28 chose to breast-feed their infants. Breast-feeding problems were reported by 11 of the 28 mothers with implants (39%), and 8 of these women reported problems related to lactation insufficiency (28%): 4 nipple problems and 4 milk production problems. Seven of these women had periareolar incisions. (About 30% of breast implant augmentations are carried out through a periareolar incision; ASPRS, 1997.) The women who chose not to breast-feed (18 out of 46) reported fear of lactation insufficiency and other complications due to the implants as the primary reason (Strom et al., 1997). In addition to these reports, Peters et al. (1997) noted in a study of 100 consecutive women who were having silicone gel implants removed, that 19 of 75 women responding to a questionnaire reported successful breast feeding;

it was not clear how many of the 75 had completed pregnancies and attempted breast feeding, however.

These studies primarily describe retrospectively small cohorts of mothers with implants. Only one study involved a matched comparison group, and the type of implant was specified in only one study, although most of the women in the other two reports probably had gel-filled implants, given the usage of implants for augmentation at the time of the study. These studies did not measure the frequency of infections or mastitis, either, although Hurst (1996) reported on multiple correlates of lactation insufficiency. These studies suggest that there is no difference in age, ethnicity, delivery type, smoking history, or breast-feeding experience among women with breast implants and those without implants, but as many as 64% of women with implants may have lactation insufficiency compared to less than 10% of women without implants (Hurst, 1996). Based on these studies, the relative risk of lactation insufficiency is at least three times greater in women who have a history of breast surgery, and the risk of lactation insufficiency increases with a periareolar incision (Hurst, 1996; Neifert et al., 1990; Strom et al., 1997). Periareolar incisions may be more likely to sever lactiferous ducts, depending on operative technique.

Breast-feeding problems appear to be common in women with either silicone or saline implants. The frequency of lactation insufficiency ranges from 28 to 64% for both silicone gel- and saline-filled implants. Women with breast implants have also been less likely to attempt breast feeding due to their fear of problems stemming from the implant (Crase, 1996). Although the data on periareolar incisions and lactation are suggestive, the mechanism of increased lactation problems due to implants remains uncertain; Hurst (1996a) suggests that pressure exerted by an implant may be detrimental to milk production. Increased intramammary pressure, when prolonged and unrelieved, may cause atrophy of the alveolar cellular wall and diminished milk production. The location of the implant might also be a factor. Implants in the submuscular position might exert less pressure or in other ways interfere less with functioning glandular tissue.

In addition to the reports discussed above, six studies report eight cases of abnormal lactation or lactation complications (mastitis, galactorrhea, or galactocele formation) after breast implant surgery (DeLoach et al., 1994; Hartley and Schatten, 1971; Johnson and Hanson, 1996; Luhan, 1979; Mason et al., 1991; Menendez-Graino et al., 1990). Galactocele and galactorrhea after breast augmentation surgery are uncommon complications based on these reports published over a 14-year time span. The eight cases included both saline implants and gel-filled implants. Although these case reports describe complications related to lactation, the prevalence of these complications cannot be adequately assessed. Furthermore, information is lacking in a number of studies, such as the type of breast implant or the type of surgical incision.

Based on the information available, the type of implant does not appear to be related to postpartum breast infection or abnormal lactation. The cause of galactoceles remains unknown, but postoperative breast congestion around the implant may trigger the release of lactogenic hormone and thereby stimulate milk production and secretion. Oxytocin or prolactin release may be stimulated either hormonally, by direct pressure on the breast, or both, and substantial increases in serum prolactin have been measured in women after breast stimulation (Kolodny et al., 1972). The majority of these women will require removal and replacement of their implants along with hormonal medication to suppress the galactorrhea.

Breast Feeding in the United States: Prevalence and Advantages

In the United States, the prevalence of breast feeding at one week postpartum was 52% for hospital-born infants in 1989, and only 18% still were receiving breast milk by 6 months of age (Riordan and Auerbach, 1993). In general, breast feeding is more common among older Caucasian women of higher socioeconomic status. The World Health Organization, the UNICEF, and the U.S. Public Health Service (Surgeon General) have established national and international goals to promote and support breast feeding (Riordan and Auerbach, 1993; U.S. DHHS, 1991). The Surgeon General's nationwide objective proposes to increase the proportion of women who are breast feeding their infants at hospital discharge to 75% and the percentage of women still breast feeding infants at 6 months of age to 50% by the year 2000. One study provides data on the prevalence of breast feeding in women with breast implants (Strom et al., 1997). In this survey discussed earlier, 61% of women with breast implants chose to breast feed, suggesting that the prevalence of attempted breast feeding by women with implants approximates its prevalence in the general population.

The distinct advantages of breast feeding and breast milk are widely appreciated. Breast feeding plays an important role in human infant development. Breast milk provides not only essential nutrition for the infant but also protection against infections and other immunologic disorders. Gastrointestinal disease, respiratory ailments and asthma, otitis media, and allergies occur less frequently in breast-feeding infants (Castello, 1986; Lawrence, 1989; Riordan and Auerbach, 1993). Although more speculative, breast feeding is also said to provide protection against obesity, arteriosclerosis, celiac disease, and other metabolic disorders (Hanson et al., 1985; Lawrence, 1989; Mayer et al., 1988). With respect to the mother, breast feeding creates a psychological bond between infant and mother, which ultimately may lead to a socially healthier child (Newton and Newton, 1967). In addition, lactation enhances maternal postpartum recovery, and body weight returns to prepregnancy levels more rapidly (American Academy of Pediatrics, 1997). The committee believes that breast feeding should be encouraged in all mothers when possible, including those with silicone breast implants. There is evidence that breast implantation may increase the risk of insufficient lactation, but no evidence that this poses a hazard to the infant beyond the loss of breast feeding itself. The evidence for the advantages of breast feeding to infant and mother is conclusive.

EFFECTS ON CHILDREN

In the early 1990s, claims were made that children of women with silicone breast implants might be adversely affected by transmammary or transplacental delivery of silicone during breast feeding or pregnancy (Gedalia et al., 1995; Levine and Ilowite, 1994; Teuber and Gershwin, 1994). Hypotheses were advanced that silicone transmitted in breast milk might cause an autoimmune or connective tissue disease in children of mothers with breast implants; that maternal autoantibodies resulting from exposure to silicone in breast implants might be transferred to children across the placenta or in breast milk; or that silicone-induced immunological abnormalities, other than autoantibodies, in mothers with breast implants might be transmitted to their children across the placenta or in breast milk. The committee finds no evidence for these hypotheses.

Connective Tissue or Autoimmune Disease and Esophageal Effects

Two case series from California (Teuber and Gershwin, 1994) and New York (Levine and Ilowite, 1994) proposed that signs and symptoms found in children whose mothers had silicone breast implants were suggestive of autoimmune disorders. Teuber and Gershwin (1994) described one female child of each of two mothers who had breast implants (one ruptured, one suspected to have ruptured), positive antinuclear antibodies (ANA) and arthralgia or arthritis. Both children, one 3 and one 9 years of age, had longstanding myalgia. Both were found to have antinuclear antibodies (titers of 1:40 and 1:80, respectively), and the 9-year-old girl had high-titer antibodies against denatured human type II collagen. These children were normal on physical examination except for diffuse tenderness of the lower back, abdomen, and muscles of the extremities in the 9-year-old (Teuber and Gershwin, 1994).

Levine and Ilowite (1994) suggested a link between esophageal symptoms found in breast-fed children and maternal silicone breast implants.

Although labeled as a case control study by the authors, sample reduction procedures in the experimental and control groups attenuate this study to a case series of eight breast-fed children and three bottle-fed children. (A correction making this change was published by Journal of the American Medical Association, 272 (10): 770, 1994.) Physician or support groups referred mothers with silicone breast implants who were concerned about the effects of these implants in their children. Of 67 children born to these women, 56 were breast-fed and 11 were bottle-fed. No data were provided on the health histories or status of this original sample. The sample was reduced to 43 children with recurrent abdominal pain and then, for unclear reasons, further reduced to 26 children with additional symptoms such as vomiting, dysphagia, decreased weight–height ratio or a sibling with these complaints. Family permission was not obtained for 15 of these 26 to participate in this study. The final sample included 11 children (6 boys and 5 girls), from 18 months to 13 years of age, 8 breast-fed and 3 bottle-fed. The average duration of breast-feeding was five months, and the mean interval between discontinuation of breast-feeding and evaluation was 5.7 years. The average age of the breast-fed children was 6 years (18 months to 9 years), and of the bottle-fed children was 5 years (18 months to 13 years). These 11 children were compared to patients (11 boys and 6 girls; average age, 10.7 years) from a control group of 20 patients with feeding problems reduced to 17 by excluding 3 patients with achalasia. Six of the eight breast-fed children from mothers with silicone breast implants were reported to have significantly abnormal esophageal motility with nearly absent peristalsis in the distal two-thirds and decreased lower sphincter pressure based on esophageal manometry and upper-intestinal endoscopy with esophageal biopsy. Compared to controls, the breast-fed children were said to have significantly decreased lower sphincter pressure and abnormal esophageal wave propagation. No gross endoscopic findings or histologic evidence of infection or deposits of silicone were observed among any of the children. Levine and Ilowite (1994) speculated that their findings provided support for a scleroderma-like esophageal disease in children breast-fed by mothers with silicone breast implants.

The committee notes a number of problems with this study. The unexplained reductions in the study groups raise questions of selection bias as does the refusal to participate of 15 of 26 (58%) children in the final sample. Parents and children may have been influenced to focus on esophageal symptoms by the emphasis on these symptoms in a questionnaire circulated to enlist the experimental group. Many data gaps exist in reporting signs, symptoms, and clinical laboratory findings in the original and subsequent experimental groups of children and mothers. Apparently the children did not fulfill any of the criteria for scleroderma, including positive autoantibodies; information of this sort was not given for the mothers. No data on the type or status of implants in the mothers were provided. The control group was also reduced and is inappropriately age matched, raising issues of age differences in use of technology to evaluate esophageal function and in the response to sedation used to enable examination. These may be important considerations (Hillemeier, 1986). Bartel examined one of the original breast-fed children and suggested a separate neurological cause for the esophageal findings (Bartel, 1994). One analysis of the six breast-fed cases with abnormalities suggested that they might all have come from just two families, which would limit the generalizability of these findings. Why the three original bottle-fed children in the study sample were not controls instead is not clear if the variable at issue was the effect of breast feeding, as the title of this report indicates. If the variable under study was simply the presence of breast implants, then these three children provide no evidence that breast implants are associated with abnormalities of esophageal function in children. Many of these concerns have also been noted by others (Bartel, 1994; Berlin, 1994; Brody, 1994a; Cook, 1994; Epstein, 1994, 1996; Flick, 1994; Liau et al., 1994; Placik, 1994).

The authors of both of these case reports speculated that the symptoms and findings in these children might, in fact, be due to exposure to silicone in breast milk or in utero or to transmission of some undefined immunological factor(s) from the mothers. No assays for silicon or silicone were performed, however, in any of the mothers or the children. As noted earlier in this chapter, silicon concentrations in breast milk of mothers with implants are not elevated above concentrations in lactating control women without implants. As reported in Chapter 5 as well as in this chapter, silicon concentrations in blood or serum of women with silicone breast implants are the same as concentrations in normal or lactating control women (Lugowski et al., 1998; Semple et al., 1998), with the exception of two reports of nonlactating women, which found somewhat higher than normal controls, but still quite low concentrations (Teuber et al., 1995a, 1996; Peters et al., 1995a). The highest silicon concentrations—orders of magnitude higher—are found in cows' milk and infant formula (Semple et al., 1998). If breast milk is a key factor in effects in children, these findings do not identify a cause; they provide evidence against elevated silicone as a causative agent in human breast milk.

With the exception of low- to moderate-titer, nonspecific ANAs in the mothers of the two girls reported by Teuber and Gershwin (1994), no immunological abnormalities were found in the mothers of these children. Since antinuclear antibodies are not infrequently found in normal women of childbearing age, it is difficult to assign any significance to them in these cases (see Chapter 7 of this report and, for example, Yadin et al., 1989). Some of the children reported had nonspecific ANAs, but most did not. One child had anticollagen antibodies, as noted. No other immune abnormalities were found in these children, and in the case of esophageal abnormalities as noted above, the children of mothers with breast implants who were bottle-fed did not display abnormal esophageal motility providing no evidence that some other, possibly immune factor might be at work in these mothers and children.

In a two-year follow-up to their original report, Levine et al. (1996) reported on the original eight plus three additional similarly breast-fed children. Although the children were reported to be in better general health, the esophageal findings were essentially unchanged. The original bottle-fed children were not reported again. Macrophage activation was measured by urinary nitrates and neopterin as an indication of a hypothesized silicone-induced inflammatory process, and the effect of treatment using ranitidine (4 mg/kg per day, an inhibitor of stomach acid secretion) was evaluated. Endoscopic examinations revealed mild esophagitis in eight of ten children, with four normal biopsies and six biopsies showing inflammation. Urinary nitrates were not significantly different from the initial determination, but urinary neopterin levels had decreased. The authors concluded that esophageal dysmotility was chronic in children breast-fed by mothers with silicone breast implants and that prokinetic agents (like ranitidine) might be useful in treatment (Levine et al., 1996). This follow-up study suffers from many of the problems of the first. Three new cases were added with almost no additional data. Very little information on the general health status of any of the children is provided. There is no discussion of the control of dietary nitrates, which could influence urinary nitrate measurements. Intercurrent infections and even immunizations can result in urinary neopterin concentrations an order of magnitude greater than those observed here (Fuchs et al., 1992).

An attempt was made to investigate the effect of maternal silicone gel implants on esophageal pathology in breast-fed rat pups. Silicone gel was injected beneath the nipples of Sprague-Dawley rats, which were subsequently bred. Some of the resulting pups breast-fed without further intervention, and some breast-feeding pups received an injection of 2 ml of silicone gel in the neck as a further challenge. The esophagus of each pup at intervals up to 64 weeks was examined by a variety of light and electron microscopic techniques. No silicone was found in any esophagus, and no esophageal fibrosis was observed. In this study, silicone did not accumulate in the esophagus, and no esophageal pathology was seen (Raso et al., 1997).

Since esophageal problems or decreased esophageal motility have not been found in bottle-fed children of women with silicone breast implants, any consequences for esophageal function appear to be related to breast feeding. The committee can not imagine, and finds no evidence for, any immune mechanism associated with breast milk that would produce esophageal or immune–autoimmune changes a decade after breast feeding. Also, in the absence of any finding of elevated silicon or silicone in breast milk of mothers with implants or accumulating in the esophagus or elsewhere in the bodies of these children or in the esophagus of an experimental rat model, the committee has not found evidence that silicone could produce esophageal changes years after birth. No biologically plausible mechanism for an immune or silicone effect in breast milk associated with esophageal changes is apparent to the committee or has been suggested by others. Finally, as discussed later in this chapter, a well-designed epidemiological study provides no support for an association of esophageal disease in children with silicone breast implants in their mothers.

Immunological Studies

A number of studies have proposed immune effects in children of mothers with breast implants. As noted earlier, Levine et al. (1996) measured urinary nitrites or nitrates and neopterin as proxies for macrophage activity and reported that some children breast fed by mothers with silicone implants, and in particular children with esophageal symptoms, had elevated urinary concentrations of these substances. They also reported that concentrations varied inversely with esophageal wave propagation and with age, suggesting a relationship with esophageal dysfunction and a waning of the infant effect as the children age (Levine et al., 1996). Because nitrate intake was not controlled and neopterin concentrations are intensely variable under a number of different circumstances as discussed earlier, these results are difficult to interpret in this highly selected population. There is also no evidence that the putative causative exposure to silicone actually occurs.

Maternal antibody transmission from a mother with silicone breast implants to her child, with a presumed health consequence, was reported by Gedalia et al. (1995). In this case, the infant presented with positive anti-Ro antibody and skin rash. Similar instances of neonatal systemic lupus erythematosus (SLE) with anti-Ro autoantibodies transmitted from a mother with SLE and anti-Ro antibodies were discussed. From time to time, cardiac sequelae are observed. In this infant, the antibody and rash cleared by 1 year of age (Gedalia et al., 1995). Levine et al. (1996) measured antinuclear antibodies and a wide array of other autoantibodies in 40 male and 40 female (and anticollagen antibodies in a 33-child subset of these) symptomatic children, both breast- and bottle-fed, referred by physicians, attorneys , or support groups. All children were born to mothers with breast implants and averaged 6.8 years of age. A control group of 42 symptomatic children not exposed to maternal breast implants was also tested. Although there was a relationship of antibodies to symptomatology, there was no significant difference between the control and the experimental groups (Levine et al., 1996). As noted earlier, there is a modest prevalence of antinuclear antibodies in women of childbearing age. With rare exceptions as above, this is not known to cause health problems in their infants or young children.

Shanklin et al. (1996a) and Smalley et al. (1996a) have reported studies of children born to women with silicone breast implants. Shanklin et al. reported that 127 children born to women before placement of breast implants were in better health than 93 children born after implantation. The committee noted that this study population was very probably highly selected. There was no information to confirm the specific health status of these children. T-lymphocyte mitogen tests were reported in a summary fashion to be positive in 84% of a group of 33 children born after implantation. Stimulation indexes, that is, T-cell responses on exposure to silica, were also reported as overall average values in mothers and children (Shanklin et al., 1996a). Smalley et al. (1996a) reported that children of women with silicone breast implants had a proliferative response to silica. These authors used a stimulation index that compares the reaction of cells stimulated by the antigen (in this case silicon dioxide) with the reaction of unstimulated control cells. The mean stimulation index of 15 mothers was 182, whereas that of their 24 children was 77, in comparison to an index of less than 25 in historical normal controls. Comparison of small numbers of children of mothers without implants to children of mothers with implants suggested that the latter group had a higher mean stimulation index. Smalley et al. (1996a) concluded that silicone crosses the placenta, causing T-cell responsiveness to silica in the children. As noted earlier, these children were often not in good health.

These experimental procedures have been used in a number of reports from this group. In general, they are incompletely reported. Culture conditions, cell density, and the amount of particulate silica added to the cultures are not described. Nearly all data relate to colloidal silica, and there is insufficient or flawed evidence that this is a substance to which women with silicone implants are exposed. The stimulation indices are not interpretable without quantitative knowledge of the actual cellular reactions; comparative reaction counts may provide an index that is misleading if the actual counts are all below values that indicate a reliable test. It is possible that proliferative responses reflect some non-antigen-specific reaction to silica, but the authors' conclusion that silicone crosses the placenta and causes T-cell responsiveness to silica (an entirely different molecule) in children is speculative. In an independent assessment of this test, Young (1996b) reported it to be unreliable and variable in ways that had no relationship to clinical facts or to the silicone breast implant status of the tested women. The studies reviewed here do not provide any evidence to alter conclusions on immunological effects reached earlier in the discussion of case reports.

Epidemiological Studies

Files of the Danish National Registry of Patients were used to identify all children born from 1977 to 1992 to a cohort of 1,135 women with cosmetic breast implants and to a comparison cohort of 7,071 women who had undergone breast reduction surgery. Cause-specific hospitalization rates among children, related to those of the general population, were calculated from this registry. Children were followed for the occurrence of adverse health outcomes from the time of birth to death, emigration, or until December 31, 1993. Adverse outcomes included most esophageal disorders, defined connective tissue disease, other rheumatic conditions, and congenital malformations. Findings among the 939 children of mothers with breast implants included higher numbers of esophageal disorders, but the excess was similar for children born before and after implantation. More frequent hospitalizations than expected for these conditions were also observed among 3,906 children of women who underwent breast reduction surgery. No significant increases in connective tissue diseases or congenital malformations were observed in either the breast implant or the breast reduction cohorts. Specifically, the investigators found four cases of esophageal disorders among children born after the mother's breast implantation, compared with 1.4 expected. However, the increased risk observed among children potentially exposed to silicone was similar to the excess risk found in silicone-unexposed children (12 cases observed, 4.5 expected). A slight, nonsignificantly increased risk of congenital malformation among children born after the date of the mother's implant was seen (21 cases observed, 15.9 cases expected), but was also found in the group of children born before implantation (59 cases observed, 49.4 cases expected). No cases of defined connective tissue disease or other rheumatic conditions were observed in children of mothers with breast implants, but the expected numbers were small and thus the power to detect an association was low.

The observed excess of hospitalization in Denmark for minor esophageal disorders among children of mothers with breast implants or breast reduction surgery suggests a lower threshold for seeking professional medical care for infant-feeding problems normally solved outside the hospital system. The absence of defined connective tissue disease or other rheumatic conditions in these 279 children suggests that the incidence of connective tissue diseases is not likely to be greatly elevated in children of women with implants (Kjoller et al., 1998).

Since study participants were drawn from a nationwide register of patients and children were traced through population registers, sample selection bias was unlikely. However, using hospital record data, rather than clinical data collected prospectively, may limit the interpretation of study results. Episodic symptoms of dysphagia, feeding problems, abdominal pain, or vomiting are probably evaluated outside the hospital setting and escape recognition by the national registry. The average time of five years between the date of implantation and the birth of a child may be too short to appropriately evaluate the effect of implant gel fluid diffusion or rupture. Few data were available on breast-feeding history, and the type of breast implant was not specified in 16% of the sample. Nevertheless this study has moderately large numbers of women and children and is well designed.

CONCLUSIONS

The committee concludes on the basis of the studies reviewed in this chapter that evidence for an association of maternal silicone breast implants and children's health effects is insufficient or flawed. No biologically plausible causation has been suggested. Convincing evidence is available that silicon concentrations in breast milk are the same in mothers with and without breast implants, and thus there are no data to support transmission of silicone to infants in breast milk of mothers with implants. A modest number of normal mothers are positive for ANAs. Except for rare instances, as noted, evidence that this or similar situations in mothers with silicone breast implants have deleterious effects on children is lacking. Evidence for children's esophageal disease caused by maternal breast implants is insufficient or flawed.

12

Silicone Implants and Breast Imaging

Women with silicone breast implants undergo imaging evaluations to detect early breast cancer just as women without breast implants. In addition, women undergo imaging to assess the integrity of these implants. Several characteristics of implants and the techniques of their placement affect imaging evaluations. These include the major types of prostheses (e.g., silicone elastomer shells and fillers of silicone gel, saline, both gel and saline mixed, or multiple lumens), the great variety of implants of current and historical manufacturers (described in Chapter 3), and the different placement of implants (subcutaneous), subglandular, or submammary, above the chest wall muscles, and submuscular or subpectoral under those muscles, as described in Chapter 5).

IMPLANT INTEGRITY ASSESSMENT

Implant rupture is defined in Chapter 5 as silicone gel detectable on the outer implant and/or capsular surface. This does not necessarily imply a complete disruption of the implant shell, but indicates only loss of shell integrity and movement of silicone gel outside the elastomer shell. As discussed earlier, rupture, which includes what some have termed leakage, is different from gel fluid diffusion, which refers to the diffusion of the lower molecular weight silicone fluid that permeates the silicone gel through the implant shell into the capsule or surrounding tissues.

Breast implants are encased by a fibrous capsule, and a potential or actual fluid-filled space is produced between the implant shell and the surrounding capsule, as described in Chapters 3 and 5. Rupture involving only the silicone shell, with free silicone gel still contained by the surrounding fibrous capsule, are defined as intracapsular rupture. Disruption of both the implant shell and fibrous capsule allows silicone access to breast tissue and is defined as an extracapsular rupture. Normal silicone fluid diffusion is detectable only rarely by imaging examinations.

Other terms associated with loss of shell or fibrous capsule integrity are also in common usage. Herniation indicates focal bulging of an intact implant through a defect in the surrounding fibrous capsule. Extrusion implies a sudden flow of silicone gel through defects in the implant shell and fibrous capsule, which may occur with traumatic events. Infiltration is a slow movement of extracapsular silicone gel into surrounding breast or other tissue. Extravasation is an inclusive term encompassing extrusion and infiltration, whereas migration refers to extracapsular silicone gel movement away from the implant.

The frequency of implant rupture is unknown. Chapter 5 discusses the reasons for this, which include such factors as the changing composition of implants, the decades-long observation required in some cases, the study of nonrepresentative groups of women with implants, and incomplete or imprecise detection of rupture. Some confusion is also occasionally caused by the separation of rupture into leakage and rupture or disruption categories. Estimates of implant rupture prevalence range from 0.3 to 77%, as reported earlier. Rupture prevalence depends at least in part on implant characteristics such as elastomer shell thickness and strength; thus descriptions of rupture prevalence must consider and identify the types and "generations" of implants. Breast implant integrity can be evaluated clinically; mammographically; and with computed tomography, ultrasound, and magnetic resonance imaging (MRI).

Mammography

The intact silicone gel-filled implant appears as a radiodense structure sharply circumscribed from surrounding breast tissue. At times, the implant fibrous capsule may be visible just superficially to the implant shell. Dystrophic calcification can be identified in the fibrous capsule (Benjamin and Guy, 1977). Calcification is often seen and could represent a long-term inflammatory response to the breast prosthesis (Barker et al., 1978; Cocke et al., 1985; Ginsbach et al., 1979; Inoue et al., 1983; Koide and Katayama, 1979; Peters et al., 1995d; Redfern et al., 1977; Young et al., 1989). Textured implants may disorganize capsular fibrotic reactions and decrease capsular contracture. Use of textured implants could be a source of a false-positive mammographic diagnosis of rupture. The presence of a textured implant is easily detected by its brush border (Piccoli, 1968). The capsule around a textured implant grows into and around the pores and small papillary projections of the shell surface. Silicone can be observed in these irregularities, and this may mimic implant rupture (Kasper, 1998).

Direct mammographic evidence of rupture is related to demonstration of extravasated silicone, silicone droplets, or calcified silicone in surrounding breast tissue as a result of an extracapsular rupture. Because of the radiodensity of silicone, direct evidence of intracapsular rupture contained by the intact fibrous capsule may not be possible. Indirect mammographic signs of intracapsular rupture include changed implant dimensions compared to prior studies, an ill-defined border or irregular implant density, marked bulging of an implant border, and silicone in mammary gland ducts or lymphatics (Destouet et al., 1992; Ganott et al., 1992; Gorczyca et al., 1994a; Peters et al., 1995d; Reynolds et al., 1994; Theophelis and Stevensen, 1986).

Reporting of the sensitivity and specificity of detection of implant rupture varies depending on the way rupture is defined mammographically. Accurate sensitivity and specificity also depend on an accurate verification of rupture. As discussed in Chapter 5, careful direct visual examination of a breast implant on explantation is considered the most reliable standard. In the reports reviewed in Chapter 5, this standard was generally (but not always; see, for example, Peters and Pugash, 1993, Table I) used to determine the performance of imaging technologies in diagnosing rupture (i.e., their sensitivity and specificity). Even the explantation standard is occasionally imperfect, however, because intact implants may inadvertently and unknowingly be torn during explantation, leading to a mistaken diagnosis of rupture, or tiny holes that allow gel through the shell may not be seen, leading to a mistaken diagnosis that the implant is intact.

Handel et al. (1992) described two levels of concern in the mammographic detection of ruptures. Suspicious findings included major bulges, anteroposterior flattening, and irregular, ill-defined margins of the implant, while silicone outside the implant was considered diagnostic. If signs considered diagnostic defined a mammogram as a true positive for rupture, the sensitivity was only 15% but specificity was 100%. However, if both suspicious and diagnostic findings were included, then sensitivity and specificity were 69 and 82%, respectively (Handel et al., 1992). Everson et al. (1994) demonstrated a 23% mammographic sensitivity with a 98% specificity. These authors also felt that mammography was specific for the detection of extracapsular implant rupture but was of limited use for intracapsular rupture. Ahn et al. (1994a) noted an 11% sensitivity and 89% specificity. They reported a high false-negative rate of 33.3%. These authors also confirmed the ability of mammography to detect free silicone, indicating an extracapsular rupture, but found that free silicone in the posterior aspect and intrapectoralis muscular areas was difficult to identify (Ahn et al., 1994a). Andersen et al. (1989) also found that mammograms were excellent for detecting free silicone in the breast, demonstrating an accuracy of 90%. However, if a mammogram with any findings (in addition to free silicone) suggestive of rupture was called positive, the sensitivity fell to 67% (Andersen et al., 1989). Other authors have reported varying sensitivities in series and reviews of various size, for example, 89% (Cohen et al., 1997); 62% (Nemecek, cited in Samuels et al., 1995); 16.2% (Robinson et al., 1995); and 45%–67% (Samuels et al., 1995).

Ultrasound

Ultrasound is used routinely as an adjunct to film mammography for evaluating palpable breast masses or clinically occult masses detected by x-ray. Ultrasound evaluation of silicone gel implants can be a sensitive technique for the evaluation of implant integrity. Since the examination is highly operator dependent, sensitivity and specificity are more variable than with other imaging techniques and depend on the experience of the radiologist in performing and interpreting the examination and on the scanning techniques utilized. A high-resolution linear array transducer of 7–10 MHz should be used, and real-time scanning by the interpreting physician is strongly recommended to eliminate confusion due to artifacts that commonly occur (Gorczyca et al., 1994b). Artifactual echoes that are anteriorly positioned in the silicone gel implant, as well as echoes produced behind the implant in the chest wall and pictured within the lumen of the implant, may be confused with implant rupture. These are effects of the varying speed of sound in silicone gel and breast tissue. If the operator and interpreter are inexperienced, these artifacts can be confused with findings of loss of implant integrity (Forsberg et al., 1996).

There are several sonographic signs relating to the evaluation of implant integrity. The interface of the breast with the implant may contain highly echogenic signals obscuring posterior breast tissue. This has been termed the "snowstorm" sign and represents free silicone gel adjacent to the implant (Harris et al., 1993). The presence of hypoechoic nodules that may be associated with this snowstorm sign is thought to represent larger conglomerates of silicone within breast tissue (Herzog, 1989; Van Wingerden and Van Staden, 1989) and also to indicate an extracapsular rupture. Echogenic material within the implant lumen (Berg et al., 1993; DeBruhl et al., 1993) as well as the presence of either single, multiple and continuous, multiple and discontinuous, or parallel ("stepladder" sign) echogenic lines or bands may correspond to a disrupted and collapsed implant shell contained within an intact fibrous capsule, i.e., an intracapsular rupture (DeBruhl et al., 1993; Gorczyca et al., 1992).

A wide range in the sensitivity and specificity of ultrasound detection of rupture is reported in the literature. The sensitivities range from 25 to 100%, and specificities range from 50 to 99% (Ahn et al., 1994a; Berg et al., 1995; Caskey et al., 1994; Chilcote et al., 1994; Chung et al., 1996; DeBruhl et al., 1993; Everson et al., 1994; Harris et al., 1993; Liston et al., 1994; Medot et al., 1997; Palmon et al., 1994; Peters and Pugash, 1993; Petro et al., 1994; Reynolds et al., 1994; Venta et al., 1996). However, the majority of these studies report a sensitivity of 48–74% (Ahn et al., 1994a; Berg et al., 1995; Caskey et al., 1994; Chung et al., 1996; DeBruhl et al., 1993; Everson et al., 1994; Harris et al., 1993; Palmon et al., 1994; Peters and Pugash, 1993; Reynolds et al., 1994; Venta et al., 1996) and a specificity of 50–90% (Berg et al., 1995; Caskey et al., 1994; Chilcote et al., 1994; Chung et al., 1996; Everson et al., 1994; Medot et al., 1997; Palmon et al., 1994; Reynolds et al., 1994; Venta et al., 1996). A low sensitivity reported in one article (Chilcote et al., 1994) was associated with separation of data into ruptures and all implant failures. The ruptures were defined as tears greater than 10 cm in diameter. When this definition was used, sensitivity was 50%. When rents less than 0.5 cm were included in the definition, sensitivity dropped to 25%. The article reporting 100% sensitivity used both wall redundancy and "atypical silicone," neither of which was described. However, the sensitivity is based on only seven ruptured implants (Petro et al., 1994). The study reporting a 99% specificity (Peters and Pugash, 1993) was a retrospective study of 150 consecutive office patients with only 8 going on to surgery. Diagnoses were based on a combination of ultrasound and clinical analysis; one woman with abnormal ultrasound turned out to have intact implants at surgery.

Although sensitivity and specificity show wide variation, it appears that ultrasound is more specific than it is sensitive. Several authors calculated the sensitivity and specificity of the various ultrasound signs of altered implant integrity. Caskey et al. (1994) demonstrated that low-level echoes within the implant were the most sensitive sign of rupture (55%), while adjacent echogenic noise had the highest specificity (97%). Echogenic noise surrounding an implant had a 97% correlation with rupture, but this sign was seen in only 5% of ruptures. DeBruhl et al. (1993) found the presence of internal parallel echogenic lines to be the most sensitive sign, occurring in 70% of ruptured implants. Palmon et al. (1994), however, demonstrated that linear echoes can be seen in most silicone breast implants, and their presence or absence is not useful in predicting rupture. Medot et al. (1997) analyzed the detection of implant integrity with ultrasound based on the presence or absence of capsular contracture. The sensitivity and specificity for rupture was 41 and 70%, respectively, with capsular contracture, and 69 and 74%, respectively, without capsular contracture. They concluded that ultrasound is reliable only for indicating rupture in the absence of capsular contracture.

Magnetic Resonance Imaging

Silicone gel can be differentiated from breast tissue by taking advantage of its unique nuclear magnetic resonance properties. The basis of magnetic resonance imaging and chemical characterization is detection of a resonance signal from perturbed protons within the body. Since protons are the most abundant nuclear elements, a detectable resonance signal can be expected. Protons perturbed by radiofrequency waves in a homogeneous magnetic field emit a second radiofrequency wave when the stimulating frequency is discontinued. The properties of this emitted resonance frequency depend on the molecule to which the protons are attached and the nature of the disturbing input radiofrequency. Through a judicious use of sequence parameters, the protons in breast tissue (i.e., in water) and those in silicone can be separated (Derby et al., 1993).

Although a detailed analysis of the various MRI sequences is not within the scope of this report, a brief description of basic principles will improve understanding of MRI examinations of women with breast implants. T1 and T2 imaging refer to imaging sequences that can enhance signal from protons in various biochemical compounds. Silicone, on a T1-type image, will have a low signal and, on a T2-type image, a high signal. Protons associated with fat will also have a high signal on T2 images, although lower than silicone. There are several techniques that are successful in separating proton resonance signals emanating from fat, water, and silicone. The three-point Dixon technique (Schneider and Chan, 1993) produces an image that demonstrates a signal only from silicone and nullifies signals from fat and water. The RODEO (rotating delivery of excitation off-resonance) technique can selectively eliminate signals within the proton resonance range of silicone (Harms et al., 1995), allowing silicone detection by determining which signals are lost after the RODEO technique is applied.

The accuracy of MRI in evaluating the integrity of breast implants derives from its ability to detect rupture of the implant shell contained by an intact fibrous capsule, that is, intracapsular rupture. Several signs of rupture have been described with MRI. The "linguine sign" (Gorczyca et al., 1994c) is a series of low-signal curvilinear lines within the high-signal silicone gel and represents segments of free-floating implant shell. In instances of intracapsular rupture without complete collapse of the implant shell, silicone is present both within and outside the shell. This silicone may invaginate a portion of the implant shell producing the so-called keyhole, teardrop, or noose sign (Berg et al., 1994, 1995; Gorczyca, 1994c;

Mund et al., 1993). The "subcapsular line" sign is also an indication of a ruptured implant without complete disruption of the implant shell. Silicone completely surrounds the shell and highlights the implant envelope as a low-signal line subtended by intra- and extracapsular silicone gel closely paralleling the intact fibrous capsule (Benjamin and Guy, 1977).

As noted earlier, the various types of breast implants and surgical procedures must be considered to avoid false-positive diagnoses of implant rupture. The most prevalent pitfall is the presence of radial folds, which are normal invaginations of the periphery of the implant shell. These folds appear thicker than the low-signal lines seen with shell disruption since they represent two adjacent portions of the implant shell. They rarely traverse the implant on all images and when imaged in plane may present a sheetlike appearance that is unusual in true implant shell disruption (Benjamin and Guy, 1977). Double-lumen devices have an inner shell containing silicone gel and a surrounding compartment of saline. The outer saline-containing shell may rupture, resulting in the image of a normal single-lumen implant. This can be a source of confusion when placement of a double-lumen implant was recorded. At times, an intact single-lumen implant surrounded by reactive fluid contained by the fibrous capsule can be mistaken for a normal double-lumen device. Water droplets within the silicone gel can be detected by MRI and may also indicate loss of implant shell integrity. This finding may be deceptive since saline or saline with antibiotics or steroids may have been injected into the implant at the time of placement (Berg et al., 1994).

The sensitivity and specificity of MRI for implant rupture is greater than that of mammography or ultrasound. This is especially true when magnetic resonance coils specifically designed for the breast are utilized. Soo et al. (1997) reported a sensitivity of 88% utilizing the linguine sign and any two signs indicative of silicone on the surface of the implant (keyhole, subcapsular, or teardrop). The specificity of the examination was 92%, with a positive predictive value (PPV) of 43% and a negative predictive value (NPV) of 85% (Soo et al., 1997). Gorczyca et al. (1992) demonstrated a 76% sensitivity and 97% specificity utilizing a shoulder coil, and in 1994, they demonstrated an 89% sensitivity and 97% specificity using a dedicated breast coil (Gorczyca et al., 1994a). Several studies report a low sensitivity of MRI for detection of implant integrity. Weizer et al. (1995) described a sensitivity of 46%; the authors state that the use of a body coil was a major reason for the low sensitivity. Reynolds et al. (1994) used a shoulder coil for most of their implant examinations and recorded a sensitivity of 69%; this study involved only 13 patients and 24 implants. Ahn et al. (1993) demonstrated a 76% sensitivity and Middleton (1998b) a 74% sensitivity. All of the examinations in the former study were done with a body or surface coil not dedicated for breast imaging, and the latter study used a mixture of dedicated and nondedicated coils. Modern MRI scanning is a highly sensitive and specific test for the detection of implant ruptures with the use of proper equipment and imaging parameters.

There are advantages and disadvantages to all imaging modalities used in the evaluation of implant integrity. Mammography is rapid and inexpensive, but it is very inaccurate for intracapsular rupture and will reliably detect extruded silicone only in an extracapsular rupture. Ultrasound has the potential to detect both intra- and extracapsular ruptures, is inexpensive, and uses no ionizing radiation. However, it is a highly operator-dependent study that is less accurate in the presence of capsular contracture and is unable to visualize the posterior surface of the implant. The sensitivity of the examination is greater than mammography, however. MRI has the highest sensitivity and specificity for evaluation of implant integrity and has none of the limitations of mammography or ultrasound, but it is expensive and time-consuming. MRI requires modern dedicated breast-imaging coils, and necessitates a thorough knowledge of implants and of potential diagnostic pitfalls. When these conditions are present, the interoperator agreement may be excellent, however (Brown et al., 1999).

Although the sequence of modalities used to evaluate implant integrity will vary, the committee has concluded based on current information, that the following steps are reasonable. A clinical suspicion of loss of implant integrity such as a sudden size change, pain, or asymmetry should initiate the imaging sequence. Mammography and ultrasonography can be the initial imaging examinations. If both are normal, the clinician may wish to follow the patient. If these examinations are unequivocally abnormal, then explantation may be considered on a case-by-case basis. Any equivocal or suspicious result of mammography or ultrasound study should be followed by MRI evaluation. If this examination is positive for rupture, explantation may be considered. Some have suggested MRI on all clinically suspicious cases or for routine examination of women with implants and clinical signs suggestive of loss of implant integrity (Samuels et al., 1995). The committee finds that there is no convincing evidence to support routine screening of asymptomatic women for implant rupture. Data on the cost/benefit of routine screening for rupture are lacking, however. Studies that provided such data and analysis might allow a firm conclusion on whether screening for rupture is indicated or not indicated in asymptomatic women with silicone breast implants, either as a routine procedure, or in specific situations such as women with rupture prone implants or in circumstances of changing technologies or certain clinical comorbidities. To justify routine screening of the general population of asymptomatic women with silicone breast implants, such studies would have to provide convincing scientific data showing that routine screening and a consequent intervention effectively reduced complications and morbidity secondary to implant rupture. Table 12-1 reviews reports on the evaluation of implant integrity.

MAMMOGRAPHY AND IMPLANTS

Technique

Modern mammography is divided into screening and diagnostic examinations. Screening mammography is an x-ray examination to detect unsuspected breast cancer at an early stage in asymptomatic women. It usually consists of two views of each breast, a mediolateral oblique (MLO) and a craniocaudal (CC) view. The examination is performed by a qualified technologist, often in the absence of the interpreting physician. Diagnostic mammography is an x-ray examination to evaluate abnormal physical findings in the breast or abnormal findings detected with a screening mammogram. Diagnostic mammography is performed under the on-site supervision of a qualified interpreting physician.

The presence of silicone gel-filled breast implants may interfere with standard mammography since silicone is radiopaque, and the physical presence of the implant compresses fat and glandular tissues, creating more homogeneous dense tissue that frequently lacks the contrast needed to detect subtle early features associated with breast cancer. Eklund et al. (1988) described a modified compression technique that permits more effective imaging of breasts with implants. The prosthesis is displaced posteriorly and superiorly against the chest wall while the breast tissue is gently pulled anteriorly onto the image receptor and held in place by the compression device. This maneuver should be used for both the CC and the MLO views, and such views are termed implant-displaced views. Breast implants are surrounded by a fibrous capsule that may be soft or hard. If the capsule is hard and immobile, it may be impossible to perform the implant-displaced views. The MLO view may be replaced by the 90-degree lateral view if the latter depicts more breast tissure in individual patients. When there is clinical concern for lesions cephalad to the implant between the 11 and 1 o'clock positions or caudad to the implant between the 5 and 7 o'clock positions, the 90 degree lateral view can be helpful (Heinlein and Bassett, 1997). Thus, the current standard for mammography of women with implants is both a nondisplaced and an implant-displaced view for each of the routine views. This examination results in four views per breast, the CC and MLO views in both the implant-displaced and the standard modes.

The augmented breast presents unique imaging problems depending on the experience and expertise of the technologist and interpreting physician, surgical techniques, and characteristics of the implant. Even with the modified technique described above, the amount of breast tissue visualized will be limited by the implant. Discussion of the utility of mammography with implants began as early as 1968 when Mendes-Filho and Ludovici advocated preimplant mammography to facilitate later comparison. In 1974, Rintala and Svinhufvud concluded that the prosthesis did not hamper the technical performance of the examination. Cohen et al. (1977) disagreed, concluding that gel implants did obscure portions of the breast. In one of the first actual estimates, Wolfe (1978) reported breast tissue nonvisibility in the presence of silicone gel implants at about 25%. Hayes et al. (1988) examined six sets of mammograms in the CC and MLO views and subtracted the calculated volume of the implant from the calculated volume of both the implant and the visualized tissue. They found that the proportion of obscured glandular tissue ranged from 15 to 100%, with an average of 41%. Silverstein et al. (1990a) calculated the area of mammographically visualized breast tissue before and after augmentation mammaplasty using a transparent grid to measure surface area. Women whose implants were placed in a subglandular position had a mean decrease in measurable tissue of 49% with nondisplaced mammography and 39% with implant-displaced views. The decrease in measurable tissue was 28 and 9% in nondisplaced and displaced views, respectively, in patients with subpectoral implants (Silverstein et al., 1990a). More qualitatively, Destouet et al. (1992) rated the quality of implant-displaced views from excellent to poor based on an estimate of improved breast tissue visualization with these views compared to standard views in 252 women. They found the subpectoral position of the implant provided implant-displaced views uniformly rated as excellent, compared to only 7% so rated for the subglandular position (Destouet et al., 1992). Jensen and Mackey (1985) also found part of the breast obscured to mammography by implants. Lindbichler et al. (1996), using qualitative assessments rating mammograms as good, acceptable, and limited, found that examinations in 29% of subpectoral and 22% of subglandular silicone gel implanted breasts were of limited quality.

The finding of reduced visualization in mammograms of women with breast implants has spurred interest in utilizing radiolucent implant fillers. Young et al. (1993a) tested the biocompatibility of peanut oil (a medium-chain triglyceride) and also tested the radiographic properties of oil-filled versus saline-filled prostheses implanted in rabbits. With silicone gel as a control, 10 ml of sterile peanut oil was injected into rats. These rats demonstrated a rapid absorption of peanut oil with no abnormalities at histologic evaluation of the lungs, liver, kidneys, and tissues adjacent to the injection sites. Radiography of the two types of implants

TABLE 12-1 Implant Integrity Determination

Study	No. (patients/ breasts)	Study Design	Technique
Soo et al., 1996	37/72	Surgical proof,[a] retrospective	MRI
Soo et al., 1997	44/86	Surgical proof, retrospective	MRI
Gorczyca et al., 1992	70/140	Surgical proof, retrospective	MRI
Gorczyca et al., 1994	41/81	Surgical proof, retrospective	MRI
Monticciolo et al., 1994	23/38	Surgical proof, prospective	MRI Mammography
Quinn et al., 1996	54/108	Surgical proof, prospective/ retrospective	MRI/
Ahn et al., 1993	80/—	Surgical proof, retrospective	MRI
Andersen et al., 1989	24/—	Surgical proof, retrospective	Mammography
Chung et al., 1996	98/192	Surgical proof, prospective	US
Caskey et al.,1994	31/59	Surgical proof, prospective	US
Chilcote et al., 1994	25/42	Surgical proof prospective	US
Medot et al., 1997	65/122	Surgical proof, retrospective	US
DeBruhl et al., 1993	28/57	Surgical proof, prospective	US
Venta et al., 1996	43/78	Surgical proof, prospective	US
Harris et al., 1993	22/29	Medical records, surgical proof	US Mammography Clinical exam
Palmon et al., 1997	33/64	Prospective, evaluation only sign of echo lines in implant	US—thick lines US—thin lines US—commas
Ahn et al., 1994a	29/59	Surgical proof, prospective	US Mammography MRI

Sensitivity	Specificity	PPV (%)	NPV (%)	Accuracy
TD—48% of rupture	0	0	0	0
Linguine—48% of rupture				
Folds—4% of rupture				
Linguine—44%	100%	100	58	0
Subcap, L, or KS, 94%	87%	90	92	
L or any two of SC, KS				
TD, 88%	92%	93	85	
76%	97%	84	96	94
3-point Dixon, 60%	3-point Dixon, 97%	0	0	0
FSE, 89%	FSE, 97%			
94%	100%	0	0	0
81%	100%			
87%	78%	0	0	0
93%	92%	0	0	0
76%	97%	0	0	0
67%	0	0	0	0
74%	89%	77	88	0
55%	84%	0	0	0
All implant failures, 25%	75%	0	0	54
Rupture only, 50%	75%			71
With CC, 41.2%	70%	53.9	58.3	0
Without CC, 68.7%	73.6%	61.1	79.6	0
70%	92%	82	85	0
50%	55%	58	91	0
65%	0	0	0	0
45%				
50%				
48%	50%	0	0	0
48%	50%			
43%	50%			
70%	92%	0	0	0
11%	89%			
81%	92%			

Continued

TABLE 12-1 Continued

Study	No. (patients/ breasts)	Study Design	Technique
Petro et al., 1994	0/22	Surgical proof, prospective	US, wall redundancy US, atypical silicone US, both
Middleton, 1998b	877/1626	Surgical proof, retrospective	MRI
Dobke et al., 1994	39/74	Surgical proof, retrospective	MRI
Berg et al., 1995	—/144	Surgical proof, prospective	MRI—rupture MRI—leak US—rupture US—leak
Weizer et al., 1995	81/160	Surgical proof, prospective	US MRI
Reynolds et al., 1994	13/24	Surgical proof	Mammography US MRI
Peters and Pugash, 1993	150/—	Some surgical, some clinical, retrospective	US
Ahn et al., 1994b	—/22	Surgical proof, retrospective	CT

NOTE: FSE = fast spin echo; KS = keyhole sign; L = linguine; TD = teardrop; and US = ultrasound.

[a]Imaging verified at explant.

placed in 21 rabbits showed the peanut oil-containing implants to be radiolucent while those filled with saline obscured surrounding soft tissue (Young et al., 1993a). Using an American College of Radiology (ACR) phantom to simulate microcalcifications and soft tissue masses, Gumucio et al. (1989) placed various implant fillers over the ACR phantom and then evaluated the phantom scores produced with each. The shells filled with silicone gel or a mixture of saline and silicone gel completely obscured the phantom. Shells filled with gelatin allowed limited visibility of the simulated calcifications but obscured the masses. Peanut oil and sunflower oil allowed the best resolution of the artifacts within the ACR phantom.

Beisang and Geise (1991) reported polyvinylpyrrolidone (PVP), known as Bio-Oncotic gel, as a filler whose radiographic properties were close to normal breast tissue. Young et al. (1993a) found peanut oil to allow imaging of the ACR phantom most clearly; the oil was four times

Sensitivity	Specificity	PPV (%)	NPV (%)	Accuracy
81%	71%			
29%	87%	0	0	0
100%	71%			
74%	98%	0	0	0
100%	91%	0	0	0
98%	91%			
50%				
65%				
25%	57%	0	0	0
47%	83%	55	83	0
46%	88%	60	83	
69%	82%	0	0	0
54%	64%			
69%	55%			
67%	99%	0	0	0
94%	100%	0	0	0

more radiolucent than saline or Bio-Oncotic gel and about 45 times more radiolucent than silicone gel. In a unique study conducted by Handel et al. (1993b), a patient scheduled to undergo a mastectomy consented to a series of CC views utilizing implant shells filled with various filler materials interposed between the breast and the film cassette. Lesions were best seen through the triglyceride solution. Lesions were observed best with Bio-Oncotic gel when it was at 10% concentration in saline. No lesions could be visualized through silicone gel (Handel et al., 1993b). Implants of polyester fiber commonly used in vascular grafts were reported not to obscure mammographic detail, although no clinical and little experimental experience with breast implants made of this material is available (Yager and Chaglassian, 1998). The committee has not found enough information to support any conclusions about these and other (e.g., soybean oil) fillers. Bio-Oncotic gel was approved for marketing in the United States for several years about ten years ago, and the new U.S. company,

Nova Med, which is introducing a saline implant to the domestic market, markets PVP filled implants in Europe and plans to do so in the United States at some time in the future (see Chapter 3). Soybean oil is under investigation but was recently taken off the market in the United Kingdom because of some reports of adverse reactions.

The adverse publicity regarding silicone implants has caused increasing numbers of women (approaching 40,000 annually in 1994, ASPRS) to have their implants removed. Data on the frequency of implant removal (explantation) are presented in Chapter 1 of this report. Explantation, at times associated with a mastopexy (breast-lifting procedure), produces mammographic changes that must be recognized. Although imaging findings associated with explantation are not common, architectural distortion from scarring or spiculated masses from residual silicone granulomas can occur and simulate malignancy (Hayes et al., 1993). The presence of bilateral symmetric soft-tissue masses posterior to the glandular tissue, as well as coarse plaque-like calcification from residual calcified capsules left behind, should suggest the possibility of a prior explantation (Peters et al., 1996d; Stewart et al., 1992; Young et al., 1989). At times, residual fibrous capsule remaining after explantation may be particularly thick walled, especially if calcified, and seromas may form within these capsules. They present on mammograms as large, oval, soft-tissue masses with either circumscribed or ill-defined margins (Soo et al., 1995).

Women with breast implants frequently ask whether the compressive forces used during the mammographic examination can cause a loss of implant integrity. There is only rare and anecdotal information in the literature regarding the loss of implant integrity after mammography; this has been discussed in Chapter 5. The subglandular position is the most common location of implants that seem to rupture during mammography. Women usually experience pain and a change in implant shape. In one case, the woman described a "popping" sensation at the time of compression. However, as noted, this is said to be a rare complication. It is now recommended that the nondisplaced mammographic views use only enough compressive force to maintain a movement-free breast, not the force one would normally use in the nonaugmented breast. The implant-displaced view places no compressive force on the implant but merely displaces the implant posteriorly and superiorly (Beraka, 1995; DeCamara et al., 1993; Hawes, 1990; Williams, 1991). As noted earlier, the committee has concluded that a concern about implant rupture should definitely not discourage properly performed mammography.

CANCER DETECTION IN A SCREENING SITUATION

Since the introduction of silicone gel breast prostheses in 1962, about

2 million American women have had breast implants. Studies have suggested that breast cancer may be discovered at an advanced stage in women with breast implants and thus have a poorer prognosis. This is ascribed to difficulty in performing mammography which occurs, although to a lesser extent, even with implant-displaced views. The efficacy of mammography in significantly decreasing the mortality from breast cancer has been demonstrated by randomized controlled trials (Kerlikowske, 1997; Smart et al., 1995). The key to the success of mammography is early detection of breast cancer when the tumor is not yet palpable. A review of the cumulative survival by tumor size from the Swedish two-county screening trial undertaken from 1977 to 1985 demonstrates this association. A total of 1,705 cancers were detected in women 40–74 years of age. Fifty-six percent were less than 2 cm in diameter, and the mortality rate from breast cancer in this group was 13% (tumors 1–1.5 cm in diameter are generally not palpable). Tumors 2.0 cm and greater had a mortality rate of 46%, three to fourfold higher (Swedish National Board of Health and Welfare, 1996).

The committee reviewed 12 relevant studies of women with breast implants and cancer detection. This information is summarized in Table 12-2 (Cahan et al., 1995; Carlson et al., 1993; Clark et al., 1993; Dershaw and Chaglassian, 1989; Douglas et al., 1991; Fajardo et al., 1995; Fornage et al., 1994; Grace et al., 1990; Leibman and Kruse, 1993; Schirber et al., 1993; Silverstein et al., 1988, 1992). The accrual dates in these studies, when provided, ranged from 1978 to 1992. Since the majority of the patient accrual took place prior to the establishment of implant-displaced views by Eklund et al. (1988), most of the women studied did not have this maneuver performed. These articles reported 320 women, 278 of whom had mammography with the detection of 264 malignancies. Mammography as the only method of detecting the malignancy occurred in only 38, or 14%, of the women. Palpation as the only method of detection occurred in 126, or 48%, of women, and both mammography and palpation were used in 98, or 37%. (The method of detection was not known in two cases.) Because of the relatively young age of these women, mammography may not have been done routinely and, when done, may have been in response to a clinical indication.

Since it was impossible to determine how many of these women had screening mammography, it is difficult to properly evaluate cancer detection with mammography. Thus, these studies may not represent the detection capabilities of mammography for preclinical disease in women with silicone breast implants. In some of these studies, women with implants had larger primary tumors, more positive axillary nodes, or a lower percentage of palpable tumors visible on mammography than comparison groups of women without breast implants (for example, Carlson et

TABLE 12-2 Augmentation and Breast Cancer Detection

Study	Patient Accrural Dates	No. of Patients/ Mammo/ Cancers	Mammo Only	Palpable Only
Douglas et al., 1991	1978–1988	8/6/8	1	6
Schirber et al, 1993	6 years (no dates given)	9/7/9	0	8
Silverstein et al., 1988	1981–1989	36/36/36	1	13
Fornage et al., 1994	Retrospective, no dates given	7/?/22	7	1
Cahan et al., 1995	1977–1992	22/22/23	4	17
Fajardo et al., 1995	1985–1992	18/18/18	2	13
Carlson et al., 1993	No dates given	35/31/37	2	16
Dershaw and Chaglassian, 1989	1984–1987	59/59/5	1	3
Silverstein et al., 1992	1981–1990	42/42/42	2	19

Both Mammo and Palpable	ID Views	Cancer Statistics	Implant Location
1	No	Augmented: Mammography with palpable mass, 0% Nonaugmented: Mammography with palpable mass, 92%	Subglandular—6 Subpectoral—2
1	?	Augmented: 4/9 Stage II, 5/9 Stage I	0
22	32/36	Augmented: Stage similar to nonmammography detection	Subglandular—15 Subpectoral—17 Not mentioned—4
?	"Most no"	Augmented: 8 cysts, 6 cancers, 6 fibroadenomas, 1 granuloma, and 1 fat necrosis	0
?	?	Augmented: Mammography without palpable mass, 17% 16 IDC 2 ILC 5 DCIS 7 nodes positive	Subglandular—18
3	12/18	Mammography only 1 DCIS, node negative 1 IDC palp +/or mammography 14 IDC, 7 nodes positive 1 mets 1 DCIS	Subglandular—17 Subpectoral—1
19	None	Augmented: 3 DCIS 33 IDC lesions 1 ILC 16 nodes positive 2 distant mets	Subglandular—29 Subpectoral—6
1	None	0	Subglandular—40 Subpectoral—14 Free—5
21	7	Augmented: 4 DCIS 34 IDC 4 ILC 19 nodes positive	Subglandular—37 Subpectoral—5

Continued

TABLE 12-2 Continued

Study	Patient Accrural Dates	No. of Patients/ Mammo/ Cancers	Mammo Only	Palpable Only
Clark et al., 1993	1982–1991	33/29/33	8	14
Leibman and Kruse, 1993	1980–1990	25/22/25	9	4
Grace et al., 1990	1975–1988	6/6/6	1	1

NOTE: DCIS = ductal carcinoma in situ; IDC = infiltrating ductal carcinoma; and ILC = infiltrating lobular carcinoma.

al., 1993; Fajardo et al., 1975; Silverstein et al., 1988). Reintgen et al. (1993) in reviewing the effectiveness of mammography in women with breast cancer also supported these findings. Others, however, found no difference in detection, tumor size, or positive axillary nodes between women with or without breast implants (Cahan et al., 1995; Leibman and Kruse, 1993). The committee has found no data on the relative effectiveness of screening for cancer by physical examination of the implanted breast, although descriptions of examination techniques have been reported (Mann, 1995). Studies are needed to determine whether, among women who routinely undergo screening mammography, there are differences in the stage of breast cancers diagnosed in women with and without silicone breast implants.

A study by Deapen et al. (1997) reported cancer staging in a large group of women with implants. This study included 3,182 women who received cosmetic breast implants between 1953 and 1980. In the study group, 31 breast cancer cases were observed compared to 49 expected. The median follow-up was 14.4 years. The authors found that the stage of

Both Mammo and Palpable	ID Views	Cancer Statistics	Implant Location
11	Done post-1988	Augmented: Tumor size < 2 cm, 82% Lymph node positive, 19% Stage 0/I, 70% Stage II/II, 30% Nonaugmented: Tumor size < 2 cm, 63% Lymph node positive, 41%	0
12	Done post-1988	Augmented: 18 IDC 5 DCIS 2 LCIS 7 nodes positive	0
4	None	Augmented: 6 IDC 1 DCIS	0

breast cancer among women with implants was essentially the same as among women without implants. Women with reconstruction after mastectomy for cancer were not included in this study, so the authors included only first breast cancers in the control group. Since women with implants placed primarily in the 1960s and 1970s formed the study population, the effectiveness of mammography must also be evaluated. Mammographic technique prior to 1980 was inferior to modern mammography.

Some authors have raised concerns that calcification in implant capsules, either with the implant in place or after explantation, might lead to false-positive diagnoses of malignancy and unnecessary additional diagnostic or even therapeutic interventions. Worse, false-negative assumptions that calcifications are capsular instead of cancer associated might be made (see Chapter 5; see also Douglas et al., 1991; Fajardo et al., 1995; Gumucio et al., 1989; Leibman and Kruse, 1993; Peters and Smith, 1995; Peters et al., 1995d; Reynolds et al., 1994; Silverstein et al., 1990b, 1992; Stewart et al., 1992). Peters et al. (1998), Raso et al. (1999) and Rolland et al. (1989b) analyzed capsular calcifications and found them to be calcium phosphate, similar to cancerous calcifications. Rolland et al. (1989b) also reported zinc, which they speculated came from the implants, but Peters et al. (1998) and Raso et al. (1999) did not find this and pointed out that surrounding tissue probably contains much more zinc as a source for possible zinc-containing deposits than a breast implant. Consideration of whether calcifications are low or high density and comparison (in explanted breasts) with preexplant mammograms, among other things, may help to differentiate capsular from cancer-associated calcification (Raso et al., 1999; Rolland et al., 1989b). The above suggests that capsular calcification would constitute a strong indication for capsulectomy at the time of explantation (Peters et al., 1995d).

Although silicone breast implants definitely obscure some of the breast tissue which in theory at least might reduce visualization of breast tumors, the committee noted that some studies of cancer detection in women with silicone breast implants found the implants hindering and some studies found them not hindering detection. Special attention to detection is required in women with silicone breast implants. No studies have addressed whether there is differential mortality from breast cancer due to any differences in detection in women with or without breast implants.

CONCLUSIONS

The committee finds magnetic resonance imaging to be the most accurate imaging modality for the detection of intra- and extracapsular rupture. Mammography is of limited usefulness in detecting implant rupture in women with silicone implants. There is scant anecdotal evidence of rupture during mammography, and there are no data to support limiting screening or diagnostic mammography which would otherwise be indicated because of this concern. Implants placed in a subpectoral position do not interfere with mammography to the same extent as subglandular implants. Data on whether cancer detection is impaired by implants do not allow definite conclusions, although it is clear that implants do interfere with screening mammography by obscuring a variable part of breast tissue, distorting breast architecture, and especially in the presence of firm contractures, making a proper examination with proper compression of the breast more difficult and occasionally impossible.

Reference Lists

These reference lists were prepared in response to the sponsor's request for a comprehensive bibliography through 1998, although some 1999 references are also included. Many references here are not cited in the text of this report, though all were reviewed. They are included because they are responsive to the charge for comprehensiveness. The Committee on the Safety of Silicone Breast Implants gave priority to full reports in peer-reviewed publications in the open scientific literature, and these references are listed separately first. Other references—such as letters, discussions, abstracts, book chapters, and industry technical reports—are included in a second list. This arrangement should not be taken to imply that reports listed first are all of equal quality or that the subsequent list does not contain useful, scientifically valid information. References need to be judged individually on their merits. Staff categorized references by keywords to allow computer sorting. These keywords are at the bottom of each citation. (Note that the use of all capital or lowercase letters for these keywords is merely a device employed by the project staff to locate the appropriate records in its filing system; it carries no further meaning.) The keywords are provided as further information and as a suggestion of the reference content, but they should not be taken to indicate the specific usefulness or content of a report.

LIST OF PEER-REVIEWED SCIENTIFIC REPORTS

Aalto, M., Potila, M., and Kulonen, E. The effect of silica-treated macrophages on the synthesis of collagen and other proteins in vitro. Exper. Cell Res. 1975, 97, 193-202. SILICA.

Aaron, A. D., O'Mara, J. W., Lengendre, K. E., Evans, S. R. T., Attinger, C. E., and Montgomery, E. A. Chest wall fibromatosis associated with silicone breast implants. Surgical Oncology. 1996, 5, (2): 93-99. LOCAL COMPLICATIONS.

Aaron, L. A., Bradley, L. A., Alarcón, G. S., Alexander, R. W., Triana-Alexander, M., Martin, M. Y., and Alberts, K. Psychiatric diagnoses in patients with fibromyalgia are related to health care-seeking behavior rather than to illness. Arthritis and Rheumatism. 1996, 39, (3): 436-445. AI-CTD BACKGROUND/psychosocial.

Abelson, P. H. Exaggerated risks of chemicals. J Clin Epidemiol. 1995, 48, (2): 173-178. GENERAL.

Ablaza, V. J., and LaTrenta, G. S. Late infection of a breast prosthesis with Enterococcus avium. Plast. Reconstr. Surg. 1998 Jul, 102, (1): 227-230. INFECTION/local complications.

Abraham, J. L. Diagnostic applications of scanning electron microscopy and microanalysis in pathology. Israel J. Med. Sci. 1979 Aug 8, 15, (8): 716-723. SILICON MEASUREMENT.

Abraham, J. L., and Etz, E. S. Molecular microanalysis of pathological specimens in situ with a laser-raman microbe. Science. 1979 Nov 9, 206, (9): 716-718. SILICON MEASUREMENT.

Achauer, B. M. A serious complication following medical-grade silicone injection of the face. Plast. Reconstr. Surg. 1983 Feb, 71, (2): 251-253. SILICONE INJECTION.

Adams, Jr. W. P., Robinson, Jr. J. B., and Rohrich, R. J. Lipid infiltration as a possible biologic cause of silicone gel breast implant aging. Plast. Reconstr. Surg. 1998 Jan, 101, (1): 64-68. RUPTURE/local complications.

Addington, D. B., and Mallin, R. E. Closed capsulotomy causing fractures of the scar capsule and the silicone bag of a breast implant. Plast. Reconstr. Surg. 1978, 62, (2): 300-301. CAPSULE CONTRACTURE/CLOSED CAPSULOTOMY/RUPTURE/local complications.

Adler, A. J., and Berlyne, G. M. Silicon metabolism. II. Renal handling in chronic renal failure patients. Nephron. 1986 Jan, 44, 36-39. SILICON MEASUREMENT.

Aggarwal, S. K., Gemma, N. W., Kinter, M., Nicholson, J., Shipe, J. R., and Herold, D. A. Determination of platinum in urine, ultrafiltrate, and whole plasma by isotope dilution gas chromatography-mass spectrometry compared to electrothermal atomic absorption spectrometry. Analytical Biochemistry. 1993, 210, 113-118. PLATINUM.

Agnew, W. F., Todd, E., Richmond, H., and Chronister, W. Biological evaluation of silicone rubber for surgical prosthesis. J Surg Res. 1962 Nov, 11, (6): 357. TOXICOLOGY/ SILICONE CHARACTERIZATION.

Ahn, C. Y., DeBruhl, N. D., Gorczyca, D. P., Bassett, L. W., and Shaw, W. W. Silicone implant rupture diagnosis using computed tomography: A case report and experience with 22 surgically removed implants. Annals of Plastic Surgery. 1994b Dec, 33, (6): 624-628. MAMMOGRAPHY/local complications/rupture.

Ahn, C. Y., DeBruhl, N. D., Gorczyca, D. P., Shaw, W. W., and Bassett, L. W. Comparative silicone breast implant evaluation using mammography, sonography, and magnetic resonance imaging: Experience with 59 implants. Plast. Reconstr. Surg. 1994a Oct, 94, (5): 620-627. MAMMOGRAPHY/local complications/rupture.

Ahn, C. Y., Ko, C. Y., Wagar, E. A., Wong, R. S., and Shaw, W. W. Clinical significance of intracapsular fluid in patients' breast implants. Annals of Plastic Surgery. 1995a, 35, (5): 455-457. INFECTION.

Ahn, C. Y., Ko, C. Y., Wagar, E. A., Wong, R. S., and Shaw, W. W. Microbial evaluation: 139 implants removed from symptomatic patients. Plast. Reconstr. Surg. 1996 Dec, 98, (7): 1225-1229. INFECTION/local complications/capsule-contracture/pain.

Ahn, C. Y., Narayanan, K., Gorczyca, D. P., DeBruhl, N. D., and Shaw, W. W. Evaluation of autogenous tissue breast reconstruction using MRI. Plast. Reconstr. Surg. 1995, 95, (1): 70-76. MAMMOGRAPHY.

Ahn, C. Y., Shaw, W. W., Narayanan, K., Gorczyca, D. P., DeBruhl, N. D., and Bassett, L. W. Residual silicone detection using MRI following previous breast implant removal: Case reports. Aesthetic Plastic Surgery. 1995, 19, (4): 361-367. MAMMOGRAPHY/rupture/local complications/capsule-contracture/granulomas.

Ahn, C. Y., Shaw, W. W., Narayanan, K., Gorczyca, D. P., Sinha, S., Debruhl, N. D., and Bassett, L. W. Definitive diagnosis of breast implant rupture using magnetic resonance imaging. Plast. Reconstr. Surg. 1993 Sep, 92, (4): 681-691. MAMMOGRAPHY/rupture/local complications.

Ahn, C., and Shaw, W. W. Regional silicone gel migration in patients with ruptured implants. Annals of Plastic Surgery. 1994 Aug, 33, (2): 201-208. RUPTURE/local complications/migration/connective tissue disease.

Aho, K., Koskela, R., Makitalo, M. K., Heliovarra, M., and Palouso, T. Antinuclear antibodies heralding the onset of systemic lupus erythematosus. J. Rheumatol. 1992, 19, 1377-1380. AI-CTD BACKGROUND.

Al-Janadi, M., al-Balla, S., al-Dalaan, A., and Raziuddin, S. Cytokine profile in systemic lupus erythematosus, rheumatoid arthritis, and other rheumatic diseases. Journal of Clinical Immunology. 1993, 13, (1): 58-67. AI-CTD BACKGROUND/immune effects/connective tissue disease.

Alarcón-Segovia, D., and Cardiel, M. H. Comparison of three diagnostic criteria for mixed connective tissue disease. Study of 593 patients. J Rheumatol. 1989, 16, (3): 328-334. AI-CTD BACKGROUND.

Albores-Saavedra, J., Vuitch, F., Delgado, R., Wiley, E., and Hagler, H. Sinus histiocytosis of pelvic lymph nodes after hip replacement: A histiocytic proliferation induced by cobalt-chromium and titanium. American Journal of Surgical Pathology. 1994 Jan, 18, (1): 83-90. LOCAL COMPLICATIONS.

Alexandrides, I. J., Shestak, K. C., and Noone, R. B. Thermal injuries following TRAM flap breast reconstruction. Annals of Plastic Surgery. 1997 Apr, 38, (4): 335-341. SENSATION/local complications/reconstruction.

Allwork, S. P., and Norton, R. Surface ultrastructure of silicone rubber aortic valve poppets after long-term implantation. Thorax. 1976, 31, 742-752. SILICONE CHARACTERIZATION.

Alonso-Ruiz, A., Zea-Mendoza, A. C., Salazar-Vallinas, J. M., Rocamora-Ripoll, A., and Beltrán-Gutiérrez. Toxic oil syndrome: A syndrome with features overlapping those of various forms of scleroderma. Seminars in Arthritis and Rheumatism. 1986 Feb, 15, (3): 200-212. AI-CTD BACKGROUND.

American Academy of Neurology, Ad Hoc Subcommittee. Research criteria for diagnosis of chronic inflammatory demyelinating polyneuropathy (CIDP). Neurology. 1991 May, 41, 617-618. AI-CTD BACKGROUND/neurologic disease.

American Academy of Pediatrics. Breastfeeding and the use of human milk: Policy statement. Pediatrics. 1997, 100, (6): 1035-1039. CHILDREN'S EFFECTS/breast feeding.

American Medical Women's Association. Silicone Gel Breast Implants [position paper]. JAMWA. 1998 Winter, 53, (1): 33-35. GENERAL.

American Rheumatism Association Diagnostic and Therapeutic Criteria Committee, Subcommittee for Scleroderma Criteria (Masi A. T., Rodnan, G. P., Medsger, Jr. T. A., Altman, R. D., D'Angleo, W. A., Fries, J. F., and et al.). Preliminary criteria for the classification of system sclerosis (scleroderma). Arthritis and Rheumatism. 1980 May, 23, (5): 581-590. AI-CTD BACKGROUND.

Amin, P., Wille, J., Shah, K., and Kydonieus, A. Analysis of the extractive and hydrolytic behavior of microthane poly(ester-urethane) foam by high pressure liquid chromatography. Journal of Biomedical Materials Research. 1993, 27, 655-666. POLYURETHANE/carcinogenicity.

Andersen, B., Hawtof, D., Alani, H., and Kapetansky, D. The diagnosis of ruptured breast implants. Plast. Reconstr. Surg. 1989 Dec, 84, (6): 903-907. RUPTURE/local complications.

Anderson, A. M., Niven, H., Pelagalli, J., Olanoff, L. S., and Jones, R. D. The role of the fibrous capsule in the function of implanted drug-polymer sustained release systems. Journal of Biomedical Materials Research. 1981, 15, (6): 889-902. CAPSULE-CONTRACTURE/local complications.

Anderson, D. R., Schwartz, J., Cottrill, C. M., McClain, S. A., Ross, J. S., Magidson, J. G., Klainer, A., and Bisaccia, E. Silicone granuloma in acral skin in a patient with silicone-gel breast implants and systemic sclerosis. International Journal of Dermatology. 1996 Jan, 35, (1): 36-38. CONNECTIVE TISSUE DISEASE.

Anderson, J. M. Inflammatory response to implants. Transactions of the American Society of Artifical Internal Organs. 1988, 34, 101-107. IMMUNE EFFECTS/capsule-contracture.

Anderson, J. M. Mechanisms of inflammation and infection with implanted devices. Cardiovascular Pathology. 1993, 2, (3 (Supplement)): 33S-41S. IMMUNE EFFECTS/infection/local complications.

Anderson, J. M., Bonfield, T. L., and Ziats, N. P. Protein adsorption and cellular adhesion and activation on biomedical polymers. The International Journal of Artificial Organs. 1990, 13, (6): 375-382. TOXICOLOGY.

Anderson, J. M., Ziats, N. P., Azeez, A., Brunstedt, M. R., Stack, S., and Bonfield, T. L. Protein adsorption and macrophage activation on polydimethysiloxane and silicone rubber. J Biomater Sci Polymer Ed. 1995, 7, (2): 159-169. IMMUNE EFFECTS.

Anderson, S. G., Rodin, J., and Ariyan, S. Treatment considerations in postmastectomy reconstruction: Their relative importance and relationship to patient satisfaction. Annals of Plastic Surgery. 1994, 33, (3): 263-270. PSYCHOSOCIAL/reconstruction.

Andjelkovish, D. A., Mathew, R. M., Richardson, R. B., and Levine, R. J. Mortality of Iron Foundry Workers: I. Overall Findings. Journal of Occupational Medicine. 1990 Jun, 32, (6): 529-540. SILICA.

Andrews, J. Cellular behavior to injected silicone fluid: A preliminary report. Plast. Reconstr. Surg. 1966 Dec, 38, (6): 581-583. TOXICOLOGY/SILICONE INJECTION.

Angell, M. Evaluating the health risks of breast implants: the interplay of medical science, the law, and public opinion. Special Article. The New England Journal of Medicine. 1996 Jun 6, 334, (23): 1513-1518. GENERAL.

Antonyshyn, O., Gruss, J. S., Mackinnon, S. E., and Zuker, R. Complications of soft tissue expansion. British Journal of Plastic Surgery. 1988, 41, 239-250. EXPANDER/local complications/capsule-contracture/rupture/pain/hematomas.

Aoki, A., Sirai, A., Sakamoto, H., Igarashi, T., Matsunaga, K., Ishigatsubo, Y., Tani, K., and Okubo, T. A case of silicosis associated with polymyositis and benign monoclonal gammopathy. Ryumachi (Japan). 1988 Oct, 28, (5): 373-378. SILICA/myeloma.

Apesos, J. Pope Jr. T. L. Silicone granuloma following closed capsulotomy of mammary prosthesis. Annals of Plastic Surgery. 1985 May, 14, (5): 403-406. GRANULOMAS/ local complications/closed capsulotomy.

Appleton, B. E., and Lee, P. The development of systemic sclerosis (scleroderma) following augmentation mammoplasty. J Rheumatol. 1993, 20, (6): 1052-1054. CONNECTIVE TISSUE DISEASE.

Aptekar, R. G., Davie, J. M., and Cattell, H. S. Foreign body reaction to silicone rubber: Complication of a finger joint implant. Clinical Orthopaedics and Related Research. 1974, 98, 231-232. IMMUNE EFFECTS.

Archer, C., and Gordon, D. A. Silica and progressive systemic sclerosis (Scleroderma): Evidence for workers' compensation policy. American Journal of Industrial Medicine. 1996, 29, 533-538. SILICA.

Arend, W. P. Book reviews: Science on Trial. Arthritis and Rheumatism. 1996 Oct 10, 39, (10): 1771-1772. GENERAL.

Argenta, L. C. Controlled tissue expansion in reconstructive surgery. British Journal of Plastic Surgery. 1984a, 3, 520-529. EXPANDER/RECONSTRUCTION.

Argenta, L. C. Migration of silicone gel into breast parenchyma following mammary prothesis rupture. Aesthetic Plastic Surgery. 1983, 7, 253-254. MIGRATION/local complications/rupture.

Argenta, L. C. Reconstruction of the breast by tissue expansion. Clinics in Plastic Surgery. 1984b, 11, (2): 257-264. EXPANDER/reconstruction.

Argenta, L. C and Grabb, W. G. Studies on the endogenous flora of the human breast and their surgical significance. Plast Surg Forum. 1981, 4, 55. INFECTION/local complications.

Argenta, L. C., Marks, M. W., and Grabb, W. G. Selective use of serial expansion in breast reconstruction. Annals of Plastic Surgery. 1983 Sep, 11, (3): 188-195. EXPANDER/ reconstruction.

Argenta, L. C., Marks, M. W., and Pasyk, K. A. Advances in tissue expansion. Clinics in Plastic Surgery. 1985a Apr, 12, (2): 159-171. EXPANDER.

Argenta, L. C., Vanderkolk, C., Friedman, R. J., and Marks, M. W. Refinements in reconstruction of congenital breast deformities. Plast. Reconstr. Surg. 1985b Jul, 76, (1): 73-80. EXPANDER/reconstruction.

Arion, H. G. Retromammary prosthesis. C.R. Soc. Fr. Gynecol. 5, 1965. GENERAL/saline.

Armstrong, B. K., McNulty, J. C., Levitt, L. J., Williams, K. A., and Hobbs, M. S. T. Mortality in gold and coal miners in Western Australia with special reference to lung cancer. British Journal of Industrial Medicine. 1979, 36, 199-205. SILICA.

Armstrong, R. W., Berkowitz, R. L., and Bolding, F. Infection following breast reconstruction. Annals of Plastic Surgery. 1989 Oct, 23, (4): 284-288. INFECTION/local complications.

Arons, M. S., Sabesin, S. M., and Smith, R. R. Experimental studies with Etheron sponge: Effect of implantation in tumor-bearing animals. Plast. Reconstr. Surg. 1961 Jul, 28, (1): 72-80. GENERAL/carcinogenicity.

Aronsohn, R. B. A 22-year experience with the use of silicone injections. American Journal of Cosmetic Surgery. 1996, 1, 21-28. SILICONE INJECTION.

Arroyave, E. The ban on breast implants medical or political issue? The rest of the story. Journal of the Florida Medical Association. 1994, 81, (7): 479-483. GENERAL.

Artz, J. S., Dinner, M. I., Foglietti, M. A., and Sampliner, J. Breast reconstruction utilizing subcutaneous tissue expansion followed by polyurethane-covered silicone implants: A six-year experience. Plast. Reconstr. Surg. 1991 Oct, 88, (4): 635-639. EXPANDER/ local complications/polyurethane.

Ashley, F. L. Further studies on the Natural Y breast prosthesis. Plast. Reconstr. Surg. 1972 Apr, 49, (4): 414-419. POLYURETHANE/local complications.

Ashley, F. L. A new type of breast prosthesis. Preliminary report. Plast. Reconstr. Surg. 1970 May, 45, (5): 421-424. POLYURETHANE.

Ashley, F. L., Braley, S., and McNall, E. G. The current status of silicone injection therapy. Symposium on Cosmetic Surgery, Surg. Clin. North. Amer. 1971, 51, (2): 501-509. SILICONE INJECTION.

Ashley, F. L., Braley, S., Rees, T. D., Goulian, D., and Ballantyne, Jr. D. L. The present status of silicone fluid in soft tissue injection. Plast. Reconstr. Surg. 1967 Apr, 39, (4): 411-420. SILICONE INJECTION/SILICONE CHARACTERIZATION.

Ashley, F. L., Rees, T. D., Ballantyne, Jr. D. L., Galloway, D., Machida, R., Grazer, F., McConnell, D. V., Edgington, T., and Kiskaden, W. An injection technique for the treatment of facial hemiatrophy. Plast. Reconstr. Surg. 1965 Jun, 35, (6): 640-648. SILICONE INJECTION.

Ashley, F. L., Thompson, D., and Henderson, T. Augmentation of surface contour by subcutaneous injections of silicone fluid: A current report. Plast. Reconstr. Surg. 1973 Jan, 51, (1): 8-13. SILICONE INJECTION.

Asken, M. J. Psychoemotional aspects of mastectomy: a review of recent literature. American Journal of Psychiatry. 1975 Jan, 132, (1): 56-59. PSYCHOSOCIAL.

Aslam, M., and Rahman, Q. Cytotoxic and genotoxic effects of calcium silicates on human lymphocytes in vitro. Mutation Research. 1993 Jan, 300, 45-48. SILICON MEASUREMENT/silica.

Asplund, O. Breast reconstruction with submuscular prosthesis after modified radical or simple mastectomy. Surgical technique and early complications. Scandinavian Journal of Plast Reconstr Surg. 1983, 17, (2): 141-146. RECONSTRUCTION.

Asplund, O. Capsular contracture in silicone gel and saline-filled breast implants after reconstruction. Plast. Reconstr. Surg. 1984 Feb, 73, (2): 270-275. CAPSULE-CONTRACTURE/saline/local complications/reconstruction.

Asplund, O. Nipple and areola reconstruction—A study in 79 mastectomized women. Scandinavian Journal of Plastic and Reconstructive Surgery. 1983, 17, 233-240. RECONSTRUCTION.

Asplund, O., Gylbert, L., Jurell, G., and Ward, C. Textured or smooth implants for submuscular breast augmentation: A controlled study. Plast. Reconstr. Surg. 1996 May, 97, (6): 1200-1206. CAPSULE-CONTRACTURE/local complications.

Asplund, O., and Körlof, B. Late results following mastectomy for cancer and breast reconstruction. Scandinavian Journal of Plast. Reconstr. Surg. 1984, 18, (2): 221-225. PSYCHOSOCIAL/pain/local complications.

Asplund, O., and Nilsson, O. Interobserver variation and cosmetic result of submuscular breast reconstruction. Scandinavian Journal of Plast. Reconstr. Surg. 1984, 18, (2): 215-220. RECONSTRUCTION/local complications.

Atabek, U., Barot, L., Matthews, M., Brown, A. S., Spence, R. K., Mossberg, L., and et al. Immediate breast reconstruction after mastectomy. The New England Journal of Medicine. 1993, 90, 379-382. RECONSTRUCTION.

Atwood, H. D., Bates, R., Beckman, J. S., Bixe, R. N., Franz, P. F., Goodman, R. C., Lehmberg, R. W., McCutcheon, F. B., Moffett, T. R., Pope, N. A., Pullman, N. K., Shewmake, K. B., Still, E. F., Stuckey, J. G., Talbert, G. E., Walley, L. R., and Yuen, J. C. The silicone gel breast implant controversy: Current status and clinical implications. Journal of the Arkansas Medical Society. 1994 Feb, 90, (9): 427-434. GENERAL.

August, D. A., Wilkins, E., and Rea, T. Breast reconstruction in older women. Surgery. 1994, 115, (6): 663-668. RECONSTRUCTION.

Austad, E. D., Pasyk, K. A., McClatchey, K. D., and Cherry, G. W. Histomorphologic evaluation of guinea pig skin and soft tissue after controlled tissue expansion. Plast. Reconstr. Surg. 1982 Dec, 70, (6): 704-710. EXPANDER.

Austad, E. D., and Rose, G. L. A self-inflating tissue expander. Plast. Reconstr. Surg. 1982 Nov, 70, (5): 588-593. EXPANDER.

Austad, E. D., Thomas, S. B., and Pasyk, K. Tissue expansion: Dividend or loan? Plast. Reconstr. Surg. 1986 Jul, 78, (1): 63-67. EXPANDER.

Autian, J. Toxicological problems and untoward effects from plastic devices used in medical applications. Essays In Toxicology. first edition ed. McMillan, 1975a, pp. 1-33. TOXICOLOGY/carcinogenicity.

Autian, J., Singh, A. R., Turner, J. E., Hung, G. W. C., Nunez, L. J., and Lawrence, W. H. Carcinogenesis from polyurethanes. Cancer Research. 1975 Jun, 35, 1591-1596. POLYURETHANE/carcinogenicity.

Autian, J., Singh, A. R., Turner, J. E., Hung, G. W. C., Nunez, L. J., and Lawrence, W. H. Carcinogenic activity of a chlorinated polyether polyurethane. Cancer Research. 1976, 36, 3973-3977. CARCINOGENICITY/POLYURETHANE.

Azizsoltani E., Myryk, Q., Foster, L., Gindhar, G., and Gristina, A. Simple technique for the preparation of silicone gel particles: The effect of silicone gel particles on oxidative responses of macrophages. Journal of Biomedical Materials Research. 1995, 29, 101-105. IMMUNE EFFECTS.

Badley, E. M., Rasooly, I., and Webster, G. K. Relative importance of musculoskeletal disorders as a cause of chronic health problems, disability, and health care utilization: Findings from the 1990 Ontario Health Survey. Journal of Rheumatology. 1994, 21, (3): 505-514. AI-CTD BACKGROUND.

Badwin, B. et al. Cosmetic saline breast implants. Plast. Surg. Forum. 1995, 18, 275. SALINE.

Baek, H.-S., and Yoon, J.-W. Direct involvement of macrophages in destruction of ß-cells leading to development of diabetes in virus-infected mice. Diabetes. 1991 Dec, 40, (12): 1586-1597. SILICA/immune effects.

Bagnall, R. D. Adsorption of plasma proteins on hydrophobic surfaces I. Albumin and gammaglobulin. Journal of Biomedical Materials Research. 1977, 11, 947-977. SILICONE CHARACTERIZATION.

Bailey, M. H., Smith, J. W., Casas, L., and et al. Immediate breast reconstruction: Reducing the risks. Plast. Reconstr. Surg. 1989 May, 83, (5): 845-851. RECONSTRUCTION/local complications.

Baines, C. J., McFarlane, D. V., Miller, A. B., and et al. Sensitivity and specificity of first screen mammography in 15 NBSS centres. J Can Assoc Rad. 1988 Dec, 39, 273-276. MAMMOGRAPHY.

Baker, D. E., Breiting, V., and Christensen, L. Five years experience using silicone gel prostheses with emphasis on capsule shrinkage. Scand. J. Plast. Reconstr. Surg. 1984, 18, 311. CAPSULE CONTRACTURE.

Baker, Jr. J. L. The effectiveness of alpha-tocopherol (vitamin E) in reducing the incidence of spherical contracture around breast implants. Plast. Reconstr. Surg. 1981 Nov, 68, (5): 696-698. CAPSULE-CONTRACTURE/local complications.

Baker, Jr. J. L. Kolin I. Bartlett E. Psychosexual dynamics of patients undergoing mammary augmentation. Plast. Reconstr. Surg. 1974 Jun, 53, (6): 652-659. PSYCHOSOCIAL.

Baker, Jr. J. L., Bartels, R. J., and Douglas, W. M. Closed compression technique for rupturing a contracted capsule around a breast implant. Plast. Reconstr. Surg. 1976 Aug, 58, (2): 137-141. CLOSED CAPSULOTOMY.

Baker, Jr. J. L., and Donis, R. Genesis and management of the hard augmented breast. Adv Plast. Reconstr. Surg. 1990, 6, 249. CAPSULE-CONTRACTURE/local complications.

Baker, Jr. J. L., LeVier, R. R., and Spielvogel, D. E. Positive identification of silicone in human mammary capsular tissue. Plast. Reconstr. Surg. 1982 Jan, 69, (1): 56-60. SILICON MEASUREMENT/capsule-contracture/local complications.

Bakker, D., van Blitterswijk, C. A., Hesseling, S. C., and Grote, J. J. Effect of implantation site on phagocyte/polymer interaction and fibrous capsule formation. Biomaterials. 1988 Jan, 9, 14-23. CAPSULE-CONTRACTURE/local complications.

Baldt, V. M., Bankier, A., Mallek, R., Youssefzadeh, S., Freilinger, G., and Wolf, G. Long-term changes after implantation of silicone breast prostheses. Fortschr Röntgenstr. 1994, 160, (5): 441-447. SALINE/capsule-contracture/local complications.

Baldwin, J. K., and Hoover, B. K. Quality assurance for epidemiologic studies. Journal of Occupational Medicine. 1991 Dec, 33, (12): 1250-1252. GENERAL.

Baldwin, Jr. C. M., and Kaplan, E. N. Silicone-induced human adjuvant disease? Annals of Plastic Surgery. 1983 Apr, 10, (4): 270-273. CONNECTIVE TISSUE DISEASE/saline.

Ballantyne Jr., D. L. Rees T. D. Seidman I. Silicone fluid: Response to massive subcutaneous injections of dimethylpolysiloxane fluid in animals. Plast. Reconstr. Surg. 1965 Sep, 36, (3): 330-338. CARCINOGENICITY/toxicology.

Bames, H. O. Augmentation mammaplasty by lipo-transplant. Plast. Reconstr. Surg. 1953, 11, 404-414. RECONSTRUCTION.

Bames, H. O. Breast malformations and a new approach to the problem of the small breast. Plast. Reconstr. Surg. 1950, 5, 499-506. RECONSTRUCTION.

Banic, A., Boeckx, W., Greulich, M., Guelickx, P., Marchi, A., Rigotti, G., and Tschopp, H. Late results of breast reconstruction with free TRAM flaps: A prospective multicentric study. Plast. Reconstr. Surg. 1995, 95, (7): 1195-1204. RECONSTRUCTION.

Bantick, G. L., and Taggart, I. Mammography and breast implants. British Journal of Plastic Surgery. 1995, 48, (1): 49-52. MAMMOGRAPHY.

Bar-Meir, E., Teuber, S. S., Lin, H. C., Alosacie, I., Goddard, G., Terybery, J., Barka, N., Shen, B., Peter, J. B., Blank, M., Gershwin, M. E., and Shoenfeld, Y. Multiple autoantibodies in patients with silicone breast implants. Journal of Autoimmunity. 1995, 8, 267-277. CONNECTIVE TISSUE DISEASE/immune effects.

Bard, M., and Sutherland, A. M. Psychological impact of cancer and its treatment. Cancer. 1955 Jul-1955 Aug 31, 8, (4): 656-672. PSYCHOSOCIAL.

Barker, D. E. Mammometer: A New Instrument for Measuring "Pseudocapsule Firmness" after Breast Augmentation. Aesth. Plast. Surg. 1978, 2, 447-450. CAPSULE CONTRACTURE.

Barker, D. E., Retsky, M. I., and Schultz, S. "Bleeding" of silicone from bag-gel breast implants, and its clinical relation to fibrous capsule reaction. Plastic and Reconstructive Surgery. 1978 Jun, 61, (6): 836-841. LOCAL COMPLICATIONS/capsule-contracture.

Barker, D. E., Retsky, M., and Schulz, S. L. The new low bleed mammary prosthesis: An experimental study in mice. Aesthetic Plastic Surgery. 1981, 5, 85-91. CAPSULE-CONTRACTURE/local complications.

Barker, D. E., Retsky, M., and Searies, S. L. New low-bleed implant—Silastic II. Aesthetic Plastic Surgery. 1985, 9, 39-41. CAPSULE-CONTRACTURE/local complications.

Barker, D. E., and Schulz, S. L. Reaction to silicone implants in the guinea pig. Aesthetic Plastic Surgery. 1978, 1, 371-378. LOCAL COMPLICATIONS/IMMUNE EFFECTS.

Barker, D. E., and Shultz, S. L. The theory of natural capsular contraction around breast implants and how to prevent it. Aesthetic Plast. Surg. 1980, 4, 357-361. CAPSULE-CONTRACTURE/local complications.

Barloon, T. J., Young, D. C., and Bergus, G. The role of diagnostic imaging in women with breast implants. American Family Physician. 1996, 54, (6): 2029-2036. MAMMOGRAPHY.

Barlow, S. M., and Knight, A. F. Teratogenic effects of Silastic intrauterine devices in the rat with or without added medroxyprogesterone acetate. Fertility and Sterility. 1983 Feb, 39, (2): 224-230. TOXICOLOGY.

Barnard, J. J., Todd, E. L., Wilson, W. G., Mielcarek, R., and Rohrich, R. J. Distribution of organosilicon polymers in augmentation mammaplasties at autopsy. Plast. Reconstr. Surg. 1997 Jul, 100, (1): 197-203. SILICON MEASUREMENT.

Barnett, A. J., Miller, M. H., and Littlejohn, G. O. A survival study of patients with scleroderma diagnosed over 30 years (1953-1983): The value of a simple cutaneous classification in the early stages of the disease. J. Rheumatol. 1988, 15, (2): 276-283. AI-CTD BACKGROUND.

Barnett, A., Lavey, E., Pearl, R. M., and Vistnes, L. M. Toxic shock syndrome from an infected breast prosthesis. Annals of Plastic Surgery. 1983 May, 10, (5): 408-410. INFECTION/local complications.

Barney, B. B. Augmentation mammaplasty with two different kinds of prostheses. Plast. Reconstr. Surg. 1974 Sep, 54, (3): 265-267. SALINE.

Barondes, R. de R., Judge, W. D., Towne, C. G., and Baxter, M. L. New organic derivatives and some of their unique properties. The Military Surgeon. 1950 May: 379-386. TOXICOLOGY.

Barone, F. E., Perry, L., Keller, T., and Maxwell, G. P. The biochemical and histopathic effects of surface texturing with silicone and polyurethane in tissue implantation and expansion. Plast. Reconstr. Surg. 1992 Jul, 90, (1): 77. CAPSULE-CONTRACTURE/local complications/polyurethane.

Barreau-Pouhaer, L., Lê, M. G., and Rietjens, M. et al. Risk factors for failure of immediate breast reconstruction with prosthesis after total mastectomy for breast cancer. Cancer. 1992 Sep 1, 70, (5): 1145-1151. RECONSTRUCTION.

Barrett, D. M., O'Sullivan, D. C., Malizia, A. A., Reiman, H. M., and Abell-Aleff, P. C. Particle shedding and migration from silicone genitourinary prosthetic devices. Journal of Urology. 1991 Aug, 146, 319-322. LOCAL COMPLICATIONS.

Barsky, A. J. A 37-year-old man with multiple somatic complaints. J. Amer. Med. Assoc. 1997 Aug 27, 278, (8): 673-679. PSYCHOSOCIAL.

Barsky, A. J. Hypochondriasis, medical management and psychiatric treatment. Psychosomatics. 1996, 37, (1): 48-56. PSYCHOSOCIAL.

Barsky, A. J., and Borus, J. F. Somatization and medicalization in the era of managed care. J. Amer. Med. Assoc. 1995 Dec 27, 274, (24): 1931-4. PSYCHOSOCIAL.

Barthels, K. M. Decreased swimming speed following augmentation mammaplasty [discussion]. Plast. Reconstr. Surg. 1983 Feb, 72, (2): 255-256. LOCAL COMPLICATIONS.

Bartlett, P. Toxic shock syndrome associated with surgical wound infections. J. Amer. Med. Assoc. 1982 Mar 12, 247, 1448-1450. INFECTION/local complications.

Basindale, A. R., Brown, S. S. D., and Lo, P. Sterochemical nonrigidity in a chelated platinum(0)-diolefin complex. Organometallics. 1994, 13, 738-740. PLATINUM.

Bates, D. W., Schmitt, W., and Buchwald, D. et al. Prevalence of fatigue and chronic fatigue syndrome in a primary care practice. Arch Intern Med. 1993 Dec 27, 153, 2759-2765. AI-CTD BACKGROUND.

Bates, R. R., and Klein, M. Importance of a smooth surface in carcinogenesis by plastic film. Journal of the National Cancer Institute. 1966, 37, 145-151. CARCINOGENICITY.

Batich, C., and De Palma, D. Materials used in breast implants: Silicones and polyurethanes. Journal of Long-Term Effects of Medical Implants. 1992, 1, (3): 255-268. SILICONE CHARACTERIZATION/polyurethane.

Batich, C., De Palma, D., Marotta, J., Latorre, G., and Hardt, N. S. Silicone degradation reactions. Potter, M., and Rose, N., eds. Current Topics In Microbiology and Immunology - Immunology of Silicones. Heidelberg: Springer-Verlag, 1996, pp. 13-23. SILICONE CHARACTERIZATION/toxicology.

Batich, C., Williams, J., and King, R. Toxic hydrolysis product from a biodegradable foam implant. Journal of Biomed. Mater. Res. 1989, 23, (A3): 311-319. POLYURETHANE/toxicology.

Batra, M., Bernard, S., and Picha, G. Histologic comparision of breast implant shells with smooth, foam, and pillar microstructuring in a rat model from 1 day to 6 months. Plast. Reconstr. Surg. 1995 Feb, 95, (2): 354-363. CAPSULE-CONTRACTURE/local complications.

Bayet, B., Mathieu, G., Lavand Homme, P., and et al. Primary and secondary breast reconstruction with a permanent expander. European Journal of Plastic Surgery. 1991, 14, 73-79. EXPANDER/capsule-contracture/local complications.

Beale, S., Hambert, G., Lisper, H. O., and et al. Augmentation mammoplasty: The surgical and psychological effects of the operation and prediction of the result. Annals of Plastic Surgery. 1985 Jun, 14, (6): 473-493. PSYCHOSOCIAL/sensation/local complications.

Beale, S., Lisper, H. D., and Palm, B. A psychological study of patients seeking augmentation mammaplasty. British Journal of Psychiatry. 1980, 136, 133-138. PSYCHOSOCIAL.

Beckenbaugh, R. D., Dobyns, J. H., Linscheid, R. L., and Bryan, R. S. Review and analysis of silicone-rubber metacarpophalangeal implants. Journal of Bone and Joint Surgery. 1976 Jun, 58-A, (4): 483-487. LOCAL COMPLICATIONS/general.

Becker, H. Breast augmentation using the expander mammary prosthesis. Plast. Reconstr. Surg. 1987b Feb, 79, (2): 192-199. EXPANDER.

Becker, H. Breast reconstruction following mastectomy using a permanent tissue expander. Plastic Surgery Forum. 1986a, 9, 20-21. RECONSTRUCTION/expander.

Becker, H. Breast reconstruction using an inflatable breast implant with detachable reservoir. Plast. Reconstr. Surg. 1984 Apr, 73, (4): 678-683. RECONSTRUCTION/saline.

Becker, H. The expandable mammary implant. Plast. Reconstr. Surg. 1987a Apr, 79, (4): 631-637. EXPANDER/capsule-contracture/local complications/reconstruction.

Becker, H. Expansion augmentation. Clinics in Plastic Surgery. 1988 Oct, 15, (4): 587-593. EXPANDER/reconstruction/local complications.

Becker, H. The use of intradermal tattoo to enhance the final result of nipple-areola reconstruction. Plast. Reconstr. Surg. 1986b Apr, 77, (4): 673-675. RECONSTRUCTION.

Becker, H., and Hartman, J. Do saline breast implants harbor microbes? Annals of Plastic Surgery. 1996 Apr, 36, (4): 342-344. INFECTION/saline.

Beckett, W., Abraham, J., Becklake, M., Christiani, D., Cowie, R., Davis, G., Jones, R., Kreiss, K., Parker, J., and Wagner, G. Adverse effects of crystalline silica exposure. American Journal of Respiratory and Critical Care Medicine. 1997, 155, 761-765. SILICA.

Beckham, J., Caldwell, D., Peterson, B., Pippen, A. M. M., Currie, M., Keefe, F., and Weinberg, J. Disease severity in rheumatoid arthritis: relationships of plasma tumor necrosis factor-alpha, soluble interleukin 2-receptor, soluble CD4/CD8 ratio, neopterin, and fibrin D-dimer to traditional severity and functional measures. Journal of Clinical Immunology. 1992, 12, (5): 353-361. AI-CTD BACKGROUND.

Bedu, O., Gay, J., Rouffy, J., and Loeper, J. Action of silicon on cultured lymphocytes. Med. Sci. Res. 1991, 19, 317-318. IMMUNE EFFECTS.

Beebe, G. W., Simin, A. H., and Vivona, S. Long term mortality follow-up of army recruits who received adjuvant influenza virus vaccine in 1951-1953. Am. J. Epidemiol. 1972, 95, 337-345. AI-CTD BACKGROUND.

Beegle, P. H., Bostwick, J., Hargraves, H., and Hester, T. R. Evaluation of capsular contracture in submammary vs. submuscular breast augmentation. Surg. Forum. 1982, 33, 586-587. CAPSULE CONTRACTURE/local complications.

Beekman, W. H., Feitz, R., Hage, J. J., and Mulder, J. W. Life span of silicone gel-filled mammary prostheses. Plast. Reconstr. Surg. 1997b Dec, 100, (7): 1723-1726. CAPSULE-CONTRACTURE/local complications/infection/rupture/pain.

Beekman, W. H., Feitz, R., van Diest, P. J., and Hage, J. J. Migration of silicone through the fibrous capsules of mammary prostheses. Annals of Plastic Surgery. 1997a May, 38, (5): 441-445. MIGRATION/local complications/capsule-contracture/rupture.

Beekman, W. H., Scot, M. G. M., Taets van Amerongen, A. H. M., Hage, J. J., and Mulder, J. W. Silicone breast implant bleed and rupture: Clinical diagnosis and predictive value of mammography and ultrasound. Annals of Plastic Surgery. 1996, 36, (4): 345-347. MAMMOGRAPHY/rupture/local complications.

Beisang, A. A., and Geise, R. A. Radiolucent prosthetic gel. Plast. Reconstr. Surg. 1991 May, 87, (5): 855-892. MAMMOGRAPHY/general.

Ben-Hur, N. Prolonged allograft survival by partial block of the reticuloendothelial system with silicone fluid. Europ. Surg. Res. 1970, 2, 73-78. TOXICOLOGY.

Ben-Hur, N., Ballantyne, Jr. D. L., Rees, T. D., and et al. Local and systemic effects of dimethylpolysiloxane fluid in mice. Plast. Reconstr. Surg. 1970, 46, 50-56. TOXICOLOGY.

Ben-Hur, N., Ballantyne, Jr. D. L., Rees, T. D., and Seidman, I. Local and systemic effects of dimethylpolysiloxane fluid in mice. Plast. Reconstr. Surg. 1967 Apr, 39, (4): 423-426. TOXICOLOGY.

Ben-Hur, N., and Neuman, Z. Malignant tumor formation following subcutaneous injection of silicone fluid in white mice. Israel Medical Journal. 1963, 22, 15. CARCINOGENICITY/toxicology.

Ben-Hur, N., and Neuman, Z. Siliconoma—another cutaneous response to dimethylpolysiloxane. Plast. Reconstr. Surg. 1965, 36, (6): 629-631. CARCINOGENICITY/IMMUNE EFFECTS/granulomas.

Benavent, W. J. Treatment of bilateral breast carcinomas in a patient with silicone-gel breast implants. Plast. Reconstr. Surg. 1973, 51, 588-589. CANCER.

Benediktsson, K. P., Perbeck, L., Geigant, E., and Solders, G. Touch sensibility in the breast after subcutaneous mastectomy and immediate reconstruction with a prosthesis. British Journal of Plastic Surgery. 1997, 50, (6): 443-449. SENSATION/local complications/reconstruction.

Bengtsson, D., Edstrom, K., Sigurdsson, J., and Tibblin, G. Prevalence of subjectively experienced symptoms in a population sample of women with special reference to women with arterial hypertension. Scan J Prim Health Care. 1987, 5, 155-162. PSYCHOSOCIAL.

Benito, J. Breast implants: methods for reducing capsular contracture. European Journal of Plastic Surgery. 1990, 13, 198-200. CAPSULE-CONTRACTURE.

Benjamin, E., Ahmed, A., Rashid, A. T. M. F., and Wright, D. H. Silicone lymphadenopathy: A report of two cases, one with concomitant malignant lymphoma. Diagnostic Histopathology. 1982, 5, 133-141. LYMPHADENOPATHY/local complications/cancer.

Benjamin, J. L., and Guy, C. L. Calcification of implant capsules following augmentation mammoplasty. Plast. Reconstr. Surg. 1977, 59, (3): 432-433. CALCIFICATION/local complications.

Bennett, D. R., Gorzinski, S. J., and LeBeau, J. E. Structure-activity relationships of oral organosiloxanes on the male reproductive system. Toxicology and Applied Pharmacology. 1972, 21, 55-67. TOXICOLOGY.

Bennett, R. M. Fibromyalgia and the disability dilemma. Arthritis and Rheumatism. 1996 Oct, 39, (10): 1627- 1634. AI-CTD BACKGROUND.

Bennett, R. M., Clark, S. R., Campbell, S. M., and Burckhardt, C. S. Low levels of somatomedin C in patients with the fibromyalgia syndrome: A possible link between sleep and muscle pain. Arthritis and Rheumatism. 1992 Oct, 35, (10): 1113-1116. AI-CTD BACKGROUND.

Benoit, F. M. Degradation of polyurethane foam used in the Meme breast implant. Journal of Biomed. Mater. Res. 1993, 27, 1341-1348. POLYURETHANE/toxicology.

Bercowy, G. M., Vo, H., and Rieders, F. Silicon analysis in biological specimens by direct current plasma-atomic emission spectroscopy. Journal of Analytical Toxicology. 1994 Jan-1994 Feb 28, 18, 46-48. SILICON MEASUREMENT.

Berg, W. A., Anderson, N. D., Zerhouni, E. A., Chang, B. W., and Kuhlman, J. E. MR imaging of the breast in patients with silicone breast implants: Normal postoperative variants and diagnostic pitfalls. American Journal of Roentgenology. 1994, 163, (3): 575-578. MAMMOGRAPHY.

Berg, W. A., Caskey, C. I., Hamper, U. M., Anderson, N. D., Chang, B. W., Sheth, S., Zerhouni, E. A., and Kuhlman, J. E. Diagnosing breast implant rupture with MR imaging, US, and mammography. RadioGraphics. 1993, 13, 1323-1336. MAMMOGRAPHY.

Berg, W. A., Caskey, C. I., Hamper, U. M., Kuhlman, J. E., Anderson, N. D., Chang, B. W., Sheth, S., and Zerhouni, E. A. Single- and double-lumen silicone breast implant integrity: Prospective evaluation of MR and US criteria. Radiology. 1995, 197, 45-52. MAMMOGRAPHY.

Bergman, R. B., and van der Ende, A. E. Exudation of silicone through the envelope of gel-filled breast prostheses: An in vitro study. British Journal of Plastic Surgery. 1979, 32, 31-34. LOCAL COMPLICATIONS/rupture.

Berkel, H., Birdsell, D. C., and Jenkins, H. Breast augmentation: A risk factor for breast cancer. The New England Journal of Medicine. 1992 Jun 18, 326, (25): 1649-1653. CANCER.

Berkel, J., Fillius, P. M. G., Dik, E., and Deboer, A. Long term health effects of breast augmentation: A review. Pharmacoepidemiology and Drug Safety. 1994, 3, 265-273. CANCER/GENERAL/CONNECTIVE TISSUE DISEASE/mammography.

Berlin, Jr. C. M. Drugs and Chemicals: Exposure of the Nursing Mother. Clinical Pharmacology. 1989 Oct, 36, (5): 1089-1097. CHILDREN'S EFFECTS/breast feeding.

Berlin, Jr. C. M. Silicone breast implants and breastfeeding. Pediatrics. 1994 Oct, 94, (4, part 1): 547-549. BREAST FEEDING/children's effects.

Berlyne, G. M., Adler, A. K., Ferram N., Bemmett, S., and Holt, J. Silicon metabolism: some aspects of renal silicon handling in normal man. Nephron. 1986, 43, 5-9. SILICON MEASUREMENT.

Berman, D. E., Lettieri, J., Herold, D. A., Lin, Y. F., and Morgan, R. F. Steroid and benzyl alcohol diffusion through tissue expanders and double lumen breast implants. Annals of Plastic Surgery. 1991, 27, (4): 316-320. STEROIDS/local complications/expander.

Berman, D. E., Lettieri, J., Herold, D., Edlich, R. F., and Morgan, R. F. Lidocaine permability in silicone tissue expanders: An in vitro analysis. Plast. Reconstr. Surg. 1989 Oct, 84, (4): 621-623. PAIN/local complications/expander.

Bern, S., Burd, A., and May, Jr. J. W. The biophysical and histologic properties of capsules formed by smooth and textured silicone implants in the rabbit. Plast. Reconstr. Surg. 1992 Jun, 89, (6): 1037-1042. CAPSULE-CONTRACTURE/local complications.

Berrino, P., Campora, E., and Santi, P. Post quadrantectomy breast deformities: Classification and techniques of surgical correction. Plast. Reconstr. Surg. 1987 Apr, 79, (4): 567-572. RECONSTRUCTION.

Berrino, P., Casabona, F., and Santi, P. Long-term advantages of permanent expandable implants in breast aesthetic surgery. Plast. Reconstr. Surg. 1998a Jun, 101, (7): 1964-1972. EXPANDER.

Berrino, P., Franchelli, S., and Santi, P. Surgical correction of breast deformities following long lasting complications of polyurethane covered implants. Annals of Plastic Surgery. 1990 Jun, 24, (6): 481-488. POLYURETHANE/local complications.

Berrino, P., Galli, A., Rainero, M. L., and Santi, P. L. Long-lasting complications with use of polyurethane covered breast implants. British Journal of Plastic Surgery. 1986, 39, 549-553. POLYURETHANE/local complications/capsule-contracture.

Berrino, P., Leone, S., and Cicchetti, S. Umbilicated nipples eversion after breast augmentation. Plast. Reconstr. Surg. 1998b Jul, 102, (1): 231-233. LOCAL COMPLICATIONS.

Berson, M. I. Derma-fat-fascia transplants used in building up the breasts. Surgery. 1944, 35, 451-456. RECONSTRUCTION.

Bevin, A. G. On augmentation mammaplasty by the transaxillary approach. Plast. Reconstr. Surg. 1977 Jun, 59, (6): 841-844. CLOSED CAPSULOTOMY.

Biagini, R. E., Bernstein, I. L., and Gallagher, I. S. et al. The diversity of reaginic immune responses to platinum and palladium metallic salts. Journal of Allergy and Clinical Immunology. 1985 Dec 1, 76, (6): 794-802. PLATINUM/toxicology/immune effects.

Biggs, T. M., Cukier, J., and Worthing, L. F. Augmentation mammaplasty: A review of 18 years. Plast. Reconstr. Surg. 1982 Mar, 69, (3): 445-450. CAPSULE-CONTRACTURE/infection/local complications/hematomas.

Biggs, T. M., and Yarish, R. S. Augmentation mammaplasty: A comparative analysis. Plast. Reconstr. Surg. 1990 Mar, 85, (3): 368-372. CAPSULE-CONTRACTURE/local complications/steroids.

Biggs, T. M., and Yarish, R. S. Augmentation mammaplasty: Retropectoral versus retromammary implantation. Clin. Plast. Surg. 1988, 15, (4): 549-555. CAPSULE-CONTRACTURE.

Bignall, J. Silicone breast implants, breast feeding, and scleroderma. The Lancet. 1994, 343, 229. BREAST FEEDING/connective tissue disease.

Bilbey, J. H., and Connell, D. G. MRI diagnosis of a ruptured breast implant presenting as an infraclavicular mass. Canadian Association of Radiologists Journal. 1993 Jun, 44, (3): 224-226. MAMMOGRAPHY.

Bingham, H. G., Copeland, E. M., Hackett, R., and Caffee, H. H. Breast cancer in a patient with a silicone breast implant after 13 years. Annals of Plastic Surgery. 1988, 20, 236-237. CANCER.

Bircoll, M., and Novack, B. H. Autologous fat transplantation employing liposuction techniques. Annals of Plastic Surgery. 1987 Apr, 18, (4): 327-329. RECONSTRUCTION.

Birdsell, D. C., Jenkins, H., and Berkell, H. Breast cancer diagnosis and survival in women with and without breast implants. Plast. Reconstr. Surg. 1993 Oct, 92, (5): 795-800. CANCER.

Birnbaum, L. M., Hopp, D. D., and Mertens, B. The role of iodine-releasing silicone implants in prevention of spherical contractures in mice. Plast. Reconstr. Surg. 1982 Jun, 69, (6): 956-959. CAPSULE-CONTRACTURE/infection.

Birnbaum, L., and Olsen, J. A. Breast reconstruction following radical mastectomy, using custom designed implants. Plast. Reconstr. Surg. 1978, 61, (3): 355-363. RECONSTRUCTION.

Birtchnell, S., and Lacey, J. Augmentation and reduction mammoplasty: Demographic and obstetric differences in women attending a National Health Service Clinic. Postgraduate Medical Journal. 1988, 64, 587-589. PREVALENCE.

Bischoff, F. Organic polymer biocompatibility and toxicology. Clinical Chemistry. 1972, 18, (9): 869-894. CARCINOGENICITY/toxicology.

Black, C. M., Welsh, K. T., Walker, A. E., and et al. Genetic susceptibility to scleroderma-like syndrome induced by vinyl chloride. The Lancet. 1983 Jan 1, 8, 53-55. AI-CTD BACKGROUND.

Blackburn Jr., W. D., and Everson, M. P. Silicone-associated rheumatic disease: An unsupported myth. Plast. Reconstr. Surg. 1997 Apr, 99, (5): 1362-1367. IMMUNE EFFECTS/ connective tissue disease.

Blackburn Jr., W. D., Grotting, J. C., and Everson, M. P. Lack of evidence of systemic inflammatory rheumatic disorders in symtomatic women with breast implants. Plastic and Reconstructive Surgery. 1997 Apr, 99, (4): 1054-1060. IMMUNE EFFECTS/connective tissue disease.

Blair, A., Burg, J., Foran, J., Gibb, H., Greenland, S., Morris, R., Raabe, G., Savits, D., Teta, J., Wartenberg, D., Wong, O., and Zimmerman, R. Guidelines for Application of Meta-analysis in Environmental Epidemiology. Regulatory Toxicology and Pharmacology. 1995, 22, 189-197. GENERAL.

Bloch, C., and Hudson, D. Silicone and breast implants. South African Medical Journal. 1992, 81, (2): 449-450. CANCER/connective tissue disease/immune effects.

Blocksma, R. Experiences with dimethylpolysiloxane fluid in soft tissue augmentation. Plast. Reconstr. Surg. 1971 Dec, 48, (6): 564-567. SILICONE INJECTION.

Blocksma, R., and Braley, S. The silicones in plastic surgery. Plast. Reconstr. Surg. 1965 Apr, 35, (4): 366-370. GENERAL.

Boice, Jr. J. D., Friis, S., McLaughlin, J. K., Mellemkjær, L., Blot, W. J., Fraumeni, J. F., and Olsen, J. H. Cancer following breast reduction surgery in Denmark. Cancer Causes and Control. 1997, 8, 253-258. CANCER.

Bombardier, C. H. Chronic fatigue, chronic fatigue syndrome, and fibromyalgia: Disability and health-care use. Medical Care. 1996, 34, (9): 924-930. AI-CTD BACKGROUND.

Bommer, J., Gesma, D., Waldherr, R., Kessler, J., and Ritz, E. Plastic filing from dialysis tubing induces prostanoid release from macrophages. Kidney Intl. 1984, 26, 331. IMMUNE EFFECTS.

Bommer, J., Ritz, E., and Waldherr, R. Silicone-induced splenomegaly: treatment of pancytopenia by splenectomy in a patient on hemodialysis. The New England Journal of Medicine. 1981 Oct 29, 305, 1078. LOCAL COMPLICATIONS.

Bommer J., Waldherr R., Gastner M., Lemmes R., and Ritz E. Iatrogenic multiorgan silicone inclusions in dialysis patients. Klin Wochenschr. 1981 Oct 15, 59, (20): 1149-1157. SILICON MEASUREMENT/local complications.

Bon, A., and Eichmann, A. Serious long-term complication following silicone injection of the face. Dermatology. 1993, 187, 286-287. SILICONE INJECTION.

Boné, B., Aspelin, P., Isberg, B. Perbeck L., and Veress, B. Contrast-enhaced MR imaging of the breast in patients with breast implants after cancer surgery. Acta Radiologica. 1995 Mar, 36, (2): 111-116. MAMMOGRAPHY.

Bonfield, T. L., Colton, E., Marchant, R. E., and Anderson, J. M. Cytokine and growth factor production by monocytes/macrophages on protein preabsorbed polymers. Journal of Biomedical Materials Research. 1992, 26, 837-850. IMMUNE EFFECTS.

Bonfield, T., Colton, E., and Anderson, J. Plasma protein adsorbed biomedical polymers: Activation of human monocytes and induction of interleukin 1. Journal of Biomedical Materials Research. 1989a, 23, 535-548. IMMUNE EFFECTS.

Bonfield, T., Colton, E., and Anderson, J. Student research award in the graduate degree candidate category, 15th annual meeting of the society for biomaterials, Lake Buena Vista, Florida, April 28-May 2, 1989. Journal of Biomedical Materials Research. 1989b, 23, 535-548. CAPSULE CONTRACTURE.

Bonfield, T., Colton, E., and Anderson, J. M. Fibroblast stimulation by monocytes cultured on protein adsorbed biomedical polymers. I. Biomer and polydimethylsiloxane. Journal of Biomedical Materials Research. 1991, 25, (2): 165-175. CAPSULE-CONTRACTURE.

Boo-Chai, K. The complications of augmentation mammoplasty by silicone injection. British Journal of Plastic Surgery. 1969, 22, 281-286. SILICONE INJECTION.

Boone, J. L., and Braley, S. A. Resistance of silicone rubbers to body fluids. Chemistry and Technology. 1966 Sep, 39, (4): 1293-1297. SILICONE CHARACTERIZATION.

Boonstra. B. B., Cochrane, H., and Dannenberg, E. M. Reinforcement of silicone rubber by particulate silica. Rubber Chem. Technol. 1975, 48, (4): 558. SILICA.

Borgan, E. R., and Ruben, L. Injectable fluid silicone therapy, human mobility and mortality. J Amer. Med. Assoc. 1975, 234, 308-309. SILICONE INJECTION.

Bosanquet, A. G., Ishimaru, J.-I., and Goss, A. N. The effect of silastic replacement following discectomy in sheep temporomandibular joints. Journal of Oral Maxillofacial Surgery. 1991, 49, 1204-1209. LOCAL COMPLICATIONS.

Boschert, N. L. Thermoplastic vulcanizates in medical applications. Medical Plastics and Biomaterials. 1997 Jan: 28. SILICONE CHARACTERIZATION.

Bosetti, M., Navone, R., Rizzo, E., and Cannas, M. Histochemical and morphometric observations on the new tissue formed around mammary expanders coated with pyrolytic carbon. J Biomed Mater Res. 1998 May, 40, (2): 307-313. CAPSULE CONTRACTURE.

Bostwick III, J. Breast reconstruction after mastectomy. Cancer. 1990 Sep 15, 66, (6): 1402-1411. RECONSTRUCTION.

Bostwick III, J., and Jones, G. Why I choose autogenous tissue in breast reconstruction. Clinics in Plastic Surgery. 1994, 21, (2): 165-175. LOCAL COMPLICATIONS/capsule-contracture/expander.

Bostwick III, J., Nahai, F., Wallace, J. G., and Vasconez, L. O. Sixty latissimus dorsi flaps. Plast. Reconstr. Surg. 1979, 63, (1): 31-41. RECONSTRUCTION.

Bostwick III, J., Paletta, C., and Hartrampf, C. R. Conservative treatment for breast cancer: Complications requiring reconstructive surgery. Annals of Surgery. 1986 May, 203, (5): 481-489. CANCER.

Bowers, Jr. D. G., and Radlauer, C. B. Breast cancer after prophylactic subcutaneous mastectomies and reconstruction with silastic prostheses. Plast. Reconstr. Surg. 1969, 44, (4): 541-544. CANCER.

Bown, S. L., Middleton, M. S., Berg, W. A., Soo, M. S., and Pennelo, G. Silicone Gel Breast Implant Rupture Prevalence in a Population of Women in Birmingham, Alabama. J. Amer. Med. Assoc. (submitted). 1999. RUPTURE/local complications.

Boyes, D. C., Adey, C. K., Bailar, J., Baines, C., Kerrigan, C., and Langlois, P. Safety of polyurethane-covered breast implants. Canadian Medical Association Journal. 1991, 145, (9): 1125-1128. POLYURETHANE.

Bradley, S. G., Munson, A. E., McCay, J., Brown, R., Musgrove, D., Wilson, S., Stern, M., Luster, N., and White, Jr. K. L. Subchronic 10-day immunotoxicity of polydimethylsiloxane (silicone) fluid, gel and elastomer and polyurethane disks in female B6C3F1 mice. Drug and Chemical Toxicology. 1994a, 17, (3): 175-220. TOXICOLOGY/immune effects/polyurethane.

Bradley, S. G., White Jr., K. L., McCay, J. A., Brown, R. D., Musgrove, D. L., Wilson, S., Stern, M, Luster, M. I., and Munson, A. E. Immunotoxicity of 180-day exposure to polydimethylsiloxane (silicone) fluid, gel and elastomer and polyurethane disks in female B6C3F1 mice. Drug and Chemical Toxicology. 1994b, 17, (3): 221-269. TOXICOLOGY/immune effects/polyurethane.

Braley, S. The silicones as tools in biological engineering. Med. Electron. Biol. Eng. 1965, 3, 127-136. SILICONE CHARACTERIZATION.

Braley, S. The status of injectable silicone fluid for soft tissue augmentation. Plast. Reconstr. Surg. 1971 Apr, 47, (4): 343-344. SILICONE INJECTION.

Braley, S. The use of silicones in plastic surgery: A retrospective view. Plast. Reconstr. Surg. 1973, 51, (3): 280-288. GENERAL.

Bramm, E., Binderup, L., and Arrigoni-Martelli, E. Inhibition of adjuvant arthritis by intraperitoneal administration of low doses of silica. Agents and Actions. 1980 May, 10, (5): 435-438. SILICA/immune effects.

Bramwell, B. Diffuse sclerodermia: its frequency, its occurrence in stone-masons, its treatment by fibrolysin—elevations of temperature due to fibrolysin injections. Edinburgh Medical Journal. 1914, 12, (5): 387-401. AI-CTD BACKGROUND.

Brand, K. G. Do implanted medical devices cause cancer? Journal of Biomaterials Applications. 1994, 8, 325. CARCINOGENICITY.

Brand, K. G. Foam-covered mammary implants. Clinics in Plastic Surgery. 1988 Oct, 15, (4): 533-539. POLYURETHANE/local complications/infection.

Brand, K. G. Infection of mammary prostheses: A survey and the question of prevention. Annals of Plastic Surgery. 1993 Apr, 30, (4): 289-295. INFECTION/local complications.

Brand, K. G., and Brand, I. Risk assessment of carcinogenesis at implantation sites. Plast. Reconstr. Surg. 1980 Oct, 66, (4): 591-594. CARCINOGENICITY.

Brand, K. G., Buoen, L. C., and Brand, I. Foreign-body tumorigensis induced by glass and smooth and rough plastic: Comparative study of preneoplastic events. Journal of the National Cancer Institute. 1975 Aug, 55, (2): 319-322. CARCINOGENICITY.

Brand, K. G., Buoen, L. C., Johnson, K. H., and Brand, I. Etiological factors, stages, and the role of the foreign body in foreign-body tumorigenesis: A review. Cancer Research. 1975 Feb, 35, 279-286. CARCINOGENICITY.

Brandon, H. J., Peters, W., Young, V. L., Jerina, K. L., Wolf, C. J., and Schorr, M. W. Analysis of two Dow Corning breast implants removed after 28 years of implantation. Aesthetic Surgery Journal. 1999 Jan-1999 Feb 28, 19, (1): 40-48. CAPSULE CONTRACTURE.

Brandt, B., Breiting, V., Christensen, L., Nielsen, M., and Thomsen, J. L. Five years experience of breast augmentation using silicone gel prostheses with emphasis on capsule shrinkage. Scandinavian Journal of Plastic and Reconstructive Surgery. 1984, 18, (3): 311-316. CAPSULE CONTRACTURE/local complications/hematomas/infection.

Brandt, B., Breiting, V., Christensen, L., Nielsen, M., and Thomsen, J. L. Silicone granulomas mimicking malignant breast tumors. Breast. 1985, 11, (4): 6-8. GRANULOMAS/local complications.

Brantley, S. K., Davidson, S. F., Johnson, M. B., St. Arnold, P. A., and Das, S. K. The effects of prior exposure to silicone on capsular formation, histology, and pressure. Annals of Plastic Surgery. 1990a Jul, 25, (1): 44-47. CAPSULE CONTRACTURE/local complications/immune effects.

Brantley, S. K., Davidson, S. F., St. Arnold, P. A., Johnson, M. B., Tabbot, P. J., Grogan, J. B., Cuchens, M. A., Hsu, H. S., and Das, S. K. Assessment of the lymphocyte response to silicone. Plast. Reconstr. Surg. 1990b Dec, 86, (6): 1131-1137. IMMUNE EFFECTS.

Brash, J. L., and Samak, Q. M. Dynamics of interactions between human albumin and polyethylene surface. Journal of Colloid and Interface Science. 1978 Jul, 65, (3): 495-504. POLYURETHANE.

Brash, J. L., and Uniyal, S. Dependence on albumin-fibrinogen simple and competitive adsorption on surface properties of biomaterials. Journal of Polymer Science: Polymer Symposium. 1979, 66, 377-389. SILICONE CHARACTERIZATION.

Brautbar, N. Silicone implants and immune dysfunction: Scientific evidence for causation. International Journal of Occupational Medicine and Toxicology. 1995, 7, (1): 3-13. GENERAL/immune effects.

Brautbar, N., Campbell, A., and Vojdani, A. Silicone breast implants and autoimmunity: Causation, association, or myth? J Biomater Sci Polym Ed. 1995, 7, (2): 133-145. GENERAL/CONNECTIVE TISSUE DISEASE.

Brautbar, N., Vojdani, A., and Campbell, A. Silicone breast implants and autoimmunity: Causation or myth? Archives of Environmental Health. 1994 May-1994 Jun 30, 49, (3): 151-153. CONNECTIVE TISSUE DISEASE/immune effects.

Brawer, A. E. Chronology of systemic disease development in 300 symptomatic recipients of silicone gel-filled breast implants. Journal of Clean Technology, Environmental Toxicology, and Occupational Medicine. 1996 Jan, 5, (3): 223-233. CONNECTIVE TISSUE DISEASE.

Brawer, A. E. Clinical features of local breast phenomena in 300 symptomatic recipients of silicone gel-filled breast implants. Journal of Clean Technology, Environmental Toxicology, and Occupational Medicine. 1996 Jan, 5, (3): 235-247. CONNECTIVE TISSUE DISEASE/capsule-contracture/sensation.

Brem, R., Tempany, C, and Zerhouni, E. MR detection of breast implant rupture. Journal of Computer Assisted Tomography. 1992, 16, (1): 157-159. MAMMOGRAPHY/rupture.

Brenner, R. J. Breast MR imaging. An analysis of its role with respect to other imaging and interventional modalities. Magn Reson Imaging Clin N Am. 1994, 2, (4): 705-723. MAMMOGRAPHY.

Bridges, A. J. Rheumatic disorders in patients with silicone implants: A critical review. Journal Biomater Sci Polymer Edn. 1995, 7, (2): 147-157. CONNECTIVE TISSUE DISEASE/immune effects.

Bridges, A. J., Conley, C., Wang, G., Burns, D. E., and Vasey, F. B. A clinical and immunologic evaluation of women with silicone breast implants and symptoms of rheumatic disease. Annals of Internal Medicine. 1993a Jun 15, 118, (12): 929-935. CONNECTIVE TISSUE DISEASE/immune effects.

Bridges, A. J., and Vasey, F. B. Silicone breast implants: History, safety, and potential complications. Archives of Internal Medicine. 1993 Dec 13, 153, 2638-2644. GENERAL.

Bright, R. A., Jeng, L. L., and Moore, R. M. National survey of self-reported breast implants: 1988 estimates. Journal of Long-Term Effects of Medical Implants. 1993, 3, 81-89. PREVALENCE.

Bright, R. W. Operative correction of partial epiphyseal plate closure by osseous-bridge resection and silicone-rubber implant. The Journal of Bone and Joint Surgery. 1974 Jun, 56-A, (4): 655-664. SILICONE CHARACTERIZATION.

Brink, R. R. Evaluating breast parenchymal maldistribution with regard to mastopexy and augmentation mammaplasty. Plastic and Reconstructive Surgery. 1990 Oct, 86, (4): 715-719. RECONSTRUCTION/local complications.

Brink, R. R. Sequestered fluid and breast implant malposition. Plast. Reconstr. Surg. 1996 Sep, 98, (4): 670-684. LOCAL COMPLICATIONS.

Brinton, L. A., and Brown, S. L. Breast implants and cancer. Journal of the National Cancer Institute. 1997 Sep 17, 89, (18): 1341-1349. CANCER.

Brinton, L. A., Malone, K. E., Coates, R. J., Schoenberg, J. B., Swanson, C. A., Daling, J. R., and Stanford, J. L. Breast enlargement and reduction: Results from a breast cancer case-control study. Plast. Reconstr. Surg. 1996 Feb, 97, (2): 269-275. CANCER.

Brinton, L. A., Nasca, P. C., Mallin, K., Baptiste, M. S., Wilbanks, G. D., and Richart, R. M. Case-control study of cancer of the vulva. Obstet Gynecol. 1990, 75, (5): 859-866. CANCER.

Brinton, L. A., Toniolo, P., and Pasternack, B. S. Epidemiologic follow-up studies of breast augmentation patients. Journal of Clinical Epidemiology. 1995, 48, (4): 557-563. CANCER.

British Department of Health. Polyurethane-coated breast implants: Potential release of a probable carcinogenic degradation product following breakdown of the polyurethane foam *in vivo*. Safety Action Bulletin. 1994 Sep, 94, 39. POLYURETHANE/carcinogenicity.

Broadbent, T. R., and Woolf, R. M. Augmentation mammaplasty. Plast. Reconstr. Surg. 1967 Dec, 40, (6): 517-523. GENERAL.

Broadbent, T. R., and Woolf, R. M. Unsatisfactory results in augmentation mammoplasty: chest and breast asymmetry. Aesth Plast Surg. 1978, 2, 251-269. GENERAL.

Broadbent, T. R., and Woolf, R. M. Trends in plastic surgery in the United States. Ann Plast Surg. 1978 May, 1, (3): 249-251. GENERAL.

Brockhurst, R. J., Ward, R. C., Lou, P., Omerod, D., and Albert, D. Dystrophic calcification of silicone scleral buckling implant materials. American Journal of Ophthamology. 1993 Apr, 115, (4): 524-529. CALCIFICATION/local complications.

Brody, G. L., and Frey, C. F. Peritoneal response to silicone fluid. Arch Surg. 1968: 237-241. LOCAL COMPLICATIONS.

Brody, G. S. Fact and fiction about breast implant bleed. Plast. Reconstr. Surg. 1977 Oct, 60, (4): 615-616. LOCAL COMPLICATIONS/capsule contracture/rupture.

Brody, G. S. Mechanical analysis of explanted silicone breast implants [discussion]. Plast. Reconstr. Surg. 1996 Aug, 98, (2): 273-275. RUPTURE/local complications.

Brody, G. S. On the safety of breast implants. Plast. Reconstr. Surg. 1997 Oct, 100, (5): 1314-1321. GENERAL.

Brody, G. S. Risk assessment of carcinogenesis at implantation sites [discussion]. Plast. Reconstr. Surg. 1980 Oct, 66, (4): 595. CARCINOGENICITY.

Brody, G. S., Conway, D. P., Deapen, D. M., Fisher, J. C., Hochberg, M. C., LeRoy, E. C. Medsger Jr. T. A., Robson, M. C., Shons, A. R., and Weisman, M. H. Consensus statement on the relationship of breast implants to connective-tissue disorders. Plastic and Reconstructive Surgery. 1992 Dec, 90, (6): 1102-1105. CONNECTIVE TISSUE DISEASE.

Brohim, R. M., Foresmann, P. A., Hildebrandt, P. K., and Rodeheaver, G. T. Early tissue reaction to textured breast implant surfaces. Annals of Plastic Surgery. 1992, 28, (4): 354-362. POLYURETHANE/local complications/capsule-contracture.

Brooks, S. M., Baker, D. B., Gann, P. H., Jarabek, A. M., Hertzberg, V., Gallagher, J., Biagini, R. E., and Berstein, I. L. Cold air challenge and platinum skin reactivity in platinum refinery workers: Bronchial reactivity precedes skin prick response. Chest. 1990 Jun, 97, (6): 1401-1407. PLATINUM.

Brorson, T., Skarping, G., and Sangö, C. Biological monitoring of isocyanates and related amines. International Archives of Occupational and Environmental Health. 1991, 63, 253-259. CARCINOGENICITY/toxicology.

Brown, J. B., Fryer, M. P., and Ohlwiler, D. A. Study and use of synthetic materials, such as silicones and Teflon, as subcutaneous prostheses. Plast. Reconstr. Surg. 1960a Sep, 26, (3): 264-279. GENERAL.

Brown, J. B., Fryer, M. P., Ohlwiler, D. A., and Kollias, P. Dimethylsiloxane and halogenated carbons as subcutaneous prostheses. American Surgeon. 1962, 28, 146-148. GENERAL.

Brown, J. B., Fryer, M. P., Randall, P., and Lu, M. Silicones in plastic surgery. Laboratory and clinical investigations, a preliminary report. Plast. Reconstr. Surg. 1953, 12, 374-376. GENERAL.

Brown, J. B., Ohwiler, D. A., and Fryer, M. P. Investigation of and use of dimethylsiloxanes, halogenated carbons and polyvinyl alcohol as subcutaneous prostheses. Am Surg. 1960b, 152, 534. GENERAL.

Brown, J., Fryer, M., Randall, P., and Lu, M. Silicones in plastic surgery: Laboratory and clinical investigations, a preliminary report. Plast. Reconstr. Surg. 1953 May 15, 12, 374-376. TOXICOLOGY.

Brown, Jr. J. F., and Slusarczuk, J. Macrocyclic Polydimethysliloxanes. J. Am. Chem. Soc. 1965, 87, 931. SILICONE CHEMISTRY.

Brown, S. L., Langone, J. J., and Brinton, L. A. Silicone breast implants and autoimmune disease. JAMWA. 1998 Winter, 53, (1): 1-5. CONNECTIVE TISSUE DISEASE/immune effects.

Brown, S. L., Middleton, M. S., Berg, W. A., Soo, M. S., and Pennello, G. Silicone gel breast implant rupture prevalence in a population of women in Birmingham, Alabama. Unpublished Document, 1999. RUPTURE/local complications.

Brown, S. L., Parmentier, C. M., Woo, E. K., Vishnuvajjala, R. L., and Headrick, M. L. Silicone gel breast implant adverse event reports to the Food and Drug Administration, 1984-1995. Public Health Reports. 1998, 113, 535-543. PSYCHOSOCIAL/general.

Brown, S. L., Silverman, B. G., and Berg, W. A. Rupture of silicone-gel breast implants: Causes, sequelae, and diagnosis. The Lancet. 1997b Nov 22, 350, 1531-1537. RUPTURE/local complications/mammography.

Brozena, S. J., Fenske, N. A., Cruse, C. W., Espinoza, C. G., Vasey, F. B., Germain, B. F., and Espinoza, L. R. Human adjuvant disease following augmentation mammoplasty. Arch Dermatol. 1988 Sep, 124, 1383. CONNECTIVE TISSUE DISEASE.

Brozman, M., and Hostyn, L. Local response by organism to the silicon implante in experiment. Acta Chir Plast. 1971, 13, (3): 183-187. INFECTION.

Bruck, H. G. Long-term results of polyurethane-covered prostheses. Aesthetic Plast Surg. 1990, 14, 85-86. POLYURETHANE.

Brunner, C. A., Feller, A. M., Groner, R., Dees, E., Biefel, K., and Biemer, E. Increase of immunologically relevant parameters in correlation with Baker classification in breast implant recipients. Annals of Plastic Surgery. 1996 May, 36, (5): 512-518. IMMUNE EFFECTS/local complications/capsule-contracture/connective tissue disease.

Brunner, C. A., Groner, R., Biemer, E., and Johnson, J. P. Expression of CD44-v6-containing isoform on breast tissue adjacent to silicone breast implants. Annals of Plastic Surgery. 1997 Sep, 39, (3): 235-240. IMMUNE EFFECTS.

Bryant, H., and Brasher, P. M. Breast implants and breast cancer—reanalysis of a linkage study. The New England Journal of Medicine. 1995 Jun 8, 332, (23): 1535-1539. CANCER.

Bryson, G., and Bischoff, F. Silicate-Induced Neoplasms. Progr. Exp. Tumor Res. 1967, 9, 77-164. CARCINOGENICITY/toxicology/silica.

Buchwald, D., and Garrity, M. D. Comparison of patients with chronic fatigue syndrome, fibromyalgia, and multiple chemical sensitivites. Archives of Internal Medicine. 1994 Sep 26, 154, (18): 2049-2053. AI-CTD BACKGROUND.

Buchwald, D., Umali, P., Kith, P., Pearlman, T., and Komaroff, A. L. Chronic fatigue and the chronic fatigue syndrome: Prevalence in a Pacific Northwest health care system. Annals of Internal Medicine. 1995 Jul, 123, (2): 81-88. AI-CTD BACKGROUND.

Bucky, L. P., Ehrlich, H. P., Sohoni, S., and May, Jr. J. W. The capsule quality of saline-filled smooth silicone, textured silicone, and polyurethane implants in rabbits: A long-term study. Plast. Reconstr. Surg. 1994 May, 93, (6): 1123-1131. CAPSULE-CONTRACTURE/local complications/saline/polyurethane.

Bucky, L. P., and May, Jr. J. W. The capsule in various types of breast implants [letter-reply]. Plast. Reconstr. Surg. 1995 Apr, 95, (5): 937-938. CAPSULE-CONTRACTURE/local complications.

Buehler, P. K. Patient selection for prophylactic mastectomy: Who is at high risk? Plast. Reconstr. Surg. 1983 Sep, 72, (3): 324-329. CANCER.

Burda, C. D., Cox, F. R., and Osborne, P. Histocompatibility antigens in the fibrositis (fibromyaliga) syndrome. Clinical and Experimental Rheumatology. 1986, 4, 355-357. AI-CTD BACKGROUND.

Burkhardt, B. R. Capsular Contracture: Hard Breasts, Soft Data. Clinics in Plastic Surgery. 1988, 15, (4): 521-532. CAPSULE-CONTRACTURE/infection.

Burkhardt, B. R. Fibrous capsular contracture around breast implants: The role of subclinical infection. Infect Surg. 1985, 4, 469-475. INFECTION/local complications/capsule-contracture.

Burkhardt, B. R., and Demas, C. P. The effect of siltex texturing and povidone-iodine irrigation on capsular contracture around saline inflatable breast implants. Plast. Reconstr. Surg. 1994 Jan, 93, (1): 123-128. CAPSULE-CONTRACTURE/local complications.

Burkhardt, B. R., Dempsey, P. D., Schnur, P. L., and Tofield, J. J. Capsular contracture: A prospective study of the effect of local antibacterial agents. Plast. Reconstr. Surg. 1986 Jun, 77, (6): 919-930. CAPSULE-CONTRACTURE/local complications/infection.

Burkhardt, B. R., and Eades, E. The effect of Biocell texturing and povidone-iodine irrigation on capsular contracture around saline-inflatable breast implants. Plast. Reconstr. Surg. 1995 Nov, 96, (6): 1317-1325. CAPSULE-CONTRACTURE/local complications/saline.

Burkhardt, B. R., Fried, M., Schnur, P. L., and Tofield, J. J. Capsules, infection, and intraluminal antibiotics. Plast. Reconstr. Surg. 1981, 68, 43-47. INFECTION/local complications.

Burkhardt, B. R., Schnur, P. L., Tofield, J. J., and Dempsey, P. D. Objective clinical assessment of fibrous capsular contracture. Plast. Reconstr. Surg. 1982 May, 69, (5): 794-797. CAPSULE-CONTRACTURE/local complications.

Burmester, G. R., Dimitriu-Bona, A., Waters, S. J., and Winchester, R. J. Identification of the three major synovial lining cell populations by monoclonal antibodies directed to Ia antigens and antigens associated with monocytes/macrophages and fibroblasts. Scandinavian Journal of Immunology. 1983, 17, 69-82. CAPSULE-CONTRACTURE/local complications/immune effects.

Burns, C. J., Laing, T. J., Gillespie, B. W., Heering, S. G., Alcser, K. H., Mayes, M. D., Wasko, C. M., Cooper, B. C., Garabrant, D. H., and Schottenfeld, D. The epidemiology of scleroderma among women: Assessment of risk from exposure to silicone and silica. The Journal of Rheumatology. 1996, 23, (11): 1904-1911. CONNECTIVE TISSUE DISEASE/silica.

Butler, J. E., Lü, E. P., Navarro, P., and Christiansen, B. Comparative studies on the interaction of proteins with a polydimethylsiloxane elastomer. I. Monolayer protein capture capacity (PCC) as a function of protein pl, buffer pH and buffer ionic strength. Journal of Molecular Recognition. 1997, 10, (1): 36-51. IMMUNE EFFECTS.

Buyon, J. P. The effects of pregnancy on autoimmune diseases. Journal of Leukocyte Biology. 1998 Mar, 63, 281-287. AI-CTD BACKGROUND.

Buyon, J. P., Ben-Chetrit, E., Karp, S., Roubey, A. S., Pompeo, L., Revers, W. H., Tan, E. M., and Winchester, R. Acquired congenital heart block: pattern of maternal antibody response to biochemically defined antigens of the SSA/Ro-SSB/La system in neonatal lupus. J. Clin. Invest. 1989, 84, 627-634. CHILDREN'S EFFECTS/breast feeding.

Buyon, J. P., Slade, S. G., Reveille, J. D., Hamel, J. C., and Chan, E. K. L. Autoantibody responses to "native" 52k SS-A/Ro protein in neonatal lupus. J. Immunol. 1994, 152, 3675-3684. CHILDREN'S EFFECTS/breast feeding.

Byler, D. M., and Susi, H. Examination of the secondary structure of protein by convoluted FTIR spectra. Biopolymers. 1986, 25, 469-487. SILICON MEASUREMENT.

Byron, M. A., Venning, V. A., and Mowat, A. G. Post-mammoplasty human adjuvant disease. British Journal of Rheumatology. 1984, 23, 227-229. SALINE/connective tissue disease/immune effects.

Cabral, A. R., Alocer-Varela, J., Orozco-Topete, R., Reyes, E., Fernández-Domínguez, L., and Alarcón-Segovia, D. Clinical, histopathological, immunological and fibroblast studies in 30 patients with subcutaneous injections of modelants including silicone and mineral oils. La Revista De Investigación Clinica. 1994 Jul, 46, (4): 257-266. SILICONE INJECTION.

Caffee, H. H. The effects of intraprosthetic methylprenisolone on implant capsules and surrounding tissue. Annals of Plastic Surgery. 1984, 12, (4): 348-352. STEROIDS/local complications.

Caffee, H. H. External compression for the prevention of scar capsule contracture: A preliminary report. Annals of Plastic Surgery. 1982 Jun, 8, (6): 453-458. CAPSULE-CONTRACTURE/local complications.

Caffee, H. H. The influence of silicone bleed on capsule contracture. Annals of Plastic Surgery. 1986a Oct, 17, (4): 284-287. CAPSULE-CONTRACTURE/local complications.

Caffee, H. H. Measurement of implant capsules. Ann. Plast. Surg. 1983 Nov, 11, (5): 412-416. CAPSULE-CONTRACTURE.

Caffee, H. H. Textured silicone and capsular contracture. Ann. Plast. Surg. 1990, 24, 197-199. CAPSULE-CONTRACTURE/local complications.

Caffee, H. H. Vitamin E and capsule contracture. Annals of Plastic Surgery. 1987 Dec, 19, (6): 512-514. CAPSULE CONTRACTURE.

Caffee, H. H., Hardt, N. S., and La Torre, G. Detection of breast implant rupture with aspiration cytology. Plast. Reconstr. Surg. 1995, 95, (7): 1145-1149. RUPTURE/local complications.

Caffee, H. H., Mendenhall, N. P., Mendenhall, W. M., and Bova, F. J. Postoperative radiation and implant capsule contraction. Annals of Plastic Surgery. 1988 Jan, 20, (1): 35-38. RADIATION/capsule-contracture/local complications.

Cahan, A. C., Ashikari, R., Pressmen, P., Cody, H., Hoffman, S., and Sherman, J. E. Breast cancer after breast augmentation with silicone implants. Annals of Surgical Oncology. 1995, 2, (2): 121-125. MAMMOGRAPHY/cancer.

Cairns, T. S., and de Villiers, W. Capsular contracture after breast augmentation—a comparison between gel- and saline-filled prostheses. South African Medical Journal. 1980 Jun, 57, 951-953. CAPSULE-CONTRACTURE/local complications/saline/sensation.

Callery, C. D., Rosen, P. P., and Kinne, D. W. Sarcoma of the breast. A study of 32 patients with reappraisal of classifications therapy. Annals Surgery. 1985, 201, 527. CANCER.

Camilleri, I. G., Malata, C. M., and McLean, N. R. A review of 120 Becker permanent tissue expanders in reconstruction of the breast. British Journal of Plastic Surgery. 1996, 49 , (6): 346-351. EXPANDER/reconstruction/local complications/radiation/psychosocial.

Cammarata, A., Georgiou, J., Cruz, E., and et al. Inflammatory carcinoma in a patient with a breast implant. Breast, Diseases of the Breast. 1984, 10, (3): 24. CANCER.

Campbell, A. W., Brautbar, N., and Vojdani, A. Suppressed natural killer cell activity in patients with silicone breast implants: reversal upon explantation. Toxicology and Industrial Health. 1994, 10, (3): 149-154. IMMUNE EFFECTS/explantation.

Campbell, R. D., and Milner, C. M. MHC genes in autoimmunity. Current Opinion in Immunology. 1993, 5, 887-893. AI-CTD BACKGROUND.

Capozzi, A. Clinical experience with Heyer-Schulte inflatable implants in breast augmentation. Plast. Reconstr. Surg. 1986 May, 77, (5): 772-778. EXPANDER/local complications/rupture/capsule-contracture/saline.

Capozzi, A. Long-term complications of polyurethane-covered breast implants. Plast. Reconstr. Surg. 1991 Sep, 88, (3): 458-461. CAPSULE-CONTRACTURE/rupture/local complications/polyurethane.

Capozzi, A., Du Bou, R., and Pennisi, V. R. Distant migration of silicone gel from a ruptured breast implant. Plast. Reconstr. Surg. 1978, 62, 302-303. MIGRATION/local complications/rupture/granulomas.

Capozzi, A., and Pennisi, V. R. Clinical experience with polyurethane-covered gel-filled mammary prostheses. Plast. Reconstr. Surg. 1981 Oct, 68, (4): 512-518. POLYURETHANE/local complications/infection/capsule-contracture.

Carbotte, R. M., Denburg, S. D., and Denburg, J. A. Cognitive deficit associated with rheumatic diseases: Neuropsychological perspectives. Arthritis and Rheumatism. 1995 Oct, 38, (10): 1363-1374. AI-CTD BACKGROUND/psychosocial/neurologic disease.

Cardona, M. A., Simmons, R. L., and Kaplan, S. S. TNF and IL-1 generation by human monocytes in response to biomaterials. Journal of Biomedical Materials Research. 1992, 26, 851-859. IMMUNE EFFECTS/polyurethane.

Cardy, R. H. Carcinogenicity and chronic toxicity of 2,4-toluenediamine in F344 rats. Journal of the National Cancer Institute. 1979 Apr, 62, (4): 1107-1113. CARCINOGENICITY/toxicology.

Carette, S. Chronic pain syndromes. Annals of Rheumatic Diseases. 1996, 55, (8): 497-501. AI-CTD BACKGROUND.

Carlisle, E. M. Silicon as an essential element. Federation Proceedings. 1974, 33, (6): 1758-1766. GENERAL.

Carlson, G. W., Curley, S. A., Martin, J. E., Fornage, B. D., and Ames, F. C. The detection of breast cancer after augmentation mammaplasty. Plast. Reconstr. Surg. 1993 Apr, 91, (5): 837-840. MAMMOGRAPHY.

Carmen, R., and Kahn, P. Test in vitro of silicone rubber heart-valve poppets for lipid absorption. Journal of the Association for the Advancement of Medical Instrumentation. 1969, 3, (1): 14-17. SILICONE CHARACTERIZATION.

Carmen, R., and Mutha, S. C. Lipid absorption by silicone rubber heart valve poppets—in-vivo and in-vitro results. Journal of Biomedical Materials Research. 1972, 6, (5): 327-346. SILICONE CHARACTERIZATION.

Carmichael, J. B., and Winger, R. Cyclic distribution in dimethylsiloxanes. J. Polymer Sci. 1965, A3, 971. SILICONE CHEMSITRY.

Caro, X. J. Immunofluorescent detection of IgG at the dermal-epidermal junction in patients with apparent primary fibrositis syndrome. Arthritis and Rheumatism. 1984 Oct, 27, (10): 1174-1179. AI-CTD BACKGROUND.

Carpeneda, C. A. Inflammatory reaction and capsular contracture around smooth silicone implants. Aesthetic Plastic Surgery. 1997, 21, (2): 110-114. CAPSULE-CONTRACTURE/local complications.

Carpenter, J. C. Study of the degradation of polydimethylsiloxane on soil. Environmental Science and Technology. 1995, 29, (4): 864-868. SILICONE CHARACTERIZATION.

Carrico, C. J., Meakins, J. L., Marshall, J. C., Fry, D., and Maier, R. V. Multiple-organ-failure syndrome. Arch Surg. 1986 Feb, 121, 196-208. INFECTION.

Carrico, T. J., and Cohen, I. K. Capsular contracture and steroid-related complications after augmentation mammaplasty. Plast. Reconstr. Surg. 1979 Sep, 64, (3): 377-380. CAPSULE-CONTRACTURE/local complications/steroids.

Carson, S., Weinberg, M., and Oser, B. Safety evaluation of Dow Corning® 360 fluid and antifoam A. Proc Sci Sec Toilet Goods Assoc. 1966 May, 45, 8-19. TOXICOLOGY.

Caskey, C. I., Berg, W. A., Anderson, N. D., Sheth, S., Chang, B. W., and Hamper, U. M. Breast implant rupture: Diagnosis with US. Radiology. 1994, 190, 81-84. MAMMOGRAPHY/rupture.

Castello, D. Prophylactic treatment of childhood asthma. International Journal of Clinical Pharmacological Research. 1986, 6, 373-378. CHILDREN'S EFFECTS.

Cathcart, R. S., and Hagerty, R. C. Preoperative and postoperative considerations in elective breast operations. Annals of Plastic Surgery. 1989 Jun, 22, (6): 533-538. GENERAL.

Cavic-Vlasak, B. A., Thompson, M., and Smith, D. C. Silicones and their determination in biological matrixes. A review. Analyst. 1996, 121, (6): 53R-63R. SILICONE CHARACTERIZATION.

Celli, B., Textor, S., and Kovnat, D. M. Adult respiratory distress syndrome following mammary augmentation. The American Journal of the Medical Sciences. 1978, 275, (1): 81-85. SILICONE INJECTION.

Centeno, J. A., and Johnson, F. B. Microscopic identification of silicone in human breast tissues by infrared microspectroscopy and x-ray microanalysis. Applied Spectroscopy. 1993 Jan, 47, (3): 341-345. SILICON MEASUREMENT.

Centeno, J. A., Kalasinsky, V. F., Johnson, F. B., Vinh, T. N., and O'Leary, T. J. Fourier transform infrared microscopic identification of foreign materials in tissue sections. Laboratory Investigation. 1992, 66, (1): 123-131. SILICON MEASUREMENT.

Céspedes, I., Ophir, J., and Huang, Y. On the feasibility of pulse-echo speed of sound estimation in small regions: Simulation studies. Ultrasound in Medicine and Biology. 1992, 18, (3): 283-291. MAMMOGRAPHY.

Chan, S. C., Birdsell, D. C., and Gradeen, C. Y. Detection of toluenediamines in the urine of a patient with polyurethane-covered breast implants. Clin Chem. 1991a, 37, (5): 756-758. POLYURETHANE/TOXICOLOGY.

Chan, S. C., Birdsell, D. C., and Gradeen, C. Y. Urinary excretion of free toluenediamines in a patient with polyurethane-covered breast implants. Clinical Chemistry. 1991b, 37, (12): 2143-2145. TOXICOLOGY/polyurethane.

Chandler, M. L., and LeVier, R. R. Structure-activity relationships of diphenylsilanediol and similar silicon-containing anticonvulsants. The Pharmacologist. 1977. TOXICOLOGY.

Chandra, G., Lo, P. Y., Hitchcock, P. B., and Lappert, M. F. A convenient and novel route to bis(n-alkyne)platinum(0) and other platinum(0) complexes from Speler's hydrosilylation catalyst H2[PtCl6] x H2O. X-ray structure of [Pt{(n-CH2==CHSiMe2)2O}(P-t-Bu3)]. Organometrallics. 1987, 6, 191-192. PLATINUM/toxicology.

Chang, L., Caldwell, E., Reading, G., and Wray, Jr. R. C. A comparison of conventional and low-bleed implants in augmentation mammoplasty. Plast. Reconstr. Surg. 1992 Jan, 89, (1): 79-92. CAPSULE-CONTRACTURE/local complications.

Chang, Y. Adjuvanticity and arthritogenecity of silicone. Plast. Reconstr. Surg. 1993 Sep, 92, (3): 469-473. IMMUNE EFFECTS.

Chang, Y. H., Pearson, C. M., and Abe, C. IV induction by a synthetic adjuvant: immunologic, histopathologic, and other studies. Arthritis and Rheumatism. 1980 Jan, 23, (1): 62-71. AI-CTD BACKGROUND.

Chantelau, E. A., Berger, M., and Bohlken, B. Silicone oil released from disposable insulin syringes. Diabetes Care. 1986 Nov, 9, (6): 672-673. GENERAL/silicon measurement.

Chaplin, C. H. Loss of both breasts from injections of silicone (with additive). Plast. Reconstr. Surg. 1969 Nov, 44, (5): 447-450. SILICONE INJECTION/silicon measurement.

Chase, D. R., Oberg, C. K., Chase, R. L., Malott, L. R., and Weeks, D. A. Pseudoepithelialization of breast implant capsules. International Journal of Surgical Pathology. 1994a, 1, (3): 151-154. CAPSULE-CONTRACTURE/local complications.

Chase, D. R., Oberg, K. C., Cahse, R. L., Malott, R. L., and Weeks, D. A. Tissue reactions to mammary implants: a capsule summary. Advances in Anatomic Pathology. 1995, 2, (1): 24-27. CAPSULE CONTRACTURE.

Chastre, J., Basset, F., Viau, F., Dournovo, P., Bouchama, A., Akesbi, A., and Gilbert, C. Acute pneumonitis after subcutaneous injections of silicone in transsexual men. The New England Journal of Medicine. 1983a Mar 31, 308, (13): 764-767. SILICONE INJECTION.

Chastre, J., Brun, P., and Soler, P. et al. Acute and latent pneumonitis after subcutaneous injections of silicone in transexual men. Am. J. Respir. Dis. 1987, 135, 236-240. SILICONE INJECTION.

Chen, F. Induction of nitric oxide and nitric oxide synthase MRNA by silica and lipopolysaccharide in pma-primed thp-1 cells. APMIS. 1996 Jan, 104, 176-182. SILICA.

Chen, N. T., Butler, P., Hooper, D., and May, J. Bacterial growth in saline implants: In vitro and in vivo studies. Annals of Plastic Surgery. 1996 Apr, 36, (4): 337-341. INFECTION.

Chen, T. H. Silicone injection granulomas of the breast: Treatment by subcutaneous mastectomy and immediate subpectoral breast implant. British Journal of Plastic Surgery. 1995, 48, 71-76. SILICONE INJECTION/granulomas.

Chen, Y. M., Lu, C. C., and Perng, R. P. Silicone fluid-induced pulmonary embolism. American Review of Respiratory Diseases. 1993, 147, 1299-1302. SILICONE INJECTION.

Cherup, L. L., Antaki, J. F., Liang, M. D., and Hamas, R. S. Measurement of capsular contracture: The conventional breast implant and the Pittsburgh implant. Plastic Reconstructive Surgery. 1989 Dec, 84, (6): 893-901. CAPSULE-CONTRACTURE/local complications/saline.

Cheung, K. L., Blamey, R. W., Robertson, J. F., Elston, C. W., and Ellis, I. O. Subcutaneous mastectomy for primary breast cancer and ductal carcinoma in situ. European Journal of Surgical Oncology. 1997 Aug, 23, (4): 343-347. CANCER.

Chilcote, W. A., Dowden, R. V., Paushter, D. M., Hale, J. C., Desberg, A. L., Singer, A. A., Obuchowski, N., and Godec, K. Ultrasound detection of silicone gel breast implant failure: A prospective analysis. Breast Disease. 1994 Jan, 7, 307-316. MAMMOGRAPHY/rupture/local complications.

Child, G. P., Paquin, H. O., and Deichman, W. B. Chronic toxicity of the methylpolysiloxane DC antifoam A in dogs. AMA Archives of Industrial Hygiene Occupational Medicine. 1951, 3, (5): 479-482. TOXICOLOGY.

Chinn, J. A., Posso, S. E., Horbett, T. A., and Ratner, B. D. Postadsorptive transitions in fibrinogen adsorbed to polyurethanes: Changes in antibody binding and sodium dodecyl sulfate elutability. Journal of Biomedical Materials Research. 1992, 26, 757-778. TOXICOLOGY.

Chisholm, E. M., Marr, S., Macfie, J., Broughton, A. C., and Brennan, T. G. Post-mastectomy breast reconstruction using the inflatable tissue expander. British Journal of Surgery. 1986, 73, 817-820. EXPANDER/reconstruction.

Cho, S-B, Nakanishi, K., Kokubo, T., Soga, N., Ohtsuki, C., and Nakamura, T. Apatite formation on silica gel in simulated body fluid: Its dependence on structures of silica gels prepared in different media. Journal of Biomedical Materials Research. 1996 Jan, 33, 145-151. CALCIFICATION/local complications/silica.

Choi, Y., Kotzin, B., Herron, L., Callahan, J., Marrack, P., and Kappler, J. Interaction of *Staphylococcus aureus* toxin "superantigens" with human T cells. Proceedings of the National Academy of Sciences. 1989, 86, 8941-8945. IMMUNE EFFECTS/infection/local complications.

Christ, J., and Askew, J. Silicone granuloma of the penis. Plast. Reconstr. Surg. 1982 Feb, 69, (2): 337-339. GRANULOMAS/local complications.

Christie, A. J., Pierret, and Levitan. Silicone Synovitis. Seminars in Arthritis and Rheumatism. 1989, 19, 3. IMMUNE EFFECTS.

Chu, F. C. H., Kaufmann, T. P., Dawson, G. A., and et al. Radiation therapy of cancer in prosthetically augmented or reconstructed breasts. Radiology. 1992, 185, 429-433. RADIATION.

Chung, K. C., Wilkins, E. G., Beil, R. J., Helvie, M. A., Ikeda, D. M., Oneal, R. M., Forrest, M. E., and Smith, Jr. D. J. Diagnosis of silicone gel breast implant rupture by ultrasonography. Plast. Reconstr. Surg. 1996 Jan, 97, (1): 104-109. MAMMOGRAPHY/local complications/rupture.

Chung, Y-H., and Shong, Y. K. Development of thyroid autoimmunity after administration of recombinant human interferon-2b for chronic viral hepatitis. The American Journal of Gastroenterology. 1993, 88, (2): 244-247. AI-CTD BACKGROUND.

Ciapetti, G., Cenni, E., Pratelli, L., and Pizzoferrato, A. *In vitro* evaluation of cell/biomaterial interaction by mtt assay. Biomaterials. 1993, 14, (5): 359-364. IMMUNE EFFECTS/toxicology.

Ciapetti, G., Gradnhi, D., Stea, S., Cenni, E., Schiavon, P., Giallani, R., and Pizzoferrato, A. Assessement of viability and proliferation of *in vivo* silicone-primed lymphocytes after *in vitro* re-exposure to silicone. Journal of Biomedical Materials Research. 1995, 29, 583-590. IMMUNE EFFECTS.

Ciatto, S., Del Turco, M. R., Bonardi, R., Cataliotti, L., Distante, V., Cardona, G., and Bianchi, S. Nonpalpable lesions of the breast detected by mammography: Review of the 1182 consecutive histologically confirmed cases. European Journal of Cancer. 1994, 30A, (1): 40-44. MAMMOGRAPHY.

Citro, G., Galati, R., Verdina, A., Marini, S., Zito, R., and Giardina, B. Activation of 2,4-diaminotoluene to proximate carcinogens in vitro, and assay of DNA adducts. Xenobiotica. 1993, 23, (3): 317-325. CARCINOGENICITY/toxicology.

Claman, H. N., and Robertson, A. D. Antinuclear antibodies and breast implants. Western Journal of Medicine. 1994 Mar, 160, (3): 225-228. IMMUNE EFFECTS/connective tissue disease.

Clark, P., Garbe, E., Habbick, B., Lawrence, V., and Spitzer, W. O. Question on breast-Implants study. Lancet. 1998 May 2, 351, 1358-1359. GENERAL.

Clark, P., Peters, G. N., and O'Brien, K. M. Cancer in the augmented breast. Cancer. 1993 Oct 1, 72, (7): 2170-2174. CANCER/mammography.

Clauw, D. J. The pathogenesis of chronic pain and fatigue syndromes, with special reference to fibromyalgia. Medical Hypotheses. 1995, 44, 369-378. AI-CTD BACKGROUND.

Clauw, D. J., Schmidt, M., Radulovic, D., Singer, A., Katz, P., and Bresette, J. The relationship between fibromyalgia and interstitial cystitis. Journal of Psychiatric Research. 1997, 31, (1): 125-131. AI-CTD BACKGROUND.

Cleare, M. J., Hughes, E. G., Jacoby, B., and Pepys, J. Immediate (type I) allergic responses to platinum compounds. Clinical Allergy. 1976, 6, 183-195. PLATINUM.

Clegg, D. O., Williams, H. J., Singer, J. Z., Steen, V. D., Schlegel, S., Ziminski, C., Alarcón, G. S., Luggen, M. E., Polisson, R. P., Willkens, R. F., Yarboro, C., McDuffie, F. C., and Ward, J. R. Early undifferentiated connective tissue disease: II. The frequency of circulating antinuclear antibodies in patients with early rheumatic diseases. Journal of Rheumatology. 1991, 18, (9): 1340-1343. AI-CTD BACKGROUND/immune effects.

Clegg, H. W., Bertagnoll, P., Hightower, A. W., and Baine, W. B. Mammaplasty-associated mycobacterial infection: A survey of plastic surgeons. Plast. Reconstr. Surg. 1983b Aug, 72, 165-169. INFECTION/local complications.

Clegg, H. W., Foster, M. T., Sanders, W. E., and Baine, W. B. Infection due to organisms of the *Mycobacterium fortuitum* complex after augmentation mammaplasty: Clinical and epidemiologic features. Journal of Infectious Diseases. 1983a Mar, 147, (3): 427. INFECTION/local complications.

Clugston, P. A., Perry, L. C., Hammond, D. C., and Maxwell, G. P. A rat model for capsular contracture: The effects of surface texturing. Annals of Plastic Surgery. 1994 Dec, 33, (6): 595-599. CAPSULE CONTRACTURE/local complications.

Coady, M. S., Gaylor, J., and Knight, S. L. Fungal growth within a silicone tissue expander: Case report. British Journal of Plastic Surgery. 1995, 48, (6): 428-430. EXPANDER/ infection/local complications.

Cocke, Jr. W. M. A critical review of augmentation mammoplasty with saline-filled prostheses. Annals of Plastic Surgery. 1994 Mar, 32, (3): 266. SALINE/local complications/ rupture.

Cocke, Jr. W. M. Inflammation and Silicone Prostheses. Plast. Reconstr. Surg. 1984, 74, (2): 314. GENERAL.

Cocke, Jr. W. M., and Sampson, H. Silicone bleed associated with double-lumen breast prostheses. Annals of Plastic Surgery. 1987 Jun, 18, (6): 524-526. LOCAL COMPLICATIONS.

Cocke, Jr. W. M., Sampson, H. W., and Quarles, J. M. Observations of cell function and morphology in the presence of silicone gel: An in vitro study. Annals of Plastic Surgery. 1987 Nov, 19, (5): 406-408. TOXICOLOGY.

Cocke, Jr. W. M., Whie, R., Vecchione, T. R., and Sampson, W. Calcified capsule following augmentation mammoplasty. Annals of Plastic Surgery. 1985 Jul, 15, (1): 61-65. CALCIFICATION/local complications.

Cocke, W. M., Leathers, H. K., and Lynch, J. B. Foreign body reactions to polyurethane covers of some breast prostheses. Plast. Reconstr. Surg. 1975 Nov, 56, (5): 527-530. POLYURETHANE/migration/local complications.

Cohen, B. E., Biggs, T. M., Cronin, E. D., Collins, Jr., and D.R. Assessment and longevity of the silicone gel breast implant. Plast. Reconstr. Surg. 1997 May, 99, (6): 1597-1601. LOCAL COMPLICATIONS/mammography.

Cohen, B. E., Casso, D., and Whetstone, M. Analysis of risks and aesthetics in a consecutive series of tissue expansion breast reconstructions. Plast. Reconstr. Surg. 1992, 89, 840-843. GENERAL.

Cohen, D. E., Kaufman, L. D., Varma, A. A., Seibold, J. R., Stiller, M., and Gruber, B. L. Antilaminin autoantibodies in collagen vascular diseases: The use of adequate controls in studies of autoimmune responses to laminin. Annals of Rheumatic Diseases. 1994, 53, 191-193. AI-CTD BACKGROUND/immune effects.

Cohen, I. K., and Carrico, T. J. Capsular contracture and steroid-related complications in augmentation mammoplasty. Aesthetic Plast. Surg. 1980, 4, 267. STEROIDS/capsule-contracture/local complications.

Cohen, I. K., Diegelmann, R. F., and Wise, W. S. Biomaterials and collagen synthesis. Journal of Biomedical Materials Research. 1976, 10, (6): 965-970. CAPSULE-CONTRACTURE/local complications.

Cohen, I. K., Goodman, H., and Theogaraj, S. D. Xeromammography—A reason for using saline-filled breast prosthesis. Plast. Reconstr. Surg. 1977 Dec, 59, (12): 886-888. MAMMOGRAPHY/saline.

Cohen, S. B., and Rohrich, R. J. Evaluation of the patient with silicone gel breast implants and rheumatic complaints. Plast. Reconstr. Surg. 1994 Jul, 94, (1): 120-125. IMMUNE EFFECTS/CONNECTIVE TISSUE DISEASE.

Cohney, B. C., Cohney, T. B., and Hearne, V. A. Augmentation mammoplasty—A further review of 20 years using the polyuretheane-covered prosthesis. Journal of Long-Term Effects of Medical Implants. 1992, 1, (3): 269-279. POLYURETHANE/local complications/rupture/capsule-contracture/migration.

Cohney, B. C., Cohney, T. B., and Hearne, V. A. Nineteen years' experience with polyurethane foam-covered mammary prosthesis: A preliminary report. Annals of Plastic Surgery. 1991, 27, (1): 27-30. POLYURETHANE/capsule-contracture/local complications.

Cohney, B. C., and Mitchell, S. R. N. An improved method of removing polyurethane. Aesth. Plast. Surg. 1997, 21, 191-192. POLYURETHANE.

Cole-Beuglet, C., Schwartz, G., Kurtz, A. B., Patchefsky, A. S., and Goldberg, B. B. Ultrasound mammography for the augmented breast. Radiology. 1983, 146, (3): 737-742. MAMMOGRAPHY.

Coleman, D. J., Foo, I. T, and Sharpe, D. T. Textured or smooth implants for breast augmentation? A prospective controlled trial. British Journal of Plastic Surgery. 1991, 44, (6): 444-448. CAPSULE-CONTRACTURE/local complications.

Coleman, D. L., King, R. N., and Andrade, J. D. The foreign body reaction: A chronic inflammatory response. J Biomed Mater Res. 1974, 8, 199-211. GENERAL.

Coleman, E. A., Lemon, S. J., Rudick, J., Depuy, R. S., Feuer, E., and Edwards, B. Rheumatic disease among 1167 women reporting local implant and systemic problems after breast implant surgery. Journal of Women's Health. 1994 Nov, 8, (3): 165. CONNECTIVE TISSUE DISEASE.

Collins, J. D., Shaver, M. L., Disher, A. C., and Miller, T. Q. Compromising abnormalities of the brachial plexus as displayed by magnetic resonance imaging. Clin. Anat. 1995, 8, (1-16). NEUROLOGIC DISEASE.

Collis, N., and Sharpe, D. T. Breast implant controversy: an update. The Breast. 1998, 7, 61-65. GENERAL.

Collis, N., and Sharpe, D. T. Breast implants: a survey of cosmetic clinics. British Journal of Plastic Surgery. 1998, 51, 311-312. GENERAL.

Collis, N., and Sharpe, D. T. Rupture of silicone-gel breast implants. The Lancet. 1998, 351, 520. RUPTURE/local complications.

Colon, G. A. Infection after augmentation mammaplasty [letter]. Plast. Reconstr. Surg. 1986 Sep, 78, (3): 424-425. INFECTION/local complications.

Colon, G. A. Mammoscopy and endoscopic implant and breast tissue evaluation. Clinics in Plastic Surgery. 1995 Oct, 22, (4): 697-706. LOCAL COMPLICATIONS/rupture.

Colon GA. The reverse double-lumen prothesis—a preliminary report. Ann Plast Surg. 1982 Oct, 9, (4): 293-297. EXPANDER.

Compton, R. A. Silicone manufacturing for long-term implants. Journal of Long-Term Effects of Medical Implants. 1997, 7, (1): 29-54. TOXICOLOGY/silicone characterization/silica.

Comunale, S., Troiano, L., and Napolita. Augmentation mammaplasty with silicone-gel-filled implants—It's effect on mammography. The Breast Journal. 1997, 6, (5): 318. MAMMOGRAPHY.

Conant, E. F., Forsberg, F., Moore, Jr. J. H., Piccoli, C. W., Rawool, N., Greer, J., and Fox, J. W. Surgical removal of ruptured breast implants: The use of intraoperative sonography in localizing free silicone. AJR American Journal of Roentgenology. 1995 Dec, 165, 1378-1379. MAMMOGRAPHY/local complications/rupture.

Connell, E. B. The exploitation of autoimmune disease: Breast implant litigation and its dire implications for women's health. Journal of Women's Health. 1998, 7, (3): 329-338. GENERAL.

Conway, B. J., McCrohan, J. L., Rueter, F. G., and Suleiman, O. H. Mammography in the eighties. Radiology. 1990, 177, 335-339. MAMMOGRAPHY.

Conway, H., and Dietz, G. Augmentation mammaplasty. Surgery Gyn Obstetrics. 1962, 114, 573-579. GENERAL.

Conway, H., and Goulian, D. Experience with an injectable silastic RTV as a subcutaneous prosthetic material, a preliminary report. Plast. Reconstr. Surg. 1963 Sep, 32, (3): 294-302. SILICONE INJECTION.

Cook, L. S., Daling, J. R., Voigt, L. F., deHart, P. M., Malone, K. E., Stanford, J. L., Weiss, N. S., Brinton, L. A., Gammon, M. D., and Brogan, D. Characteristics of women with and without breast augmentation. J. Amer. Med. Assoc. 1997 May 28, 277, (20): 1612-1617. GENERAL/psychosocial.

Cook, P. D., Osborne, B. M., Connor, R. L., and Strauss, J. F. Follicular lymphoma adjacent to foreign body granulomatous inflammation and fibrosis surrounding silicone breast prosthesis. The American Journal of Surgical Pathology. 1995 Jun, 19, (6): 712-717. CANCER.

Cook, R. R., Delongchamp, R. R., Woodbury, M., Perkins, L. L., and Harrison, M. C. The prevalence of women with breast implants in the United States. Journal of Clinical Epidemiology. 1995, 48, (4): 519-525. PREVALENCE.

Cook, R. R., Harrison, M. C., and LeVier, R. R. The breast implant controversy. Arthritis and Rheumatism. 1994 Feb, 37, (2): 153-157. GENERAL.

Cook, R. R., and Klein, P. J. Epidemiology and causation: The breast implant controversy. Plast. Reconstr. Surg. 1998, 102, (3): 921-923. GENERAL.

Cooper, G. G., Webster, M. H., Bell, G., and et al. The results of breast reconstruction following mastectomy. British Journal of Plastic Surgery. 1984, 37, 369-372. INFECTION/local complications/capsule-contracture/reconstruction.

Copeland, M., Choi, M., and Bleiweiss, M. Silicone breakdown and capsular synovial metaplasia in textured-wall saline breast prostheses. Plast. Reconstr. Surg. 1994 Oct, 94, (5): 628-633. SALINE/capsule-contracture/local complications.

Copeland, M., Kressel, A., Spiera, H., Hermann, G., and Bleiweiss, I. J. Systemic inflammatory disorder related to fibrous breast capsules after silicone implant removal. Plast. Reconstr. Surg. 1993 Nov, 92, (6): 1179-1181. CAPSULE-CONTRACTURE/local complications/CONNECTIVE TISSUE DISEASE.

Corsico, D. N., Diena, A., and Rosselli Del Turco, B. Pharmacological evaluation on some silicon compounds. 1971 Jun 25. SILICONE CHARACTERIZATION.

Corsten, L. A., Suduikis, S. V., and Donegan, W. L. Patient satisfaction with breast reconstruction. Wisconsin Medical Journal. 1992 Mar, 91, (3): 125-126. PSYCHOSOCIAL.

Coulaud, J. M., Labrousse, J., Carli, P., Galliot, M., Vilde, F., and Lissac, J. Adult respiratory distress syndrome and silicone injection. Toxicological European Research. 1983 Jul, 34, 171-174. SILICONE INJECTION.

Council on Scientific Affairs, American Medical Association. Silicone gel breast implants. J. Amer. Med. Assoc. 1993 Dec 1, 270, (21): 2602-2606. GENERAL.

Courtiss, E. H., and Goldwyn, R. M. Breast sensation before and after plastic surgery. Plast. Reconstr. Surg. 1976 Jul, 58, (1): 1-13. SENSATION/local complications.

Courtiss, E. H., Goldwyn, R. M., and Anastasi, G. W. The fate of breast implants with infections around them. Plast. Reconstr. Surg. 1979 Jun, 63, (6): 812-816. INFECTION/granulomas/local complications.

Courtiss, E. H., Webster, R. C., and White, M. F. Selection of alternatives in augmentation mammaplasty. Plast. Reconstr. Surg. 1974 Nov, 54, (5): 552-557. GENERAL.

Coury, A. J., Slaikeu, P. C. Calahan P. T., and Stokes, K. B. Medical applications of implantable polyurethanes: Current issues. Progress in Rubber and Plastics Technology. 1987, 3, (4): 24-37. POLYURETHANE.

Cowie, R. L. Silica dust-exposed mine workers with scleroderma. Chest. 1987 Aug, 92, (2): 260-262. CONNECTIVE TISSUE DISEASE/silica.

Cowie, R. L., and Dansey, R. D. Features of systemic sclerosis (scleroderma) in South African goldminers. South African Medical Journal. 1990 Apr, 77, (8): 400-402. SILICA.

Crespo, L. D., Eberlein, T. J., O'Connor, N., Hergrueter, C. A., Pribaz, J. J., and Eriksson, E. Postmastectomy complications in breast reconstruction. Annals of Plastic Surgery. 1994 May, 32, (5): 452-456. LOCAL COMPLICATIONS/reconstruction.

Crews, H. M. A decade of ICP-MS analysis. American Laboratory. 1993 Mar, 25, 34AA-34DD. SILICON MEASUREMENT.

Crisp, A., de Juan, Jr. E., and Tiedeman, J. Effect of silicone oil viscosity on emulsification. Archives of Ophthalmology. 1987 Apr, 105, 546-550. SILICONE CHARACTERIZATION.

Crofford, L. J., and Demitrack, M. A. Evidence that abnormalities of central neurohormonal systems are key to understanding fibromyalgia and chronic fatigue syndrome. Rheumatic Disease Clinics of North America. 1996 May, 22, (2): 267-284. AI-CTD BACKGROUND.

Croft, P., Rigby, A. S., Boswell, R., Schollum, J., and Silman, A. The prevalence of chronic widespread pain in the general population. J. Rheumatol. 1993, 20, (4): 710-713. AI-CTD BACKGROUND.

Croft, P., Schollum, M., and Silman, A. Population study of tender point counts in pain as evidence of fibromyalgia. British Medical Journal. 1994, 309, 696-699. AI-CTD BACKGROUND.

Cronin, T. D., and Greenberg, R. L. Our experiences with the silastic gel breast prostheses. Plast. Reconstr. Surg. 1970 Jun, 46, (1): 1-7. GENERAL/local complications.

Cruz, G., Gillooley, J. F., and Waxman, M. Silicone granulomas of the breast. New York State Journal of Medicine. 1985 Oct, 85, (10): 599-601. SILICONE INJECTION.

Cucin, R. L., Guthrie, R. H., and Graham, M. Rate of diffusion of Solo-Medrol across the silastic membranes of breast prostheses—an in vitro study. Annals of Plastic Surgery. 1982, 9, 228-229. STEROIDS.

Cuddihy, E. F., Moacanin, J., and Roschke, E. J. In vivo degradation of silicone rubber poppets in prosthetic heart valves. J. Biomed. Mater. Res. 1976, 10, 471-481. SILICONE CHARACTERIZATION.

Cuéllar, M. L., Gluck, I., Molina, J. F., Gutierrez, S., García, C., and Espinoza, R. Silicone breast implant-associated musculoskeletal manifestations. Clinical Rheumatology. 1995a, 14, (6): 667-672. CONNECTIVE TISSUE DISEASE/immune effects.

Cuéllar, M. L., Scopelitis, E., Tenenbaum, S. A., Garry, R. F., Silveira, L. H., Cabrera, G., and Espinoza, L. R. Serum antinuclear antibodies in women with silicone breast implants. J. Rheumatol. 1995b, 22, (2): 236-240. IMMUNE EFFECTS/connective tissue disease.

Cukier, J., Beauchamp, R. A., Spindler, J. S., Spindler, S., Lorenzo, C., and Trentham, D. E. Association between bovine collagen dermal implants and a dermatomyositis or a polymyositis-like M30467 syndrome. Annals of Internal Medicine. 1993 Jun 15, 118, (12): 920-928. AI-CTD BACKGROUND.

Cumming, R., and Klineberg, R. Breastfeeding and other reproductive factors and the risk of hip fractures in elderly women. International J. Epidemiology. 1993, 22, 684-691. CHILDREN'S EFFECTS/breast feeding.

Curz-Korchin, N. I. Effectiveness of silicone sheets in the prevention of hypertrophic breast scars. Annals of Plastic Surgery. 1996, 37, (4): 345-349. LOCAL COMPLICATIONS.

Cutler, M. G., Collings, A. J., Kiss, I. S., and Sharratt, M. A lifespan study of polydimethylsiloxane in the mouse. Food and Cosmetic Toxicology. 1974, 12, 443-450. TOXICOLOGY.

Czerny, V. Plasticher Ersatz der Brust-druese durch ein Lipom. Zentrallbl. Chir. 1895, 27, 72. RECONSTRUCTION.

Dahl, C. H., Baccari, M. E., and Arfai, P. A silicone gel inflatable mammary prosthesis. Plast. Reconstr. Surg. 1974, 53, (2): 234-235. INFECTION/EXPANDER.

Dalakis, M. C. Polymyositis, dermatomyositis, and inclusion-body myositis. The New England Journal of Medicine. 1991 Nov 21, 325, (21): 1487-1498. AI-CTD BACKGROUND.

Dale, P. S., and Wardlaw, J. C. Desmoid tumor occurring after reconstruction mammaplasty for breast carcinoma. Annals of Plastic Surgery. 1995 Nov, 35, (5): 515-518. LOCAL COMPLICATIONS.

Dalinka, M. K., Rockett, J. F., and Kurth, R. J. Carcinoma of the breast following mastectomy and mammoplasty. Radiology. 1969 Oct, 93, 914. CANCER.

Dalton, E. W., Silverstein, P., and Kelly, J. M. Subcutaneous mastectomy by extended periareolar incisions. American Journal of Surgery. 1978 Dec, 136, 719-721. RECONSTRUCTION.

Darby, T. D., Johnson, H. J., and Northup, S. J. An evaluation of a polyurethane for use as a medical grade plastic. Toxicology and Applied Pharmacology. 1978, 46, 449-453. CARCINOGENICITY/polyurethane.

Das, S. K., Johnson, M., Ellsaesser, C., and et al. Macrophage interleukin 1 response to injected silicone in a rat model. Annals of Plastic Surgery. 1992 Jun, 28, (6): 535-537. IMMUNE EFFECTS/toxicology.

Das, S. K., Johnson, S. G., Brantley, S. K., and Johnson, M. The effects of injected silicone on DNA lymphocytic structure. Journal of Long-Term Effects of Medical Implants. 1992, 1, (3): 285-291. SILICONE INJECTION/immune effects.

Dauber, J. H., Rossman, M. D., Pietra, G. G., Jimenez, S. A., and Daniele, R. P. Experimental silicosis: Morphologic and biochemical abnormalities produced by instillation of quartz into guinea pig lungs. American Journal of Pathology. 1980 Dec, 101, (3): 595-612. SILICA.

Davis, P. K., and Jones, S. M. The complications of silastic implants. Experience with 137 consecutive cases. British Journal of Plastic Surgery. 1971, 24, 405-411. LOCAL COMPLICATIONS.

De Angelis, G. A., de Lange, E. E., Miller, L. R., and Morgan, R. F. MR imaging of breast implants. Radiographics. 1994, 14, 783. MAMMOGRAPHY.

De Blecourt, R. A., and et al. Capsular contracture after augmentation mammaplasty—a retrospective study. Eur. J. Plast. Surg. 1989, 12, 83-86. CAPSULE CONTRACTURE/local complications.

De Bruhl, N. D., Gorczyca, D. P., Ahn, C. Y., Shaw, W. W., and Bassett, L. W. Silicone breast implants: US evaluation. Radiology. 1993, 189, 95-98. MAMMOGRAPHY.

De Camara, D. L., Sheridan, J. M., and Kammer, B. A. Rupture and aging of silicone gel breast implants. Plast. Reconstr. Surg. 1993 Apr, 91, (5): 828-834. RUPTURE/local complications.

De Cholnoky, T. Augmentation mammaplasty: Survey of complication in 10,941 patients by 265 surgeons. Plast. Reconstr. Surg. 1970, 45, 573-577. LOCAL COMPLICATIONS.

De Fife, K. M., Jenney, C. R., McNally, A. K., Colton, E., and Anderson, J. M. Interleukin-13 induces human monocyte/macrophage fusion and macrophage mannose receptor expression. The Journal of Immunology. 1997, 158, 3385-3390. IMMUNE EFFECTS.

De Loach, E. D., Lord, S. A., and Ruf, L. E. Unilateral galactocele following augmentation mammoplasty. Annals of Plastic Surgery. 1994, 33, (1): 68-71. BREAST FEEDING/local complications.

De Lorenzi, E., Massolini, G., Macchia, M., and Caccialanza, G. HPLC determination of urinary 2,4- and 2,6-toluendiamines as potential degradation products of polyurethane breast implants. Chromatographia. 1995 Dec, 41, (11-12): 661-664. TOXICOLOGY/POLYURETHANE.

De Lustro, F., Fries, J., Kang, A., Katz, S., Kaye, R., and Reichlin, M. Immunity to injectable collagen and autoimmune disease: A summary of current understanding. Journal of Dermatology and Surgical Oncology. 1988, 14, (7 (Supplement 1)): 57-65. IMMUNE EFFECTS.

De Nicola, R. R. Permanent artifical (silicone) uretha. The Journal of Urology. 1950 Jan, 63, (1): 168-172. GENERAL.

De Saxe, B. M. Breast augmentation. Results in a series of 150 cases. South African Medical Journal. 1974, 48, 737-740. LOCAL COMPLICATIONS.

De Vlam, K., De Keyser, F., Verbruggen, G., Vandenbossche, M., Vanneuville, B., D'Hasese, D., and Veys, E. M. Detection and identification of antinuclear antibodies in the serum of normal blood donors. Clin. Exp. Rheumatol. 1993, 11, 393-397. AI-CTD BACKGROUND.

Dean, C., Chetty, U., and Forrest, A. P. M. Effects of immediate breast reconstruction on psychosocial morbidity after mastectomy. The Lancet. 1983 Feb 6, 1, 459-462. PSYCHOSOCIAL/reconstruction.

Deapen, D. M., Bernstein, L., and Brody, G. S. Are breast implants anticarcinogenic? A 14-year follow-up of the Los Angeles study. Plastic and Reconstructive Surgery. 1997 Apr, 99, (5): 1346-1353. CANCER.

Deapen, D. M., and Brody, G. S. Augmentation mammaplasty and breast cancer: A five year update of the Los Angeles study. Plast. Reconstr. Surg. 1992, 89, (4): 660-665. CANCER.

Deapen, D. M., and Brody, G. S. Augmentation mammaplasty and breast cancer: A five year update of the Los Angeles study. Journal of Clinical Epidemiology. 1995, 48, (4): 551-556. CANCER.

Deapen, D. M., Pike, M. C., Casagrande, J. T., and Brody, G. S. The relationship between breast cancer and augmentation mammaplasty: An epidemiologic study. Plast. Reconstr. Surg. 1986 Mar, 77, (3): 361-367. CANCER.

Decorato, D. Derogatis A. J. Prominent gallium uptake associated with silicone implants in an asymptomatic patient. Clinical Nuclear Medicine. 1994 Dec, 19, (12): 1107-1108. IMMUNE EFFECTS.

Degiannis, D., Seibold, J., Czarnecki, M., Raskova, J., and Raska, K. Soluble interleukin-2 receptors in patients with systemic sclerosis. Arthritis and Rheumatism. 1990 Mar, 33, (3): 375-380. CONNECTIVE TISSUE DISEASE/immune effects.

Del Junco, D. More breast implant pros and cons. Contractures and confounding: The controversy continues. J. Amer. Med. Assoc. 1997 May 28, 277, (20): 1643-1644. GENERAL.

Del Rosario, A. D., Bui, H. X., Pastore, J., Singh, J., and Ross, J. S. True synovial metaplasia of breast implant capsules: A light and electron microscopic study. Ultrastructural Pathology. 1995 Jan 1, 19, 83-93. CAPSULE-CONTRACTURE/local complications.

Delclos, K. B., Blaydes, B., Heflich, R. H., and Smith, B. A. Assessment of DNA adducts and the frequency of 6-thioguanine resistant T-lymphocytes in F344 rats fed 2,4-toluenediamine or implanted with a toluenediisocyanate-containing polyester polyurethane foam. Mutation Research. 1996, 367, 209-218. TOXICOLOGY/Polyurethane.

Dellon, A. L., Cowley, R. A., and Hoopes, J. E. Blunt chest trauma: Evaluation of the augmented breast. The Journal of Trauma. 1980, 20, (11): 982-985. RUPTURE/local complications.

Dempsey, W. C., and Latham, W. D. Subpectoral implants in augmentation mammaplasty. Plast. Reconstr. Surg. 1968, 42, 515. RECONSTRUCTION.

Dempsey, W. C., and Latham, W. D. Subpectoral implants in augmentation mammaplasty. Plast. Reconstr. Surg. 1977, 60, 325. GENERAL.

Den Braber, E. T., de Ruijter, and Jansen, J. A. The effect of a subcutaneous silicone rubber implant with shallow surface microgrooves on the surrounding tissues in rabbits. J Biomed Mater Res. 1997 Dec, 37, (4): 539-547. CAPSULE CONTRACTURE.

Derby, K. A., Frankel, S. D., Kaufman, L., Kramer, D., Carlson, J., Miniyeve, M., Occhipinti, K, and Friedenthal, R. Differentiation of silicone gel from water and fat in MR phase imaging of protons at 0.064 T. Radiology. 1993 Nov, 189, (2): 617-620. MAMMOGRAPHY.

Derby, L. D., Sinow, J. D., Bowers, L. D., and Cunningham, B. Quantitative analysis of lidocaine HCI delivery by diffusion across tissue expander membranes. Plast. Reconstr. Surg. 1992, 89, (5): 900-907. PAIN/expander.

DerHagopian, R. P., Zaworski, R. E., Sugarbaker, E. V., and Ketcham, A. S. Management of locally recurrent breast cancer adjacent to prosthetic implants. The American Journal of Surgery. 1981 May, 141, 590-592. CANCER.

Derman, G. H., Argenta, L. C., and Grabb, W. C. Delayed extrusion of inflatable breast prostheses. Annals of Plastic Surgery. 1983 Feb, 10, (2): 154-158. LOCAL COMPLICATIONS.

Dershaw, D. D. Evaluation of the breast undergoing lumpectomy and radiation therapy. Radiologic Clinics of North America. 1995 Nov, 33, (6): 1147-1160. MAMMOGRAPHY.

Dershaw, D. D., and Chaglassian, T. A. Mammography after prosthesis placement for augmentation or reconstructive mammoplasty. Radiology. 1989, 170, 69-74. MAMMOGRAPHY.

Destouet, J. M., Monsees, B. S., Oser, R. F., Nemecek, J. R., Young, V. L., and Pilgram, T. K. Screening mammography in 350 women with breast implants: prevalence and findings of implant complications. American Journal of Roentgenology. 1992 Nov, 159, 973-978. RUPTURE/capsule-contracture/mammography/local complications.

Devor, D. E., Waalkes, M. P., Goering, P., and Rehm, S. Development of an animal model for testing human breast implantation materials. Toxicologic Pathology. 1993, 21, (3): 261-273. POLYURETHANE/toxicology.

Di Lorenzo, G., Mansueto, P., Melluso, M., Sangiorgi, G., Cigna, D., Candore, G., and Caruso, C. Morphea after silicone gel breast implantation for cosmetic reasons in an HLA-B8, DR3-positive woman. International Archives of Allergy and Immunology. 1997, 112, 93-95. CONNECTIVE TISSUE DISEASE.

Dick, A. C., Deans GT, Johnston L, and Spence RAJ. Ruptured silicone breast implant: A misleading chest X-ray. Ulster Med J. 1994, 63, (2): 238-240. MAMMOGRAPHY/local complications/rupture.

Dickson, M. G., and Sharpe, D. T. The complications of tissue expansion in breast reconstruction: A review of 75 cases. British Journal of Plastic Surgery. 1987, 40, 629-635. EXPANDER/local complications.

Dillon, J. G., and Hughes, M. K. Degradation of five polyurethane gastric bubbles following *in vivo* use: SEC, ATR-IR and DSC studies. Biomaterials. 1992, 13, (4): 240-248. POLYURETHANE.

Dinner, M. I., Labandter, H. P., and Dowden, R. V. The role of the rectus abdominis myocutaneous flap in breast reconstruction. Plastic and Reconstructive Surgery. 1982 Feb, 69, (2): 209-214. RECONSTRUCTION.

Dobbie, J. W., and Smith, M. J. B. Silicate nephrotoxicity in the experimental animal: The missing factor in analgesic nephropathy. Scottish Medical Journal. 1982b, 27, 10-16. SILICON MEASUREMENT.

Dobbie, J. W., and Smith, M. J. B. The silicon content of body fluids. Scottish Medical Journal. 1982a, 27, 17-19. SILICON MEASUREMENT.

Dobke, M. K., Grzybowski, J., Stein, P., and et al. Fibroblast behavior in vitro is unaltered by products of staphylococcal cultured from silicone implants. Annals of Plastic Surgery. 1994 Feb, 32, (2): 118-125. INFECTION/local complications.

Dobke, M. K., and Middleton, M. S. Clinical impact of breast implant magnetic resonance imaging. Annals of Plastic Surgery. 1994 Sep, 33, (3): 241-246. MAMMOGRAPHY/ local complications.

Dobke, M. K., Svahn, J. K., Vastine, V. L., Landon, B. N., Stein, P. C., and Parsons, C. L. Characterization of microbial presence at the surface of silicone mammary implants. Annals of Plastic Surgery. 1995 Jun, 34, (6): 563. INFECTION/capsule contracture.

Dodd, L. G., Sneige, N., Reece, G. P., and Fornage, B. Fine-needle aspiration cytology of silicone granulomas in the augmented breast. Diagnostic Cytopathology. 1993, 9, (5): 498-502. GRANULOMAS/local complications.

Dolezel, B., Adamírová, L., Vondrácek, P., and Náprstek, Z. In vivo degradation of polymers. Biomaterials. 1989 Aug, 10, 387-392. SILICONE CHARACTERIZATION.

Dolsky, R. L. Inserting the Même prosthesis. Plast. Reconstr. Surg. 1984 Mar, 73, (3): 466-468. POLYURETHANE.

Domanskis, E. J., and Owsley, J. Q. Histological investigation of the etiology of capsule contracture following augmentation mammaplasty. Plast. Reconstr. Surg. 1976 Dec, 58, (6): 689-693. CAPSULE-CONTRACTURE/local complications.

Donahue, S. P., Friberg, T. R., and Johnson, B. L. Intraconjunctival cavitary inclusions of silicone oil complicating retinal detachment repair. American Journal of Ophthalmology. 1992 Nov, 114, (5): 639-640. GENERAL.

Dong, D. E., Andrade, J. D., and Coleman, D. L. Adsorption of low density lipoproteins onto selected biomedical polymers. Journal of Biomedical Materials Research. 1987 Jun, 21, (6): 683-700. CALCIFICATION/local complications.

Dorfman, R. F., and Berry G.J. Kikuchi's histiocytic necrotizing lymphadenitis: An analysis of 108 cases with emphasis on differential diagnosis. Seminars in Diagnostic Pathology. 1988 Nov, 5, (4): 329-345. AI-CTD BACKGROUND.

Dorne, L., Alikacem, N., Guidoin, R., and Auger, M. High resolution solid-state 29Si NMR spectroscopy of silicone gels used to fill breast prostheses. Magnetic Resonance in Medicine. 1995, 34, (4): 548-554. SILICONE CHARACTERIZATION.

Dorne, L., Stroman, P., Rolland, C., Auger, M., Alikacem, N., Bronskill, M., Grondin, P., King, M., and Guidoin, R. Magnetic resonance study of virgin and explanted silicone breast prostheses. Can proton relaxation times be used to monitor their biostability? ASAIO J. 1994, 40, (3): M625-M631. SILICONE CHARACTERIZATION/MAMMOGRAPHY.

Dougherty, S. H. Pathobiology of infection in prosthetic devices. Reviews of infectious diseases. 1988 Nov-1988 Dec 31, 10, (6): 1102-1117. INFECTION/local complications.

Douglas, K. P., Bluth, E. I., Sauter, E. R., McKinnon, W. M., Bergeron, R. B., Merritt, C. R. B., and Finley, J. M. Roentgenographic evaluation of the augmented breast. Southern Medical Journal. 1991 Jan, 84, (1): 49-51. MAMMOGRAPHY.

Dowden, R. V. Detection of gel implant rupture: A clinical test. Plast. Reconstr. Surg. 1993 Mar, 91, (3): 548-550. RUPTURE/local complications.

Dowden, R. V. Mammography after implant breast reconstruction. Plast. Reconstr. Surg. 1995 Jul, 96, (1): 119-121. MAMMOGRAPHY.

Dowden, R. V. Periprosthetic bacteria and the breast implant patient with systemic symptoms. J. Plast. Reconstr. Surg. 1994 Aug, 94, (2): 300-305. INFECTION/local complications/connective tissue disease/immune effects.

Dowden, R. V., and Anain, S. Endoscopic implant evaluation and capsulotomy. Plast. Reconstr. Surg. 1993 Feb, 91, (2): 283-287. CAPSULE CONTRACTURE/local complications.

Dowden, R. V., Blanchard, J. M., and Greenstreet, R. L. Breast reconstruction: Selection, timing and local recurrence. Annals of Plastic Surgery. 1983 Apr, 10, (4): 265-269. RECONSTRUCTION.

Drake, D. B., Miller, L., Janus, C. L., DeLange, E. E., and Morgan, R. F. Magnetic resonance imaging of in situ mammary prostheses. Annals of Plastic Surgery. 1994 Sep, 33, (3): 258-262. MAMMOGRAPHY.

Dreyfuss, D. A., Singh, S., Dowlatshahi, K., and Krizek, T. J. Silicone implants as an anticarcinogen. Surg. Forum. 1987, 38, 587-589. CARCINOGENICITY.

Duffield, F. V. P., Yoakum, A., Bumgarner, J., and Moran, J. Determination of human body burden baseline data of platinum through autopsy tissue analysis. Environmental Health Perspectives. 1976, 15, 131-134. PLATINUM.

Duffy, D. M. Silicone: a critical review. Adv Dermatol. 1990, 5, 93-110. SILICONE INJECTION.

Duffy, Jr. F. J., and May, J. W. Tissue expanders and magnetic resonance imaging: The hot breast implant. Annals of Plastic Surgery. 1995 Dec, 35, (6): 647-649. MAMMOGRAPHY/expander.

Duffy, M. J., and Woods, J. E. Health risks of failed silicone gel breast implants: A 30-year clinical experience. Plast. Reconstr. Surg. 1994 Aug, 94, (2): 295-299. CONNECTIVE TISSUE DISEASE/local complications.

Dugowson, C. E., Koepsell, T. D., Voigt, L. F., Bley, L., Nelson, J. L., and Daling, J. R. Rheumatoid arthritis in women: Incidence rates in group health cooperative, Seattle, Washington, 1987-1989. Arthritis and Rheumatism. 1991 Dec, 34, (12): 1502-1507. AI-CTD BACKGROUND.

Duigan, G. E. Solicitation of implant patients. Medical Journal of Australia. 1994, 160, (11): 732. GENERAL.

Dumble, L. J. Dismissing the evidence: The medical response to women with silicone implant-related disorders. Health Care for Women International. 1996, 17, (6): 515-525. GENERAL.

Duna, G. F., and Wilke, W. S. Diagnosis, etiology, and therapy of fibromyalgia. Comprehensive therapy. 1993, 19, (2): 60-63. AI-CTD BACKGROUND.

Dunn, K. W., Hall, P. N., and Khoo, C. T. K. Breast implant materials: Sense and safety. British Journal of Plastic Surgery. 1992, 45, 315-321. IMMUNE EFFECTS/silicone characterization.

Duvic, M., Moore, D., Menter, A., and Vonderheid, E. C. Cutaneous T-cell lymphoma in association with silicone breast implants. Journal of the American Academy of Dermatology. 1995 Jun, 32, (6): 939-942. IMMUNE EFFECTS/cancer.

Dylewski, J. R., and Beatty, C. L. In vitro characterization of silicone bleed from breast prostheses. Soc Biomat Transact. 1984, 7, 309. RUPTURE/local complications.

Eberlein, T. J., Carespo, L. P., Smith, B. L. Hergrueter C. A., Douville, L., and Eriksson, E. Prospective evaluation of immediate reconstruction after mastectomy. Annals of Surgery. 1993 Jul, 218, (1): 29-36. RECONSTRUCTION.

Eckardt, R. E., and Hindin, R. The health hazards of plastics. Journal of Occupational Medicine. 1973 Oct, 15, (10): 808-819. TOXICOLOGY.

Eckhauser, F. E., Strodel, W. E., and Girardy, J. W. Turcotte J. G. Bizarre complications of peritoneovenous shunts. Annals of Surgery. 1981 Feb, 193, (2): 180-184. CAPSULE-CONTRACTURE/local complications.

Edelman, D. A., Grant, S., and Van Os, W. A. A. Autoimmune disease following the use of silicone gel-filled breast implants: A review of the clinical literature. Seminars in Arthritis and Rheumatism. 1994 Dec, 24, (3): 183-189. CONNECTIVE TISSUE DISEASE.

Edelman, D. A., Grant, S., and van Os, W. A. A. Breast cancer risk among women using silicone gel implants. Int J Fertil Menopausal Stud. 1995 Sep, 40, (5): 274-280. CANCER.

Edgerton, M. T., and McClary, A. R. Augmentation mammaplasty: Psychiatric implications and surgical indications. Plastic and Reconstructive Surgery. 1958 Apr, 21, (4): 279. PSYCHOSOCIAL.

Edgerton, M. T., Meyer, E., and Jacobson, W. A. Augmentation mammaplasty. II. Further surgical and psychiatric evaluation. Plast. Reconstr. Surg. 1961 Mar, 27, (3): 279-302. PSYCHOSOCIAL.

Edgerton, M. T., and Wells, J. H. Indications for and pitfalls of soft tissue augmentation with liquid silicone. Plast. Reconstr. Surg. 1976 Aug, 58, (2): 157-165. SILICONE INJECTION.

Edney, J. J. Post mastectomy breast reconstruction 1995 recent advances. Nebraska Medical Journal. 1996, 81, (3): 70-72. RECONSTRUCTION.

Edwards, B. F. Teflon-silicone breast implants. Plastic and Reconstructive Surgery. 1963 Nov, 32, (5): 519-526. GENERAL.

Edworthy, S. M., Martin, L., Barr, S. G., Birdsell, D. C., Brant, R. F., and Fritzler, M. J. A clinical study of the relationship between silicone breast implants and connective tissue disease. J. Rheumatol. 1998, 25, (2): 254-260. CONNECTIVE TISSUE DISEASE.

Ehrlich, H. P., and Wyler, D. J. Fibroblast contraction of collagen lattices in vitro: Inhibition by chronic inflammatory cell mediators. Journal of Cellular Physiology. 1983, 116, 345-351. CAPSULE CONTRACTURE.

Ehrlich HP and Rajaratnam JB. Cell locomotion forces versus cell contraction forces for collagen lattice contraction: an in vitro model of wound contraction. Tissue Cell. 1990, 22, (4): 407-17. CAPSULE CONTRACTURE.

Eisenberg, D. M., Kessler, R. C., Foster, C., Norlock, F. E., Calkins, D. R., and Delbanco, T. L. Unconventional medicine in the United States: Prevalence, costs, and patterns of use. The New England Journal of Medicine. 1993 Jan 28, 328, (4): 246-252. PSYCHOSOCIAL.

Eisenberg, H. C., and Bartels, R. J. Rupture of a silicone bag-gel breast implant by closed compression capsulotomy. Plast. Reconstr. Surg. 1977 Jun, 59, 849-850. CLOSED CAPSULOTOMY/local complications/rupture.

Eisenberg, R. A., Pisetsky, D. S., Craven, S. Y., Grudier, J. P., O'Donnell, M. A., and Cohen, P. L. Regulation of the anti-Sm autoantibody response in systemic lupus erythematosus mice by monoclonal anti-Sm antibodies. J. Clin. Invest. 1990, 85, 86-92. CHILDREN'S EFFECTS/breast feeding.

Eklund, G. W., Busby, R. C., Miller, S. H., and Job, J. S. Improved imaging of the augmented breast. American Journal of Roentgenology. 1988, 151, 469-473. MAMMOGRAPHY.

Eklund, G. W., and Cardenosa, G. The art of mammographic positioning. Radiological Clinics of North America. 1992, 30, 21-53. MAMMOGRAPHY.

El-Hassan, N. D., Zaworski, R. E., Castro, A., and et al. Serum prolactin levels following augmentation mammaplasty. Plastic and Reconstructive Surgery. 1981, 68, (2): 215-217. BREAST FEEDING.

El-Jammal, A., and Templeton, D. M. Measurement of platinum in biomedical silicones by ICP-MS. Analytical Proceedings Including Analytical Communications. 1995 Aug, 32, 293-295. PLATINUM/toxicology.

El-Roeiy, A., and Gleicher, N. Definition of normal autoantibody levels in an apparently healthy population. Obstetrics and Gynecology. 1988 Oct, 72, (4): 596-602. AI-CTD BACKGROUND.

El Yousef, S. J., O'Connell, D. M., Duchnesneau, R. H., Smith, M. J., Hubay, C. A., and Guyton, S. P. Benign and malignant breast disease: Magnetic resonance and radiofrequency pulse sequences. American Journal of Roentgenology. 1985, 145, 1-8. MAMMOGRAPHY.

Elberg, J. J., Kjøller, K. H., and Krag, C. Silicone mammary implants and connective tissue disease. Scandinavian Journal of Plastic and Reconstructive and Hand Surgery. 1993, 27, (4): 243-248. CONNECTIVE TISSUE DISEASE/immune effects.

Elkowitz, A., Colen, S., Slavin, S., Seibert, J., Weinstein, M., and Shaw, W. Various methods of breast reconstruction after mastectomy: An economic comparison. Plastic and Reconstructive Surgery. 1993 Jul, 92, (1): 77-83. RECONSTRUCTION.

Ellenberg, A. H. Marked thinning of the breast skin flaps after the insertion of implants containing triamcinolone. Plast. Reconstr. Surg. 1977 Nov, 60, (5): 755-758. STEROIDS/local complications.

Ellenberg, A. H., and Braun, H. A 3 1/2-year experience with double-lumen implants in breast surgery. Plast. Reconstr. Surg. 1980 Mar, 65, (3): 307-313. LOCAL COMPLICATIONS.

Ellenberger, P., Graham, W. P., Mandwes, E. K., and Basrab, R. M. Labeled leukocyte scans for detection of retained polyurethane foam. Plast. Reconstr. Surg. 1986 Jan, 77, (1): 77-79. POLYURETHANE/infection/local complications.

Ellenbogen, R., and Rubin, L. Injectable fluid silicone therapy: Human morbidity and mortality. J. Amer. Med. Assoc. 1975, 234, (3): 308-309. SILICONE INJECTION/granulomas/local complications.

Elliott, L. F., Eskenazi, L., Beegle, Jr. P. H., Podres, P. E., and Drazan, L. Immediate TRAM flap breast reconstruction. Plastic and Reconstructive Surgery. 1993, 294, (2): 217-227. RECONSTRUCTION.

Ellis, T. M., Hardt, N. S., and Atkinson, M. A. Antipolymer antibodies, silicone breast implants, and fibromyalgia. The Lancet. 1997a Apr 19, 349, (9059): 1170-3. IMMUNE EFFECTS/connective tissue disease.

Ellis, T. M., Hardt, N. S., Campbell, L., Delmar, A., Piacentini, A., and Atkinson, M. A. Cellular immune reactivities in women with silicone breast implants: A preliminary investigation. Annals of Allergy, Asthma, and Immunology. 1997b Aug, 79, (2): 151-154. IMMUNE EFFECTS.

Emery, J. A., Spanier, S. S., Kasnic jr., G., and Hardt, N. S. The synovial structure of breast-implant-associated bursae. Modern Pathology. 1994, 7, (7): 728-733. SALINE/capsule-contracture/local complications/calcification.

Endo, L. P., Edwards, N. L., Longley, S., Corman, L. C., and Panush, R. S. Silicone and rheumatic diseases. Seminars in Arthritis and Rheumatism. 1987 Nov, 17, (2): 112-118. IMMUNE EFFECTS/connective tissue disease.

Enestrom, S., Bengtson, A., Lindstrom, F., and Johan, K. Attachment of IgG to dermal extracellular matrix in patients with fibromyalgia. Clinical and Experimental Rheumatology. 1990, 8, 127-135. AI-CTD BACKGROUND.

Engel, A., Lamm, S. H., and Lai, S. H. Human breast sarcoma and human breast implantation: A time trend analysis based on SEER data (1973-1990). Journal of Clinical Epidemiology. 1995, 48, (4): 539-544. CANCER.

Englert, H. J., and Brooks, P. Scleroderma and augmentation mammoplasty—A causal relationship? Australian and New Zealand Journal of Medicine. 1994 Feb, 24, (1): 74-80. CONNECTIVE TISSUE DISEASE.

Englert, H. J., Howe, G. B., Penny, R., and Brooks, P. Scleroderma and silicone breast implants. British Journal of Rheumatology. 1994, 33, (4): 397-399. CONNECTIVE TISSUE DISEASE.

Englert, H. J., Morris, D., and March, L. Scleroderma and silicone gel breast prostheses—The Sydney study revisited. Australia and New Zealand Journal of Medicine. 1996, 26, 349-355. CONNECTIVE TISSUE DISEASE.

Epstein, S. S. Implants pose poorly recognized risks of breast cancer. International Journal of Occupational Medicine and Toxicology. 1995, 4, (3): 315-342. CARCINOGENICITY.

Erdmann, M. W. H., Asplund, O., and Bahnasy, H. Transcutaneous extravasation of silicone following breast augmentation. British Journal of Plastic Surgery. 1992, 45, 479-480. RUPTURE/local complications/granulomas.

Ericsson, A. D. Syndromes associated with silicone breast implants: a clinical study and review. J. Nutr. Environ. Med. 1998, 8, 35-51. GENERAL.

Eriksson, L., and Westesson, P. Deterioration of the temporary silicone implant in the temporomandibular joint: A clinical and arthroscopic follow-up study. Oral Surgery. 1986 Jul, 62, (1): 2-6. LOCAL COMPLICATIONS.

Ersek, R. A. Molecular impact surface textured implants (MISTI) alter beneficially breast capsule formation at 36 months. J. Long Term Eff. Med. Implants. 1991a, 1, 155. CAPSULE-CONTRACTURE/local complications.

Ersek, R. A. Prostheses for breast augmentation: Progress in materials and design of these implants continues. Travis County Medical Society Journal. 1989, 35, 8. GENERAL.

Ersek, R. A. Rate and incidence of capsular contracture: A comparison of smooth and textured silicone double-lumen breast prostheses. Plastic and Reconstructive Surgery. 1991b May, 87, (5): 879-883. CAPSULE-CONTRACTURE/local complications.

Ersek, R. A., Burroughs, J. R., Ersek, C. L., and Navarro, A. Interrelationship of capsule thickness and breast hardness confirmed by a new measurement methods. Plastic and Reconstructive Surgery. 1991 Jun, 87, (6): 1069-1073. CAPSULE-CONTRACTURE/local complications.

Ersek, R. A., Ersek, G. A., Ersek, C. L., and Williams, J. A new biologically osmotically and oncotically balanced gel that shows calcifications blocked by silicone. Aesthetic Plastic Surgery. 1993, 17, 331. CALCIFICATION/local complications.

Ersek, R. A., Glacs, K. L., and Navarro, J. A. Results of reaugmentation with MISTI prostheses after failure of smooth silicone prostheses. Plast. Reconstr. Surg. 1992 Jan, 89, (1): 83-87. CAPSULE-CONTRACTURE/local complications.

Ersek, R. A., and Salisbury, A. V. Textured surface, nonsilicone gel breast implants: Four years' clinical outcome. Plastic and Reconstructive Surgery. 1997 Dec, 100, (7): 1729-1739. SALINE.

Ersek, R. A., and Shelton, T. O. Radiolucent gel for breast prostheses. Travis County Medical Society Journal. 1991, 37, 8. GENERAL.

Espinoza, L. R. Serum antinuclear antibodies in women with silicone breast implants. J. Rheumatol. 1995, 22, 236-240. IMMUNE EFFECTS.

Evans, G. R. D., and Baldwin, B. J. From cadavers to implants: Silicon tissue assays of medical devices. Plast. Reconstr. Surg. 1997b Nov, 100, (6): 1459-1463. SILICON MEASUREMENT.

Evans, G. R. D., and Baldwin, B. J. Silicon tissue assay: A measurement of capsular levels from chemotherapeutic Port-a-Catheter devices. Plast. Reconstr. Surg. 1997a Apr, 99, (5): 1354-1358. SILICON MEASUREMENT.

Evans, G. R. D., and Baldwin, B. J. Silicon tissue assay: Are there intracapsular variations? Annals of Plastic Surgery. 1996 Dec, 37, (6): 592-595. SILICON MEASUREMENT.

Evans, G. R. D., Netscher, D. T., Schusterman, M. A., Kroll, S. S., Robb, G. L., Reece, G. P., and Miller, M. J. Silicon tissue assays: A comparison of nonaugmented cadaveric and augmented patient levels. Plast. Reconstr. Surg. 1996 May, 97, (6): 1207-1214. SILICON MEASUREMENT.

Evans, G. R. D., Schusterman, M. A., Kroll, S. S., Miller, M. J., Reece, G. P., Robb, G. L., and Ainslie, N. Reconstruction and the radiated breasts: Is there a role for implants? Plast. Reconstr. Surg. 1995 Oct, 96, (5): 1111-1118. RADIATION/reconstruction.

Evans, G. R. D., Slezak, S., Rieters, M., and Bercowry, G. M. Silicon tissue assays in non-augmented cadaveric patients: Is there a baseline level? Plast. Reconstr. Surg. 1994 May, 93, (6): 1117—1122. SILICON MEASUREMENT.

Evans, R. C. Effect of vancomycin hydrochloride on *Staphylococcus epidermidis* biofilm associated with silicone elastomer. Antimicrobial Agents And Chemotherapy. 1987 Jun, 31, 889-894. INFECTION/local complications.

Everson, L. I., Parantainen, H., Detile, T., Stillman, A., Olson, P. N., Landis, G., Foshager, M. C., Cunningham, B., and Griffiths, H. J. Diagnosis of breast implant rupture: Imaging findings and relative efficacies of imaging. American Journal of Roentgenology. 1994 Aug, 163, (1): 57-60. MAMMOGRAPHY/local complications/rupture.

Expert Panel on the Safety of Polyurethane-covered Breast Implants (Boyes, D. C., Adey, C. K., Bailar, J., Baines, C., Kerrigan, C., and Langlois, P. Safety of polyurethane-covered breast implants. Canadian Medical Association Journal. 1991 Nov 1, 145, (9): 1125-1132. POLYURETHANE.

Eyssen, J. E., von Werssowetz, A. J., and Middleton, G. D. Reconstruction of the breast using polyurethane-coated prostheses. Plast. Reconstr. Surg. 1984 Mar, 73, (3): 415-419. POLYURETHANE/capsule-contracture/local complications/reconstruction.

Fajardo, L. L., Harvey, J. A., McAleese, K. A., Roberts, C. C., and Granstrom, P. Breast cancer diagnosis in women with subglandular silicone gel-filled augmentation implants. Radiology. 1995, 194, 859-862. MAMMOGRAPHY.

Farago, M. E., Kavanagh, P., Blanks, R., Kelly, J., Kazantizis, G., Thornton, I., Simpson, P. R., Cook, J. M., Delves, H. T., and Gwendy, E. M. Platinum concentrations in urban road dust and soil, and in blood and urine in the United Kingdom. Analyst. 1998 Mar, 123, 451-454. PLATINUM/toxicology.

Fee-Fulkerson, K., Conaway, M. R., Winer, E. P., Fulkerson, C. C., Rimer, B. K., and Georgiade, G. Factors contributing to patient satisfaction with breast reconstruction using silicone gel implants. Plast. Reconstr. Surg. 1996 Jun, 97, (7): 1420-1426. PSYCHOSOCIAL.

Fee, T. E., and Caffee, H. H. Predictors of postoperative aesthetics following explantation of the augmented breast. Annals of Plastic Surgery. 1997 Mar, 38, (3): 217-222. EXPLANTATION.

Feig, S. A. Radiation risk from mammography: Is it clinically significant? Am J Roentgenol. 1984, 143, 469-475. MAMMOGRAPHY.

Feliberti, M. C., Arrillaga, A., and Colon, G. A. Rupture of inflated breast implants in closed compression capsulotomy. Plastic and Reconstructive Surgery. 1977, 59, (6): 848-849. CLOSED CAPSULOTOMY/rupture/local complications.

Felix, K., Lin, S., Bornkamm, G.-W., and Janz, S. Tetravinyl-tetramethylcyclo-tetrasiloxane (tetravinyl D4) is a mutagen in Rat2lacI fibroblasts. Carcinogenesis. 1998, 19, (2): 315-320. CARCINOGENICITY/toxicology.

Feller, W. F., Holt, R., Spear, S., and Little, J. Modified radical mastectomy with immediate breast reconstruction. The American Surgeon. 1986, 52, (3): 129-133. RECONSTRUCTION.

Fellner, M., and Rudikoff, D. Adverse reaction following silicone injections. Int. J. Dermatol. 1979 Jun, 18, (5): 375-376. SILICONE INJECTION.

Feng, L.-J., Mauceri, K., and Berger, B. E. Autogenous tissue breast reconstruction in the silicone-intolerant patient. Cancer. 1994 Jul 1, 74, (1 (Supplement)): 440-449. RECONSTRUCTION/neurologic disease/connective tissue disease.

Fenske, T. K., Davis, P., and Aaron, S. L. Human adjuvant disease revisited: A review of eleven post-augmentation mammaplasty patients. Clinical and Experimental Rheumatology. 1994, 12, (5): 477-481. CONNECTIVE TISSUE DISEASE.

Ferguson, J. H. Breast implants redux: this time with data. Neurology. 1998, 50, 849-852. NEUROLOGIC DISEASE.

Ferguson, J. H. Silicone breast implants and neurologic disorders: Report of the Practice Committee of the American Academy of Neurology. Neurology. 1997, 48, 1504-1507. NEUROLOGIC DISEASE.

Ferreira, J. A. The various etiological factors of hard capsule formation in breast augmentation. Aesthetic Plastic Surgery. 1984, 8, 109-117. CAPSULE-CONTRACTURE/local complications/saline.

Ferreira, M. C., Spina, V., and Iriya, K. Changes in the lung following injections of silicone gel. British Journal of Plastic Surgery. 1975, 28, 173-176. SILICONE INJECTION.

Fessell, W. J. Systemic lupus erythematosus in the community: Incidence, prevalence, outcome, and first symptoms, the high prevalence in black women. Archives of Internal Medicine. 1974 Dec, 134, 1027-1035. AI-CTD BACKGROUND.

Fessenden, R. J., and Fessenden, J. The biological properties of silicone compounds. Adv. Drug Res. 1967, 4, 95-132. SILICONE INJECTION.

Fessenden, R. J., and Hartman, R. A. Metabolic fate of phenyltrimethylsilane and phenyldimethylsilane. J Med Chem. 1970 Jan, 13, (1): 52-54. TOXICOLOGY.

Fiala, T. G. S., Lee, W. P. A., and May, Jr. J. W. Augmentation mammoplasty: Results of a patient survey. Annals of Plastic Surgery. 1993 Jun, 30, (6): 503-509. CONNECTIVE TISSUE DISEASE/sensation/local complications/capsule-contracture/psychosocial.

Filiberti, A., Tamburini, M., Murru, L., Lovo, G. F., Ventafridda, V., Arioli, N., and Grisotti, A. Psychologic effects and esthetic results of breast reconstruction after mastectomy. Tumori. 1986, 72, 585-588. PSYCHOSOCIAL.

Filsinger, D. H. Formaldehyde levels based on bulk and elevated temperature evolution rate measurements of silicone materials. Am Indust Hygiene Assoc J. 1995, 56, 1201-1207. TOXICOLOGY.

Finegold, I. Allergy to silicone: Is it real? Compr Ther. 1996, 22, (6): 393-398. CONNECTIVE TISSUE DISEASE/immune effects.

Fisher, A. A. Reactions at silicone-injected sites on the face associated with silicone breast implant inflammation or rejection. Cutis. 1990 Jun, 45, 393-395. IMMUNE EFFECTS/ silicone injection/local complications.

Fisher, J. C., and Brody, G. S. Breast implants under siege: An historical commentary. Journal of Long-Term Effects of Medical Implants. 1992, 1, (3): 243-253. GENERAL.

Fisher, J. C., and Hammond, D. C. The combination of expanders with autogenous tissue in breast reconstruction. Clinics in Plastic Surgery. 1994, 21, (2): 309-320. EXPANDER/ reconstruction.

Fisher, J. C., Hammond, D. C., Barone, F. E., and Maxwell, G. P. 170 notarized consecutive breast reconstructions with textured tissue expanders in 130 patients. Plastic Surgery Forum. 1991, 14, 15. RECONSTRUCTION/capsule-contracture/local complications/ expander.

Fisher, J. C., Potchen, E. J., and Sergent, J. Office communication with breast implant patients: Radiologic and rheumatologic concerns. Perspectives in Plastic Surgery. 1992, 6, (2): 79-89. GENERAL/psychosocial.

Fitzgerald, J. B., and Malette, W. G. The physiologic effects of intravascular Antifoam A. Journal of Surgical Research. 1961, 1, (2): 104-107. TOXICOLOGY.

Flick, J. A. Silicone implants and esophageal dysmotility: Are breast-fed infants at risk? J. Amer. Med. Assoc. 1994 Jan 19, 271, (3): 240-241. BREAST FEEDING/children's effects.

Flick, J. A., Boyle, J. T., Tuchman, D. N., Athreya, B. H., and Doughty, R. A. Esophageal motor abnormalities in children and adolescents with scleroderma and mixed connective tissue disease. Pediatrics. 1988 Jul, 82, (1): 107-111. AI-CTD BACKGROUND/ children's effects.

Flint, K. P. Fibromyalgia. The Journal of the South Carolina Medical Association. 1993 Nov, 89, (11): 511-515. AI-CTD BACKGROUND.

Fock, K. M., Feng, P. H., and Tey, B. H. Autoimmune disease developing after augmentation mammoplasty: Report of 3 cases. J. Rheumatol. 1984, 11, (1): 98-100. CONNECTIVE TISSUE DISEASE.

Fodor, P. B., and Svistel, A. J. Chest wall deformity following expansion of irradiated tissue for breast reconstruction. NY State J. Med. 1989, 89, 419-429. RADIATION/reconstruction/local complications.

Foerster, D. W. False bursa concept in augmentation mammaplasty. Aesthet. Plast. Surg. 1978, 2, 419. GENERAL.

Foliart, D. E. Synovitis and silicone joint implants: A summary of reported cases. Plast. Reconstr. Surg. 1997 Jan, 99, (1): 245-252. LOCAL COMPLICATIONS.

Folkman, J. Controlled drug release from polymers. Hospital Practice. 1978: 127-133. SILICONE CHARACTERIZATION.

Folkman, J., and Long, D. M. The use of Silicone rubber as a carrier for prolonged drug therapy. JSR. 1964 Mar, IV, (3): 139-142. SILICONE CHARACTERIZATION.

Foo, I. T. H., Coleman, D. J., Holmes, J. D., Palmer, J. H., and Sharpe, D. T. Delay between expansion and expander/implant exchange in breast reconstruction—A prospective study. British Journal of Plastic Surgery. 1992, 45, (4): 279-283. EXPANDER/capsule-contracture/local complications.

Forman, D. L., Chiu, J., Restifo, R. J., Ward, B. A., Haffty, B., and Ariyan, S. Breast reconstructuion in previously irradiated patients using tissue expanders and implants: a potentially unfavorable result. Annals of Plastic Surgery. 1998 Apr, 40, (4): 360-364. RADIATION/reconstruction.

Fornage, B. D., Sneige, N., and Singletary, S. E. Masses in breast with implants: Diagnosis with US-guided fine-needle aspiration biopsy. Radiology. 1994 May, 191, 339-342. MAMMOGRAPHY/cancer.

Forsberg, F., Conant, E. F., Russell, K. M., and Moore, Jr. J. H. Quantitative ultrasonic diagnosis of silicone breast implant rupture: An in vitro feasibility study. Ultrasound in Medicine and Biology. 1996 Nov 1, 22, (1): 53-60. MAMMOGRAPHY.

Foster, W. C., Springfield, D. S., and Brown, K. L. B. Pseudotumor of the arm associated with rupture of silicone-gel breast prostheses: Report of two cases. The Journal of Bone and Joint Surgery. 1983 Apr, 65-A, (4): 548-551. CLOSED CAPSULOTOMY/rupture/ migration/local complications.

Fowell, E., and Gibbons, D. F. Effect of implant compliance and surface texture on fibrous capsule morphology and myofibroblast population. Biol. Eng. Soc. 1982: 31-37. CAPSULE-CONTRACTURE/local complications.

Fox, R. I. Clinical features, pathogenesis and treatment of Sjögren's syndrome. Current Opinion in Rheumatology. 1996, 8, 438-45. AI-CTD BACKGROUND.

Fox, R. I. Epidemiology, pathogenesis, animal models, and treatment of Sjogren's syndrome. Current Opinion in Rhematology. 1994, 6, 501-508. AI-CTD BACKGROUND.

Fox, R. I., Chan, E., and Kang, H. Laboratory evaluation of patients with Sjögren's syndrome. 1992 Jun, 25, 213-222. AI-CTD BACKGROUND.

Fox, R. I., Howell, F. V., Bone, R. C., and Michelson, P. Primary Sjögren syndrome: Clinical and immunopathologic features. Seminars in Arthritis and Rheumatism. 1984 Nov, 14, (2): 77-105. AI-CTD BACKGROUND.

Fraenkel, L., Zhang, Y., Chaisson, C. E., Maricq, H. R., Evans, S. R., Brand, F., Wilson, P. W. F., and Felson, D. T. Different factors influencing the expression of Raynaud's phenomenon in men and women. Arthritis and Rheumatism. 1999 Feb, 42, (2): 306-310. AI-CTD BACKGROUND.

Francel, T. J., Ryan, J. J., and Manson, P. N. Breast reconstruction utilizing implants: A local experience and comparison of three techniques. Plast. Reconstr. Surg. 1993 Oct, 92, (5): 786-794. RECONSTRUCTION/expander/psychosocial/saline/local complications.

Frank, C. J., McCreery, R. L., Redd, D. C., and Gransler, T. S. Detection of silicone in lymph node biopsy specimens by near-infrared Raman spectroscopy. Appl Spectrosc. 1993, 47, 387-390. SILICON MEASUREMENT.

Frank, D. H., and Robson, M. C. A pneumatic tourniquet as an aid to release of capsular contracture around a breast implant. Plastic and Reconstructive Surgery. 1978, 61, (4): 612-613. CAPSULE-CONTRACTURE/closed capsulotomy/local complications.

Frankel, A. From pioneers to profits. American Lawyer. 1992 Jun: 82-91. GENERAL.

Frankel, S. D., Occhipinti, K. A., Kaufman, L., Hunt, T. K., and Kerley, S. M. MRI of a silicone breast implant surrounded by an enlarging hemorrhagic collection. Plast. Reconstr. Surg. 1994 Nov, 94, (6): 865-868. MAMMOGRAPHY/local complications/ hematomas.

Frankel, S. D., Occhipinti, K., Kaufmam, L., Kramer, D., Carlson, J., Mineyev, M., Eshima, I., and Friedenthal, R. MRI findings in subjects with breast implants. Plast. Reconstr. Surg. 1995 Sep, 96, (4): 852-857. MAMMOGRAPHY.

Frankel, S. D., Occhipinti, K., Kaufman, L., Kramer, D., Carlson, J., Mineyev, M., and Friedenthal, R. Characteristics of magnetic resonance sequences used for imaging silicone gel, saline, and gel-saline implants at low field strengths. Investigative Radiology. 1994, 29, (8): 781-786. MAMMOGRAPHY.

Frantz, P., and Herbst, C. A. Augmentation mammoplasty, irradiation, and breast cancer. Cancer. 1975, 36, 1147. CANCER/radiation.

Franz, F. P., Blocksma, R., Brundage, S. R., and Ringler, S. L. Massive injection of liquid silicone for hemifacial surgery. Annals of Plastic Surgery. 1988 Feb, 20, (2): 140-145. SILICONE INJECTION.

Fraser, S., Phipps, R., and Perry, P. M. Breast carcinoma around a silicone prosthesis—Back to basics. J Royal College of Surgery Edinburgh. 1989 Jun, 34, 164. MAMMOGRAPHY/cancer.

Frazer, C. K., and Wylie, F. J. Mammographic appearances following breast prosthesis removal. Clinical Radiology. 1995, 50, (5): 314-317. MAMMOGRAPHY/explantation.

Freedman, A. M., and Jackson, I. T. Infections in breast implants. Infectious Disease Clinics of North America. 1989, 3, (2): 275-287. INFECTION/local complications.

Freeman, B. S. Complications of SQ mastectomy with prosthetic replacement, immediate or delayed. Southern Medical Journal. 1967, 6, 1277-1280. LOCAL COMPLICATIONS/ RECONSTRUCTION.

Freeman, B. S. Reconstruction of the breast form by Silastic gel from breast prostheses. British Journal of Plastic Surgery. 1974 Jul, 27, 284-286. RUPTURE/local complications.

Freeman, B. S. Successful treatment of some fibrous envelope contractures around breast implants. Plast. Reconstr. Surg. 1972 Aug, 50, (2): 107-113. CAPSULE-CONTRACTURE/local complications.

Freeman, B. S., Bigelow, E. L., and Braley, S. A. Experiments with injectable plastic. Use of injectible silicone and Silastic rubber in animals and its clinical use in deformities of the head and neck. American Journal of Surgery. 1966, 112, 534-536. SILICONE INJECTION.

Freeman, B. S., and Wiemer, D. R. Untoward results and complications following reconstruction after mastectomy. Clinics in Plastic Surgery. 1979 Jan, 6, (1): 93-105. RECONSTRUCTION/local complications/capsule-contracture.

Freundlich, B., Altman, C., Sandorfi, N., Greenberg, M., and Tomaszewski, J. A profile of symtomatic patients with silicone breast implants: a Sjögren's-like syndrome. Seminars in Arthritis and Rheumatism. 1994 Aug, 24, (1 (Supplement 1)): 44-53. CONNECTIVE TISSUE DISEASE/pain/rupture/local complications.

Friedland, J., Corraro, P., and Converse, J. Retrospective cephalometric analysis of mandibular bone absorption under silicone rubber chin implants. Plastic and Reconstructive Surgery. 1976 Feb, 57, (2): 144-151. LOCAL COMPLICATIONS.

Friedman, R. J. Silicone breast prostheses and implantation and explanation. Seminars in Arthritis and Rheumatism. 1994, 24, (1): 8-10. GENERAL/explantation.

Friemann, J., Bauer, M., Golz, B., Rombeck, N., Hohr, D., Erbs, G., Steinau, H.-U., and Olbrisch, R. R. Physiological and pathological reaction patterns on silicone breast implants. Zentralbl Chir. 1997, 122, 551-564. CAPSULE CONTRACTURE.

Friis, S., McLaughlin, J. K., Mellemkjær, L., Kjøller, K. H., Blot, W. J., Boice, Jr. J. D., Fraumeni, Jr. J. F., and Olsen, J. H. Breast implants and cancer risk in Denmark. International Journal of Cancer. 1997b, 71, 956-958. CANCER.

Friis, S., Mellemkjær, McLaughlin J. K., Breiting, V., Kjær, S. K., Blot, W., and Olsen, J. H. Connective tissue disease and other rheumatic conditions following breast implants in Denmark. Annals of Plastic Surgery. 1997a Jul, 39, (1): 1-8. CONNECTIVE TISSUE DISEASE.

Fritzler, M. J., Pals, J. D., Kinsella, T. D., and Bowen, T. J. Antinuclear, anticytoplasmic and anti-Sjögren's syndrome antigen A (SS-A/Ro) antibodies in female blood donors. Clinical Immunology and Immunopathology. 1985, 36, 120-128. IMMUNE EFFECTS.

Frondoza, C., Jones, I., Rose, N. R., Hatakeyama A., Phelps, R., and Bona, C. Silicone does not potentiate development of the scleroderma-like syndrome in tight skin (TSK/+) mice. Journal of Autoimmunity. 1996, 9, 473-483. IMMUNE EFFECTS/connective tissue disease.

Fuchs, D., Weiss, G., Reibnegger, G., and Wachter, H. The role of neopterin as a monitor of cellular immune activation in transplantation, inflammatory, infectious and malignant diseases. Critical Review of Clinical Laboratory Sciences. 1992, 29, 307-341. AI-CTD BACKGROUND.

Fujimoto, K., Minato, M., Tadokoro, H., and Ikada, Y. Platelet desposition onto polymeric surfaces during shunting. Journal of Biomedical Materials Research. 1993, 27, 335-343. GENERAL.

Fujino, T., Harishina, T., and Enomoto, K. Primary breast reconstruction after a standard radical mastectomy by a free flap transfer: Case Report. Plast. Reconstr. Surg. 1976 Sep, 58, (3): 371-374. RECONSTRUCTION.

Fukuda, K., Straus, S. E., Hickie, I., Hickie, I., Sharpe, M. C., Dobbins, J. G., Komaroff, A., and International Chronic Fatigue Syndrome Study Group. The chronic fatigue syndrome: A comprehensive approach to its definition and study. Annals of Internal Medicine. 1994 Dec, 121, (12): 81-88. AI-CTD BACKGROUND.

Fung, K. P., Mahantayya, M. V., Ho, C. O., and Yap, K. M. Midazolam as a sedative in esophageal manometry: A study of the effect on esophageal motility. Journal of Pediatric Gastroenterology and Nutrition. 1992, 15, (1): 85-88. CHILDREN'S EFFECTS.

Funke, M., Fischer, U., and Grabbe, E. MR-mammography: Current status and perspectives. Akt. Radiol. 1996, 6, (3): 130-135. MAMMOGRAPHY.

Furey, P. C., Macgillivray, D. C., Castiglione, C. L., and Allen, L. Wound complications in patients receiving adjuvant chemotherapy after mastectomy and immediate breast reconstruction for breast cancer. Journal of Surgical Oncology. 1994, 55, 194-197. INFECTION/local complications.

Gabriel, S. E., O'Fallon, W. M., Beard, C. M., Kurland, L. T., Woods, J. E., and Melton, III L. J. Trends in the utilization of silicone breast implants, 1964-1991, and methodology for a population-based study of outcomes. Journal of Clinical Epidemiology. 1995, 48, (4): 527-537. PREVALENCE.

Gabriel, S. E., O'Fallon, W. M., Kurland, L. T., Beard, C. M., Woods, J. E., and Melton, L. J. Risk of connective-tissue diseases and other disorders after breast implantation. The New England Journal of Medicine. 1994 Jun 16, 330, (24): 1697-1702. CONNECTIVE TISSUE DISEASE.

Gabriel, S. E., Woods, J. E., O'Fallon, M., Beard, C. M., Kurland, L. T., and Melton, III J. M. Complications leading to surgery after breast implantation. The New England Journal of Medicine. 1997 Mar 6, 336, (10): 677-682. CAPSULE-CONTRACTURE/local complications/rupture/hematomas/infection/pain.

Gaither, K. K., Fox, O. F., Yamagat, H., Mamula, M. J., Reichlin, M., and Harley, J. G. Implications of anti-Ro/Sjogren's syndrome antigen autoantibody in normal sera for autoimmunity. J. Clin. Invest. 1987, 79, 841-846. AI-CTD BACKGROUND.

Gamon, A. E.Weyenber, D. Midland, Mich.: 1983 Nov 28. PLATINUM/toxicology.

Ganczarczyk, L., Urowitz, M. B., and Gladman, D. D. Latent lupus. J. Rheumatol. 1989, 16, (4): 475-478. AI-CTD BACKGROUND.

Ganott, M. A., Kathleen, M. H., and Ilkhanipour, Z. S. Costa-Greco M. A. Augmentation mammoplasty: Normal and abnormal findings with mammography and ultrasound. Radiographics. 1992, 12, 281-295. MAMMOGRAPHY.

Garbers, S., Terry, M. B., and Toniolo, P. Accuracy of self-report of breast implants. Plast. Reconstr. Surg. 1998 Mar, 101, (3): 695-698. CONNECTIVE TISSUE DISEASE.

Garrido, L. 29Si NMR and blood silicon levels in silcone gel breast implant recipients. Mag. Res. Med. 1996, 36, 498-501. SILICONE INJECTION/silicon measurement.

Garrido, L., Pfleiderer, B., Jenkins, B. G., Hulka, C. A., and Kopans, D. B. Migration and chemical modification of silicone in women with breast prostheses. Magnetic Resonance Medicine. 1994, 31, 328-330. MIGRATION/local complications/silicon measurement.

Garrido, L., and Young, V. L. Analysis of periprosthetic capsular tissue from women with silicone breast implants by magic-angle spinning NMR. Mag. Res. Med. 1999. SILICONE CHARACTERIZATION/silicon measurement/silica.

Gasperoni, C., Salgarello, M., and Gargani, G. Polyurethane-covered mammary implants: A 12-year experience. Annals of Plastic Surgery. 1992 Oct, 29, (4): 303-308. POLYURETHANE/local complications/capsule-contracture/hematomas.

Gatti, J. E. Poland's deformity reconstruction with a customized, extrasoft silicone prosthesis. Annals of Plastic Surgery. 1997 Aug, 39, (2): 1-7. RECONSTRUCTION.

Gause, B. L., Sznol, M., Kopp, W. C., Janik, J. E., Smith, II J. W., Steis, R. G., Urba, W. J., Sharfman, W., Fenton, R. G., Creekmore, S. P., Holmlund, J., Conlon, K. C., VanderMolen, L. A., and Longo, D. L. Phase I study of subcutaneously administered interleukin-2 combination with interferon alfa-2a in patients with advanced cancer. Journal of Clinical Oncology. 1996 Aug, 14, (8): 2234-2241. AI-CTD BACKGROUND.

Gayou, R. M. A histological comparison of contracted and noncontracted capsules around silicone breast implants. Plastic and Reconstructive Surgery. 1979, 63, (5): 700-707. CAPSULE-CONTRACTURE/local complications.

Gayou, R. M., and Rudolph, R. Capsular contracture around silicone mammary prostheses. Annals of Plastic Surgery. 1979 Jan, 2, 62-71. CAPSULE-CONTRACTURE/local complications.

Geatch, DR, Ross DA, Heasman A, and Taylor JJ. Expression of T-cell receptor Vbeta2, 6 and 8 gene families in chronic adult periodontal disease. Eur J Oral Sci. 1997 Oct, 105, (5): 397-404. IMMUNE EFFECTS.

Gedalia, A., Cuéllar, M. L., and Espinoza, L. R. Skin rash and anti-Ro/SS-A antibodies in an infant from a mother with silicone breast implants. Clinical and Experimental Rheumatology. 1995, 13, (4): 521-523. CHILDREN'S EFFECTS/connective tissue disease/immune effects.

Genovese, M. C. Fever, rash, and arthritis in a woman with silicone gel breast implants. Western Journal of Medicine. 1997 Sep, 167, (3): 149-158. CONNECTIVE TISSUE DISEASE.

Georgiade, G. S., Georgiade, N., McCarty, Jr. K. S., and Siegler, H. F. Rationale for immediate reconstruction of the breast following radical mastectomy. Annals of Plastic Surgery. 1982 Jan, 8, (1): 20-28. RECONSTRUCTION/cancer.

Georgiade, G. S., Riefkohl, R., Cox, E., McCarty, K. S., Seigler, H. F., Georgiade, N. G., and Snowhite, J. C. Long-term clinical outcome of immediate reconstruction after mastectomy. Plast. Reconstr. Surg. 1985 Sep, 76, (3): 415-420. RECONSTRUCTION/cancer.

Georgiade, N. G., Serafin, D., and Barwich, W. Late development of hematoma around a breast implant, necessitating removal. Plastic and Reconstructive Surgery. 1979, 64, (5): 708-710. STEROIDS/hematomas/local complications.

Gerard, D. Sexual functioning after mastectomy: life vs. lab. Journal of Sex & Marital Therapy. 1982 Winter, 8, (4): 305-315. PSYCHOSOCIAL.

Gerashchenko, B. I. Adsorption of aerosil on erythrocyte surface by flow cytometry measurements. Cytometry. 1994, 15, 80-83. SILICA.

Germain, B. F. Silicone breast implants and rheumatic diseases. Bull Rheum Dis. 1991, 41, (6): 1-5. CONNECTIVE TISSUE DISEASE.

Gersuny, R. Uber eine subcutane Prosthese. Z. Heilk. 1900, 1, 199. GENERAL.

Gibney, J. The long-term results of tissue expansion for breast reconstruction. Clinics in Plastic Surgery. 1987 Jul, 14, (3): 509-518. EXPANDER/capsule-contracture/local complications/rupture/reconstruction.

Gibney, J. Use of a permanent tissue expander for breast reconstruction. Plast. Reconstr. Surg. 1989 Oct, 84, (4): 607. EXPANDER/local complications/infection/capsule-contracture/pain/reconstruction.

Giesecke, J., and Arnander, C. Toxic shock syndrome after augmentation mammoplasty. Annals of Plastic Surgery. 1986 Dec, 17, (6): 532-533. INFECTION/local complications.

Gifford, G. H., Merrill, E. W., and et al. *In vivo* tissue reactivity of radiation cured silicone rubber implants. Journal of Biomedical Materials Research. 1976, 10, 857-865. TOXICOLOGY/radiation.

Giles, Jr. A. L., Chung, C. W., and Kommineni, C. Dermal carcinogencity study by mouse-skin painting with 2,4-toluenediamine alone or in representative hair dye formulations. Journal of Toxicology and Environmental Health. 1976, 1, 433-440. CARCINOGENICITY/toxicology.

Gilliland, M. D., Larson, D. L., and Copeland, E. M. Appropriate timing for breast reconstruction. Plast. Reconstr. Surg. 1983 Sep, 72, (3): 335-337. RECONSTRUCTION.

Giltay, E. J., Moens, H. J. B., Riley, A. H., and Tan, R. G. Silicone breast prostheses and rheumatic symptoms: A retrospective follow-up study. Ann Rheum Dis. 1994, 53, 194-196. CONNECTIVE TISSUE DISEASE.

Ginsbach, G., Busch, L., and Kuhnel, W. The nature of the collagenous capsules around breast implants, light and electron microscopic investigations. Plast. Reconstr. Surg. 1979 Oct, 64, (4): 456-464. CAPSULE-CONTRACTURE/local complications.

Gitelman, H. J., and Alderman, F. R. Silicon accumulation in dialysis patients. American Journal of Kidney Diseases. 1992 Feb, 14, (2): 140-143. SILICON MEASUREMENT.

Glenn, E. M. Adjuvant-induced polyarthritis in rats: Biologic and histologic background. American Journal of Veterinary Research. 1965 Sep, 26, (114): 1180-1194. AI-CTD BACKGROUND/immune effects.

Glicksman, C. A., Glicksman, A. S., and Courtiss, E. H. Breast imaging for plastic surgeons. Plast. Reconstr. Surg. 1992 Dec, 90, (6): 1106-1111. MAMMOGRAPHY.

Gnanadesigan, N., Pechter, E. A., and Mascola, L. Listeria infection of silicone breast implant. Plast. Reconstr. Surg. 1994 Sep, 94, (3): 531-535. INFECTION/local complications.

Godfrey, P. M., and Godfrey, N. V. Response of locoregional and systemic symptoms to breast implant replacement with autologous tissues: Experience in 37 consecutive patients. Plastic and Reconstructive Surgery. 1996 Jan, 97, (1): 110-116. CONNECTIVE TISSUE DISEASE/local complications/explantation.

Gogolewski, S. Leading contribution: selected topics in biomedical polyurethanes. A review. Colloid Polym Sci. 1989, 267, 757-785. POLYURETHANE.

Goin, J. M. High pressure injection of silicone gel into an axilla—a complication of closed compression capsulotomy of the breast. Plast. Reconstr. Surg. 1978 Dec, 62, (6): 891-895. MIGRATION/closed capsulotomy/rupture/capsule-contracture/local complications.

Goin, M. K., and Goin, J. Psychological reactions to prophylactic mastectomy synchronous with contralateral breast reconstruction. Plast. Reconstr. Surg. 1982 Sep, 70, (3): 355-359. PSYCHOSOCIAL/reconstruction.

Goin, M. K., and Goin, J. M. Midlife reactions to mastectomy and subsequent breast reconstruction. Archives of General Psychiatry. 1981 Feb, 38, 225-227. PSYCHOSOCIAL/reconstruction.

Goin, M. K., Goin, J. M., and Gianini, M. H. The psychic consequences of a reduction mammaplasty. Plast. Reconstr. Surg. 1977 Apr, 59, (4): 530-534. PSYCHOSOCIAL.

Goldberg, P, Stolzman, M, and Goldberg, H. Psychological considerations in breast reconstruction. Annals of Plastic Surgery. 1984, 13, (1): 38-43. PSYCHOSOCIAL.

Goldblum, R. M., Pelley, R. P., O'Donell, A. A., Pyron, D., and Heggers, J. P. Antibodies to silicone elastomers and reactions to ventriculoperitoneal shunts. The Lancet. 1992 Aug 29, 340, 510-513. IMMUNE EFFECTS.

Goldenberg, D. L., Simms, R. W., Geiger, A., and Komaroff, A. K. High frequency of fibromyalgia in patients with chronic fatigue seen in a primary care practice. Arthritis and Rheumatism. 1990, 33, (3): 381. AI-CTD BACKGROUND.

Goldman, J. A., Greenblatt, J., Joines, R., White, L., Aylward, B., and Lamm, S. H. Breast implants, rheumatoid arthritis, and connective tissue diseases in a clinical practice. Journal of Clinical Epidemiology. 1995, 48, (4): 571-582. CONNECTIVE TISSUE DISEASE.

Goldman, L. D., and Goldwyn, R. M. Some anatomical considerations of subcutaneous mastectomy. Plast. Reconstr. Surg. 1973 May, 51, (5): 501-505. GENERAL.

Goldsmith, H. S., and Alday, E. S. Role of the surgeon in the rehabilitation of the breast cancer patient. Cancer. 1971, 28, (6): 1672. RECONSTRUCTION/cancer.

Goldsmith, J. R., and Goldsmith, D. F. Fiberglass or silica exposure and increased nephritis or ESRD (end stage renal disease). American Journal of Industrial Medicine. 1993, 23, 873-881. SILICA.

Goldstein, R., Duvic, M., Targoff, I. N., Reichlin, M., McMenemy, A. M., Reveille, J. D., Warner, N. B., Pollack, M. S., and Arnett, F. C. HLA-D region genes associated with autoantibody responses to histidyl-transfer RNA synthetase (Jo-1) and other translation-related factors in myositis. Arthritis and Rheumatism. 1990 Aug, 33, (8): 1240-1248. AI-CTD BACKGROUND.

Goldwyn, R. M. Breast reconstruction after mastectomy. The New England Journal of Medicine. 1987 Dec 31, 317, (27): 1711-1714. GENERAL/reconstruction.

Goldwyn, R. M. An unusual complication of the use of the cronin implant for augmentation mammoplasty. British Journal of Plastic Surgery. 1969, 22, 167-168. RUPTURE/local complications.

Goodman, S. B., Fornasier, V. L., and Kei, J. The effects of bulk *versus* particulate polymethylmethacrylate on bone. Clinical Orthopaedics and Related Research. 1988, 232, 255-262. LOCAL COMPLICATIONS.

Gorczyca, D. P. MR imaging of breast implants. MRI Clinics of North America. 1994, 2, (4): 659-672. MAMMOGRAPHY.

Gorczyca, D. P., Debruhl, N. D., Ahn, C. Y., Hoyt, A., Sayre, J. W., Nudell, P., Mccombs, M., Shaw, W., and Bassett, L. W. Silicone breast implant ruptures in an animal model: Comparison of mammography, MR imaging, US, and CT. Radiology. 1994b, 190, 227-232. MAMMOGRAPHY/local complications/rupture.

Gorczyca, D. P., DeBruhl, N. D., Mund, D,.F., and Bassett, L. W. Linguine sign at MR imaging: Does it represent the collapsed silicone implant shell? Radiology. 1994c May, 191, 576-577. MAMMOGRAPHY/local complications/rupture.

Gorczyca, D. P., Schneider, E., DeBruhl, N. D., Foo, T. K. F., Ahn, C. Y., Sayre, J. W., Shaw, W. W., and Bassett, L. W. Silicone breast implant rupture: Comparison between Three-Point Dixon and Fast Spin-Echo MR imaging. American Journal of Roentgenology. 1994a Feb, 162, 305-310. MAMMOGRAPHY.

Gorczyca, D. P., Sinha, S., Ahn, C. Y., DeBruhl, N. D., Hayes, M. K., Gausche, VC. R., Shaw, W. W., and Bassett, L. W. Silicone breast implants in vivo: MR imaging. Radiology. 1992 Nov, 185, (2): 407-410. MAMMOGRAPHY.

Gorney, M. Justice and publicity: A question of responsibility. Plast. Reconstr. Surg. 1993 Nov 16, 93, (7): 1500-1503. GENERAL.

Gottlieb, V., Muench, A. G., Rich, J. D., and Pagadala, S. Carcinoma in augmented breasts. Annals of Plastic Surgery. 1984 Jan, 12, (1): 67-69. MAMMOGRAPHY/cancer.

Goulian, D. Current status of liquid injectable silicone. Aesthetic Plastic Surgery. 1978 Jan. SILICONE INJECTION.

Gower, D. J., Lewis, J. C., and Kelly, D. L. Sterile shunt malfunction: A scanning electron microscopic perspective. J Neurosurg. 1984, 61, 1079-1084. IMMUNE EFFECTS.

Grace, G. T., Roberts, C., and Cohen, I. K. The role of mammography in detecting breast cancer in augmented breasts. Annals of Plastic Surgery. 1990 Aug, 25, (2): 119-123. MAMMOGRAPHY.

Granchi, D., Cavadagna, D., Ciapetti, G., Stea, S., Shiavon, P., Giuliani, R., and Pizzoferrato, A. Silicone breast implants: The role of the immune system on capsular contracture formation. Journal of Biomedical Materials Research. 1995, 29, 197-202. CAPSULE-CONTRACTURE/local complications/immune effects.

Grant, E., Mascatello, V. J., and Cigtay, O. Irregularity of silastic breast implants mimicking a soft tissue mass. American Journal of Roentgenology. 1978 Mar, 130, 461-462. MAMMOGRAPHY.

Grant, S., and Edelman, D. A. Pregnancy, lactation and the use of silicone breast implants. Advances in Contraception. 1994, 10, 187-193. BREAST FEEDING.

Grasso, P., Fairweather, F. A., and Golberg, L. A short-term study of epithelial and connective tissue reactions to subcutaneous injection of silicone fluid. Fd Cosmet Toxicol. 1965 Aug, 3, (2): 263-269. TOXICOLOGY/immune effects.

Green, J., and et al. Clinical cognitive impairment and brain mapping in a series of 93 patients exposed to silicone breast implants. Disability. 1996 Jan. NEUROLOGIC DISEASE.

Greene, W. B., and Raso, D. et al. Migration of silicone gel from breast implants. USA Microscopy and Analysis. 1995b May, 12, (29). MIGRATION/local complications.

Greene, W. B., Raso, D. S., Walsh, L. G., Harley, R. A., and Silver, R. M. Electron probe microanalysis of silicon and the role of the macrophage in proximal (capsule) and distant sites in augmentation mammaplasty patients. Plast. Reconstr. Surg. 1995a Mar, 95, (3): 513-519. SILICON MEASUREMENT.

Greenland, S., and Finkle, W. D. A case-control study of prosthetic implants and selected chronic diseases. Annals of Epidemiology. 1996 Jan, 6, (6): 530-540. CONNECTIVE TISSUE DISEASE.

Greenwald, D. P., Randolph, M., and May, Jr. J. W. Mechanical analysis of explanted silicone breast implants. Plast. Reconstr. Surg. 1996 Aug, 98, (2): 269-272. RUPTURE/local complications.

Groff, G. D., Schned, A. R., and Taylor, T. H. Silicone-induced adenopathy eight years after metacarpophalangeal arthroplasty. Arthritis and Rheumatism. 1981 Dec, 24, (12): 1578-1581. LYMPHADENOPATHY/local complications.

Grossman, A. R. The current status of augmentation mammaplasty. Plast. Reconstr. Surg. 1973 Jul 1, 52, (1): 1-7. GENERAL.

Gruber, A. D., Matthews, S., and Gruber, R. P. Attempted improvement in mammography by inducing a phase transition in silicone gel. Annals of Plastic Surgery. 1993 Sep, 31, (3): 283-285. MAMMOGRAPHY.

Gruber, R. P., and Friedman, G. The pressures generated by closed capsulotomies of augmented breasts. Plastic Reconstructive Surgery. 1978 Sep, 6, 379-380. CLOSED CAPSULOTOMY.

Gruber, R. P., and Friedman, G. D. Periareolar subpectoral augmentation mammaplasty. Plast. Reconstr. Surg. 1981 Apr, 67, (4): 453-457. CAPSULE-CONTRACTURE/local complications.

Gruber, R. P., and Jones, H. W. Review of closed capsulotomy complications. Annals of Plastic Surgery. 1981 Apr, 6, (4): 271. CAPSULE-CONTRACTURE/local complications/closed capsulotomy.

Gruber, R. P., Kahn, R. A., Lash, H., Maser, M. R., Apfelberg, D. B., and Laub, D. R. Breast reconstruction following mastectomy: A comparison of submuscular and subcutaneous techniques. Plast. Reconstr. Surg. 1981, 67, (3): 312-317. RECONSTRUCTION.

Guenther, J. M., Tokita, K. M., and Giuliano, A. E. Breast-conserving surgery and radiation after augmentation mammoplasty. Cancer. 1994 May 15, 73, (10): 2613-2618. RADIATION/reconstruction.

Guidoin, R. et al. A non-destructive investigation to identify the failure mechanisms of 313 retrieved mammary prostheses. Proc Soc Biomaterials. 1992: 48. RUPTURE/local complications.

Guidoin, R. et al. The polyurethane foam covering the Même breast prosthesis: A biomedical breakthrough or a biomaterial tar baby? Annals of Plastic Surgery. 1992, 29, 477-478. POLYURETHANE.

Guillaume, J. C., Roujeau, J. C., and Touraine, R. Systemic lupus after breast prosthesis. Ann Dermatol Venerel. 1984, 111, 703-704. CONNECTIVE TISSUE DISEASE.

Guldner, H. H., Lakomek, H. J., and Bautz, F. A. Anti-(U1)RNP and anti-Sm autoantibody profiles in patients with systemic rheumatic diseases: Differential detection of immunoglobulin G and M by immunoblotting. Clinical Immunology and Immunopathology. 1986, 40, 532-538. AI-CTD BACKGROUND.

Gumucio, C. A., Pin, P., Young, V. L., Destouet, J., Monsees, B., and Eichling, J. The effect of breast implants on the radiographic detection of microcalcification and soft-tissue masses. Plast. Reconstr. Surg. 1989 Nov, 84, (5): 772-778. MAMMOGRAPHY/calcification.

Guo, W., Willen, R., Liu, X., Odelius, R., and Carlen, B. Splenic response to silicone drain material following intraperitoneal implantation. Journal of Biomedical Materials Research. 1994 Dec, 28, (12): 1433-1438. TOXICOLOGY.

Gur, E. N., Hanna, W., Andrighetti, L., and Semple, J. L. Light and electron microscopic evaluation of the pectoralis major muscle following tissue expansion for breast reconstruction. Plast. Reconstr. Surg. 1998 Sep, 102, (4): 1046-1051. EXPANDER.

Gurdin, M., and Carlin, G. A. Complications of breast implantations. Plast. Reconstr. Surg. 1967 Dec, 40, (6): 530-533. LOCAL COMPLICATIONS/infection/hematomas/capsule-contracture.

Gussler, J., and Briesemeister, L. The insufficient milk syndrome: a biocultural explantation. Medical Anthropology. 1980, 4, (2): 145-174. BREAST FEEDING.

Guthrie, J. L., and McKinney, R. W. Determination of 2,4- and 2,6-diaminotoluene in flexible urethane foams. Annals of Chemistry. 1977, 49, (12): 1676-1680. POLYURETHANE/toxicology.

Guthrie, R. H., and Cucin, R. L. Breast reconstruction after mastectomy: Problems in position, size and shape. Plast. Reconstr. Surg. 1980, 65, (5): 595-602. RECONSTRUCTION/local complications/capsule contracture.

Gutiérrez, F. J., and Espinoza, L. R. Progressive systemic sclerosis complicated by severe hypertension reversal after silicone implant removal. The American Journal of Medicine. 1990 Sep, 89, 390-392. CONNECTIVE TISSUE DISEASE/explantation.

Gutowski, K. A., Mesna, G. T., and Cunningham, B. L. Saline-filled breast implants: A plastic surgery educational foundation multicenter outcomes study. Plast. Reconstr. Surg. 1997 Sep, 100, (4): 1019-1027. SALINE/local complications/capsule-contracture/psychosocial/rupture.

Gylbert, L. O. Applanation tonometry for the evaluation of breast compressibility. Scandinavian Journal of Plastic and Reconstructive and Hand Surgery. 1989, 23, (3): 223-229. CAPSULE-CONTRACTURE/local complications.

Gylbert, L. O., Asplund, O., Berggren, A., Jurell, G., Ransjö, U., and Östrup, L. Preoperative antibiotics and capsular contracture in augmentation mammaplasty. Plastic and Reconstructive Surgery. 1990b Aug, 86, (2): 260-267. CAPSULE-CONTRACTURE/local complications/infection.

Gylbert, L. O., Asplund, O., and Jurell, G. Capsular contracture after breast reconstruction with siliocone-gel and saline-filled implants: a 6-year follow-up. Plast. Reconstr. Surg. 1990a Mar, 85, (3): 373-377. CAPSULE-CONTRACTURE/local complications/saline.

Gylbert, L. O., Asplund, O., Jurell, G., and Olenius, M. Results of subglandular breast augmentation using a new classification method—18-year follow-up. Scandinavian Journal of Plastic and Reconstructive Surgery and Hand Surgery. 1989, 23, (2): 133-136. CAPSULE-CONTRACTURE/local complications.

Gylbert, L. O., and Berggren, A. Constant compression caliper for objective measurement of breast capsular contracture. Scandinavian Journal of Plastic and Reconstructive and Hand Surgery. 1989, 23, (2): 137-142. CAPSULE-CONTRACTURE/local complications.

Habal, M. B. The biologic basis for the clinical application of the silicones: a correlate to their biocompatibility. Archives of Surgery. 1984 Jul, 119, 843-848. SILICONE CHARACTERIZATION/general.

Habal, M. B. Biophysical evaluation of the tumorigenic response to implanted polymers. Journal of Biomedical Materials Research. 1980, 14, 447-454. CARCINOGENICITY.

Habal, M. B. Current status of biomaterial's clinical applications in plastic and reconstructive surgery. Biomat Med Devices Artif Organs. 1979, 7, 229-741. GENERAL.

Habal, M. B. Personal considerations on the long-term effects of enlargement of the woman's breast with silicone implants. J Long-Term Eff Med Imp. 1993, 3, 351-364. LOCAL COMPLICATIONS.

Habal, M. B., Powell, M. L., and Schimpff, R. D. Immunological evaluation of the tumorigenic response to implanted polymers. Journal of Biomedical Materials Research. 1980, 14, 455-466. IMMUNE EFFECTS/carcinogenicity.

Habal, M. B., Quigg, J. M., Peck, L. S., Lin, T. L., Martin, P., Hattori, H., Ohmstede, D., Farnworth, S., and Goldberg, E. P. Evaluation of silicone gel mammary prostheses in a rabbit implant model. Society for Biomaterials Transactions. 1993, 16, 230. SILICON MEASUREMENT/capsule-contracture/local complications.

Hagerty, R. F., and McIver, F. A. Subcutaneous mastectomy with delayed subpectoral reconstruction. Southern Medical Journal. 1978, 71, (5): 525-529. RECONSTRUCTION/local complications.

Hagmar, L. H., Welinder, H., and Mikoczy, Z. Cancer incidence and mortality in the Swedish polyurethane foam manufacturing industry. British Journal of Industrial Medicine. 1993, 50, 537-543. CANCER/polyurethane.

Hahn, R. A. The nocebo phenomenon: concept, evidence, and implications for public health. Preventive Medicine. 1997, 26, 607-611. GENERAL.

Hakelius, L., and Ohlsen, L. A clinical comparison of the tendency to capsular contracture between smooth and textured gel-filled silicone mammary implants. Plast. Reconstr. Surg. 1992 Aug, 90, (2): 247-254. CAPSULE-CONTRACTURE/local complications.

Hakelius, L., and Ohlsen, L. Tendency to capsular contracture around smooth and textured gel-gilled silicone mammary implants: A five-year follow-up. Plast. Reconstr. Surg. 1997 Nov, 100, (6): 1566-1569. CAPSULE-CONTRACTURE/local complications.

Haleblian, J., Runkel, R., Mueller, N., Christopherson, J., and Ng, K. Steroid release from silicone elastomer containing excess drug in suspension. Journal of Pharmaceutical Sciences. 1971 Apr, 60, (4): 541-545. STEROIDS/local complications.

Hall, C. L., Colvin, R. B., Carey, K., and McCluskey, R. T. Passive transfer of autoimmune disease with isologous IgG1 and IgG2 antibodies to the tubular basement membrane in strain XIII guinea pigs. Loss of self-tolerance induced by autoantibodies. J. Exp. Med. 1977, 146, 1246-1260. CHILDREN'S EFFECTS/breast feeding.

Hallock, G. Maximum overinflation of tissue expanders. Plastic and Reconstructive Surgery. 1987 Oct, 80, (4): 567-569. EXPANDER/saline.

Hallock, G., and Rice, D. C. Objective monitoring for safe tissue expansion. Plast. Reconstr. Surg. 1986, 77, (3): 416-420. EXPANDER.

Halpern, J., McNeese, M. D., Kroll, S. S., and Ellerbroek, N. Irradiation of prosthetically augmented breasts: A retrospective study on toxicity and cosmetic results. Int J Radiat Oncol Biol Phys. 1990, 18, 189-191. RADIATION/capsule-contracture/local complications.

Hameed, M. R., Erlandson, R., and Rosen, P. P. Capsular synovial-like hyperplasia around mammary implants similar to detritic synovitis: A morphologic and immunohistochemical study of 15 cases. The American Journal of Surgical Pathology. 1995, 19, 433-438. CAPSULE-CONTRACTURE/local complications.

Hammar, C.-G., Freij, G., Strömberg, S., and Vessman, J. Mass fragmentographic determination of 2,6-*cis*-diphenylhexamethylcyclotetrasiloxane in human serum. Acta Pharmacologica et Toxicologica. 1975 Jan 1, Vol 36, Supp. III, 33-39, Chapter IV. SILICON MEASUREMENT.

Hammer, M., and Krippner, H. Three cases of chronic polyarthritis after silicone implantation (breast augmentation): Causal relationship? Immun. Infekt. 1991, 19, (2): 62-63. IMMUNE EFFECTS/CONNECTIVE TISSUE DISEASE.

Hammerstad, M., Dahl, B. H., Rindal, R., Kveim, M. R., and Roald, H. E. Quality of the capsule in reconstructions with textured or smooth silicone implants after mastectomy. Scandinavian Journal of Plastic and Reconstructive Surgery and Hand Surgery. 1996 Mar, 30, (1): 33-36. CAPSULE-CONTRACTURE.

Hammond, E. Some preliminary findings on physical complaints from a perspective survey of 1,064,004 men and women. American Journal of Public Health. 1964 Jan, 54, (1): 11-23. AI-CTD BACKGROUND.

Handel, N., Jensen, J. A., Black, Q., Waisman, J. R., and Silverstein, M. J. The fate of breast implants: A critical analysis of complications and outcomes. Plast. Reconstr. Surg. 1995 Dec, 96, (7): 1521-1533. GENERAL/capsule-contracture/rupture/infection/connective tissue disease/local complications.

Handel, N., Lewinsky, B., Jensen, J. A., and Silverstein, M. J. Breast conservation therapy after augmentation mammaplasty: Is it appropriate? Plast. Reconstr. Surg. 1996 Dec, 98, (7): 1216-1224. RADIATION/mammography/cancer.

Handel, N., Lewinsky, B., Silverstein, M. J., Gordon, P., and Zierk, K. Conservation therapy for breast cancer following augmentation mammaplasty. Plast. Reconstr. Surg. 1991b May, 87, (5): 873-878. CAPSULE-CONTRACTURE/local complications/radiation/cancer.

Handel, N., Silverstein, M. J., Gamagami, P., and Collins, A. An in vivo study of the effect of various breast implant filler materials on mammography. Plastic and Reconstructive Surgery. 1993b May, 91, (6): 1057-1062. MAMMOGRAPHY/general.

Handel, N., Silverstein, M. J., Gamagami, Jensen, J. A., and Collins, A. Factors affecting mammographic visualization of the breast after augmentation mammaplasty. J. Amer. Med. Assoc. 1992 Oct 14, 268, (14): 1913-1917. MAMMOGRAPHY.

Handel, N., Silverstein, M. J., Jensen, J. A., Collins, A., and Zierk, K. Comparative experience with smooth and polyurethane breast implants using the Kaplan-Meier Method of Survival Analysis. Plastic and Reconstructive Surgery. 1991a Sep, 88, (3): 475-481. POLYURETHANE/capsule-contracture/local complications/infection.

Handel, N., Silverstein, M. J., Waisman, E., and Waisman, J. R. Reasons why mastectomy patients do not have breast reconstruction. Plast. Reconstr. Surg. 1990 Dec, 86, (6): 1118-1122. RECONSTRUCTION/psychosocial.

Handel, N., Wellisch, D., Silverstein, M. J., Jensen, J. A., and Waisman, E. Knowledge, concern, and satisfaction among augmentation mammaplasty patients. Annals of Plastic Surgery. 1993a Jan, 30, (1): 13-20. PSYCHOSOCIAL.

Hanson, L., Ahlstedt, S., Anderson, B., Carlsson, B., Fallstrom, S., Melander, L., Porras, O., Soderstrom, T., and Eden, C. Protective factors in milk and the development of the immune system. Pediatrics. 1985, 75 (supplement), 172-176. BREAST FEEDING.

Harbut, M. R., and Churchill, B. C. Asthma in patients with silicone breast implants: Report of a case series and identification of hexachloroplantinate contaminant as a possible etiologic agent. Israel Journal of Occupational Health. 1999, 3, 73-82. TOXICOLOGY/platinum.

Hardin, J. R. The lupus autoantibodies and pathogenesis of system lupus erythematosus. Arthritis and Rheumatism. 1986 Apr, 29, (4): 456-460. AI-CTD BACKGROUND.

Hardt, N. S., Emery, J. A., Steinbach, B. G., Latorre, G., and Caffee, H. Cellular transport of silicone from breast prostheses. International Journal of Occupational Medicine and Toxicology. 1995b, 4, 127-133. MIGRATION.

Hardt, N. S., Yu, L. T., Latorre, G., and Steinbach, B. Fourier transform infrared microspectroscopy used to identify foreign materials related to breast implants. Methods in Pathology. 1994 Aug, 7, (6): 669-676. CAPSULE-CONTRACTURE/local complications/silicon measurement.

Hardt, N. S., Yu, L., LaTorre, G., and Steinbach, B. Complications related to retained breast implant capsules. Plast. Reconstr. Surg. 1995a Feb, 95, (2): 364-371. CAPSULE-CONTRACTURE/local complications/explantation.

Hardy, T. S., and Weill, H. Crystalline silica: Risks and policy. Environmental Health Perspectives. 1995 Feb, 103, (2): 152-155. SILICA.

Harman-Boehm, I., and Boehm, R. Breast augmentation: a new therapeutic use for insulin. Diabetes Care. 1989 Sep, 12, (8). GENERAL.

Harms, S. E., Flamig, D. P., Evans, W. P., Harries, S. A., and Bown, S. MR imaging of the breast: Current status and future potential. AJR American Journal of Roentgenology. 1994, 163, 1039-1047. MAMMOGRAPHY.

Harms, S. E., Flamig, D. P., Hesley, K. I., Meiches, M. D., Jensen, R. A., Evans, W. P., Savino, D. A., and Wells, R. V. MR imaging of the breast with rotating delivery of excitation off resonance: Clinical experience with pathologic correlation. Radiology. 1993, 187, (2): 493-501. MAMMOGRAPHY.

Harms, S. E., Jensen, R. A., Meiches, M. D., Flamig, D. P., and Evans, W. P. Silicone-suppressed 3D MRI of the breast using rotating delivery of off-resonance excitation. J Comput Assist Tomogr. 1995, 19, (3): 394-399. MAMMOGRAPHY.

Harris, H. I. Augmentation of the breast with silicone injections or prostheses. Journal of the International College of Surgeons. 1965 Feb, 43, (2): 202-210. SILICONE INJECTION.

Harris, H. I. Survey of breast implants from the point of view of carcinogenesis. Plast. Reconstr. Surg. 1961 Jul, 28, (1): 81. CANCER.

Harris, K. M., Ganott, M. A., Shestak, K. C., Losken, H. W., and Tobon, H. Silicone implant rupture: Detection with US. Radiology. 1993 Jun, 187, (3): 761-768. RUPTURE/mammography/local complications.

Hartley, J. H., and Shatten, W. E. Postoperative complications of lactation after augmentation mammoplasty. Plast. Reconstr. Surg. 1971 Feb, 47, (2): 150-153. BREAST FEEDING/local complications.

Hartley Jr., J. H. Specific applications of double lumen prosthesis. Clinics in Plastic Surgery. 1976 Apr, 3, (2): 247. CAPSULE-CONTRACTURE/local complications.

Hartrampf, C. R., Scheflan, M., and Black, P. W. Breast reconstruction with a transverse abdominal island flap. Plast. Reconstr. Surg. 1982, 69, (2): 216-224. RECONSTRUCTION.

Hartrampf Jr., C. R. Abdominal wall competence in transverse abdominal island flap operations. Annals of Plastic Surgery. 1984 Feb, 12, (2): 139-146. RECONSTRUCTION.

Hartwell Jr., S. W., Anderson, R., Hall, M. D., and Esselstyn Jr., C. Reconstruction of the breast after mastectomy for cancer. Plast. Reconstr. Surg. 1976 Feb, 57, (2): 152-157. RECONSTRUCTION.

Harving, S., Ravnsbæk, J., and Johansen, L. V. Salvage of exposed implants. Scandinavian Journal of Plastic and Reconstructive and Hand Surgery. 1989, 23, (2): 143-144. INFECTION/expander/local complications.

Hatcher, C., Brooks, L., and Love, C. Breast cancer and silicone implants: Psychological consequences for women. Journal of the National Cancer Institute. 1993 Sep, 85, (17): 1361-1365. GENERAL/cancer/psychosocial.

Hattevig, G., and Kjellman, B. Bjorksten B. Clinical symptoms and IgE responses to common food proteins and inhalants in the first 7 years of life. Clinical Allergy. 1987, 17, 571-578. CHILDREN'S EFFECTS.

Hausner, R. J., Schoen, F. J., Mendez-Fernandez, M. A., Henly, W. S., and Geis, R. C. Migration of silicone gel to auxillary lymph nodes after prosthetic mammoplasty. Archives of Pathology & Laboratory Medicine. 1981, 105, 371-372. MIGRATION/local complications/lymphadenopathy.

Hausner, R. J., Schoen, F. J., and Pierson, K. K. Foreign-body reaction to silicone in axillary lymph nodes after augmentation mammaplasty. Plast. Reconstr. Surg. 1978 Sep, 62, 381-384. MIGRATION/local complications/lymphadenopathy.

Haustein, U.-F., Ziegler, V., and Hermann, K. Chemically induced scleroderma. Hautartzt. 1992, 43, 469-474. AI-CTD BACKGROUND.

Hawthorne, G. A., Ballantyne, D., Rees, T., and Seidman, I. Hematological effects of dimethylpolysiloxane fluid in rats. Journal of Reticuloendothelial Society. 1970, 7, (5): 586-593. TOXICOLOGY.

Hayashi, K., Matsuda, T., Takano, H., and Umezu, M. Effects of immersion in cholesterol-lipid solution on the tensile and fatigue properties of elastomeric polymers for blood pump applications. Journal of Biomedical Materials Research. 1984 Oct, 18, (8): 939-951. SILICONE CHARACTERIZATION.

Hayashi, N., Tamaki, N., Senda, M., Yammamoto, K., Yonekura, Y., Torizuka, K., Ogawa, T., Katakura, K., Umemura, C., and Kodama, M. A new method of measuring in vivo sound speed in the reflection mode. J Clin Ultrasound. 1988 Feb, 16, 87-93. MAMMOGRAPHY.

Hayden, J. F., and Barlow, S. A. Structure-activity relationships of organosiloxanes in the female reproductive system. Toxicology and Applied Pharmacology. 1972 Jan, 21, (1): 68-79. TOXICOLOGY.

Hayes Jr., H., and McLeod, P. Indentation tonometry of the breasts. Plast. Reconstr. Surg. 1979 Jan, 63, (1): 13-18. CAPSULE-CONTRACTURE/local complications.

Hayes Jr., H., Vandergrit, J., and Diner, W. C. Mammography and breast implants. Plast. Reconstr. Surg. 1988 Jul, 82, (1): 1-6. MAMMOGRAPHY.

Hayes, M. K., Gold, R. H., and Bassett, L. W. Mammographic findings after the removal of breast implants. American Journal of Roentgenology. 1993 Mar, 160, 487-490. MAMMOGRAPHY/explantation.

Heggers, J. P., Kossovsky, N., Parsons, R. W., Robson, M. C., Pelley, R. P., and Raine, T. J. Biocompatibility of silicone implants. Annals of Plastic Surgery. 1983 Jul, 11, (1): 38-45. GENERAL.

Helal, B., Cozen, L., and Kramer, L. Silicone injection of joints: experimental and clinical trials. International Surgery. 1970 Nov, 54, (5): 317-322. TOXICOLOGY/silicone injection.

Helbich, T. H., Wunderbaldinger, P., Plenk, H., Deutinger, M., Bretenseher, M., and Mostbeck, G. H. The value of MRI in silicone granuloma of the breast. European Journal of Radiology. 1997, 24, (2): 155-158. MAMMOGRAPHY/granulomas/silicone injection.

Henderson, I. C. Appropriate timing for breast reconstruction [discussion]. Plast. Reconstr. Surg. 1983 Sep, 72, (3): 338-339. RECONSTRUCTION.

Henderson, J., Culkin, D., Mata, J., Wilson, M., and Venable, D. Analysis of immunological alterations associated with testicular prostheses. The Journal of Urology. 1995 Nov, 154, 1748-1751. IMMUNE EFFECTS.

Henly, D. R. et al. Particulate silicone for use in periurethral injections: Local tissue effects and search for migration. Journal of Urology. 1995 Jun 1, 153, (6): 2039-2043. TOXICOLOGY.

Hennekens, C. H., Lee, I.-M., Cook, N. R., Hebert, P. R., Karlson, E. W., LaMotte, F., Manson, J. E., and Buring, J. E. Self-reported breast implants and connective tissue diseases in female health professionals. J. Amer. Med. Assoc. 1996 Feb 28, 275, (8): 616-621. CONNECTIVE TISSUE DISEASE.

Henriksson, K. G., and Linvall, B. Polymyositis and dermatomyositis 1990—diagnosis, treatment and prognosis. Progress in Neurobiology. 1990 Jan, 35, 181-193. AI-CTD BACKGROUND.

Henrotte, J.-G., Viza, D., Vich, J. M., and Gueyne, J. The regulatory role of silicon on the cell cycle. C.R. Acad. Sci. Paris. 1988, 306, 525-528. SILICA.

Heredero, F. X. S., and Semper, E. M. Polyarthralgia after augmentation mammaplasty with saline-filled implants. European Journal of Plastic Surgery. 1992, 15, 1-8. SALINE/connective tissue disease/immune effects.

Herman, S. The Même implant. Plast. Reconstr. Surg. 1984 Mar, 73, (3): 411-414. POLYURETHANE.

Hester, Jr. T. R. The polyurethane-covered mammary prosthesis: Facts and fiction. Perspect. Plastic Surg. 1988, 2, 135. POLYURETHANE.

Hester, Jr. T. R., and Cukic, J. Use of stacked polyurethane-covered mammary implants in aesthetic and reconstructive surgery. Plast. Reconstr. Surg. 1991 Sep, 88, (3): 503-509. POLYURETHANE.

Hester, Jr. T. R., Ford, N. F., Gale, P. J., Hammett, J. L., Raymond, R., Turnbull, D., Frankos, V. H., and Cohen, M. B. Measurement of 2,4-toluenediamine in urine and serum samples from women with Même or Replicon breast implants. Plast. Reconstr. Surg. 1997 Oct, 100, (5): 1291-1298. CARCINOGENICITY/polyurethane/toxicology.

Hester, Jr. T. R., Nahai, F., Bostwick, J., and Cukic, J. A 5-year experience with polyurethane-covered mammary prostheses for treatment of capsular contracture, primary augmentation mammoplasty, and breast reconstruction: Plastic and reconstructive breast surgery. Clinics in Plastic Surgery. 1988 Oct, 15, (4): 569-585. CAPSULE-CONTRACTURE/local complications.

Hetter, G. P. Satisfactions and dissatisfactions of patients with augmentation mammaplasty. Plast. Reconstr. Surg. 1979, 64, (2): 151-155. PSYCHOSOCIAL.

Hetter, GP. Improved patient satisfaction with augmentation mammoplasty: the transaxillary subpectoral approach. Aesthetic Plast Surg. 1991 Spring, 15, 123-127. PSYCHOSOCIAL.

Heywang-Köbrunner, S. H. Contrast-enhanced magnetic resonance imaging of the breast. Investigative Radiology. 1994, 29, (1): 94-104. MAMMOGRAPHY.

Heywang-Köbrunner, S. H., Viehweg, P., Heinig, A., and Küchler, Ch. Contrast-enhanced MRI of the breast: Accuracy, value, controversies, solutions. European Journal of Radiology. 1997, 24, (2): 94-108. MAMMOGRAPHY.

Heywang, S. H., Eiermann, W., Bassermann, R., and et al. Carcinoma of the breast behind a prosthesis—A comparison of ultrasound, mammography, and MRI (case report). Computerized Radiology. 1985, 9, (5): 283-286. MAMMOGRAPHY/CANCER.

Heywang, S. H., Fenzl, G., Hahn, D., Krischke, I., Edmaier, M., Eiermann, W., and Basserman, R. MR imaging of the breast: Comparison with mammography and ultrasound. Journal of Computer Assisted Tomography. 1986, 10, (4): 615-620. MAMMOGRAPHY.

Heywang, S. H., Hilbertz, T., Beck, R., Bauer, W. M., Eiermann, W., and Permanetter, W. Gd-DTPA enhanced MR imaging of the breast in patients with postoperative scarring and silicon implants. Journal of Computer Assisted Tomography. 1990 May-1990 Jun 30, 14, (3): 348-356. MAMMOGRAPHY.

Hicken, N. F. Mastectomy: A clinical pathologic study demonstrating why most mastectomies result in incomplete removal of the mammary gland. Archives of Surgery. 1940, 40, 6-14. CANCER.

Higuchi, H., and et al. Abnormalities of the autonomic nervous system in chemically sensitive patients with silicone breast implants. Intl. J. Occup. Med. Immunol. Toxicol. 1996, 5, (1): 11-23. NEUROLOGIC DISEASE.

Hill, P., and Schatten, W. Potential indicators of insufficient milk supply syndrome. Research in Nursing and Health. 1991, 14, 11-19. BREAST FEEDING.

Hillemeier, C. Esophageal manometrics in children. Journal of Pediatric Gastroenterology and Nutrition. 1986, 5, (6): 840-842. CHILDREN'S EFFECTS.

Hinderer, U. T., and Escalona, J. Dermal and subdermal tissue filling with fetal connective tissue and cartilage, collagen, and silicone: Experimental study in the pig compared with clinical results. A new technique of dermis mini-autograft injections. Aesthetic Plastic Surgery. 1990, 14, 239-248. RECONSTRUCTION/silicone injection.

Hine, C. H., Elliott, E. W., Wright, R. R., Cavalli, R. D., and Porter, C. D. Evaluation of a silicone lubricant injected spinally. Toxicology and Applied Pharmacology. 1969, 15, (3): 566-573. NEUROLOGIC DISEASE.

Hipps, C. J., Raju, D. R., and Straith, R. E. Influence of some operative and post operative factors on capsular contracture around breast prostheses. Plast. Reconstr. Surg. 1978, 61, (3): 384-389. CAPSULE-CONTRACTURE/local complications/infection/steroids/closed capsulotomy.

Hirakawa, K., Bauer, T. W., Culver, J. E., and Wilde, A. H. Isolation and quantitation of debris particles around failed silicone orthopedic implants. The Journal of Hand Surgery. 1996 Sep, 21A, (5): 819-827. GENERAL.

Hirmand, H., Hoffman, L. A., and Smith, J. P. Silicone migration to the pleural space associated with silicone-gel augmentation mammaplasty. Annals of Plastic Surgery. 1994 Jun, 32, (6): 645-647. MIGRATION/local complications/rupture.

Hirmand, H., Latrenta, G. S., and Hoffman, L. A. Autoimmune disease and silicone breast implants. Journal of Oncology. 1993 Jul, 7, (7): 17-30. GENERAL/CONNECTIVE TISSUE DISEASE.

Hirohata, T., Nomura, A. M. Y., and Kolonel, L. N. Breast size and cancer. British Medical Journal. 1977 Sep 3, 2, 641. CANCER.

Hitoshi, S., Ito, Y., Takehara, K., Fujita, T., and Ogata, E. A case of malignant hypertension and scleroderma after cosmetic surgery. Japanese Journal of Medicine. 1991, 30, 97-100. SILICONE INJECTION/connective tissue disease.

Hobbs, E. J., Fancher, O. E., and Clandra, J. C. Effect of selected organopolysiloxanes on male rat and rabbit reproductive organs. Toxicology and Applied Pharmacology. 1972, 21, (1): 45- 54. TOXICOLOGY.

Hobbs, E. J., Keplinger, M. L., and Calandra, J. C. Toxicity of polydimethylsiloxanes in certain environmental systems. Environmental Research. 1975, 10, (3): 397-406. CHILDREN'S EFFECTS/silicone characterization/toxicology.

Hochberg, M. C. Adult and juvenile rheumatoid arthritis: Current epidemiologic concepts. Epidemiologic Review. 1981, 3, 27-41. AI-CTD BACKGROUND.

Hochberg, M. C. Cosmetic surgical procedures and connective tissue disease: the Cleopatra Syndrome revisited. Annals of Internal Medicine. 1993 Jun 15, 118, (12): 981-983. CONNECTIVE TISSUE DISEASE.

Hochberg, M. C., Miller, R., and Wigley, F. M. Frequency of augmentation mammoplasty in patients with systemic sclerosis: data from the Johns Hopkins–University of Maryland Scleroderma Center. Journal of Clinical Epidemiology. 1995, 48, (4): 565-569. PREVALENCE/CONNECTIVE TISSUE DISEASE.

Hochberg, M. C., Perlmutter, D. L., Medsger Jr., T. A., Nguyen, K., Steen, V., Weisman, M. H., White, B., and Wigley, F. M. Lack of association between augmentation mammoplasty and systemic sclerosis (scleroderma). Arthritis and Rheumatism. 1996 Jul, 39, (7): 1125-1131. CONNECTIVE TISSUE DISEASE.

Hoefflin, S. M. Extensive experience with polyurethane breast implants. Plast. Reconstr. Surg. 1990 Jul, 86, (1): 166-167. POLYURETHANE.

Hoffman, et al. Neurocognitive symptoms and quantitative EEG results in women presenting with silicone-induced autoimmune disorder. International Journal of Occupational Medicine and Toxicology. 1995. NEUROLOGIC DISEASE.

Hoffman, J. P., Kusiak, J., Bornas, M., and et al. Risk factors for immediate prosthetic postmastectomy reconstruction. Am Surg. 1991, 57, 514-521. RECONSTRUCTION.

Hoffman, S. Correction of established capsular contractures with polyurethane implants. Aesthetic Plastic Surgery. 1989, 13, (1): 33-40. POLYURETHANE/capsule-contracture/local complications.

Hoffman, S. The management of severe capsular contractures following breast augmentation. Aesth. Plast. Surg. 1983, 7, 109-112. CAPSULE CONTRACTURE/local complications.

Hoffman, S. Treatment of breast contractures with open capsulotomy and replacement of gel prostheses with polyurethane-covered implants. Plast. Reconstr. Surg. 1991, 97, (4): 808. CAPSULE-CONTRACTURE/local complications/polyurethane.

Hoflehner, H., Pierer, G., and Rehak, P. Mammacompliance: An objective technique for measuring capsular fibrosis. Plast. Reconstr. Surg. 1993 Nov, 92, (6): 1078-1084. CAPSULE-CONTRACTURE/local complications.

Holcombe, R, Baethge, B., Wolf, R., Betzing, K., Stewart, R., Hall, V., and Fukuda, M. Correlation of serum interleukin-8 and cell surface lysosome-associated membrane protein expression with clinical disease activity in systemic lupus erythematosus. Lupus. 1994, 3, 97-102. AI-CTD BACKGROUND.

Holley, D. T., Tourarkissian, B., Vasconez, H. C., and et al. The ramifications of immediate reconstruction in the management of breast cancer. The American Surgeon. 1995 Jan, 61, (1): 60-65. RECONSTRUCTION.

Hollos, P. Breast augmentation with autologous tissue: An alternative to implants. Plast. Reconstr. Surg. 1995 Aug, 96, (2): 381-384. GENERAL.

Holm, C., and Mühlbauer, W. Toxic shock syndrome in plastic surgery patients: Case report and review of the literature. Aesthetic Plastic Surgery. 1998, 22, 180-184. INFECTION/local complications.

Holmes, J. D. Capsular contracture after breast reconstruction with tissue expansion. British Journal of Plastic Surgery. 1989, 42, 591-594. CAPSULE-CONTRACTURE/local complications/reconstruction/expander.

Holt, R. W., and Spear, S. L. Cancer in the augmented breast: Diagnosis and treatment. Breast Dis Breast. 1984, 10, (3): 16. CANCER.

Holten, I. W. R., and Barnett, R. A. Intraductal migration of silicone from intact gel breast prostheses. Plast. Reconstr. Surg. 1995 Mar, 95, (3): 563-566. MIGRATION/local complications.

Hong, R. Autoimmunity: Present-day concepts and future prospects. Current Problems in Pediatrics. 1991 Jul, 21, 253-258. AI-CTD BACKGROUND.

Hooper, B., Whittingham, S., Matthews, J. D., Mackay, I. R., and Curnow, D. H. Autoimmunity in a rural community. Clin. Exp. Immunol. 1972, 12, 79-87. AI-CTD BACKGROUND.

Hoopes, J. E., Edgerton, M. T., and Shelly, W. Organic synthetics for augmentation mammoplasty: Their relation to breast cancer. Plastic and Reconstructive Surgery. 1967, 39, (3): 263. CANCER/carcinogenicity.

Horning, P., and Alexander, E. S. Observations on the Oppenheimer method of inducing tumors by subcutaneous implantation of plastic films. In. Symposium on Carcinogenesis Mechanisms of Action. 1959, p. 12-25. CARCINOGENICITY.

Hørven, S., Stiles, T. C., Holst, A., and Moen, T. HLA antigens in primary fibromyalgia syndrome. Journal of Rheumatology. 1992, 19, 1269-1270. AI-CTD BACKGROUND.

Hosokawa, S., and Yoshida, O. Silicon transfer during haemodialysis. Int. Urol. Nephrol. 1990, 22, 373-378. SILICON MEASUREMENT.

Houpt, K. R., and Sontheimer, R. D. Automimmune connective tissue disease and connective tissue-disease-like illnesses after silicone gel augmentation mammoplasty. Journal of the American Academy of Dermatology. 1994 Oct, 31, (4): 626-642. CONNECTIVE TISSUE DISEASE.

Houpt, P., Dijkstra, R., and Storm van Leeuwen, J. B. The result of breast reconstruction after mastectomy for breast cancer in 109 patients. Annals of Plastic Surgery. 1988, 21, 516-525. RECONSTRUCTION.

Howie, P. W., Forsyth, J. S., Ogston, S. A., Clark, A., and Florey, C. D. Protective effect of breast feeding against infection. Brit. Med. J. 1990, 300, (6716): 11-16. BREAST FEEDING.

Hsieh, C. C., and Trichopoulos, D. Breast size, handedness and breast cancer risk. European Journal of Cancer. 1991, 27, (2): 131-135. GENERAL/cancer.

Huang, T. T. Breast and subcapsular pain following submuscular placement of breast prostheses. Plast. Reconstr. Surg. 1990 Aug, 86, (2): 275-280. PAIN/local complications.

Huang, T. T., Blackwell, S., and Lewis, S. Migration of silicone gel after the 'squeeze technique' to rupture a contracted breast capsule: Case report. Plast. Reconstr. Surg. 1978 Feb, 61, (2): 277-280. CAPSULE CONTRACTURE/MIGRATION/local complications/closed capsulotomy.

Huang, T. T., Parks, D. H., and Lewis, S. R. Outpatient breast surgery under intercostal block anesthesia. Plast. Reconstr. Surg. 1980 Feb: 239-240. PAIN.

Hubbard, A. K. Role for T-lymphocytes in silica-induced pulmonary inflammation. Laboratory Investigation. 1989, 61, (1): 46-51. SILICA.

Hudson, J. I., Hudson, M. S., Pliner, L. F., Goldenberg, D. L., and Pope, H. G. Jr. Fibromyalgia and major affective disorder: A controlled phenomenology and family history study. American Journal of Psychiatry. 1985, 142, 441. AI-CTD BACKGROUND.

Hueper, W. C. Cancer induction by polyurethane and polysilicane plastics. Journal of the National Cancer Institute. 1964 Dec, 33, (6): 1005-1027. CARCINOGENICITY/polyurethane.

Hueper, W. C. Carcinogenic studies on water-insoluble polymers. Path. Microbiol. 1961, 24, 77-106. TOXICOLOGY/carcinogenicity.

Hueper, W. C. Carcinogenic studies on water-soluble and insoluble macromolecules. A.M.A. Arch. Path. 1959, 67, 589. TOXICOLOGY/carcinogenicity.

Hueper, W. C. Experimental production of cancer by means of implanted polyurethane plastic. American Journal of Clinical Pathology. 1960 Oct, 34, (4): 328-333. POLYURETHANE/carcinogenicity/toxicology.

Hueper, W. C. Polyurethane plastic foam for fractures. J. Amer. Med. Assoc.. 1960 Jun 18: 196. POLYURETHANE.

Hueston, J. T., and Hare, W. S. C. Rupture of subpectoral prostheses during closed compression capsulotomy. Australian and New Zealand Journal of Surgery. 1979 Oct, 49, (5): 564-567. CAPSULE-CONTRACTURE/local complications/closed capsulotomy/rupture.

Hueston, J. T., and McKenzie, G. Breast reconstruction after radical mastectomy. Australian and New Zealand Journal of Surgery. 1970 May, 39, (4): 367-370. RECONSTRUCTION.

Hughes, K. C. Unusual masses found within ruptured silicone gel prostheses. Plast. Reconstr. Surg. 1997 Aug, 100, (2): 525-528. HEMATOMAS/local complications/rupture.

Humphrey, L. J. Subcutaneous mastectomy is not a prophylaxis against carcinoma of the breast: Opinion or knowledge? The American Journal of Surgery. 1983 Mar, 145, (3): 311-312. CANCER.

Hunter, J. G., Padilla, M., and Cooper-Vastola, S. Late *Clostridium perfringens* breast implant infection after dental treatment. Annals of Plastic Surgery. 1996 Mar, 36, (3): 309-312. INFECTION/local complications.

Hurst, N. M. Lactation after augmentation mammoplasty. Obstetrics and Gynecology. 1996 Jan, 87, (1): 30-34. BREAST FEEDING/local complications.

Hutson, M. M., and Blaha, J. D. Patients' recall of preoperative Instruction for Informed Consent for an Operation. The Journal of Bone and Joint Surgery. 1991 Feb, 73-A, (2): 160-162. GENERAL.

Hyams, K. C. Developing case definitions for symptom-based conditions: the problem of specificity. Epidemiologic Reviews. 1998, 20, 148-156. CONNECTIVE TISSUE DISEASE.

Hyde, J. F. Chemical background of silicones. Science. 1965 Feb 19, 147, (3660): 829-836. SILICONE CHARACTERIZATION/silicone chemistry.

Iannello, S., and Belfiore, F. Silicone breast prosthesis and rheumatoid arthritis: a new systemic disease: siliconosis. A case report and a critical review of the literature. Minerva Med. 1998, 89, (4): 117-130. CONNECTIVE TISSUE DISEASE.

Imai, M., Yamada, C., Saga, S., Nagayoshi, S., and Hoshino, M. Immunological cross reaction between sera from patients with breast cancer and mouse mammary tumor virus. Gann. 1979 Feb, 70, (1): 63-74. AI-CTD BACKGROUND.

Imber, G., Schwager, R. G., Guthrie, R. H. Jr., and Gray, G. F. Fibrous capsule formation after subcutaneous implantation of synthetic materials in experimental animals. Plast. Reconstr. Surg. 1974 Aug, 54, (2): 183-186. CAPSULE-CONTRACTURE/local complications.

Inoue, U., Wanibuchi, Y., and Nishi, T. Is foreign body calcification a late reaction after augmentation mammaplasty? Fortschr. Roentgenstr. 1983, 138, 74-80. CALCIFICATION/local complications.

International Agency for Research on Cancer. IARC Monographs on the Evaluation of the Carcinogenic Risk of Chemicals to Humans. World Health Organization, 1985. TOXICOLOGY.

International Agency for Research on Cancer. IARC Monographs on the Evaluation of the Carcinogenic Risk of Chemicals to Humans: Silica, Some Silicates, Coal Dust and *para*-Aramid Fibrils. Vol. 68 ed. United Kingdom: World Health Organization, 1997. SILICA/cancer.

International Agency for Research on Cancer. IARC Monographs on the Evaluation of the Carcinogenic Risk of Chemicals to Humans: Some Chemicals Used in Plastics and Elastomers. Vol. 39 ed. Switzerland: World Health Organization, 1986. CANCER/toxicology/polyurethane.

Irving, I., Hall, C., Castilla, P., and Rickham, P. P. Tissue reaction to pure and impregnated silastic. Journal of Pediatric Surgery. 1971 Dec, 6, (6): 724-729. LOCAL COMPLICATIONS.

Irwin, M., Mascovich, A., Gillin, J. C., and et al. Partial sleep derivation reduces natural killer cell activity in humans. Psychosom. Med. 1994, 56, 493-498. AI-CTD BACKGROUND.

Irwin, M., McClintick, J., Costlow, C., and et al. Partial night sleep deprivation reduces natural killer and cellular immune responses in human. FASEB J. 1996, 10, 643-653. AI-CTD BACKGROUND.

Ishii, Jr. C. H., Bostwick, III J., Raine, T. J., and Coleman, III J. J. Hester T. R. Double-pedicle transverse rectus abdominis myocutaneous flap for unilateral breast and chest-wall reconstruction. Plast. Reconstr. Surg. 1985, 76, (6): 901-907. RECONSTRUCTION.

Isobe, T., and Osserman, E. F. Pathologic conditions associated with plasma cell dyscrasias: a study of 806 cases. Annals New York Academy of Sciences. 1971 Dec 31, 190, 507-518. AI-CTD BACKGROUND.

Isquith, A. J., Matheson, D., and Slesinski, R. Genotoxicity studies on selected organosilicon compounds: *In vitro* assays. Food and Cosmetics Toxicology. 1988, 26, (3): 255 -261. TOXICOLOGY.

Ito, N., Hiasa, Y., Konishi, Y., and Marugami, M. The development of carcinoma in liver of rats treated with m-toluylenediamine and the synergistic and antagonistic effects with other chemicals. Cancer Res. 1969, 29, 1137-1145. POLYURETHANE.

Iverson, G. L., Anderson, K. W., and McCracken, L. M. Research methods for investigating causal relations between SLE disease variables and psychiatric symptomatology. Lupus. 1995, 4, (4): 349-354. AI-CTD BACKGROUND/psychosocial.

Iwuagwu, F. C., and Frame, J. D. Silicone breast implants: complications. British Journal of Plastic Surgery. 1997, 50, 632-636. LOCAL COMPLICATIONS.

Jabaley, M. E., and Das, S. K. Late breast pain following reconstruction with polyurethane-covered breast implants. Plast. Reconstr. Surg. 1986 Sep, 78, (3): 390-395. POLYURETHANE/pain/local complications.

Jacobs, J. C., Hensle, T. W., Kwan, D., Imundo, L. F., Hauser, A., and Tan, E. M. Do silicone testicular implants increase the risk of systemic lupus erythematosus (SLE) in children? (1) Do boys with silicone implants develop antinuclear antibodies with greater frequency than age/sex matched healthy controls? [abstract]. Pediatric Research. 1995, 39, (4): 393A. IMMUNE EFFECTS/connective tissue disease.

Jacobs, J. C., Imundo, L., Robinson, O. G., Bradley, E. L., and Wilson, D. S. Analysis of explanted silicone implants: A report of 300 patients. Annals of Plastic Surgery. 1995, 34, 1-7. RUPTURE/local complications/explantation.

Jacobson, G. M., Sause, W. T., Thomson, J. W., and Plenk, H. P. Breast irradiation following silicone gel implants. International Journal of Radiation Oncology Biol Phys. 1986, 12, 835-838. RADIATION/general.

Jacobsson, L., Axell, T., Hansen, B., Henricsson, V., Larsson, A., Lieberking, K., Lilja, B., and Manthorpe, R. Dry eyes or mouth —An epidemiological study in Swedish adults, with special reference to primary Sjögren's syndrome. Journal of Autoimmunity. 1989, 2, (4): 521-527. AI-CTD BACKGROUND.

James, R. T. Psychiatric aspects of mastectomy. Australian and New Zealand Journal of Surgery. 1979 Oct, 49, (5): 519-520. PSYCHOSOCIAL.

James, S. J., Pogribna, M., Miller, B. J., Bolon, B., and Muskhelishvili, L. Characterization of cellular response to silicone implants in rats: Implications for foreign-body carcinogenesis. Biomaterials. 1997, 18, (9): 667-675. TOXICOLOGY/carcinogenicity/immune effects.

Janson, R. A. Implant arm: Axillary compression from breast prosthesis. Plast. Reconstr. Surg. 1985 Mar, 75 (3), 420-422. PAIN/local complications.

Jarrett, J. R., Cutler, R. G., and Teal, D. Subcutaneous mastectomy in small, large, or ptotic breasts with immediate submuscular placement of implants. Plast. Reconstr. Surg. 1978, 62, (5): 702-705. RECONSTRUCTION.

Jarrett, J. R., Cutler, R. G., and Teal, D. F. Aesthetic refinements in prophylactic subcutaneous mastectomy with submuscular reconstruction. Plast. Reconstr. Surg. 1982 Apr, 69, (4): 624-631. CAPSULE-CONTRACTURE/local complications/expander/reconstruction.

Jasty, M., and Smith, E. Wear particles of total joint replacements and their role in periprosthetic osteolysis. Current Opinion in Rheumatology. 1992, 4, 204-209. LOCAL COMPLICATIONS/general.

Jenkins, M. E., Friedman, H. I., and von Recum, A. F. Breast implants: Facts, controversy, and speculations for future research. Journal of Investigative Surgery. 1996, 9, (1): 1-12. GENERAL.

Jennings, D. A., Morykwas, M. J., Burns, W. W., Crook, M. E., Hudson, W. P., and Argenta, L. C. In vitro adhesion of endogenous skin microorganism to breast prostheses. Ann. Plast. Surg. 1991a, 27, (3): 216-220. INFECTION.

Jennings, D. A., Morykwas, M. J., DeFranzo, A. J., and Argenta, L. C. Analysis of silicon in human breast and capsular tissue surrounding prostheses and expanders. Annals of Plastic Surgery. 1991b, Dec, 27, (6): 553-558. SILICON MEASUREMENT/expander.

Jennings, T. A., Peterson, L., Axiotis, C. A., Friedlaender, G. E., Cooke, R. A., and Rosai, J. Angiosarcoma associated with foreign body material. A report of three cases. Cancer. 1988 Dec 1, 62, (11): 2436-2444. CANCER.

Jenny, H., and Smahel, J. Clinicopathological correlations in pseudocapsule formation after breast augmentation. Aesth Plast Surg. 1981, 5, (1): 63-68. CAPSULE-CONTRACTURE/local complications.

Jensen, S and Mackey, J. Xeromammography after augmentation mammoplasty. Am. J. Roentgenol. 1985, 144, 629-633. MAMMOGRAPHY.

Jewett, S. T., and Mead, J. H. Extra-abdominal desmoid arising from a capsule around a silicone breast implant. Plast. Reconstr. Surg. 1979 Apr, 63, (4): 577-579. LOCAL COMPLICATIONS.

Jimenez, D. F. Silicone allergy in ventriculoperitoneal shunts. Child's Nervous System. 1994, 10, 59-63. IMMUNE EFFECTS.

Johanson, T. R. M., Lowe, L., Brown, M. D., Sullivan, M. J., and Nelson, B. R. Histology and physiology of tissue expansion. J. Dermatol. Surg. Oncol. 1993, 19, 1074. EXPANDER.

Johnson, C. H., van Heerden, J. A., Donohue, J. H., Marlin, J. K., Jackson, I. T., and Ilstrup, D. M. Oncological aspects of immediate breast reconstruction following mastectomy for malignancy. Archives of Surgery. 1989 Jul, 124, 819-824. CANCER/reconstruction.

Johnson, H. A. Silastic breast implants: Coping with complications. Plast. Reconstr. Surg. 1969 Dec, 44, (6): 588-591. GENERAL/local complications.

Johnson, M., and Lloyd, H. E. D. Bilateral breast cancer 10 years after an augmentation mammaplasty. Plast. Reconstr. Surg. 1974, 55, 88-90. CANCER.

Johnson, P. E., and Hanson, K. D. Acute puerperal mastitis in the augmented breast. Plast. Reconstr. Surg. 1996 Sep, 98, (4): 723-725. BREAST FEEDING/infection.

Jones, R. N., Turner-Warwick, M., and et al. High prevalence of antinuclear antibodies in sandblasters' silicosis. American Review of Respiratory Disease. 1976, 113, 393-395. SILICA.

Jonsson, C.-O., Engman, K., and Asplund, O. Psychological aspects of breast reconstruction following mastectomy. Scandinavian Journal of Plastic and Reconstructive Surgery. 1984, 18, (3): 317-325. PSYCHOSOCIAL/reconstruction.

Jordan, D. R., and Nerad, J. A. An acute inflammatory reaction to silicone stents. Ophthal Plast Reconstr Surg. 1987, 3, 147. IMMUNE EFFECTS/general.

Jovanovic-Peterson, L., Sparks, S., Palmer, J. P., and Petterson, C. M. Jet-injected insulin is associated with decreased antibody production and postpranial glucose variability when compared with needle-injected insulin in gestational diabetic women. Diabetes Care. 1993 Nov, 16, (11): 1479-1484. IMMUNE EFFECTS.

Juby, A. G., Davis, P., McElhaney, J. E., and Gravenstein, S. Prevalence of selected auto antibodies in different elderly subpopulations. Br. J. Rheumatol. 1994, 33, 1121-1124. AI-CTD BACKGROUND.

Kacew, S. Adverse effects of drugs and chemical in breast milk on the nursing infant. J Clin Pharmacol. 1993, 33, 213-221. CHILDREN'S EFFECTS/breast feeding.

Kacew, S. Current issues in lactation: Advantages, environment, silicone. Biomedical and Environmental Sciences. 1994, 7, (4): 307-319. BREAST FEEDING/children's effects.

Kacprzak, J. L. Atomic absorption spectroscopic determination of dimethylpolysiloxane in juices and beer. Journal of the Association of Official Analytical Chemists. 1982, 65, (1): 148-150. SILICON MEASUREMENT.

Kagan, H. D. Sakurai injectable silicone formula. Archives of Otolaryngology. 1963 Nov, 78, 53-58. SILICONE INJECTION.

Kahn, P., and Carmen, R. Reduction of ball variance in silicone rubber occluders. Annals of Thoracic Surgery. 1989, 48, S10-S11. SILICONE CHARACTERIZATION/general.

Kaiser, J. Breast-implant ruling sends a message. Science. 1997 Jan, 275, (5296): 21. GENERAL.

Kaiser, W. A., Biesenbach, G., Stuby, U., Grafinger, P., and Zazgornik, J. Human adjuvant disease: Remission of silicone induced autoimmune disease after explantation of breast augmentation. Annals of Rheumatic Diseases. 1990, 49, 937-938. CONNECTIVE TISSUE DISEASE/explantation.

Kaiser, W. A., and Zargornik, J. Does silicone induce automimmune diseases? Review of the literature and case reports. Z Rheumatol. 1992, 51, (1): 31-34. CONNECTIVE TISSUE DISEASE.

Kaiser, W. A., and Zeitler, E. MR imaging of the breast: Fast imaging sequences with and without Gd-DTPA: Preliminary observations. Radiology. 1989 Mar, 170, 681-686. MAMMOGRAPHY.

Kala, S. V., and et al. Low molecular weight silicones are widely distributed after a single subcutaneous injection in mice. Am. J. Pathol. 1998, 152, 645-649. TOXICOLOGY.

Kala, S. V., Lykissa, E. D., and Lebovitz, R. M. Detection and characterization of poly(dimethylsiloxane)s in biological tissues by GC/AED and GC/MS. Analytical Chemistry. 1997 Apr 1, 69, (7): 1267-1272. SILICON MEASUREMENT/toxicology.

Kallenberg, C. G. M. Overlapping syndromes, undifferentiated connective tissue disease, and other fibrosing conditions. Current Opinions in Rheumatology. 1994, 6, 650-654. AI-CTD BACKGROUND.

Kalman, P. G., Ward, C. A., McKeown, N. B., and et al. Improved biocompatability of silicone rubber by removal of surface entrapped air nuclei. Journal of Biomedical Materials Research. 1991 Feb, 25, 199-211. TOXICOLOGY.

Kao, C. C., Rand, R. P., Holt, C. A., Pierce, R. H., Timmons, J. H., and Wood, D. E. Internal mammary silicone lymphadenopathy mimicking recurrent breast cancer. Plast. Reconstr. Surg. 1997 Jan, 99, (2): 225-229. LYMPHADENOPATHY/local complications.

Kao, W. J., McNally, A. K., Hiltner, A., and Anderson, J. M. Role for interleukin-4 in foreign-body giant cell formation on a poly(etherurethane urea) *in vivo*. Journal of Biomedical Materials Research. 1995, 29, 1267-1275. IMMUNE EFFECTS.

Kao, W. J., Zhao, Q. H., Hiltner, A., and Anderson, J. M. Theoretical analysis of in vivo macrophage adhesion and foreign body giant cell formation on polydimethylsiloxane, low density polyethylene, and polyurethanes. Journal of Biomedical Materials Research. 1994, 28, (1): 73-79. IMMUNE EFFECTS/general.

Kamel, M., Fornasier, V.L., and Peters, W. Cartilaginous metaplasia in the capsule of a Dacron-backed silicone gel breast prosthesis. Ann. Plast. Surg. 1999 Feb, 42, (2): 202-206. LOCAL COMPLICATIONS.

Kaplan, H. S. A neglected issue: The sexual side effects of current treatments for breast cancer. Journal of Sex & Marital Therapy. 1992, 18, (1): 3-19. PSYCHOSOCIAL.

Karfík, V., and Šmahel, J. Subcutaneous silicone granuloma. Acta Chirugiae Plasticae. 1968, 10, (4): 328-332. GRANULOMAS/local complications.

Karimeddini, M. K., and Spencer, R. P. Silicone breast implants and renal contrast agent: Iatrogenic sources of increased bone density. Clinical Nuclear Medicine. 1996 Nov, 21, (11): 889-890. GENERAL.

Karlson, E. W., Hankinson, S. E., Liang, M. H., Sanchez-Guerrero, J., Colditz, G. A., Rosenau, B. J., Speizer, F. E., and Schur, P. H. Association of silicone breast implants with immunologic abnormalities: a prospective study. Am J Med. 1999, 106, 11-19. IMMUNE EFFECTS/connective tissue disease.

Karlson, E. W., Sanchez-Guerrero, J., Wright, E. A., Lew, R. A., Daltroy, L. H., Katz, J. N., and Liang, M. H. A connective tissue disease screening questionnaire (CSQ) for population studies. Annals of Epidemiology. 1995 Jul, 5, (4): 297-302. CONNECTIVE TISSUE DISEASE.

Kasper, C. S. Histologic features of breast capsules reflect surface configuration and composition of silicone bag implants. American Journal of Clinical Pathology. 1994 Nov, 102, (5): 655-659. CAPSULE-CONTRACTURE/local complications.

Kasper, C. S., and Chandler, Jr. P. J. Talc deposition in skin and tissues surrounding silicone gel-containing prosthetic devices. Arch Dermatol. 1994 Jan, 130, 48-53. CAPSULE CONTRACTURE.

Kasper, M. E., Harrell, E. H., Jones, W. B., and Krusz, J. C. Neuropsychological profile associated with silicone-gel breast implants. Journal of Nutritional & Environmental Medicine. 1998, 8, 7-17. PSYCHOSOCIAL.

Katzin, W. E., Feng, L.-J., Abbuhl, M., and Klein, M. A. Phenotype of lymphocytes associated with the inflammatory reaction to silicone gel breast implants. Clinical and Diagnostic Laboratory Immunology. 1996 Mar, 3, (2): 156-161. IMMUNE EFFECTS.

Kaufman, L. D., Varga, J., Gomez-Reino, J. J., Jimenez, S., and Targoff, I. N. Autoantibodies in sera from patients with l-tryptophan-associated eosinophilia-myalgia syndrome. Clinical Immunology and Immunopathology. 1995 Aug, 76, (2): 115-111. AI-CTD BACKGROUND/immune effects.

Kaufman, R. L., Tong, I., and Beardmore, T. D. Prosthetic synovitis: Clinical and histologic characteristics. J. Rheumatol. 1985, 12, (6): 1066-1074. IMMUNE EFFECTS.

Keesey, J., Lindstrom, J., Cokely, H., and Herrmann, C. Anti-acetylcholine receptor antibody in neonatal myasthenia gravis. N. Engl. J. Med. 1977, 296, 55. CHILDREN'S EFFECTS/breast feeding.

Kelly Jr., A. P., Jacobson, H. S., Fox, J. I., and Jenny, H. Complications of subcutaneous mastectomy and replacement by the Cronin silastic mammary prosthesis. Plastic and Reconstructive Surgery. 1966, 37, (5): 438-445. RECONSTRUCTION.

Kelsey, J. L. Breast cancer epidemiology: Summary and future directions. Epidemiologic Reviews. 1993, 15, 256-263. CANCER.

Kennan, J. J., Peters, Y. A., Swarthout, D. E., Owen, M. J., Namkanisorn, A., and Chaudhury, M. K. Effect of saline exposure on the surface and bulk properties of medical grade silicone elastomers. J Biomed Mater Res. 1997, 36, 487-497. SILICONE CHARACTERIZATION/toxicology.

Kennedy, C., and Swinger, H. Eosinophilia of the cerebrospinal fluid: Late reaction to a silicone shunt. Developmental Medicine Child Neurology. 1988, 30, 378-390. IMMUNE EFFECTS/neurologic disease/children's effects.

Kennedy, G. L., Keplinger, M. L., and Calandra, J. C. Reproductive, teratologic and mutagenic studies with some polydimethylsiloxanes. Journal of Toxicology and Environmental Health. 1976 Jul, 1, 909-920. TOXICOLOGY/children's effects.

Kent, K., Ziegel, R. F., Kent, K., Frost, A. L., and Schaaf, N. G. Controlling the porosity and density of silicone rubber prosthetic materials. The Journal of Prosthetic Dentistry. 1983 Aug, 50, (2): 230-236. SILICONE CHARACTERIZATION.

Kerlikowske, K. Efficacy of screening mammography among women 48-49 years and 50-59 years: Comparison of relative and absolute benefit. Natl. Cancer Inst., Monogr. 1997, 22, 79-86. MAMMOGRAPHY.

Kern, K. A., Flannery, J. T., and Kuehn, P. G. Carcinogenic potential of silicone breast implants: A Connecticut statewide study. Plast. Reconstr. Surg. 1997 Sep, 100, (3): 737-747. CANCER.

Kern, S. F., Anderson, R. C., and Harris, P. N. Observations on the toxicity of methylsilicone. Journal of Am. Pharm. Assoc. 1949, 38, (10): 575-576. TOXICOLOGY.

Kessler, D. A. Special Report: The basis of the FDA's decision on breast implants. New England Journal of Medicine. 1992 Jun 18, 326, (25): 1713-1715. GENERAL.

Khan, A., Hill, J. M., Grater, W., Loeb, E., MacLellan, A., and Hill, N. Atopic hypersensitivity to *cis*-dichlorodiammineplatinum (II) and other platinum complexes. Cancer Research. 1975 Oct, 35, 2766-2770. PLATINUM/toxicology.

Khoo, A., Kroll, S. S., Reece, G. P., Miller, M. J., Evans, G. R. D., Robb, G. L., Baldwin, B. J., Wang, B., and Schusterman, M. A. A comparison of resource costs of immediate and delayed breast reconstruction. Plast. Reconstr. Surg. 1998 Apr, 101, (4): 964-968. RECONSTRUCTION.

Kidder, L. H., Kalasinsky, V. F., Luke, J. L., Levin, I. W., and Lewis, E. N. Visualization of silicone gel in human breast tissue using new infrared imaging spectroscopy. Nature Medicine. 1997 Feb, 3, (2): 235-237. SILICON MEASUREMENT/migration.

Kilodny, R. C., Jacobs, L. S., and Daughaday, W. H. Mammary stimulation causes prolactin secretion in non-lactating women. Nature. 1972, 238, 284. BREAST FEEDING/local complications.

Kim, D. W., and Harris, J. P. Risk of progressive sensorineural hearing loss and Menier's disease after breast implantation. Otolaryngology-Head and Neck Surgery. 1998 Jun, 118, (6): 747-750. NEUROLOGIC DISEASE.

Kim, K. S., Hong, C., and Futress, J. W. Histomorphologic changes in expanded skeletal muscle in rats. Plast. Reconstr. Surg. 1993, 92, 710. EXPANDER.

Kimura, W. K., Treon, J. F., and Bensen, T. R. Therapeutic use of methylpolysiloxane. Cur. Ther. Res. 1964, 6, 202. TOXICOLOGY.

Kincaid, S. B. Breast reconstruction: A Review. Annals of Plastic Surgery. May1984, 12, (5): 431-448. GENERAL.

King, E. J., Mohanty, G. P., Harrison, C. V., and Nagelschmidt, G. The action of different forms of pure silica on the lungs of rats. British Journal of Industrial Medicine. 1953, 10, 9017. SILICA.

Kircher, T. Silicone lymphadenopathy: A complication of silicone elastomer finger joint prostheses. Human Pathology. 1980 May, 11, (3): 240-244. LYMPHADENOPATHY/local complications.

Kirsner, R. S., and Falanga, V. Features of an autoimmune process in mid-dermal elastolysis. Journal of the American Academy of Dermatology. 1992, 27, (5 (Part 2)): 832-834. IMMUNE EFFECTS.

Kissin, M. W., and Kark, A. E. Late leakage of saline-filled breast prosthesis. Archives of Surgery. 1983 Jun, 118, (6): 769. CAPSULE-CONTRACTURE/rupture/local complications.

Kitazawa, T., Shuman, H., and Somlyo, A. P. Quantitative electron probe analysis: Problems and solutions. Ultramicroscopy. 1983, 11, 251-262. SILICON MEASUREMENT.

Kitchen, S. B., Paletta, C. E., Shehadi, S. I., and Bauer, W. C. Epithelialization of the lining of a breast implant capsule. Cancer. 1994 Mar 1, 73, (5): 1449-1452. CAPSULE-CONTRACTURE/local complications/granulomas/cancer.

Kjøller, K. H., Krag, C., and Friis, S. Silicone breast implants and breast cancer. Ugeskr Laeger. 1997, 159, (12): 1744-1748. CANCER.

Kjoller, K., McLaughlin, J. K., Friis, S., Blot, W. J., Mellemkjar, L., Hogsted, C., Winther, J. F., and Olsen, J. H. Health outcomes in offspring of mothers with breast implants. Pediatrics. 1998 Nov, 102, (5): 1112-1115. CHILDREN'S EFFECTS.

Klajman, A., Kafri, B., Shobat, J., Drucher, I., Moalem, T., and Jaretzky, A. The prevalence of antibodies to histones induced by procainamide in old people, in cancer patients, and in rheumatoid-like disease. Clin. Immunol. Immunopathol. 1983, 27, (1): 1-83. AI-CTD BACKGROUND.

Klamer, T. W., Donegan, W. L., and Max, M. H. Breast tumor incidence in rats after partial mammary resection. Archives of Surgery. 1983 Aug, 118, 933-935. CANCER.

Klein, E. E., and Kuske, R. R. Changes in photon dose distributions due to breast prostheses. I. J. Radiation Oncology. 1993, 25, (3): 541-549. RADIATION.

Kling, E., Bieg, S., Boehme, M., and Scherbaum, W. Circulating intercellular adhesion molecule 1 as a new activity marker in patients with systemic lupus erythematosus. The Clinical Investigator. 1993, 71, 299-304. AI-CTD BACKGROUND.

Klockars, M., Koskela, R-S., Jarvinen, E., Kolari, P. J., and Rossi, A. Silica exposure and rheumatoid arthritis: A follow up study of granite workers 1940-81. British Medical Journal. 1987 Apr 18, 294, 997-1000. SILICA.

Kneafsey, B., Crawford, D. S., Khoo, C. T., and Saad, M. N. Correction of developmental breast abnormalities with a permanent expander/implant. British Journal of Plastic Surgery. 1996 Jul, 49, (5): 302-306. EXPANDER.

Knize, D. M. Silicone breast implants—a cancer threat? Colorado Medicine. 1988 Dec 1: 487. CANCER.

Ko, C. Y., Ahn, C. Y., Ko, J., Chopra, W., and Shaw, W. W. Capsular synovial metaplasia as a common response to both textured and smooth implants. Plast. Reconstr. Surg. 1996 Jun, 97, (7): 1427-1433. PAIN/capsule-contracture/local complications/polyurethane.

Ko, C. Y., Ahn, C. Y., and Markowitz, B. L. Injected liquid silicone, chronic mastitis, and undetected breast cancer. Annals of Plastic Surgery. 1995 Feb, 34, (2): 176-179. SILICONE INJECTION/cancer.

Kobayashi, S., Isase, H., Karamatsu, S., and et al. A case of stromal sarcoma of the breast occurring after augmentation mammaplasty. Japanese Journal of Cancer Clinics. 1988, 34a, 467-472. CANCER.

Koch, A., Kunkel, S., Burrows, J., Evanoff, H., Haines, G., Pope, R., and Strrieter, R. Synovial tissue macrophage as a source of the chemotactic cytokine IL-8. Journal of Immunology. 1991 Oct 1, 147, (7): 2187-2195. CONNECTIVE TISSUE DISEASE/immune effects.

Koeger, A. C., Alcaix, D., Milleron, B., and et al. Silica and connective tissue diseases: A study of twenty-four cases. Medicine. 1995, 74, 221. SILICA.

Koeger, A. C., and Bourgeois, P. Systemic manifestations after silicone breast implants. Revue du Rhumatisme. 1993 Feb, 60, 120-126. CONNECTIVE TISSUE DISEASE.

Koeger, A.-C., Lang, T., Alcaix, D., Milleron, B., Rozenberg, S., Chaibi, P., Arnaud, J., Mayaud, C., Camus, J.-P., and Bourgeois, P. Silica-associated connective tissue disease. Medicine. 1995, 74, (5): 221-237. SILICA/connective tissue disease.

Koeger, A. C., Wrona, N., Sitbon, E., and Nicoletis, C. Maladies auto-immunes associees aux protheses mammaires en silicone. Chirurgie. 1993, 119, 618-625. IMMUNE EFFECTS/CONNECTIVE TISSUE DISEASE.

Koide, T., and Katayama, H. Calcification in augmentation mammoplasty. Radiology. 1979 Feb, 130, (2): 337-338. CALCIFICATION/mammography.

Kolodny, R. C., Jacobs, L. S., and Daughaday, W. H. Mammary stimulation causes prolactin secretion in non-lactating women. Nature. 1972 Aug 4, 238, 284-286. BREAST FEEDING/local complications.

Konstantinov, K., von mikecz, A., Buchwald, D., Jones, J., Gerace, L., and Tan, E. M. Autoantibodies to nuclear envelope antigens in chronic fatigue syndrome. Journal Of Clinical Investigation. 1996 Oct, 98, (8): 1888-1896. AI-CTD BACKGROUND/immune effects.

Kopans, D. B. Problems with the American College of Radiology *Standard for Diagnostic Mammography*. AJR American Journal of Roentgenology. 1995 Dec, 165, 1367-1369. MAMMOGRAPHY.

Kopans, D. B. Screening for breast cancer and mortality reduction among women 40-49 years of age. Cancer. 1994 Jul 1, 74, (1 (Supplement)): 311-322. CANCER/mammography.

Kopans, D. B., Meyer, J. E., and Lindfors, K. K. Whole breast US imaging: Four-year follow-up. Radiology. 1985, 157, (2): 505-507. MAMMOGRAPHY.

Kopans, D. B., Moore, R. H., McCarthy, K. A., Hall, D. A., Hulka, C. A., Whitman, G. J., Slanetz, P. J., and Halpern, E. F. Should women with implants or a history of treatment for breast cancer be excluded from mammography screening programs? AJR American Journal of Roentgenology. 1997 Jan, 168, (1): 29-31. MAMMOGRAPHY.

Kopf, E. H. Injectable silicones. Rocky Mountain Medical Journal. 1966 Mar, 63, (3): 34-36. SILICONE INJECTION.

Kopf, E. H., Vinnik, C. A., and Bongiovi, J. J. et al. The complications of silicone injections. Rocky Mountain Medical Journal. 1976, 22, 281-285. SILICONE INJECTION.

Korman, N. J., Sudilovsky, O., and Gibbons, D. F. A model for the production of large volume exudate from the implant-tissue interface. Journal of Biomedical Materials Research. 1982, 16, 87-91. SILICONE CHARACTERIZATION/toxicology.

Kossoff, G., Fry, E. K., and Jelllins, J. Average velocity of ultrasound in the human female breast. The Journal of the Acoustical Society of America. 1973, 53, (6): 1730-1736. MAMMOGRAPHY.

Kossovsky, N. The demise of the non-specific foreign body giant cell reaction. Trends in Polymer Science. 1993, 1, 190-191. IMMUNE EFFECTS.

Kossovsky, N. Ventricular shunt failure: Evidence of immunologic sensitization. Surgical Forum. 1983, 34, 527-528. IMMUNE EFFECTS.

Kossovsky, N., Cole, P., and Zackson, D. A. Giant cell myocarditis associated with silicone: an unusual case of biomaterials pathology discovered at autopsy using X-ray energy spectroscopic techniques. Am J Clin Pathol. 1990, 93, (1): 148-152. TOXICOLOGY.

Kossovsky, N., and Dujovny, M. Reporting the failure of medical devices. The New England Journal of Medicine. 1985 Feb, 312, (7): 447. GENERAL.

Kossovsky, N., Freeman, C. J., Stassi, J. B., and Mena, E. Cytokine expression in response to biomaterials. Immunomethods. 1993, 3, 43-49. IMMUNE EFFECTS.

Kossovsky, N., and Freiman, C. J. Immunology of silicone breast implants. Journal of Biomaterials Applications. 1994, 8, (3): 237-246. IMMUNE EFFECTS.

Kossovsky, N., and Freiman, C. J. Physicochemical and immunological basis of silicone pathophysiology. Journal of Biomater. Sci. Polym. Ed. 1995, 7, (2): 101-113. IMMUNE EFFECTS.

Kossovsky, N., and Freiman, C. J. Review—physiochemical and immunological basis of silicone pathophysiology. Journal of Biomaterials Science Polymer Edition. 1995, 7, (2): 101-113. IMMUNE EFFECTS.

Kossovsky, N., and Freiman, C. J. Silicone breast implant pathology: Clinical data and immunologic consequences. Archives of Pathology and Laboratory Medicine. 1994 Jul, 118, (7): 686-693. GENERAL/immune effects.

Kossovsky, N., Gornbein, J. A., Zeidler, M., Stassi, J., Chun, G., Papasian, N., Nguyen, R., Ly, K., and Rajguru, S. Self-reported signs and symptoms in breast implant patients with novel antibodies to silicone surface associated antigens [anti-SSAA(x)]. Journal of Applied Biomaterials. 1995, 6, (4): 153-160. CONNECTIVE TISSUE DISEASE/immune effects.

Kossovsky, N., Heggers, J. P., Parsons, R. W., and Robson, M. C. Acceleration of capsule formation around silicone implants by infection in a guinea pig model. Plast. Reconstr. Surg. 1984 Jan, 73, (1): 91-96. INFECTION/capsule-contracture/local complications.

Kossovsky, N., Heggers, J. P., and Robson, M. C. Experimental demonstration of the immunogenicity of silicone-protein complexes. J Biomed Materials Research. 1987, 21, 1125-1133. IMMUNE EFFECTS.

Kossovsky, N., Heggers, J. P., Robson, M. C., and Ellis, J. T. Delayed hypersensitivity to silicone products. Materials Sciences and Implant Orthopedic Surgery. 1998, 116, 283-305. IMMUNE EFFECTS.

Kossovsky, N., and Papasian, N. Mammary implants: A clinical review. Journal of Applied Biomaterials. 1992 Sep, 3, 239-242. GENERAL.

Kossovsky, N., and Stassi, J. A pathophysiologic examination of the biophysics and bioreactivity of silicone breast implants. Seminars in Arthritis and Rheumatism. 1994 Aug, 24, (1 (Supplement 1)): 18-21. GENERAL.

Kossovsky, N., and Zeidler, M. Protein denaturation by silicone adjuvant in humans: Human serum IgG show high avidity to matrix proteins following in vivo exposure to silicone. 1993 Apr 19. IMMUNE EFFECTS.

Kossovsky, N., Zeidler, M., Chun, G., and et al. Surface dependent antigens identified by high binding avidity of serum antibodies in a subpopulation of patients with breast prostheses. J Appl Biomaterials. 1993 Dec, 4, 281-288. IMMUNE EFFECTS.

Kotzin, B. L. Twins and t-cell responses. Nature 364:(15):187-188. 1993 Jul. IMMUNE EFFECTS.

Kozeny, G. A., Barbato, a. L., Bansal, V. K., Vertuno, L. L., and Hano, J. E. Hypercalcemia associated with silicone-induced granulomas. The New England Journal of Medicine. 1984 Oct 25, 311, (17): 1103-1105. GRANULOMAS/local complications.

Kraemer, O., Andersen, M., and Siim, E. Breast reconstruction and tissue expansion in irradiated versus not irradiated women after mastectomy. Scand. J. Plast. Reconstr. Hand Surg. 1996, 30, 201-206. RADIATION/reconstruction.

Krishnan, L., and Krishnan, E. C. Electronic beam irradiation after reconstruction with silicone gel implant in breast cancer. American Journal of Clinical Oncology. 1986, 9, (3): 223-226. RADIATION/cancer/reconstruction.

Krishnan, L., Krishnan, E. C., Wolf, C. D., and Jewell, W. R. Preservation of augmented breasts in patients with breast cancer. RadioGraphics. 1993, 13, (4): 831-839. RADIATION/reconstruction.

Krishnan, L., St. George, F. J., Mansfield, C. M., and Krishnan, E. C. Effect of silicone gel breast prosthesis on electron and photon dose distribution. Medical Physics. 1983 Jan-1983 Feb 28, 10, (1): 96-99. RADIATION/reconstruction.

Kroll, S. S., and Baldwin, B. A. A comparison of outcomes using three different methods of breast reconstruction. Plast. Reconstr. Surg. 1992 Sep, 90, (3): 455-462. RECONSTRUCTION/expander.

Kroll, S. S., Evans, G. R. D., Reece, G. P., Miller, M. J., Robb, G., Baldwin, B. J., and Schusterman, M. A. Comparison of resource costs between implant-based and TRAM flap breast reconstruction. Plast. Reconstr. Surg. 1996 Feb, 97, (2): 364-373. RECONSTRUCTION.

Kroner, K., Knudsen, U. B., Lundby, L., and Hvid, H. Long-term phantom breast syndrome after mastectomy. The Clinical Journal of Pain. 1992, 8, 346-350. PAIN.

Ksander, G. A. Effects of diffused soluble steroid on capsules around experimental breast prostheses in rats. Plast. Reconstr. Surg. 1979 May, 63, (5): 708. STEROIDS/local complications/capsule-contracture.

Ksander, G. A., and Gray, L. Reduced capsule formation around soft silicone rubber prostheses coated with solid collagen. Annals of Plastic Surgery. 1985, 14, 351-358. CAPSULE-CONTRACTURE/local complications.

Ksander, G. A., and Vistnes, L. M. Collagen and glycosaminoglycans in capsules around silicone implants. Journal of Surgical Research. 1981, 31, 433-439. CAPSULE-CONTRACTURE/local complications.

Ksander, G. A., and Vistnes, L. M. The incidence of experimental contracture varies with the source of the prosthesis. Plast. Reconstr. Surg. 1985 May, 75, (5): 668-676. CAPSULE-CONTRACTURE/local complications.

Ksander, G. A., Vistnes, L. M., and Fogarty, D. C. Experimental effects on surrounding fibrous capsule formation from placing steroid in a silicone bag-gel prosthesis before implantation. Plast. Reconstr. Surg. 1978, 62, (6): 873-884. CAPSULE-CONTRACTURE/local complications/steroids.

Ksander, G. A., Vistnes, L. M., and Kosek, J. Effect of implant location on compressibility and capsule formation around miniprostheses in rats, and experimental capsule contracture. Annals of Plastic Surgery. 1981 Mar, 6, 182-193. CAPSULE-CONTRACTURE/local complications.

Kuhn, D. C., and Demers, L. M. Influence of mineral dust surface chemistry on eicosanoid production by the alveolar macrophage. Journal of Toxicology and Environmental Health. 1992, 35, 39-50. SILICA.

Kuiper, D. H. Silicone granulomatous disease of the breast simulating cancer. Michigan Medicine. 1973 Mar: 215-218. SILICONE INJECTION/cancer/granulomas/local complications.

Kulber, D. A., Mackenzie, D., Steiner, J. H., Glassman, H., Hopp, D., Hiatt, J. R., and Hoffman, L. Monitoring the axilla in patients with silicone gel implants. Annals of Plastic Surgery. 1995 Dec, 35, (6): 580-584. MIGRATION/local complications/mammography/lymphadenopathy.

Kumagai, Y., Abe, C., Hirano, T., Fukuda, Y., and Shiokawa, Y. Mixed connective tissue disease after breast augmentation which terminated in scleroderma kidney: an autopsy case report of human adjuvant disease. The Ryumachi. 1981, 21 (Suppl), 171-176. CONNECTIVE TISSUE DISEASE.

Kumagai, Y., Abe, C., and Shiokawa, Y. Scleroderma after cosmetic surgery: Four cases of human adjuvant disease. Arthritis and Rheumatism. 1979 May, 22, (5): 532-537. SILICONE INJECTION/connective tissue disease.

Kumagai, Y., Shiokawa, Y., Medsger Jr., T. A., and Rodnan, G. P. Clinical spectrum of connective tissue disease after cosmetic surgery: Observations on eighteen patients and a review of the Japanese literature. Arthritis and Rheumatism. 1984 Jan, 27, (1): 1-12. CONNECTIVE TISSUE DISEASE/silicone injection.

Kuske, R. R., Schuster, R., Klein, E., Young, L., Perez, C. A., and Fineberg, B. Radiotherapy and breast reconstruction: Clinical results and dosimetry. Int J Radiation Oncology Biol Phys. 1991 Jul, 21, (2): 339-346. RADIATION/pain/capsule-contracture/local complications/reconstruction.

Kyle, R. A. Benign monoclonal gammopathy—After 20 to 35 years of follow-up. Mayo Clinic Proceedings. 1993, 68, 26-36. MYELOMA.

Laban, E., and Kon, M. Lesion of the long thoracic nerve during the axillary breast augmentation: An unusual complication. Plastic and Reconstructive Surgery. 1990, 24, 445-446. SENSATION/local complications.

Labow, R. S., Meek, E., and Santerre, J. P. Differential synthesis of cholesterol esterase by monocyte-derived macrophages cultured on poly(ether or ester)-based poly(urethanes)s. J Biomed Mater Res. 1998, 39, 469-477. TOXICOLOGY.

Ladin, D. A., Saed, G. M., and Fivenson, D. P. T-cell response in silicone gel breast implant capsules. Surgical Forum. 1994, 45, 730-731. IMMUNE EFFECTS.

Lafreniere, R., and Ketcham, A. S. Breast carcinoma post-augmentation mammaplasty: Therapy with limited surgery and radiation. Journal of Surgical Oncology. 1987, 35, 99-103. CANCER.

Lahey, F. H. Further experiences with injured bile ducts. Journal of Medicine. 1949, 240, (5): 161-168. GENERAL.

Lai, Y-F, Chao, T-Y, and Wong, S-L. Acute pneumonitis after subcutaneous injections of silicone for augmentation mammaplasty. Chest. 1994, 106, (4): 1152-1155. SILICONE INJECTION.

Laitung, J. K. G., McClure, J., and Shuttleworth, C. A. The fibrous capsules around static and dynamic implants: Their biochemical, histological, and ultrastructural characteristics. Annals of Plastic Surgery. 1987 Sep, 19, (3): 208-214. CAPSULE-CONTRACTURE/local complications.

Lamm, S. H. Silicone breast implants and long-term health effects: When are data adequate? Journal of Clinical Epidemiology. 1995, 48, (4): 507-511. GENERAL.

Lamm, S. H. Silicone breast implants, breast cancer and specific connective tissue diseases: A systematic review of the data in the epidemiological literature. International Journal of Toxicology. 1998, 17, 497-527. CONNECTIVE TISSUE DISEASE/cancer.

Lamm, S. H., and Engel, A. Human breast sarcoma incidence and silicone breast implantation rates: A comparison. J Clin Res Drug Dev. 1989, 3, 218-219. CANCER/prevalence.

Landon, B. N., Dobke, M. K., Grzybowski, J., Virden, C. P., Dobak, J., and Steinsapir, E. S. Enhanced activity of lyosomal beta-galactosidase following silicone implantation: An experimental study in rats. J Lab Clin Med. 1993, 121, (6): 742-750. IMMUNE EFFECTS.

Lantieri, L. A., Roudot-Thoraval, F., Collins, E. D., Raulo, Y., and Baruch, J. P. Influence of underfilling on breast implant deflation. Plast. Reconstr. Surg. 1997 Dec, 100, (7): 1740-1744. RUPTURE/local complications/saline.

Lapin, R., Daniel, D., Hutchins, H., and Justice, G. Primary breast reconstruction following mastectomy using a skin-expander prosthesis. Diseases of the Breast. 1980, 6, (2): 20-24. EXPANDER/reconstruction.

Lappe, M. A. Causal inference in syndromes associated with silicone breast implants: Psychogenic and environmental factors. International Journal of Occupational Medicine and Toxicology. 1995, 4, (1): 165-175. IMMUNE EFFECTS/PSYCHOSOCIAL.

Lappe, M. A. Silicone-reactive disorder: A new autoimmune disease caused by immunostimulation and superantigens. Medical Hypotheses. 1993, 41, 348-352. CONNECTIVE TISSUE DISEASE/immune effects.

Lappert, M. F., and Scott, F. P. A. Preliminary communication. The reaction pathway from Speier's to Karstedt's hydrosilylation catalyst. The Journal of Organometallic Chemistry. 1995, 492, C11-C13. PLATINUM.

Larson, D. L., Anderson, R. C., Maksud, D., and Grunert, B. K. What influences public perceptions of silicone breast implants? Plastic and Reconstructive Surgery. 1994 Aug, 94, (2): 318-325. PSYCHOSOCIAL.

Laughlin, R. A., Raynor, A. C., and Habal, B. M. Complications of closed capsulotomies after augmentation mammoplasty. Plast. Reconstr. Surg. 1977, 60, (3): 362-363. CLOSED CAPSULOTOMY/local complications.

Lavey, E. B., and Pearl, R. M. Inflammation in a silicone-induced granuloma caused by a tuberculosis skin test. Annals of Plastic Surgery. 1981 Aug, 7, (2): 152-154. SILICONE INJECTION/immune effects/granulomas.

Lavine, D. M. Saline inflatable prostheses: 14 years' experience. Aesthetic Plastic Surgery. 1993, 17, 325-330. CAPSULE-CONTRACTURE/local complications/hematomas/rupture/saline.

Lawrence, R. Breastfeeding and medical disease. Medical Clinics of North America. 1989, 73, 583-603. BREAST FEEDING.

Lawrence, R. C., Hochberg, M. C., Kelsey, J. L., and et al. Estimates of the prevalence of selected arthritic and musculoskeletal diseases in the United States. Journal of Rheumatology. 1989, 16, (4): 427-441. AI-CTD BACKGROUND.

Lawrie, S., and Pelosi, A. Chronic fatigue syndrome in the community. Prevalence and associations. British Journal of Psychiatry. 1995, 166, (6): 793-797. AI-CTD BACKGROUND.

Lazaro, M. A., Morteo, D. G., DeBenyacar, M. A., Paira, S. O., Lema, B., Morteo, O. G., and Cocco, M. Lymphadenopathy secondary to silicone hand joint prostheses. Clinical and Experimental Rheumatology. 1990, 8, 17-22. LYMPHADENOPATHY/local complications.

Le Fevre, R., Coulston, F., and Goldberg, L. Action of a copolymer of mixed phenylmethylcyclosiloxanes on reproduction in rats and rabbits. Toxicology and Applied Pharmacology. 1972, 21, 29-44. TOXICOLOGY.

Le Vier, R. R., Bennett, D. R., and Hunter, M. J. Effects of oral 2,6-*cis*-diphenylhexamethylcyclotetrasiloxane on the reproductive system of the male *Macaca mulatta*. Acta Pharmacologica et Toxicologica. 1975 Jan 1, Vol 36, Supp. III, 68-80, Chapter VIII. TOXICOLOGY.

Le Vier, R. R., and Jankowiak, M. E. The hormonal and antifertility activity of 2,6-*cis*-diphenylhexamethylcyclotetrasiloxane in the female rat. Acta Pharmacologica et Toxicologica. 1975 Jan 1, Vol 36, Supp. III, 81-92, Chapter Viii. TOXICOLOGY.

Lebovic, G. S. Silicone autoimmune disease. Diseases of the Breast. 1996: 620-628, Ch. 19. GENERAL/CONNECTIVE TISSUE DISEASE.

Lee, C. L., Polmanteer, K. E., and King, E. G. Flow behavior of narrow-distribution polydimethylsiloxane. J. Polymer. Sci. A2. 1970, 8, 1909. SILICONE CHARACTERIZATION.

Lee, D., Goldstein, E. J., and Zarem, H. A. Localized *Mycobacterium avium*-intracellulare mastitis in an immunocompetent woman with silicone breast implants. Plastic and Reconstructive Surgery. 1995, 95, (1): 142-144. INFECTION/local complications.

Lee, S.-L., Tsay, G. J., and Tsai, R.-T. Anticentromere antibodies in subjects with no apparent connective tissue diseases. Ann. Rheum. Dis. 1993, 52, 586-589. AI-CTD BACKGROUND.

Lees-Haley, P. R. Contamination of neuropsychological testing by litigation. Forensic Reports. 1990, 3, 421-426. PSYCHOSOCIAL.

LeFevre, R., Coulston, F., and Goldberg, L. Action of a copolymer of mixed phenylmethylcyclosiloxanes on reproduction in rats and rabbits. Toxicology and Applied Pharmacology. 1972, 21, 29-44. TOXICOLOGY.

Leff, R. L., Burgess, S. H., Miller, F. W., Love, L. A., Targoff, I. N., Dalakas, M. C., Joffe, M. M., and Plotz, P. H. Distinct seasonal patterns in the onset of adult idiopathic inflammatory myopathy in patients with anti-Jo-1 and anti-signal recognition particle autoantibodies. Arthritis and Rheumatism. 1991, 34, (11): 1391-1396. IMMUNE EFFECTS/CONNECTIVE TISSUE DISEASE.

Lefkowitz, D. L., Mills, K., Lefkowitz, S. S., Bollen, A., and Moguilvesky, N. Neutrophil-macrophage interaction: A paradigm for chronic inflammation. Medical Hypotheses. 1995 Jan, 44, 58-62. AI-CTD BACKGROUND.

Leibman, A. J. Imaging of complications of augmentation mammaplasty. Plast. Reconstr. Surg. 1994 May, 93, (6): 1134-1139. MAMMOGRAPHY.

Leibman, A. J., Kossoff, M. B., and Kruse, B. D. Intraductal extension of silicone from a ruptured breast implant. Plast. Reconstr. Surg. 1992, 89, (3): 546-547. RUPTURE/local complications/closed capsulotomy/migration.

Leibman, A. J., and Kruse, B. Breast cancer: Mammographic and sonographic findings after augmentation mammoplasty. Radiology. 1990, 174, 195. MAMMOGRAPHY.

Leibman, A. J., and Kruse, B. D. Imaging of breast cancer after augmentation mammaplasty. Annals of Plastic Surgery. 1993 Feb, 30, (2): 111-115. MAMMOGRAPHY/cancer.

Leibman, A. J., and Sybers, R. Mammographic and sonographic findings after silicone injection. Annals of Plastic Surgery. 1994 Oct, 33, (4): 412-414. SILICONE INJECTION/mammography.

Leighton, W. D., Russel, R. C., Feller, A. M., Eriksson, E., Mathur, A., and Zook, D. G. Experimental pretransfer expansion of free-flap donor sites: II physiology, histology, and clinical correlation. Plast. Reconstr. Surg. 1988, 82, 76. EXPANDER.

Leininger, R. I., Mirkovitch, V., Peters, A., and Hawks, W. A. Change in properties of plastics during implantation. Trans. Amer. Soc. Artif. Int. Organs. 1964, 10, 320-322. SILICONE CHARACTERIZATION.

Lemen, J. K. Rabbit Teratology Study via Surgical Implant. Vienna, Va.: 1991 Apr 29. TOXICOLOGY.

Lemperle, G. Unfavorable results after breast reconstruction with silicone breast. Acta Chirurgica Belgica. 1980 Mar, 79, (2): 159-160. STEROIDS/local complications/reconstruction.

Lemperle, G., and Exner, K. Effect of cortisone on capsular contracture in double-lumen breast implants: Ten years' experience. Aesthetic Plastic Surgery. 1993 Jan, 17, 317-323. CAPSULE-CONTRACTURE/local complications/steroids.

Leong, A. Pathologic findings in silicone spallation: Autopsy and biopsy studies. Annals Academy of Medicine. 1983 Apr, 12, (2): 304-310. LOCAL COMPLICATIONS.

Leong, A. S. Y., Disney, A. P. S., and Gove, D. W. Spallation and migration of silicone from blood-pump tubing in patients on hemodialysis. The New England Journal of Medicine. 1982 Jan 21, 306, (3): 135-140. SILICONE CHARACTERIZATION/granulomas/local complications/general.

Lerner, M. R., and Steitz, J. A. Antibodies to small nuclear RNAs complexed with proteins are produced by patients with systemic lupus erythematosus. Proceedings of the National Academy of Sciences USA. 1979, 76, 5495-5497. AI-CTD BACKGROUND.

LeRoy, E. C., Maricq, H. R., and Kahaleh, M. B. Undifferentiated connective tissue syndromes. Arthritis and Rheumatism. 1980 Mar, 23, (3): 341-343. AI-CTD BACKGROUND.

Lesesne, C. B. Textured surface silicone breast implants: Histology in the human. Aesthetic Plastic Surgery. 1997, 21, (2): 93-96. CAPSULE-CONTRACTURE/local complications.

Lesser, M. Silicones in medicine and pharmacy. Drug Cosmetic Ind. 1953, 72, (5): 516. SILICONE CHARACTERIZATION.

Letterman, G. S., and Schurter, M. Total mammary gland excision with immediate breast reconstruction. The American Surgeon. 1955, 21, (8): 835-844. RECONSTRUCTION.

Leung, F. Y., and Edmond, P. Determination of silicon in serum and tissue by electrothermal atomic absorption spectrometry. Clinical Biochemistry. 1997 Jul, 30, (5): 399-403. SILICON MEASUREMENT.

Levenson, T., Greenberger, P. A., and Murphy, R. Peripheral blood eosinophilia, hyperimmunoglobulinemia A and fatigue: Possible complications following rupture of silicone breast implants. Ann Allergy Asthma Immunol. 1996 Aug, 77, (2): 119-122. CONNECTIVE TISSUE DISEASE/rupture/local complications.

LeVier, R. R. Distribution of silicon in the adult rat and rhesus monkey. Bioinorganic Chemistry. 1975, 4, 109-115. SILICON MEASUREMENT.

LeVier, R. R., Bennett, D. R., and Hunter, M. J. Effects of oral 2,6-cis-diphenylhexamethylcyclotetrasiloxane on the reproductive system of the male *Macaca mulata*. Acta Pharmacologica et Toxicologica. 1975, 36, (Supplement III): 68-80. TOXICOLOGY.

LeVier, R. R., and Boley, W. F. The antigonadotrophic activity of an organosiloxane in the male rat: 2,6-cis-diphenylhexamethylcyclotetrasiloxane. Acta Pharmacologica et Toxicologica. 1975, 36, (Supplement III): 55-67. TOXICOLOGY.

LeVier, R. R., Harrison, M. C., Cook, R. R., and Lane, T. H. What is Silicone? Plast. Reconstr. Surg. 1993 Jul, 92, (1): 163-167. SILICONE CHARACTERIZATION/silica.

LeVier, R. R., Harrison, M. C., Cook, R. R., and Lane, T. H. What is Silicone? Journal of Clinical Epidemiology. 1995, 48, (4): 513-517. SILICONE CHARACTERIZATION/silica.

LeVier, R. R., and Jankowiak, M. E. The hormonal and antifertility activity of 2,6-cis-diphenylhexamethylcyclotetrasiloxane in the female rat. Acta Pharmacologica et Toxicologica. 1975, 36, (Supplement III): 81-92. TOXICOLOGY.

Levine, J. J., and Ilowite, N. T. Sclerodermalike esophageal disease in children breast-fed by mothers with silicone breast implants. J. Amer. Med. Assoc. 1994 Jan 19, 271, (3): 213-216. CHILDREN'S EFFECTS/breast feeding/connective tissue disease.

Levine, J. J., Ilowite, N. T., Pettei, M. J., and Trachtman, H. Increased urinary NO(3)- + NO(2)- and Neopterin excretion in children breast fed by mothers with silicone breast implants: Evidence for macrophage activation. The Journal of Rheumatology. 1996, 23, (6): 1083-1087. BREAST FEEDING/children's effects.

Levine, J. J., Lin, H. C., Rowley, M., Cook, A., Teuber, S. S., and Illowite, N. T. Lack of autoantibody expression in children born to mothers with silicone breast implants. Pediatrics. 1996 Feb, 97, (2): 243-245. CHILDREN'S EFFECTS/immune effects/breast feeding.

Levine, J. J., Trachtman, H., Gold, D. M., and Pettei, M. J. Esophageal dysmotility in children breast-fed by mothers with silicone breast implants. Digestive Diseases and Sciences. 1996 Aug, 41, (8): 1600-1603. CHILDREN'S EFFECTS.

Levine, N. S., and Buchanan, R. T. Decreased swimming speed following augmentation mammaplasty. Plast. Reconstr. Surg. 1983 Feb, 72, (2): 255-256. GENERAL.

Levine, R. A., and Collins, T. L. Definitive diagnosis of breast implant rupture by ultrasonography. Plast. Reconstr. Surg. 1991 Jun, 87, (6): 1126-1128. MAMMOGRAPHY/local complications/rupture.

Lewin, S. L., and Miller, T. A. A review of epidemiologic studies analyzing the relationship between breast implants and connective tissue diseases. Plast. Reconstr. Surg. 1997 Oct, 100, (5): 1309-1313. CONNECTIVE TISSUE DISEASE.

Lewis, C. M. Inflammatory carcinoma of the breast following silicone injections. Plast. Reconstr. Surg. 1980 Jul, 66, (1): 134-136. CANCER/silicone injection.

Lewis, Jr. J. R. The augmentation mammoplasty (with special reference to alloplastic materials). Plast. Reconstr. Surg. 1965 Jan, 35, (1): 51-59. GENERAL/silicone injection.

Lewis, L. N. On the mechanism of metal colloid catalyzed hydrosilylation: Proposed explanations for electronic effects and oxygen cocatalysis. Journal of the American Chemical Society. 1990, 112, 5998-6004. SILICONE CHEMISTRY.

Lewis, L. N. Platinum-catalyzed hydrosilylation—colloid formation as the essential step. Journal of the American Chemical Society. 1986, 108, (23): 7228-7231. PLATINUM/silicone chemistry.

Lewis, L. N. et al. The effect of metal colloid morphology on catalytic activity: Further proof of the intermediacy of colloids in the rhodium-catalyzed hydrosilylation reaction. Journal of Molecular Catalysis. 1991, 66, 105-113. PLATINUM/silicone chemistry.

Lewis, L. N. et al. Platinum-catalyzed hydrosilylation of alkynes. Organometallics. 1991, 10, 3750-3759. PLATINUM/silicone chemistry.

Lewis, L. N. et al. Platinum catalyzed hydrosilylation of alkynes: Comparison of rates of addition of terminal olefins to internal alkynes. Journal of Organometallic Chemistry. 1992, 427, 165-172. PLATINUM/silicone chemistry.

Lewis, L. N., and Lewis, N. Preparation and structure of platinum group metal colloids: Without solvent. Chemistry of Materials. 1989, 1, 106-114. PLATINUM/silicone chemistry.

Lewis, L. N., Stein, J., Gao, Y., Colborn, R. E., and Hutchines, G. Platinum catalysts used in the silicones industry, their synthesis and activity in hydrosilation. Platinum Metals Review. 1997, 41, (2): 66-75. PLATINUM/toxicology/silicone chemistry.

Lewis, L. N., Uriarte, R. J., and Lewis, N. Metal colloid morphology and catalytic activity: Further proof of the intermediacy of colloids in the platinum-catalyzed hydrosilylation reaction. Journal of Catalysis. 1991, 127, 67-74. SILICONE CHEMISTRY/PLATINUM.

Lewis, L. N., and Uriate, R. J. Hydrosilylation catalyzed by metal colloids: a relative activity study. Organometallics. 1990, 9, 621-625. SILICONE CHEMISTRY/platinum.

Lewold, S., Olsson, H., Gustafson, Rydholm A., and Lidgren, L. Overall cancer incidence not increased after prosthetic knee replacement: 14,551 Patients followed for 66,662 person-years. Int. J Cancer. 1996, 68, 30-33. CANCER.

Liang, M. D., Narayanan, K., Ravilochan, K., and Roche, K. The permeability of tissue expanders to bacteria: An experimental study. Plast. Reconstr. Surg. 1993, 92, 1294. INFECTION/local complications/expander.

Lieberman, M. W., Lykissa, E. D., Barrios, R., Ou, C. N., Kala, G., and Kala, S. V. Cyclosiloxanes produce fatal liver and lung damage in mice. Environmental Health Perspectives. 1999 Feb, 107, (2). TOXICOLOGY.

Lilla, J. A., and Vistnes, L. M. Long-term study of reactions to various silicone breast implants in rabbits. Plast. Reconstr. Surg. 1976 May, 57, (5): 637-649. POLYURETHANE/toxicology.

Lin, K., Bartlett, S. P., Matsuo, K., LiVolsi, V. A., Parry, C., Hass, B., and Whitaker, L. A. Hyaluronic acid-filled mammary implants: An experimental study. Plast. Reconstr. Surg. 1994 Aug, 94, (2): 306-315. GENERAL.

Lin RP, DiLeonardo M, and Jacoby RA. Silicone lymphadenopathy. A case report and review of the literature. Am J Dermatopathol. 1993 Feb, 15, (1): 82-84. LYMPHADENOPATHY/local complications.

Lindbichler, F., Hoflehner, H., Schmidt, F., Pierer, G. R., Raith, J., Umschaden, J., and Preidler, K. W. Comparison of mammographic image quality in various methods of reconstructive breast surgery. European Radiology. 1996, 6, (6): 925-928. MAMMOGRAPHY/reconstruction.

Lipshutz, H. A clinical evaluation of subdermal and subcutaneous silicone implants. Plast. Reconstr. Surg. 1966 Mar, 37, (3): 249-250. GENERAL.

Liston, J. C., Malata, C. M., Varma, S., Scott, M., and Sharpe, D. T. The role of ultrasound imaging in the diagnosis of breast implant rupture: A prospective study. British Journal of Plastic Surgery. 1994, 47, 477-482. MAMMOGRAPHY/rupture/local complications.

Little, G., and Baker, J. L. Results of closed compression capsulotomy for treatment of contracted breast implant capsules. Plast. Reconstr. Surg. 1980 Jan, 65, (1): 30-33. CAPSULE-CONTRACTURE/local complications/closed capsulotomy.

Little, J. W. III, Golembe, E. V., and Fisher, J. B. The living bra in immediate and delayed reconstruction of the breast following mastectomy for malignant and nonmalignant disease. Plast. Reconstr. Surg. 1981 Sep, 68, (3): 392-403. RECONSTRUCTION.

Little, J. W., Munasifi, T., and McCulloch, D. T. One-stage reconstruction of a projecting nipple: the quadrapod flap. Plast. Reconstr. Surg. 1983 Jan, 71, (1): 126-132. RECONSTRUCTION.

Little, K., and Parkhouse, S. Tissue reactions to polymers. The Lancet. 1962 Oct 27, 2, 857-861. SILICONE CHARACTERIZATION/toxicology.

Liu, Le-Wen and Truong, L. D. Morphologic characterization of polyvinyl sponge (Ivalon) breast prosthesis. Arch. Pathol. Lab. Med. 1996 Sep, 120, 876-878. GENERAL.

Lloyd, A. R. Chronic fatigue and chronic fatigue syndrome: shifting boundaries and attributions. The American Journal of Medicine. 1998 Sep 28, 105, (3A): 7S-10S. AI-CTD BACKGROUND.

Loeng, A. S. Y., and Gove, D. W. Pathological findings in silicone spallation *in vitro* studies. Pathology. 1983, 15, 189-192. SILICON MEASUREMENT.

Loeser, E. Long-term toxicity and carcinogencitiy studies with 2,4/2,6-toluene-diisocyanate (80/20) in rats and mice. Toxicology Letters. 1983, 15, 71-81. TOXICOLOGY/carcinogenicity.

Logothetis, M. L. Women's reports of breast implant problems and silicone-related illness. J Obstet Gynecol Neonatal Nurs. 1995 Sep, 24, 609-616. CONNECTIVE TISSUE DISEASE/psychosocial.

Looney, R. J., Frampton, M. W., Byam, J., Kenaga, C., Speers, D. M., Cox, C., Mast, R., Klykken, P. C., Morrow, P. E., and Utell, M. J. Acute respiratory exposure of human volunteers to octamethylcyclotetrasiloxane (D4): absence of immunological effects. Toxicological Sciences. 1998, 44, 214-220. TOXICOLOGY.

Lorenz, R. The value of sonography for the discovery of complications after the implantation of silicone gel prostheses for breast augmentation or reconstruction. Rofo Fortschr Geb Rontgenstr Neuen Bildgeb Verfahr. 1997, 166, (3): 233-237. MAMMOGRAPHY/rupture/local complications.

Lossing, C., Elander, A., and Holmström, H. Capsular contracture after breast reconstruction with the lateral thoracodorsal flap. Aesthetic Plastic Surgery. 1989, 13, 81-84. RECONSTRUCTION/capsule-contracture/local complications.

Lossing, C., and Hansson, H. A. Peptide growth factors and myofibroblasts in capsules around human breast implants. Plast. Reconstr. Surg. 1993 Jun, 91, 1277-1286. CAPSULE-CONTRACTURE/local complications.

Lu, L. B., Ostermeyer Shoaib, B., and Patten, B. M. Atypical chest pain syndrome in patients with breast implants. Southern Medical Journal. 1994 Oct, 87, (10): 978-984. PAIN/local complications.

Ludgate, S. M. Silicone gel breast implants. Br J Theatre Nurs. 1994 Feb 1, 3, (11): 25. GENERAL.

Lugano, E. M., Dauber, J. H., Elias, J. A., Bashey, R. I., Jimenez, S. A., and Daniele, R. P. The regulation of lung fibroblast proliferation by alveolar macrophages in experimental silicosis. American Review of Respiratory Diseases. 1984, 129, 767-771. SILICA.

Lugowski, S. J., Smith, D. C., Lugowski, J. Z., Peters, W., and Semple, J. A review of silicon and silicone determination in tissue and body fluids—a need for standard reference materials. Fresenius Journal of Analytical Chemistry. 1998, 360, 486-488. SILICON MEASUREMENT/children's effects/breast feeding.

Luhan, J. E. Giant galactoceles, one month after bilateral augmentation mammoplasty, abdominoplasty, and tubal ligation: case study. Aesthetic. Plast. Surg. 1979, 3, 161-164. BREAST FEEDING.

Luke, J. L., Kalasinsky, V. F., Turnicky, R. P., Centeno, J. A., Johnson, F. B., and Mullick, F. G. Pathological and biophysical findings associated with silicone breast implants: A study of capsular tissues from 86 cases. Plast. Reconstr. Surg. 1997 Nov, 100, (6): 1558-1565. CAPSULE-CONTRACTURE/local complications/saline/polyurethane.

Lund, K., Ewertz, M., and Schou, G. Breast cancer incidence subsequent to surgical reduction of the female breast. Scandinavian Journal of Plastic and Reconstructive Surgery. 1987, 21, 209-212. CANCER.

Luo, Z.-J., and Lu, S.-B. Selective reinnervation of regenerating mixed nerve fibers across a silicone tube gap. Journal of Hand Surgery. 1996, 21, (5): 660-663. SILICONE CHARACTERIZATION/neurologic disease.

Luria, L. W., Carter, W. L., Kent, K., Mician, M., and Habal, M. B. Regarding the safety of silicone implants. Journal of the Florida Medical Association. 1991 Jun, 78, (6): 349-350. GENERAL.

Luster, A. D. Chemokines—chemotactic cytokines that mediate inflammation. The New England Journal of Medicine. 1998 Feb 12, 338, (7): 436-445. IMMUNE EFFECTS.

Luu, H., Biles, J., and White, K. D. Characterization of polyesterurethane degradation products. J. Appl. Biomat. 1994, 5, 1-7. POLYURETHANE/toxicology.

Lykissa, E. D., Kala, S. V., Hurley, J. B., and Lebovitz, R. M. Release of low molecular weight silicones and platinum from silicone breast implants. Analytical Chemistry. 1997 Dec, 69, (23): 4912-4916. PLATINUM/toxicology/silicon measurement.

Lyon, M. G., Bloch, D. A., Hollak, B., and Fries, J. F. Predisposing factors in polymyositis-dermatomyositis: Results of a nationwide survey. J. Rheumatol. 1989, 16, (9): 1218-1224. AI-CTD BACKGROUND.

MacDonald, K. L., Osterholm, M. T., LeDell, K. H., White, K. E., Schenck, C. H., Chao, C. C., Persing, D. H., Johnson, R. C., Barker, J. M., and Peterson, P. K. A case-control study to assess possible triggers and cofactors in chronic fatigue syndrome. American Journal of Medicine. 1996, 100, (5): 548-554. AI-CTD BACKGROUND.

Macdonald, P., Plavac, N., Peters, W., Lugowski, S., and Smith, D. Failure of 29Si NMR to detect increased blood silicone levels in silicone gel breast implant recipients. Analytical Chemistry. 1995, 67, 3799-3801. SILICON MEASUREMENT.

MacDonald, W. B., Lanier, G. E., and Deichmann, W. B. The subacute oral toxicity to the rat of certain polydimethylsiloxanes. Arch Indust Health. 1960 Jun, 21, 514. TOXICOLOGY.

Mackel, A., Delustro, F., Harper, F., and Leroy, E. C. Antibodies to collagen in scleroderma. Arthritis And Rheumatism. 1982 May. AI-CTD BACKGROUND/immune effects.

Maddison, P. J., Skinner, R. P., Pereira, R. S., Black, C. B., Ansell, B. M., Jayson, IV M., Rowell, N. R., and Welsh, K. I. Antinuclear antibodies in the relatives and spouses of patients with systemic sclerosis. Annals of the Rheumatic Diseases. 1986, 45, 793-799. AI-CTD BACKGROUND.

Maddox, A., Schoenfeld, A., Sinnett, H. D., and Shousha, S. Breast carcinoma occuring in association with silicone augmentation. Histopathology. 1993, 23, 379-382. CANCER.

Maekawa, A., Ogiu, T., Onodera, H., Furuta, K., Matsuoka, C., Ohno, Y., Tanigawa, H., Salmo, G. S., Matsuyama, M., and Hayashi, Y. Foreign-body tumorigenesis in rats by various kinds of plastics—induction of malignant fibrous histiocytomas. Journal of Toxicological Sciences. 1984, 9, 263-272. CARCINOGENICITY/toxicology.

Maekawa, A., Ogiu, T., Onondera, H., Furuta, K., Matsuoka, C., Ohno, Y., Tanigawa, H., Salmo, G. S., Matsuyama, M., and Hayashi, Y. Malignant fibrous histiocytomas induced in rats by polymers. Journal of Cancer Research and Clinical Oncology. 1984, 108, (3): 364-365. CARCINOGENICITY.

Magid, S. K., and Kagen, L. J. Serologic evidence for acute toxoplasmosis in polymyositis-dermatomyositis: Increased frequency of specific antitoxoplasma IgM antibodies. American Journal of Medicine. 1983 Aug, 75, 313-320. AI-CTD BACKGROUND.

Maguire, G. P., Lee, E. G., Bevington, D. J., Kuchemann, C. S., Crabtree, R. J., and Cornell, C. E. Psychiatric problems in the first year after mastectomy. British Medical Journal. 1978, 15, 963-965. PSYCHOSOCIAL.

Mahdi, S., Jones, T., and McGeorge, D. D. Expandable anatomical implants in breast reconstructions: a prospective study. British Journal of Plastic Surgery. 1998, 51, 425-430. RECONSTRUCTION.

Mahler, D., and Hauben, D. J. Retromammary versus retropectoral breast augmentation. A comparative study. Annals of Plastic Surgery. 1981 May, 8, (5): 370-374. CAPSULE CONTRACTURE/local complications.

Mäkelä, M., and Heliövaara, M. Prevalence of primary fibromyalgia in the Finnish population. British Medical Journal. 1991, 303, 216-219. AI-CTD BACKGROUND.

Malata, C. M., Feldberg, L., Coleman, D. J., Foo, I. T., and Sharpe, D. T. Textured or smooth implants for breast augmentation. British Journal of Plastic Surgery. 1997, 50, (2): 99-105. CAPSULE-CONTRACTURE/local complications.

Malata, C. M., and Sharpe, D. T. On the safety of breast implants. The Breast. 1992, 1, 62-75. GENERAL.

Malata, C. M., Varma, S., Scott, M., Liston, J. C., and Sharpe, D. T. Silicone breast implant rupture: Common/serious complication? Medical Progress through Technology. 1994a, 20, 251-260. RUPTURE/granulomas/local complications/silicon measurement.

Malia, R. G., Greaves, M., Rowlands, L. M., Lawrence, A. C. K., Hume, A., Rowell, N. R., Moult, J., Holt, C. M., Lindsey, N., and Hughes, P. Anticardiolipin antibodies in systemic sclerosis immunological and clinical associations. Clinical and Experimental Immunology. 1988, 73, 456-460. AI-CTD BACKGROUND.

Mancino, D., and Bevilacqua, N. Adjuvant effects of amorphous silica on the immune response to various antigens in guinea pigs. International Archives of Allergy and Applied Immunology. 1977, 53, 97-103. IMMUNE EFFECTS/toxicology/silica.

Mancino, D., Buono, G., Cusano, M., and Minucci, M. Adjuvant effects of a crystalline silica on IgE and IgG1 antibody production in mice and their prevention by the macrophage stabilizer poly-2-vinylpyridine N-oxide. International Archives of Allergy and Applied Immunology. 1983, 71, 279-281. SILICA/toxicology.

Mandel, M. A., and Gibbons, D. F. The presence of silicone in breast capsules. Aesthetic Plastic Surgery. 1979, 3, 219-225. SILICON MEASUREMENT/capsule-contracture/local complications.

Manders, E. K., Schenden, M. J., Furrey, J. A., Hetzler, P. T., Davis, T. S., and Graham, W. P. Soft tissue expansion: Concepts and complications. Plast. Reconstr. Surg. 1984, 74, (4): 493-507. EXPANDER.

Mandrekas, A. D., Zambacos, G. J., and Katsanton, P. N. Immediate and delayed breast reconstruction with permanent tissue expanders. British Journal of Plastic Surgery. 1995, 48, (8): 572-578. EXPANDER/reconstruction.

Mann, L. C. Physical examination of the augmented breast: Description of a displacement technique. Obstetrics and Gynecology. 1995 Feb, 85, (2): 290-292. CANCER.

Mansel, R. E., Horgan, K., Webster, D. J. T., Sarotria, S., and Hughes, L. E. Cosmetic results of immediate breast reconstruction post-mastectomy: A follow-up study. British Journal of Surgery. 1986, 73, 813-816. RECONSTRUCTION.

Mansel, R. E., Horgan, K., Webster, D. J. T., Shrotria, S., and Hughes, L. E. Mastectomy: A follow-up study. British Journal of Surgery. 1986, 73, (10): 813-816. CANCER/reconstruction.

Marceau, D., Rolland, C., Bronskill, M., Cardou, A., Paynter, R., and Guidoin, R. Nondestructive testing of virgin mammary prostheses: first step in an attempt to characterize the changes that occur with these implants *in vivo*. 125-139. SILICONE CHARACTERIZATION/rupture.

Marco-Franco, J. E., Torres, V. E., Nixon, D. E., Wilson, D. M., James, E. M., Bergstralh, E. J., and McCarthy, J. T. Oxalate silicon and vanadium in acquired cystic kidney disease. Clin Nephrol. 1991, 35, (2): 52-58. SILICON MEASUREMENT.

Marcus, D. M. An analytical review of silicone immunology. Arthritis and Rheumatism. 1996 Oct, 39, (10): 1619-1626. IMMUNE EFFECTS.

Marder, W. D., Meenan, R. F., Felson, D. T., and et al. The present and future adequacy of rheumatology manpower: A study of health care needs and physician supply. Arthritis and Rheumatism. 1991 Oct, 34, (10): 1209-1217. AI-CTD BACKGROUND.

Margolis, R. E. Medical device regulation: Silicone breast implant dangers. Health Span. 1991 Jan, 8, (1): 20. GENERAL.

Maricq, H. R., Weinrich, M. C., Keil, J. E., Smith, E. A., Harper, F. E., Nussbaum, A. I., LeRoy, C., McGregor, A. R., Diat, F., and Rosal, E. J. Prevalence of scleroderma spectrum disorders in the general population of South Carolina. Arthritis and Rheumatism. 1989 Aug, 32, (8): 998-1006. AI-CTD BACKGROUND.

Marik, P. E., Kark, A. L., and Zabakides, A. Scleroderma after silicone augmentation mammoplasty: A report of 2 cases. South African Medical Journal. 1990 Feb, 77, 212-213. CONNECTIVE TISSUE DISEASE.

Mark, R. J., Zimmerman, R. P., and Greif, J. M. Capsular contracture after lumpectomy and radiation therapy in patients who have undergone uncomplicated bilateral augmentation mammoplasty. Radiology. 1996 Sep, 200, (3): 621-625. RADIATION/capsule contracture.

Marks, M. W., Argenta, L. C., and Thornton, J. W. Rapid expansion: Experimental and clinical experience. Clinics in Plastic Surgery. 1987, 14, 455-463. EXPANDER.

Marotta, J.S., Widenhouse, C.W., Habal, M.B., Goldberg, E.P. Silicone gel breast implant failure and frequency of additional surgeries: Analysis of 35 studies reporting examination of more than 8,000 explants. J. Biomed. Mater. Res. (Appl. Biomater.) 1999, 48, 354-64 RUPTURE/local complications.

Marpeau, L., Rhimi, Z., Jault, T., Barrat, J., and Milliez, J. The local and general long-term risks of silicone breast implants. J Gynecol Obstet Biol Reprod. 1993, 22, 351-355. GRANULOMAS/migration/local complications.

Marques, A. F., Brenda, E., Saldiva, P. H. N., and Andrews, J. M. Capsular hematoma as a late complication in breast reconstruction with silicone gel prosthesis. Plastic Reconstructive Surgery. 1992 Mar, 89, (3): 543-545. HEMATOMAS/local complications/reconstruction.

Marques, A., Brenda, E., Amarante, MTJ, Pereira, M. D., and Castro, M. Haddad A. Findings in the removal of silicone gel breast implants: A correlation between time of implantation and rupture. European Journal of Plastic Surgery. 1997, 20, (1): 15-18. EXPLANTATION/rupture.

Marshall, T. C., Clark, C. R., Brewster, D. W., and Henderson, R. R. Toxicological assessment of heat transfer fluids proposed for use in solar energy applications, II. Toxicology and Applied Pharmacology. 1981, 58, 31-38. TOXICOLOGY.

Marshall, W. R. Amelioration of capsular contracture by motion restriction. Annals of Plastic Surgery. 1986 Mar, 16, (3): 211-218. CAPSULE-CONTRACTURE/local complications.

Marshall, W. R., Godfrey, M., Hollister, D. W., Balkocich, M. E., and Lindgren, V. V. Types of collagen in breast capsules. Annals of Plastic Surgery. 1989 Nov, 23, (5): 401-405. CAPSULE-CONTRACTURE/local complications.

Marshall, W. R., and Leggett, J. E. Misdiagnosis: A timely reminder. Annals of Plastic Surgery. 1992, 29, 444-445. CONNECTIVE TISSUE DISEASE/local complications/infection.

Martinazzoli, A., Cangemi, V., Cammarata, A., Ceccobelli, M., Costanzo, F., Lombardi, A., Gazzanelli, S., and Spallone, G. Breast reconstruction with the use of tissue expanders in outpatient treatment. Giorn. Chir. 1996, 17, (4): 195-196. EXPANDER/reconstruction.

Marzoni, F. A., Upchurch, S. E., and Lambert, C. J. An experimental study of silicone as a soft tissue substitute. Plast. Reconstr. Surg. 1959 Dec, 24, (6): 600-608. TOXICOLOGY.

Mason, J. C., Kapahi, P., and Haskard, D. O. Detection of increased levels of circulating intercellular adhesion molecule 1 in some patients with systemic lupus erythematosus. Arthritis and Rheumatism. 1993 Apr, 36, (4): 519-527. AI-CTD BACKGROUND.

Mason, J., and Apisarnthanarax, P. Migratory silicone granuloma. Archives of Dermatology. 1981 Jun, 117, 366-367. GRANULOMAS/local complications/migration.

Mason, T. C. Hyperprolactinemia and galactorrhea associated with mammary prostheses and unresponsive to bromocriptine. The Journal of Reproductive Medicine. 1991 Jul, 36, (7): 541-542. BREAST FEEDING/local complications.

Mason, T., Rabinovich, C., Fredrickson, D., and et al. Breast feeding and the development of juvenile rheumatoid arthritis. Journal of Rheumatology. 1995 Jun, 22, (6): 1166-1170. AI-CTD BACKGROUND/breast feeding/children's effects.

Masson, C. L., Dessapt, B., and Rochet, M. Migration of silicone gel following rupture of a breast implant during closed compression capsulotomy. Ann Chir Plast. 1982, 27, (4): 369-373. MIGRATION/local complications/rupture/closed capsulotomy.

Mathew, O., and Bhatia, F. Sucking and breathing patterns in breast- and bottle-feeding in term neonates: effects of nutrient delivery and composition. American Journal of Diseases in Children. 1989, 143, 588-592. BREAST FEEDING.

Matlaga, B. F., Yasenchak, L. P., and Salthouse, T. N. Tissue response to implanted polymers: The significance of sample shape 1. Journal of Biomedical Materials Research. 1976, 10, 391-397. TOXICOLOGY.

Matory, W. E., D'Orsi, C., and Moss, L. Improved mammographic imaging using tissue expanders for breast augmentation. Annals of Plastic Surgery. 1994 Aug, 33, (2): 119-127. MAMMOGRAPHY/local complications/capsule-contracture/saline/expander.

Matsushima, K., and Oppenheim, J. J. Interleukin 8 and MCAF: Novel inflammatory cytokines inducible by IL 1 and TNF. Cytokine. 1989, 1, (1): 2-13. IMMUNE EFFECTS.

Matti, B. A., and Nicolle, F. V. A simple technique for removing a silastic gel-filled breast implant through the axillary approach. British Journal of Plastic Surgery. 1989, 42, 613-614. EXPLANTATION.

Mattioli, M., and Reichlin, M. Heterogeneity of RNA protein antigens reactive with sera of patients with systemic lupus erythematosus. Description of a cytoplasmic nonribosomal antigen. Arthritis Rheum. 1974 Jul-1974 Aug 31, 17, (4): 421-429. AI-CTD BACKGROUND.

Mauras, Y., Riberi, P., and Cartier, F. Increase in blood silicon concentration in patients with renal failure. Biomedicine. 1980, 33, 228-230. SILICON MEASUREMENT.

Maxwell, G. P., and Tornambe, R. Management of mammary subpectoral implant distortion. Clinics in Plastic Surgery. 1988, 15, (4): 601-611. RECONSTRUCTION.

May, J. W., Atwood, J., and Bartlett, S. Staged use of soft-tissue expansion and lower thoracic advancement flaps in breast reconstruction. Plast. Reconstr. Surg. 1987 Feb, 79, (2): 272-275. EXPANDER/reconstruction.

May Jr., J. W., Bucky, L. P., Sohoni, S., and Ehrlich, H. P. Smooth versus textured expander implants: A double-blind study of capsule quality and discomfort in simultaneous bilateral breast reconstruction patients. Annals of Plastic Surgery. 1994 Mar, 32, (3): 225-232. CAPSULE-CONTRACTURE/local complications/saline/reconstruction.

Mayer, E., Hamman, R., Gay, E., Lezotte, D., Savitz, D., and Klingensmith, G. Reduced risk of IDDM among breast fed children. Diabetes. 1988, 37, 1625-1632. BREAST FEEDING.

McCarthy, E. J., Merkatz, R. B., and Bagley, G. P. A descriptive analysis of physical complaints from women with silicone breast implants. Journal of Women's Health. 1993, 2, 111-115. PSYCHOSOCIAL.

McCauley, R. L., Riley, Jr. W. B., Juliano, R. A., Brown, P., Evans, M. J., and Robson, M. C. In vitro alterations in human fibroblast behavior secondary to silicone polymers. Journal of Surgical Research. 1990 Jul, 49, (1): 103. CAPSULE-CONTRACTURE/local complications.

McConnell, J. P., Moyer, T. P., Nixon, D. E., Schnur, P. L., Salomao, D. R., Crotty, T. B., Weinzweig, J., Harris, J. B., and Petty, P. M. Determination of silicon in breast and capsular tissue from patients with breast implants performed by inductively coupled plasma emission spectroscopy: Comparison with tissue histology. American Journal of Clinical Pathology. 1997 Feb, 107, (2): 236-246. SILICON MEASUREMENT/saline/capsule contracture/local complications.

McCoy, B. J., Person, P., and Cohen, I. K. Collagen production and types in fibrous capsules around breast implants. Plast. Reconstr. Surg. 1984 Jun, 73, (6): 924-927. CAPSULE-CONTRACTURE/local complications.

McCraw, J. B., Horton, C. E., Grossman, J. A., Kaplan, I., and McMellin, A. An early appraisal of the methods of tissue expansion and the transverse rectus abdominus musculocutaneous flap in reconstruction of the breast following mastectomy. Annals of Plastic Surgery. 1987 Feb, 18, (2): 93-113. RECONSTRUCTION/expander.

McCraw, J. B., and Maxwell, G. P. Early and late capsular deformation as a cause of unsatisfactory results in the latissimus dorsi breast reconstruction. Clinics in Plastic Surgery. 1988 Oct, 15, (4): 717-726. CAPSULE-CONTRACTURE/local complications/reconstruction.

McCurdy, H. H and Solomons, E. T. Forensic examination of toxicological specimens for dimethylpolysiloxane (silicone oil). Journal of Analytical Toxicology. 1977, 1, 221-223. SILICONE INJECTION/silicon measurement/toxicology.

McCurdy, Jr. J. A. Relationships between spherical fibrous capsular contracture and mammary prosthesis type: A comparison of smooth and textured implants. The American Journal of Cosmetic Surgery. 1990, 7, (4): 235-239. CAPSULE CONTRACTURE/local complications.

McDermott, M. M., Dolan, N. C., Huang, J., Reifler, D., and Rademaker, A. W. Lump detection is enhanced in silicone breast models simulating postmenopausal breast tissue. Journal of General Internal Medicine. 1996 Feb 11, 11, 112-114. GENERAL/cancer.

McDermott, M., and McDevitt, H. The immunogenetics of rheumatic diseases. Bulletin on Rheumatic Diseases. 1988, 38, (1): 1-10. AI-CTD BACKGROUND/immune effects.

McDonald, A. H., Weir, K., Schneider, M. M., Gudenkauf, L., and Sanger, J. R. Silicone gel enhances the development of autoimmune disease in New Zealand black mice but fails to induce it in BALB/cAnPt mice. Clinical Immunology and Immunopathology. 1998 Jun, 87, (3): 248-255. IMMUNE EFFECTS/toxicology.

McDonald, J. W., Roggli, V. L., and Shelburne, J. D. Microprobe analysis: Diagnostic applications in pulmonary medicine. Microbeam Analysis. 1995, 4, 261-276. SILICON MEASUREMENT.

McDowell. Complications with silicones— What grade of silicone? How do we know it was silicone? Plast. Reconstr. Surg. 1978 Jun, 61, (6): 892-895. GENERAL.

McEwen, B. S. Protective and damaging effects of stress mediators. Seminars in Medicine of the Beth Israel Deaconess Medical Center. 1998 Jan 15, 338, (3): 171-179. GENERAL.

McFayden, P. Determination of free toluene diisocyanate in polyurethane prepolymers by high-performance liquid chromatography. Journal of Chromatography. 1976, 123, 468-473. POLYURETHANE/toxicology.

McGeorge, D. D., Mahdi, S., and Tsekouras, A. Breast reconstruction with anatomical expanders and implants: Our early experience. British Journal of Plastic Surgery. 1996, 49, 352-357. EXPANDER/reconstruction.

McGinley, P. H., Powell, W. R., and Bostwick, J. Dosimetry of a silicone breast prosthesis. Radiology. 1980, 135, 223-224. RADIATION.

McGrath, M. H., and Burkhardt, B. R. The safety and efficacy of breast implants for augmentation mammoplasty. Plast. Reconstr. Surg. 1984 Oct, 74 , (4): 550-560. GENERAL.

McGrath, M. H., and Hundahl, S. A. The spatial and temporal quantification of myofibroblasts. Plast. Reconstr. Surg. 1982, 69, 975. CAPSULE-CONTRACTURE/local complications.

McGregor, R. R. Toxicology of certain silicone fluids. Bull Dow Corning Cent. 1960, 2, 15. TOXICOLOGY.

McHenry, M. M., Smeloff, E. A., Fong, W. Y., Miller, G. E., and Ryan, P. M. Critical obstruction of prosthetic heart valves due to lipid adsorption by Silastic. The Journal of Thoracic and Cardiovascular Surgery. 1970 Mar, 59, (3): 413-425. SILICONE CHARACTERIZATION.

McHugh, N. J., Whyte, J., Harvey, G., and Haustein, U. F. Anti-topoisomerase I antibodies in silica-associated systemic sclerosis: A model for autoimmunity. Arthritis and Rheumatism. 1994 Aug, 37, (8): 1198-1205. SILICA.

McKim, Jr. J. M., Kolesar, G. B., and Dochterman, L. W. et al. Effects of octamethylcyclotetrasiloxane (D4) on liver size and cytochrome P450 in Fisher rats. A 28 day whole body inhalation study. Toxicologist. 1995, 15, 17. TOXICOLOGY.

McKinney, P., Edelson, R., Terrasse, A., and Zukowski, M. Chest-wall deformity following soft tissue expansion for breast reconstruction. Plast. Reconstr. Surg. 1987, 80, (3): 442-444. EXPANDER/local complications.

McKinney, P., and Tresley, G. Long-term comparison of patients with gel and saline mammary implants. Plast. Reconstr. Surg. 1983 Jul, 72, (1): 27-29. CAPSULE-CONTRACTURE/local complications/infection/saline.

McLaughlin, J. K., Nyrén, O., Blot, W. J., Yin, L., Josefsson, S., Fraumeni Jr., J. F, and Adami, H.-O. Cancer risk among women with cosmetic breast implants: A population-based cohort study in Sweden. Journal of the National Cancer Institute. 1998 Jan, 90, (2): 156-158. CANCER.

McNally, A. K., and Anderson, J. M. Complement C3 participation in monocyte adhesion to different surfaces. Proceedings of the National Academy of Sciences. 1994 Oct, 91, 10119-10123. IMMUNE EFFECTS.

McNally, A. K., and Anderson, J. M. Interleukin-4 induces foreign body giant cells from human monocytes/macrophages. American Journal of Pathology. 1995 Nov, 147, (5): 1487-1499. IMMUNE EFFECTS.

McTiernan, A., and Thomas, D. Evidence for a protective effect of lactation on risk of breast cancer in young women: results from a case control study. American Journal of Epidemiology. 1986, 124, 353-358. BREAST FEEDING/children's effects.

Medot, M., Landis, G. H., McGregor, C. E., Gutowski, K. A., Foshager, M. C., Griffiths, H. J., and Cunningham, B. L. Effects of capsular contracture on ultrasonic screening for silicone gel breast implant rupture. Annals of Plastic Surgery. 1997 Oct, 39, (4): 337-341. MAMMOGRAPHY/local complications/capsule-contracture/rupture.

Meester, W. D., and Swanson, A. B. In vivo testing of silicone rubber joint implants for lipid absorption. J. Biomed. Mat. Res. 1972, 6, 193-199. SILICONE CHEMISTRY/silicone characterization.

Megumi, Y. Immediate breast reconstruction with subpectoral implantation after trans-axillary subcutaneous mastectomy for siliconoma. Aesthetic Plastic Surgery. 1989, 13, 27-32. SILICONE INJECTION/reconstruction/granulomas.

Meier, L. G., Barthel, H. R., and Seidl, C. Development of polyarthritis after insertion of silicone breast implants followed by remission after implant removal in 2 HLA-identical sisters bearing rheumatoid arthritis susceptibility genes. J. Rheumatol. 1997, 24, (9): 1838-1841. CONNECTIVE TISSUE DISEASE/explantation.

Melloni, B. Partial characterization of the proliferative activity for fetal lung epithelial cells produced by silica-exposed alveolar macrophages. Journal of Leukocyte Biology. 1994 May, 55, 574-580. SILICA.

Melmed, E. P. Polyurethane implants: A 6-year review of 416 patients. Plast. Reconstr. Surg. 1988 Aug, 82, (2): 285-290. POLYURETHANE.

Melmed, E. P. A review of explantation in 240 symptomatic women: A description of explantation and capsulectomy with reconstruction using a periareolar technique. Plast. Reconstr. Surg. 1998 Apr, 101, (5): 1364-1373. EXPLANTATION/polyurethane/capsule-contracture/local complications/rupture.

Melmed, E. P. Silicone implants: Aesthetic triumph or surgical disaster? Plast. Reconstr. Surg. 1996 Nov, 98, (6): 1071-1073. GENERAL.

Melmed, E. P. Treatment of breast contractures with open capsulotomy and replacement of gel prostheses with polyurethane-covered implants. Plast. Reconstr. Surg. 1990 Aug, 86, (2): 270-274. CAPSULE-CONTRACTURE/local complications/polyurethane.

Melnikow, J. K., and Bedinghaus, J. Management of common breast-feeding problems. J. Family Practice. 1994, 39, (1): 56-64. BREAST FEEDING.

Mena, E. A., Kossovsky, N., Chu, C., and Hu, C. Inflammatory intermediates produced by tissues encasing silicone breast prostheses. Journal of Investigative Surgery. 1995, 8, (1): 31-42. IMMUNE EFFECTS.

Mendelson, E. B. Silicone implants present mammographic challenge. Diagnostic Imaging. 1992, 14, 70. MAMMOGRAPHY.

Mendes Filho, A., and Ludovici, C. O. Importancia demammographiu nos plasticas mamarios. Rev. Lat. Am. Cis. Plast. 1968, 12, 131. MAMMOGRAPHY.

Mendez-Fernandez, M. A. Subacute torsion of periprosthetic capsular tissue presenting as a painful breast tumor. Plast. Reconstr. Surg. 1997 Sep, 100, (3): 750-752. LOCAL COMPLICATIONS.

Mendez-Fernandez, M. A., Henly, W. S., Geis, R. C., Schoen, F. J., and Hausner, R. J. Paget's Disease of the breast after subcutaneous mastectomy and reconstruction with a silicone prosthesis. Plast. Reconstr. Surg. 1980 May, 65, (5): 683-685. CANCER.

Mendlovic, S., Segal, R., Shoenfeld, Y., and Mozes, E. Anti-DNA idiotype- and anti-idiotype-specific T cell responses in patients with systemic lupus erythematosus and their first-degree relatives. Clin. Exp. Immunol. 1990, 82, 504-508. CHILDREN'S EFFECTS/breast feeding.

Menendez-Graino, F, Fernandez, C. P., and Burrieza, P. L. Galactorrhea after reduction mammoplasty. Plast. Reconstr. Surg. 1990, 85, 645-646. BREAST FEEDING.

Merkatz, R. B., Bagley, G. P., and McCarthy, J. E. A qualitative analysis of self-reported experiences among women encountering difficulties with silicone breast implants. Journal of Women's Health. 1993, 2, (2): 105-108. PSYCHOSOCIAL.

Merle, M., Dellon, A. L., Campbell, J. N., and Chang, P. S. Complications from silicon-polymer intubation of nerves. Microsurgery. 1989 Jan, 10, (2): 130-133. NEUROLOGIC DISEASE.

Merritt, K., Shafer, J. W., and Brown, S. A. Implantation site infection rates with porous and dense materials. J. Biomat. Res. 1979, 13, 101-112. INFECTION.

Merwin, R. M., and Redmon, L. W. Induction of plasma cell tumors and sarcomas in mice by diffusion chambers placed in the peritoneal cavity. Journal of the National Cancer Institute. 1963, 31, (4): 997-1017. MYELOMA.

Meydan, D., Lambert, B., and Hellgren, D. Frequency and cell specificity of t-cell receptor interlocus recombination in human cells. Environmental and Molecular Mutagenesis. 1997, 30, 245-253. IMMUNE EFFECTS.

Meyer, J. E., Kopans, D. B., Stomper, P. C., and Linfors, K. K. Occult breast abnormalities: Percutaneous needle localization. Radiology. 1984 Feb, 150, (2): 335-337. MAMMOGRAPHY.

Middleton, M. S. Magnetic resonance evaluation of breast implants and soft-tissue silicone. Topics in Magnetic Resonance Imaging. 1998b, 9, (1 & 2): 1-45/92-137. MAMMOGRAPHY.

Middleton, M. S., and McNamara, Jr. M. P. Increased rupture rate of polyurethane-coated breast implants. Radiology. 1995 Nov, 197(P), 371. RUPTURE/local complications/polyurethane.

Mikuz, G., Hastings, G. W., and Ducheyne, P. Tissue reactions with silicone rubber implants (morphological, microchemical and clinical investigations in humans and laboratory animals). Macromolecular Biomaterials. 1984: 239-249. IMMUNE EFFECTS.

Mikuz, G., Hoinkes, G., Propst, A., and Wilflingseder, P. Silicone lymphadenopathy following augmentation mammoplasty. Chir Plast. 1982, 6, 209. LYMPHADENOPATHY/local complications.

Milauskas, A. T. Posterior capsule opacification after silicone lens implantation and its management. Journal of Cataract Refract. Surg. 1987 Nov, 13, (6): 644-648. GENERAL.

Millard, D. R., and Maisels, D. Silicon granuloma of the skin and subcutaneous tissues. American Journal of Surgery. 1966 Jul, 112, 119-123. GRANULOMAS/local complications.

Miller, A. Talc pneumoconiosis-significance of sublight microscopic mineral particles. American Journal of Medicine. 1971 Mar, 50, (3): 395-402. SILICA.

Miller, A. B., Baines, C. J., To, T., and Wall, C. Canadian national breast screening study 2. Breast cancer detection and death rates among women aged 50-59 years. Canadian Medical Association Journal. 1992, 147, (10): 1477-1488. MAMMOGRAPHY/cancer.

Miller, A. S., Willard, V., Kline, K., Tarpley, S., Guillott, J., Lawler, F. H., and Pendell, G. M. Absence of longitudinal changes in rheumatologica parameters after silicone breast implantation: a prospective 13-year study. Plast. Reconstr. Surg. 1998 Dec, 102, (7): 2299-2303. CONNECTIVE TISSUE DISEASE/immune effects.

Miller, E. J. Biochemical characteristics and biological significance of the genetically-distinct collagens. Molecular and Cellular Biochemistry. 1976 Dec 10, 13, (3): 165-192. GENERAL.

Miller, F. Classification and prognosis of inflammatory muscle disease. Rheumatic Disease Clinics of North America. 1994 Nov, 20, (4): 811-826. AI-CTD BACKGROUND.

Miller, K. M., and Anderson, J. In vitro stimulation of fibroblast activity by factors generated from human monocytes activated by biomedical polymers. J. Biomed. Mater. Res. 1989, 23, (9): 1007-1026. IMMUNE EFFECTS/capsule contracture.

Miller, K. M., Rose-Caprara, V., and Anderson, J. M. Generation of IL-1-like activity in response to biomedical polymer implants: A comparison of in vitro and in vivo models. Journal of Biomedical Materials Research. 1989, 23, 1007-10026. IMMUNE EFFECTS.

Miller, M. J., Rock, C. S., and Robb, G. L. Aesthetic breast reconstruction using a combination of free transverse rectus abdominis musculocutaneous flaps and breast implants. Annals of Plastic Surgery. 1996 Sep, 37, (3): 258-264. RECONSTRUCTION.

Miller, T. A. Capsulectomy. Plast. Reconstr. Surg. 1998, 102, (3): 882-883. RUPTURE/capsule contracture/local complications.

Miller, T. A. Silicone and plastic surgery. Plast. Reconstr. Surg. 1997 Oct, 100, (5): 1307-1308. GENERAL.

Milojevic, B. Complications after silicone injection therapy in aesthetic plastic surgery. Aesthetic Plastic Surgery. 1982, 6, 203-206. SILICONE INJECTION.

Milojevic, B. Unilateral fibrous contracture in augmentation mammoplasty. Aesth. Plast. Surg. 1983, 7, 117-119. CAPSULE CONTRACTURE/local complications.

Miranda, R. Peritoneal silicosis. Arch. Pathology and Laboratory Medicine. 1996 Mar, 120, 300-302. SILICA.

Missotten, F. E. M. Giant cyst formation in a fibrous capsule following breast augmentation: A case report. British Journal of Plastic Surgery. 1985, 38, 579. LOCAL COMPLICATIONS.

Mitnick, J. S., Harris, M. N., and Roses, D. F. Mammographic detection of carcinoma of the breast in patients with augmentation prostheses. Surgery, Gynecology and Obstetrics. 1989 Jan, 168, 30-33. MAMMOGRAPHY/cancer.

Mitnick, J. S., Vazquez., M. F., Colen, S. R., Plesser, K., and Roses, D. F. Localization of nonpalpable masses in patients with breast implants. Annals of Plastic Surgery. 1993 Sep, 31, (3): 238-240. GRANULOMAS/local complications/mammography/rupture.

Mitnick, J. S., Vazquez., M. F., Plesser, K., Pressman, P., Harris, M. N., and Roses, D. F. Fine needle aspiration biopsy in patients with augmentation prostheses and a palpable mass. Annals of Plastic Surgery. 1993 Sep, 31, (3): 241-244. GRANULOMAS/mammography/cancer/local complications/rupture.

Mitnick, J. S., Vazquez, M. F., Roses, D. F., Harris, M. N., Colen, S. R., and Colen, H. S. Stereotactic localization for fine needle aspiration biopsy in patients with augmentation prostheses. Annals of Plastic Surgery. 1992 Jul, 29, (1): 31-35. MAMMOGRAPHY.

Miyoshi, K., Miyamura, T., and Kobayashi, Y. Hypergammaglobulinemia by prolonged adjuvanticity in man: Disorders developed after augmentation mammaplasty. Jpn J Med. 1964, 9, 2122. CONNECTIVE TISSUE DISEASE/immune effects.

Miyoshi, K., Shiragami, H., and Yoshida, K. Adjuvant disease of man. Clin Immunol. 1973, 5, 785-794. CONNECTIVE TISSUE DISEASE.

Mladick, R. A. No-touch submuscular saline breast augmentation technique. Aesthetic Plastic Surgery. 1993, 17, 183-192. SALINE/capsule-contracture/rupture/infection/local complications.

Mladick, R. A. Treatment of the firm augmented breast by capsular stripping and inflatable implant exchange. Plast. Reconstr. Surg. 1977 Nov, 60, (5): 720-724. CAPSULE-CONTRACTURE/local complications.

Moacanin, J., Lawson, D. D., Chin, H. P., Harrison, E. C., and Blankenhorn, D. H. Prediction of lipid uptake by prosthetic heart valve poppets from solubility parameters. Biomater Med Devices Artif Organs. 1973, 1, 183-190. SILICONE CHARACTERIZATION/general.

Modzelewski, J., Greene, W., Sobieski, M., and Raso, D. Silicon detection in fat globules in pericapsular tissue of women and rats augmented with silicone gel. Breast Journal 2(4): 275-280. 1996 Nov 4, 2, (4): 275-280. LOCAL COMPLICATIONS/capsule contracture.

Mofid, M. M., Thompson, R. C., Pardo, C. A., Manson, P. N., and Vander Kolk, C. A. Biocompatibility of fixation materials in the brain. Plast. Reconstr. Surg. 1997 Jul, 100, (1): 14-20. LOCAL COMPLICATIONS/general.

Mohr, C., Gemsa, D., Graebner, C., Hemenway, D. R., Leslie, K. O., Absher, F. M., and Davis, G. S. Systemic macrophage stimulation in rats with silicosis: Enhanced release of tumor necrosis factor-α from alveolar and peritoneal macrophages. American Journal of Respiratory Cell and Molecular Biology. 1991 Jan, 5, 395-402. SILICA.

Moizhess, T. G., and Vasiliev, J. M. Early and late stages of foreign-body carcinogenesis can be induced by implants of different shapes. International Journal of Cancer. 1989, 44, 449-453. CARCINOGENICITY.

Mokuno, K., Kiyosawa, K., Honda, H., Hirose, Y., Murayama, T., Yoneyama, S., and Kato, K. Elevated serum levels of manganese superoxide dismutase in polymyositis and dermatomyositis. Neurology. 1996 May, 46, (5): 1445-1447. AI-CTD BACKGROUND.

Mongey, A.-B., and Hess, E. V. Antinuclear antibodies and disease specificity. Advances in Internal Medicine. 1991, 36, 151-169. IMMUNE EFFECTS/ai-ctd background.

Monsees, B. S., and Destouet, J. M. Mammography in aesthetic and reconstructive breast surgery. Perspect Plast Surg. 1991, 5, 103-119. MAMMOGRAPHY.

Monticciolo, D. L., Nelson, R. C., Dixon, W. T., Bostwick, III J., Mukundan, S., and Hester, T. R. MR detection of leakage from silicone breast implants: Value of a silicone-selective pulse sequence. American Journal of Roentgenology. 1994 Jul, 163, 51-56. MAMMOGRAPHY.

Moor, E. V., Wexler, M. R., Bar-Ziv, Y., Weinberg, A., Chaouat, M., Ad-El, D., Raveh, T., Alfie, M., Caspi, R., and Neuman, A. Chest wall deformity following maximal tissue expansion for breast reconstruction. Annals of Plastic Surgery. 1996 Feb, 36, (2): 129-132. LOCAL COMPLICATIONS/expander.

Moore, J. R. Applanation tonometry of breasts. Plast. Reconstr. Surg. 1979, 63, (1): 9-12. CAPSULE CONTRACTURE/local complications.

Morain, W. D., and Vistnes, L. M. Iondinated silicone—an antibacterial alloplastic material. Plast. Reconstr. Surg. 1977, 59, (2): 216-222. INFECTION/local complications.

Morgan, D. E., Kenney, P. J., Meeks, M. C., and Pile, N. S. MR imaging of breast implants and their complications. American Journal of Roentgenology. 1996 Nov, 167, (5): 1271-1275. MAMMOGRAPHY.

Morgan, R. W., and Elcock, M. Artificial implants and soft tissue sarcomas. Journal of Clinical Epidemiology. 1995, 48, (4): 545-549. CANCER.

Morgenstern, L., Gleischman, S. H., Michel, S. L., and et al. Relation of free silicone to human breast carcinoma. Archives of Surgery. 1985 May, 120, 573. CANCER.

Mori, T. Superoxide anions in the pathogenesis of talc-induced cerebral vasocontraction. Neuropathology and Applied Neurobiology. 1995 Jan, 21, 378-385. GENERAL.

Morse, J. H., Fotino, M., Zhang, Y., Flaster, E. R., Peebles, C. L., and Spiera, H. Position 26 of the first domain of the HLA-DQB1 allele in post-silicone implant scleroderma. J. Rheumatol. 1995, 22, (10): 1872-1875. CONNECTIVE TISSUE DISEASE.

Morykwas, M. J., Argenta, L. C., Oneal, R. M., and Kaiser, D. G. The fate of soluble steroids within breast prostheses in humans. Annals of Plastic Surgery. 1990 May, 24, (5): 427-430. STEROIDS/local complications.

Morykwas, M. J., and Rouchard, R. A. Argenta L. C. Silicon levels in treated drinking water. Plast. Reconstr. Surg. 1991, 88, (5): 925-926. SILICON MEASUREMENT.

Moucharafieh, B. C., and Wray Jr., R. C. The effects of steroid instillations and hematomas on the pseudosheaths of miniature breast implants in rats. Plast. Reconstr. Surg. 1977 May, 59, (5): 720-723. STEROIDS/capsule-contracture/local complications/hematomas.

Moufarrege, R., Beauregard, G., Bosse, J. P., Pappillon, J., and Perras, C. Outcome of mammary capsulotomies. Annals of Plastic Surgery. 1987, 19, 62-64. LOCAL COMPLICATIONS/capsule-contracture.

Muir, V. Y., and Dumonde, D. C. Different strains of rats develop different clinical forms of adjuvant disease. Annals of Rheumatic Diseases. 1982, 41, 538-543. IMMUNE EFFECTS.

Mukundan, S., Dixon, W. T., Nelson, R. C., Kruse, B. D., Monticciolo, D. L., and Nelson, R. C. MR imaging of silicone gel-filled breast implants *in vivo* with a method that visualizes silicone selectively. Journal of Magnetic Resonance Imaging. 1993, 3, 713-718. MAMMOGRAPHY.

Mulder, J. W., and Nicolai, J-P. A. Breast Tonometry—a practical device for accurate measurement of capsule-formation. Eur. J. Plast. Surg. 1990, 13, 274-277. CAPSULE CONTRACTURE/local complications.

Mullison, E. G. Current status of silicones in plastic surgery. Archives Otolaryng. 1966 Jan, 83, 85-89. GENERAL.

Mund, D. F., Farria, D. M., Gorczyca, D. P., DeBruhl, N. D., Ahn, C. Y., Shaw, W. W., and Bassett, L. W. MR imaging of the breast in patients with silicone-gel implants: Spectrum of findings. American Journal of Roentgenology. 1993, 161, 773-778. MAMMOGRAPHY.

Murakata, L. A., and Rangwala, A. F. Silicone lymphadenopathy with concomutant malignant lymphoma. J. Rheumatol. 1989, 16, (11): 1480-1483. LYMPHADENOPATHY/local complications/cancer.

Murphy, E. J. Cytotoxicity of aluminum silicates in primary neuronal cultures. Neuroscience. 1993 Jan, 57, (2): 483-490. NEUROLOGIC DISEASE/silica.

Nachbar, J. M., and Orrison, W. W. Validation of quantification of breast implant capsule surface area and volume using magnetic resonance imaging. Annals of Plastic Surgery. 1991 Oct, 27, (4): 321-326. CAPSULE-CONTRACTURE/local complications/mammography.

Naidu, S. H., Beredjiklian, P., Adler, L., Bora, Jr. F. W., and Baker, D. G. In vivo inflammatory response to silicone elastomer particulate debris. The Journal of Hand Surgery. 1996 May, 21, (3): 496-500. IMMUNE EFFECTS/general/local complications.

Naim, J. O., Ippolito, K. M. L., Lanzafame, R. J., and van Oss, C. J. The effect of molecular weight and gel preparation of humoral adjuvancy of silicone oil and silicone gel. Immunological Investigations. 1995c, 24, (3): 537-547. IMMUNE EFFECTS.

Naim, J. O., Ippolito, K. M. L., and van Oss, C. J. Adjuvancy effect of different types of silicone gel. J Biomed Mater Res. 1997 Dec, 37, (4): 534-538. IMMUNE EFFECTS.

Naim, J. O., Ippolito, K. M., Lanzafame, R. J., and van Oss, C. J. Induction of type II collagen arthritis in the DA rat using silicone gels and oils as adjuvant. Journal of Autoimmunity. 1995b, 8, 751-761. IMMUNE EFFECTS/toxicology.

Naim, J. O., Lanzafame, R. J., and van Oss, C. J. The effect of silicone-gel on the immune response. J Biomaterials Sci. 1995a, 7, 123-132. IMMUNE EFFECTS.

Naim, J. O., and van Oss, C. J. The effect of hydrophilicity-hydrophobicity and solubility on the immunogenicity of some natural and synthetic polymers. Immunological Investigations. 1992, 21, (7): 649-662. IMMUNE EFFECTS.

Naim, J. O., van Oss, C. J., Ippolito, K. M. L., Shang, J.-W., Jin, L. P., Fortuna, R., and Buehner, N. A. In vitro activation of human monocytes by silicones. Colloids and Surface Biointerfaces. 1998, 11, 79-86. IMMUNE EFFECTS.

Naim, J. O., van Oss, C. J., and Lanzafame, R. J. The induction of autoantibodies to thyroglobulin in rats with silicone gel as adjuvant. Surg Forum. 1993, 44, 676-678. IMMUNE EFFECTS.

Nakamura, A., Kawasaki, Y., Takada, K., Aida, Y., Kurokama, Y., Kojima, S., Shintani, H., Matsui, M., Nohmi, T., Matsuoka, A., Sofuni, T., Kurihara, M., Miyata, N., Uchima, T., and Fujimaki, M. Difference in tumor incidence and other tissue responses to polyesterurethanes and polydimethysiloxane in long-term subcutaneous implantation into rats. Journal of Biomed. Mater. Res. 1992, 26, 631-650. CARCINOGENICITY/connective tissue disease/polyurethane.

Nakamura, K., Refojo, J. F., and Crabtree, D. V. Factors contributing to the emulsification of intraocular silicone and fluorosilicone oils. Investigative Ophthamology and Visual Science. 1990 Apr, 31, (4): 647-656. SILICONE CHARACTERIZATION/toxicology/general.

Nakamura, K., Refojo, J. F., and Crabtree, D. V. Leong F. Analysis and fractionation of silicone and fluorosilicone oils for intraocular use. Investigative Ophthamology and Visual Science. 1990 Oct, 31, (10): 2059-2069. SILICONE CHARACTERIZATION/toxicology/general.

Nanki T, Kohsaka H, and Miyasaka N. Development of human peripheral TCRBJ gene repertoire. J Immunol. 1998 Jul, 161, (1): 228-33. IMMUNE EFFECTS.

Narini, P. P., Semple, J. L., and Hay, J. B. Repeated exposure to silicone gel can induce delayed hypersensitivity. Plast. Reconstr. Surg. 1995 Aug, 96, (2): 371. IMMUNE EFFECTS.

National Institutes of Health. Treatment of early-stage breast cancer: NIH Consensus Conference. J. Amer. Med. Assoc. 1991 Jan 16, 265, (3): 391-395. CANCER.

Nedelman, C. I. Oral and cutaneous tissue reactions to injected fluid silicones. Journal of Biomedical Materials Research. 1968, 2, 131-143. TOXICOLOGY.

Needelman, L. The microscopic interaction between silicone and the surrounding tissues. Clinics in Podiatric Medicine and Surgery. 1995, 12, (3): 415-423. CAPSULE-CONTRACTURE/local complications.

Needleman, B., Wigley, F., and Stair, R. Interleukin-1, interleukin-2, interleukin-4, interleukin-6, tumor necrosis factor alpha, and interferon-γ levels in sera from patients with scleroderma. Arthritis and Rheumatism. 1992 Jan, 35, (1): 67-72. IMMUNE EFFECTS/ai-ctd background.

Neifert, M., DeMarzo, S., Seacat, J., Young, D., Leff, M., and Orleans, M. The influence of breast surgery, breast appearance, and pregnancy-induced breast changes in lactation sufficiency as measured by infant weight gain. Birth. 1990 Mar, 17, (1): 31-38. BREAST FEEDING/children's effects.

Neill, K. M., Armstrong, N., and Burnett, C. B. Choosing reconstruction after mastectomy: a qualitative analysis. Oncol Nurs Forum. 1998, 25, (4): 743-750. PSYCHOSOCIAL/reconstruction.

Nelson, G. D. A comparative study of complications of open capsulotomies versus closed compression rupture of augmentation mammoplasties. Plastic Surg Forum. 1980b, 3, 78. CLOSED CAPSULOTOMY/capsule-contracture/rupture/local complications.

Nelson, G. D. Complications from the treatment of fibrous capsular contracture of the breast. Plast. Reconstr. Surg. 1981 Dec, 68, (6): 969-970. CAPSULE-CONTRACTURE/local complications/closed capsulotomy/rupture.

Nelson, G. D. Complications of closed compresssion after augmentation mammaplasty. Plast. Reconstr. Surg. 1980a Jul, 66, (1): 71-73. CAPSULE CONTRACTURE/closed capsulotomy/local complications/rupture.

Nelson, J. L., Furst, D. E., Maloney, S., Gooley, T., Evans, P. C., Smith, A., Bean, M. A., Ober, C., and Bianchi, D. W. Microchimerism and HLA-compatible relationships of pregnancy in scleroderma. The Lancet. 1998 Feb 21, 351, 559-541. AI-CTD BACKGROUND.

Nemecek, J. A. R., and Young, V. L. How safe are silicone breast implants? Southern Medical Journal. 1993 Aug, 86, (8): 932-944. GENERAL.

Netscher, D. T., Sharma, S., Thornby, J., Peltier, M., Lyos, A., Fater, M., and Mosharrafa, A. Aesthetic outcome of breast implant removal in 85 consecutive patients. Plast. Reconstr. Surg. 1997 Jul, 100, (1): 206-219. EXPLANTATION/local complications.

Netscher, D. T., Walker, L. E., Weizer, G., Thornby, J., Wigoda, P., and Bowen, D. A review of 198 patients (389 implants) who had breast implants removed. Journal of Long Term Effects of Medical Implants. 1995a, 5, (1): 11-18. RUPTURE/explantation/local complications.

Netscher, D. T., Weizer, G., Wigoda, P., Walker, L. E., Thornby, J., and Bowen, D. Clinical relevance of positive breast periprosthetic cultures without overt infection. Plast. Reconstr. Surg. 1995b Oct, 96, (5): 1702-1708. CAPSULE-CONTRACTURE/local complications/infection.

Neu, T. R., Van Der Mei, H. C., and Busscher, H. J. Biodeterioration of medical-grade silicone rubber used for voice prostheses: A SEM study. Biomaterials. 1993 May, 14, (6): 459. GENERAL.

Newcomb, P., Storer, B., Longnecker, M., and et al. Lactation and a reduced risk of premenopausal breast cancer. New England J. Medicine. 1994, 330, 81-87. CHILDREN'S EFFECTS/breast feeding.

Newton, N., and Newton, M. Psychologic aspects of lactation. New England Journal of Medicine. 1967, 277, 1179-1188. BREAST FEEDING.

Ng, T. P., Ng, Y. L., Lee, H. S., Chia, K. S., and Ong, H. Y. A study of silica nephroroxicity in exposed silicone and non-silicone workers. British Journal of Industrial Medicine. 1992, 49, 35-37. SILICA.

Niazi, Z. B. M., Salzberg, C. A., and Montecalvo, M. *Candida albicans* infection of bilateral polyurethane-coated silicone gel breast implants. Annals of Plastic Surgery. 1996, 37, 91-93. INFECTION/polyurethane/local complications.

Nicander, L. Changes produced in the male genital organs of rabbits and dogs by 2,6-*cis*-diphenylhexamethylcyclotetrasiloxane (KABI 1774). Acta Pharmacologica et Toxicologica. 1975, 36, Supp. III, 40-54. TOXICOLOGY.

Nicholson III, J. J., Hill, S. L., Frondoza, C. G., and Rose, N. R. Silicone gel and octamethylcylotetrasiloxane (D4) enhances antibody production to bovine serum albumin in mice. Journal of Biomedical Materials Research. 1996, 31, (3): 345-353. IMMUNE EFFECTS.

Nicolle, F. V. Capsular contracture and ripple deformity of breast implants. Aesthetic Plastic Surgery. 1996 Jul, 20, (4): 311-314. CAPSULE-CONTRACTURE/local complications.

Niezborala, M., and Garnier, R. Allergy to complex platinum salts: A histological prospective cohort study. Occupational and Environmental Medicine. 1996, 53, (4): 252-257. PLATINUM/toxicology/immune effects.

Nobunaga, M., Oribe, K., and Ohishi, S. A case of scleroderma with Sjögren's syndrome developed after mammoplasty. Clinical Rheumatology. 1984, 3, (3): 375-379. CONNECTIVE TISSUE DISEASE.

Noone, R. B., Frazier, T. G., Hayward, C. Z., and Skiles, M. S. Patient acceptance of immediate reconstruction following mastectomy. Plast. Reconstr. Surg. 1982 Apr, 69, (4): 632-638. PSYCHOSOCIAL/reconstruction.

Noone, R. B., Frazier, T. G., Noone, G. C., Blanchet, N. P., Murphy, J. B., and Rose, D. Recurrence of breast carcinoma following immediate reconstruction: A 13-year review. Plast. Reconstr. Surg. 1994a, 93, (1): 96-104. CANCER.

Noone, R. B., Murphy, J. B., Spear, S. L., and Little, J. W. A 6-year experience with immediate reconstruction after mastectomy for cancer. Plast. Reconstr. Surg. 1985 Aug, 76, (2): 258-269. RECONSTRUCTION.

Nordström, R. E. A., Pietilä, J. P., Voutilainen, P. E. J., Lilius, G. P. S., Virkkunen, P. J., and Rintala, A. E. Tissue expander injection dome leakage. Plast. Reconstr. Surg. 1988, 81, (1): 26-29. EXPANDER/local complications.

Nosanchuk, J. S. Injected dimethylpolysiloxane fluid: A study of antibody and histologic response. Plast. Reconstr. Surg. 1968a Dec, 42, (6): 562-566. IMMUNE EFFECTS/silicone injection.

Nosanchuk, J. S. Silicone granuloma in breast. Archives of Surgery. 1968b Oct, 97, 583-585. INFECTION/granulomas/local complications.

Nose, Y. Do breast implants really produce negative impacts to recipients. Artificial Organs. 1994, 18, (10): 717. GENERAL.

NRC Committee on Toxicology. ZnCdS Report. National Academy Press, Washington DC. 1997. TOXICOLOGY.

Nyrén, O., Josefsson, S., McLaughlin, J. K., Blot, W. J., Engquist, M., Hakelius, L., Boice, Jr. J. D., and Adami, H.-O. Risk of connective tissue disease and related disorders among women with breast implants: A nation-wide retrospective cohort study in Sweden. British Medical Journal. 1998a, 31, (7129): 417-421. CONNECTIVE TISSUE DISEASE.

Nyrén, O., McLaughlin, J. K., Gridley, G., Ekbom, A., Johnell, O., Fraumeni, J. F., and Adami, H. O. Cancer risk after hip replacement with metal implants: A population-based cohort study in Sweden. Journal of the National Cancer Institute. 1995 Jan 4, 87, (1): 28-33. CANCER.

Nyrén, O., McLaughlin, J. K., Yin, L., Josefsson, S., Engquist, M., Hakelius, L., Blot, W. J., and Adami, H.-O. Breast implants and risk of neurologic disease. Neurology. 1998c Apr, 50, 956-961. NEUROLOGIC DISEASE.

O'Boyle, M. K., Wechsler, R. J., Conant, E. F., Lev-Toaff, A. S., and Sagerman, J. Breast implants: Incidental findings on CT. American Journal of Roentgenology. 1994, 162, 311-313. MAMMOGRAPHY.

O'Brien, W., Hasselgren, P. O., Hummel, R. P., Coith, R., Huam, D., Kurtzman, L., and Neale, H. W. Comparison of postoperative wound complications and early cancer recurrence between patients undergoing mastectomy with or without immediate breast reconstruction. American Journal of Surgery. 1993, 166, 1-5. RECONSTRUCTION/cancer/local complications.

O'Donnell, M. The National Breast Implant Registry. Br J Theatre Nurs. 1994 Feb 1, 3, (11): 24. GENERAL.

O'Keeffe, P. J. The steroid-adjustable mammary implant. Aesthetic Plastic Surgery. 1981, 5, 129-135. CAPSULE-CONTRACTURE/local complications/steroids.

O'Mara, E. M., Pennes, D. R., and Argenta, L. C. Combination gel-inflatable mammary prosthesis: Appearance at CT. Radiology. 1989, 170, 78. MAMMOGRAPHY.

O'Rourke, E. J., Halstead, S. B., Allison, A. C., and Platts-Mills, T. A. E. Specific lethality of silica for human peripheral blood mononuclear phagocytes *in vitro*. Journal of Immunological Methods. 1978, 19, 137-151. SILICA.

Oellinger, H., Heins, S., Sander, B., and et al. Gd-DTPA enhanced MRI of breast. The most sensitive method for detecting multicentric carcinomas in female breast. Eur Radiol. 1993, 3, 223-227. MAMMOGRAPHY/cancer.

Ohbayashi, N., Inagawa, T., Katoh, Y., Kumano, K., Nagasako, R., and Hada, H. Complication of silastic dural substitute 20 years after dural plasty. Surgical Neurology. 1994, 41, 338-341. LOCAL COMPLICATIONS/general.

Ohlsen, L., Ponten, B., and Hamberg, G. Augmentation mammaplasty: A surgical and psychiatric evaluation of the results. Annals of Plastic Surgery. 1979, 2, (1): 42. PSYCHOSOCIAL.

Ohtake, N., Kogenei, Y., Itoh, M., and Shoya, N. Postoperative sequelae of augmentation mammaplasty by injection method in Japan. Aesthetic Plastic Surgery. 1989, 13, 67-74. SILICONE INJECTION.

Ojo-Amaize, E. A., Conte, V., Lin, H-C, Brucker, R. F., Agopian, M. S., and Peter, J. B. Silicone-specific blood lymphocyte response in women with silicone breast implants. Clinical Diagnostic Laboratory Immunology. 1994 Nov, 1, (6): 689-695. IMMUNE EFFECTS.

Ojo-Amaize, E. A., Lawless, O. J., and Peter, J. B. Elevated concentrations of interleukin-1 beta and interleukin-1 receptor antagonist in plasma of women with silicone breast implants. Clinical and Diagnostic Laboratory Immunology. 1996 May, 3, (3): 257-259. IMMUNE EFFECTS.

Okada, T., and Ikada, Y. *In vitro* and *in vivo* digestion of collagen covalently immobilized onto the silicone surface. Journal of Biomedical Materials Research. 1992, 26, 1569-1581. SILICONE CHARACTERIZATION.

Okada, T., and Ikada, Y. Tissue reactions to subcutaneously implanted, surface-modified silicones. Journal of Biomedical Materials Research. 1993, 27, 1509-1518. CAPSULE CONTRACTURE/immune effects.

Okano, Y., Nishikai, M., and Sato, A. Scleroderma, primary biliary cirrhosis, and Sjogren's syndrome after cosmetic breast augmentation with silicone injection: A case report of possible human adjuvant disease. Ann Rheum Dis. 1984, 43, 520-522. CONNECTIVE TISSUE DISEASE/silicone injection.

Okkerse, C., and de Boer, J. H. Reactivity of amorphous silica in aqueous solutions. Silicates Industriels. 1960: 195-202. SILICA.

Oksenberg J.R., Stavir G.T., Jeong M.C., Garovoy N., Salisbury J.R., and Erusalimsky J.D. Analysis of the T-cell receptor repertoire in human atherosclerosis. Cardiovasc Res. 1997 Nov, 36, 256†67. IMMUNE EFFECTS.

Okubo, M., Hyakusoku, H., Kouji, K., and Fumirir, M. Complications after injection mammaplasty. Aesthetic Plastic Surgery. 1992, 16, 181-187. CANCER/silicone injection.

Okunski, W., and Chowdary, R. P. Infected Même implants: Salvage reconstruction with latissimus dorsi myocutaneous flaps and silicone implants. Aesthetic Plastic Surgery. 1987, 11, (1): 49-51. INFECTION/polyurethane/local complications.

Olenius, M., Forslind, B., and Johansson, O. Morphometric evaluation of collagen fibril dimensions in expanded human breast skin. Int J Biol Macromol. 1991, 13, 162. EXPANDER/capsule contracture.

Olenius, M., and Jurell, G. Breast reconstruction using tissue expansion. Scandinavian Journal of Plastic and Reconstructive and Hand Surgery. 1992, 26, (1): 83-90. EXPANDER/reconstruction/capsule-contracture/local complications.

Olesen, L. L., Ejlertsen, T., and Nielsen, J. Toxic shock syndrome following insertion of breast prostheses. British Journal of Surgery. 1991 May, 78, (5): 585-586. INFECTION/ local complications.

Olivari, N. The latissimus flap. British Journal of Plastic Surgery. 1976, 29, 126-128. RECONSTRUCTION.

Olsen, M., O'connor, S., Arnett, F., Rosenbaum, D., Grotta, J. C., and Warner, N. B. Autoantibodies and rheumatic disorders in a neurology inpatient population: A prospective study. The American Journal of Medicine. 1991 Apr, 90, 479-488. NEUROLOGIC DISEASE/ai-ctd background.

Olson, K. J. Preface—series of papers relating reproductive activity to selected organosiloxane chemicals. Toxicology and Applied Pharmacology. 1972, 21, 12-14. TOXICOLOGY/children's effects.

Ombredanne, L. Restauration autoplastique du sein apres amputation totale. Trb. Med. 1906, 4, 325. RECONSTRUCTION.

Oneal, R. M. High pressure injection of silicone gel into an axilla—a complication of closed compression capsulotomy of the breast. Plast. Reconstr. Surg. 1979 Nov, 64, (5): 700. CLOSED CAPSULOTOMY/migration/local complications.

Oneal, R. M., and Argenta, L. C. Late side effects related to inflatable breast prostheses containing soluble steroids. Plast. Reconstr. Surg. 1982 Apr, 69, (4): 641-645. STEROIDS/local complications/capsule-contracture.

Opitz, P. G., and Young, V. L. Experience with soybean oil-filled breast implants in a Swedish surgical practice. Aesthetic Surgery Journal. 1998: 183-197. MAMMOGRAPHY/ local complications/general.

Oppenheimer, B. S., Oppenheimer, E. T., and Stout, A. P. Sarcomas induced in rats by implanting cellophane. Proc. Soc. Exp. Biol. Med. 1948, 67, 33-34. CARCINOGENICITY/toxicology.

Oppenheimer, B. S., Oppenheimer, E. T., and Stout, A. P. Sarcomas induced in rodents by imbedding various plastic films. Proc. Soc. Exp. Biol. Med. 1952, 79, 366-369. CARCINOGENICITY.

Oppenheimer, B. S., Oppenheimer, E. T., Stout, A. P., and Danishefsky, I. Malignant tumors resulting from embedding plastics in rodents. Science. 1953, 118, 305-307. CARCINOGENICITY.

Oppenheimer, B. S., Oppenheimer, E. T., Stout, A. P., Willhite, M., and Danishefsky, I. The latent period in carcinogenesis by plastics in rats and to the presarcomatous stage. Cancer. 1958, 11, 204-214. CARCINOGENICITY.

Oppenheimer, B. S., Oppenheimer, I. D., and Stout, P. S. Further studies of polymers as carcinogenic agents in animals. Cancer research. 1955, 15, 333-340. TOXICOLOGY/ CARCINOGENICITY.

Oppenheimer, E. T., Willhite, M., Danishefsky, I., and Stout, A. P. Observations on the effects of powdered polymer in the carcinogenic process. Cancer Research. 1961 Jan, 21, 132-135. CARCINOGENICITY.

Oppenheimer, E. T., Willhite, M., Stout, A. F., Danishefsky, I., and Fishmann, M. M. A comparative study of the effects of imbedding cellophane and polystyrene files in rats. Cancer Research. 1964, 24, 379. CARCINOGENICITY.

Orel, S. G. High-resolution MR imaging of the breast. Semin Ultrasound CT MR. 1996 Oct, 17, (5): 476-493. MAMMOGRAPHY.

Orel, S. G., Fowble, B. L., Solin, L. J., and Schultz, D. J. Breast cancer recurrence after lumpectomy and radiation therapy for early-stage disease: Prognostic significance of detection method. Radiology. 1993, 188, 189-194. MAMMOGRAPHY/cancer.

Orel, S. G., Troupin, R. H., Patterson, E. A., and Fowble, B. L. Breast cancer recurrence after lumpectomy and irradiation: Role of mammography in detection. Radiology. 1992, 183, 201-206. MAMMOGRAPHY.

Orentreich, N. Soft tissue augmentation with medical-grade fluid silicone. Biomater Skin Surg. 1983, 56, 859-881. SILICONE INJECTION.

Orrah, D. J., Semlyn, J. A., and Ross-Murphy, S. B. Polymer. 1988, 29, 1452. SILICONE CHARACTERIZATION.

Ortiz-Monasterio, F., and Trigos, I. Management of patients with complications from injections of foreign materials into the breasts. Plast. Reconstr. Surg. 1972 Jul, 50, (1): 42-47. SILICONE INJECTION/cancer.

Osorio, A. M., Thun, M. J., Novak, R. F., Cura J.V., and Avner, E. D. Silica and glomerulonephritis: Case report and review of the literature. American Journal of Kidney Diseases. 1987 Mar, 9, (3): 224-230. SILICA.

Osteen, R. T. Reconstruction after mastectomy. Cancer. 1995 Nov 15, 76, (10 (Supplement)): 2070-2074. PSYCHOSOCIAL/cancer/reconstruction.

Osteen, R. T., Cady, B., Friedman, M., Kraybill, W., Doggett, S., Hussey, D., and et al. Patterns of care for younger women with breast cancer. Journal of the National Cancer Institute Monographs. 1994, 16, 43-46. GENERAL.

Ostermeyer-Shoaib, B., and Patten, B. M. An atypical multiple sclerosis-like syndrome in women with silicone breast implants or silicone fluid injections into the breast. Canadian Journal of Neurological Science. 1993a, 20, 156. NEUROLOGIC DISEASE.

Ostermeyer-Shoaib, B., and Patten, B. M. Human adjuvant disease: Presentation as a multiple sclerosis-like syndrome. Southern Medical Journal. 1996a Feb, 89, (2): 179-188. NEUROLOGIC DISEASE/connective tissue disease.

Ostermeyer-Shoaib, B., Patten, B. M., and Calkins, D. S. Adjuvant breast disease: An evaluation of 100 symptomatic women with breast implants or silicone fluid injections. Keio Journal of Medicine. 1994 Jun, 43, (2): 79-87. CONNECTIVE TISSUE DISEASE/immune effects/silicone injection.

Pabst, H., and Spady, D. Effect of breast feeding on antibody response to conjugate vaccine. The Lancet. 1990, 336, (8710): 269-270. BREAST FEEDING.

Palazzolo, R. J., Mchard, J. A., Hobbs, E. J., Fancher, O. E., and Calandra, J. C. Investigation of the toxicological properties of a phenylmethylcyclosiloxane. Toxicology and Applied Pharmacology. 1972, 21, 15-28. TOXICOLOGY.

Palcheff-Wiemer, M., Concannon, M. J., Conn, V. S., and Puckett, C. L. The impact of the media on women with breast implants. Plast. Reconstr. Surg. 1993 Oct, 92, (5): 779-785. GENERAL/psychosocial.

Paletta, C. E., Bostwick, III J., and Nahai, F. The inferior gluteal free flap in breast reconstruction. Plast. Reconstr. Surg. 1989 Dec, 84, (6): 875-883. RECONSTRUCTION.

Paletta, C., Paletta, Jr. F. X., and Paletta, Sr. F. X. Sqamous cell carcinoma following breast augmentation. Annals of Plastic Surgery. 1992 Nov, 29, (5): 425-432. CANCER.

Palley, H. A. The evolution of FDA policy on silicone breast implants: A case study of politics, bureaucracy, and business in the process of decision-making. International Journal of Health Services. 1995, 25, (4): 573-591. GENERAL.

Palmon, L. U., Foshager, M. C., Parantainen, H., Everson, L. I., and Cunningham, B. Ruptured or intact: What can linear echoes within silicone breast implants tell us? AJR American Journal of Roentgenology. 1997 Jun, 168, (6): 1595-1598. MAMMOGRAPHY/local complications/rupture.

Pandurangi, R. S., Seehra, M. S., Razzaboni, B. L., and Bolsaitis, P. Surface and bulk infrared modes of crystalline and amorphous silica particles: A study of the relation of surface structure to cytotoxicity of respirable silica. Environmental Health Perspectives. 1990, 86, 327-336. SILICA.

Pangman, W. J. Breast trauma—Surgical and psychic: Its repair and prevention. Journal of the International College of Surgeons. 1965 Nov, 44, (5): 515-522. PSYCHOSOCIAL.

Pankowsky, D. A., Ziats, N. P., Tophan, N. S., Ratnoff, O. D., and Anderson, J. M. Morphological characteristics of adsorbed human plasma proteins on vascular grafts and biomaterials. Journal of Vascular Surgery. 1990 Apr, 11, (4): 599-606. TOXICOLOGY.

Papillon, J. Pros and cons of subpectoral implantation. Clinics in Plastic Surgery. 1976 Apr, 3, (2): 321. CAPSULE-CONTRACTURE/local complications.

Park, A. J., Black, R. J., Sarhadi, N. S., Chetty, U., and Watson, A. C. H. Silicone gel-filled breast implants and connective tissue disease. Plast. Reconstr. Surg. 1998 Feb, 101, (2): 261-267. CONNECTIVE TISSUE DISEASE/immune effects.

Park, A. J., Black, R. J., and Watson, A. C. H. Silicone gel breast implants, breast cancer and connective tissue disorders. British Journal of Surgery. 1993, 80, (9): 1097-1100. GENERAL/connective tissue disease/cancer.

Park, A. J., Chetty, U., and Watson, A. C. H. Patient satisfaction following insertion of silicone breast implants. British Journal of Plastic Surgery. 1996a, 17, (23): 2265-2272. PSYCHOSOCIAL.

Park, A. J., Walsh, J., Reddy, P. S. V., Chetty, U., and Watson, A. C. H. The detection of breast implant rupture using ultrasound. British Journal of Plastic Surgery. 1996b, 49, 299-301. MAMMOGRAPHY/local complications/rupture.

Parsons, C. L. Subclinical infection of penile prostheses. Infection and Urology. 1995, 8, (5): 148-150. INFECTION/local complications/general.

Parsons, C. L., Stein, P. C., Dobke, M. K., and et al. Diagnosis and therapy of subclinically infected prostheses. Surg Gynecol Obstet. 1993 Nov, 177, 504-506. INFECTION/local complications.

Parsons, R. W., and Thering, H. R. Management of the silicone injected breast. Plast. Reconstr. Surg. 1977 Oct, 60, (4): 534-538. SILICONE INJECTION/local complications/migration/cancer/capsule-contracture.

Pasteris, J. D., Wopenka, N. B., Freeman, J. J., Young, V. L., and Brandon, H. J. Analysis of breast implant capsular tissue for crystalline silica and other refractile phases. Plast. Reconstr. Surg. 1999, 103, (4): 1273-1276. SILICA/silicon measurement.

Pasyk, K. A., Austad, E. D., and Cherry, G. W. Intracellular collagen fibers in the capsule around silicone expanders in guinea pigs. Journal of Surgical Research. 1984, 36, 125-133. EXPANDER/capsule-contracture/local complications.

Pasyk, K. A., Austad, E. D., McClatchey, K., and Cherry, G. W. Electron microscopic evaluation of guinea pig skin and soft tissue expanded with a self-inflating silicone implant. Plast. Reconstr. Surg. 1982 Jul, 70, (1): 37-45. EXPANDER.

Patel, R. T., Webster, DJ. T., Mansel, R. E., and Hughes, L. E. Is immediate postmastectomy reconstruction safe in the long-term? European Journal of Surgical Oncology. 1993, 19, 372-375. RECONSTRUCTION.

Patten, B. M., and Ostermeyer-Shoaib, B. O. Disquisition on human adjuvant disease. Perspectives in Biology and Medicine. 1995 Winter, 38, (2): 274-290. GENERAL/connective tissue disease.

Patten, B., Jung, S., and Mata, K. Muscle biopsy histochemistry: A useful tool for evaluating patients who have neuromuscular disease. 1977 Aug. NEUROLOGIC DISEASE.

Pay, A. D., and Kenealy, J. Breast implant rupture following contralateral mammography. Plast. Reconstr. Surg. 1997, 99, (6): 1734-1735. MAMMOGRAPHY/rupture.

Peacock, D. J., and Cooper, C. Epidemiology of the rheumatic diseases. Current Opinion in Rheumatology. 1995, 7, 82-86. AI-CTD BACKGROUND.

Pearl, R. M., Laub, D. R., and Kaplan, E. N. Complications following silicone injections for augmentation of the face. Plast. Reconstr. Surg. 1978 Jun, 61, (6): 888-891. SILICONE INJECTION.

Pearson, C. M. Experimental joint disease: Observations on adjuvant-induced arthritis. Journal of Chronic Disease. 1963, 16, 863-874. AI-CTD BACKGROUND.

Pedersen, B. K., and Beyer, J. M. Characterization of the in vitro effects of glucocorticoids in NK cell activity. Allergy. 1986, 41, 220-224. AI-CTD BACKGROUND.

Pedersen, B. K., and Ullum, H. NK cell response to physical activity: possible mechanisms of action. Med. Sci. Sports Exer. 1994, 26, 140-146. AI-CTD BACKGROUND.

Peimer, C. A., Medige, J., Eckert, B. S., Wright, J. R., and Howard, C. S. Reactive synovitis after silicone arthroplasty. The Journal of Hand Surgery. 1986, 11A, (5): 624-638. GENERAL/local complications.

Peled, I. J. Wexler M. R. Shoshan S. Moshe S. B., Gazit, D., Bab, I., and Ticher, S. Capsule around silicone implants in diabetic rats: Histological and biochemical study. Annals of Plastic Surgery. 1986 Oct, 17, (4): 288-291. CAPSULE-CONTRACTURE/local complications.

Pellenbarg, R. Environmental Poly(organosiloxanes) (Silicones). Environmental Science and Technology. 1979 May, 13, (5): 565-569. TOXICOLOGY.

Pennington, J. Silicon in foods and diets. Food Addit Contam. 1981, 8, (1): 107-118. SILICON MEASUREMENT.

Pennisi, V. R. Long-term use of polyurethane breast prostheses: A 14-year experience. Plast. Reconstr. Surg. 1990 Aug, 86, (2): 368-371. POLYURETHANE/local complications/rupture/capsule-contracture/infection/granulomas/hematomas.

Pennisi, V. R. Making a definite inframammary fold under a reconstructed breast. Plast. Reconstr. Surg. 1977, 60, (4): 523-525. RECONSTRUCTION.

Pennisi, V. R. Obscure carcinoma encountered in subcutaneous mastectomy in silicone and paraffin-injected breasts: Two patients. Plast. Reconstr. Surg. 1984 Oct, 74, (4): 535-538. CANCER/silicone injection.

Pennisi, V. R. Polyurethane-covered silicone-gel mammary prosthesis for successful breast reconstruction. Aesthet Plast Surg. 1985, 9, 73-77. POLYURETHANE/reconstruction.

Pennisi, V. R., Lozada, G., and Capozzi, A. Minimizing complications of subcutaneous mastectomy. Breast. 1980, 6, 22. LOCAL COMPLICATIONS.

Pepys, J. Allergy of the respiratory tract to low molecular weight chemical agents. Handbook of Experimental Pharmacology. 1983, 63, 163-185. PLATINUM/toxicology.

Pepys, J., Parish, W. E., Cromwell, O., and Hughes, E. G. Specific IgE and IgG antibodies to platinum salts in sensitized workers. Monogr Allergy. 1979, 14, 142-145. PLATINUM/toxicology.

Perkins, L. L., Clark, B. D., Klein, P. J., and Cook, R. R. A meta-analysis of breast implants and connective tissue disease. Annals of Plastic Surgery. 1995 Dec, 35, (6): 561-570. CONNECTIVE TISSUE DISEASE.

Perras, C. The prevention and treatment of infections following breast implants. Plast. Reconstr. Surg. 1965 Jun, 35, (6): 649-656. LOCAL COMPLICATIONS/infection.

Perras, C., and Camirand, A. Subcutaneous mastectomy. American Journal of Nursing. 1973, 73, (9). GENERAL.

Perras, C., and Papillon, J. The value of mammography in cosmetic surgery of the breasts. Plast. Reconstr. Surg. 1973 Aug, 52, (2): 132-137. MAMMOGRAPHY.

Perrelli, G., and Piolatto, G. Tentative reference values for gold, silver and platinum: Literature data analysis. The Science of the Total Environment. 1992, 120, 93-96. PLATINUM.

Perrin, E. R. The use of soluble steroids with inflatable breast prostheses. Plast. Reconstr. Surg. 1976, 57, (2): 163-166. STEROIDS/expander/saline.

Perry, R. R., Jacques, D. P., Lesar, M. S. L., d'Avis, J. C., and Peterson, H. D. *Mycobacterium avium* infection in a silicone-injected breast. Plast. Reconstr. Surg. 1985 Jan, 75, (1): 104-106. SILICONE INJECTION/infection/local complications.

Persellin, S. T., Vogler, J. B., Brazis, P. W., and Moy, O. J. Silicone gel breast implants. Mayo Clinic Proceedings. 1993, 68, 96. GENERAL.

Persellin, S., Vogler, J. B., and Moy, O. J. Detection of migratory silicone pseudotumor with use of magnetic resonance imaging. Mayo Clinic Proceedings. 1992 Sep, 67, 891-895. MAMMOGRAPHY/migration/local complications.

Persoff, M. M. Expansion-augmentation of the breast. Plast. Reconstr. Surg. 1993 Mar, 91, (3): 393-403. EXPANDER.

Persson, B., Dahlander, A.-M., Fredriksson, M., Brage, H. N., Ohlson, C.-G., and Axelson, O. Malignant lymphomas and occupational exposures. British Journal of Industrial Medicine. 1989, 46, 516-520. CARCINOGENICITY.

Peters, C. R., Shaw, T. E., and Raghavu, R. D. The influence of vitamin E on capsule formation and contracture around silicone implants. Annals of Plastic Surgery. 1980 Nov, 5, (5): 347-352. CAPSULE-CONTRACTURE/local complications.

Peters, W. J. Current status of silicone gel breast implants. Canadian Journal of Plastic Surgery. 1994 Spring, 2, (1): 18-23. GENERAL/rupture/local complications.

Peters, W. J. Failure properties of leaf valve inflatable saline breast implants. Can J Plast Surg. 1997, 4, 241-245. RUPTURE/saline.

Peters, W. J. The mechanical properties of breast prostheses. Annals of Plastic Surgery. 1981 Mar, 6, 179-181. RUPTURE/local complications/closed capsulotomy/capsule-contracture.

Peters, W. J. The rupture of silicone gel breast implants. Ann Plast Surg. 1994a, 33, 462-463. RUPTURE/local complications.

Peters, W. J. Rupture of silicone-gel breast implants. The Lancet. 1998, 351, 521. RUPTURE/local complications.

Peters, W. J. Silicone breast implants and autoimmune connective tissue disease. Annals of Plastic Surgery. 1995 Jan, 34, (1): 103-109. SILICON MEASUREMENT/local complications/rupture/connective tissue disease/immune effects.

Peters, W. J., Keystone, E., and Smith, D. Factors affecting the rupture of silicone-gel breast implants. Annals of Plastic Surgery. 1994a May 1, 32, (5): 449-451. RUPTURE/capsule-contracture/local complications/explantation.

Peters, W. J., Keystone, E., Snow, K., Rubin, L., and Smith, D. Is there a relationship between autoantibodies and silicone-gel implants? Annals of Plastic Surgery. 1994b Jan, 32, (1): 1-7. IMMUNE EFFECTS/connective tissue disease.

Peters, W. J., and McEwan, P. Capsular contracture simulating myocardial infarction on ECG. Plast. Reconstr. Surg. 1993, 91, 529-532. CAPSULE-CONTRACTURE/pain/local complications.

Peters, W. J., and Pritzker, K. P. H. Massive heterotopic ossification in breast implant capsules. Aesthetic Plastic Surgery. 1985 Jan, 9, 43-45. CALCIFICATION/local complications.

Peters, W. J., Pritzker, K., and Smith, K. et al. Capsular Calcification associated with silicone breast implants: incidence, determinants and characterization. Ann. Plast. Surg. 1998, 41, (4): 348-360. CALCIFICATION/local complications.

Peters, W. J., and Pugash, R. Ultrasound analysis of 150 patients with silicone gel breast implants. Annals of Plastic Surgery. 1993 Jul, 31, (1): 7-9. MAMMOGRAPHY.

Peters, W. J., and Smith, D. Calcification of breast implant capsules: Incidence, diagnosis, and contributing factors. Annals of Plastic Surgery. 1995 Jan, 34, (1): 8-11. CALCIFICATION/local complications.

Peters, W. J., and Smith, D. C. Ivalon breast prostheses: Evaluation 19 years after implantation. Plast. Reconstr. Surg. 1981 Apr, 67, (4): 514-518. LOCAL COMPLICATIONS/general.

Peters, W. J., Smith, D., Fornasier, V., Lugowski, S., and Ibanez, D. An outcome analysis of 100 women after explantation of silicone gel breast implants. Annals of Plastic Surgery. 1997 Jul, 39, (1): 9-19. GENERAL/psychosocial/local complications/connective tissue disease/capsule-contracture/pain/sensation/rupture/explantation.

Peters, W. J., Smith, D., Grosman, H., and Fornasier, V. Role of mammography to assess complications of silicone gel breast implants. Can. J. Plast. Surg. 1995d, 3, (3): 150-156. MAMMOGRAPHY.

Peters, W. J., Smith, D., and Lugowski, S. Failure properties of 352 explanted silicone-gel breast implants. Canadian Journal of Plastic Surgery. 1996 Spring, 4, (1): 55-58. RUPTURE.

Peters, W. J., Smith, D., Lugowski, S., McHugh, A., and Baines, C. Do patients with silicone gel breast implants have elevated levels of serum silicon compared to control patients? Annals of Plastic Surgery. 1995b Apr, 34, (6): 343-347. SILICON MEASUREMENT.

Peters, W. J., Smith, D., Lugowski, S., McHugh, A., Kereteci, A., and Baines, C. Analysis of silicon levels in capsules of gel and saline breast implants and of penile prostheses. Annals of Plastic Surgery. 1995a Jun, 34, (6): 578-584. SILICON MEASUREMENT.

Peterson, H. D., and Burt, G. B. The role of steroids in prevention of circumferential capsular scarring in augmentation mammaplasty. Plast. Reconstr. Surg. 1974 Jul, 54, (1): 28-30. STEROIDS/local complications/capsule-contracture.

Peterson, R. D., Bowen, D., Netscher, D. T., and Wigoda, P. Capsular compliance: A measure of a hard prosthesis. Annals of Plastic Surgery. 1994 Apr, 32, (4): 337-341. CAPSULE-CONTRACTURE/local complications.

Petillo, O., Peluso, G., and Ambrosio, L. *In vivo* induction of macrophage Ia antigen (MHC class II) expression by biomedical polymers in the cage implant system. Journal of Biomedical Materials Research. 1994, 28, 635-646. IMMUNE EFFECTS.

Petit, J. Y. Primary and secondary breast reconstruction with special emphasis on the use of prostheses. Recent Results in Cancer Research. 1996, 140, 169-175. RECONSTRUCTION.

Petit, J. Y., Lê, M. G., Mouriesse, H., Rietjens, M., Gill, P., Contesso, G., and Lehmann, A. Can breast reconstruction with gel-filled silicone implants increase the risk of death and second primary cancer in patients treated by mastectomy for breast cancer? Plast. Reconstr. Surg. 1994 Jul, 94, (1): 115-119. CANCER.

Petro, J. A., Klein, S. A., Niazi, Z., Salzberg, C. A., and Byrne, D. Evaluation of ultrasound as a tool in the follow-up of patients with breast implants: A preliminary prospective study. Annals of Plastic Surgery. 1994 Jun, 32, (6): 581-587. MAMMOGRAPHY.

Pettersson, I., Wang, G., Smith, E., Wigzell, H., Hedfors, E., Horn, J., and Sharp, G. C. The use of immunoblotting and immunoprecipitation of (U) small nuclear ribonucleoproteins in the analysis of sera of patients with mixed connected tissue disease and systemic lupus erythematosus. Arthritis and Rheumatism. 1986, 29, (8): 986-996. IMMUNE EFFECTS/ai-ctd background.

Pfleiderer, B., Ackerman, J. L., and Garrido, L. In vivo 1H chemical shift imaging of silicone implants. Magn Reson Med. 1993c, 29, 656-659. MAMMOGRAPHY/silicon measurement.

Pfleiderer, B., Ackerman, J. L., and Garrido, L. In vivo localized proton NMR spectroscopy of silicone. Magn Reson Med. 1993b, 30, 149-154. MAMMOGRAPHY/silicon measurement.

Pfleiderer, B., Ackerman, J. L., and Garrido, L. Migration and biodegradation of free silicone from silicone gel-filled implants after long-term implantation. Magn Reson Med. 1993a, 30, 534-543. MIGRATION/local complications/silicon measurement.

Pfleiderer, B., Campbell, T., Hulka, C. A., Kopans, D. B., Lean, C. L., Ackerman, J. L., Brady, T. J., and Garrido, L. Silicone gel-filled breast implants in women: Findings at H-1 MR spectroscopy. Radiology. 1996, 201, (3): 777-783. SILICON MEASUREMENT/migration/local complications.

Pfleiderer, B., and Garrido, L. Migration and accumulation of silicone in the liver of women with silicone gel-filled breast implants. Magnet Resonance in Med. 1995, 33, 8-17. MIGRATION/local complications/silicon measurement.

Pfleiderer, B., Moore, J., Ackerman, J. L., and et al. Study of the aging process of PDMS implants in vivo and ex vivo by nuclear magnetic resonance spectroscopy and imaging. Polymer Preprints. 1992, 33, 767-768. MAMMOGRAPHY/silicon measurement.

Pfleiderer, B., Moore, J., Ackerman, J. L., and Garrido, L. NMR imaging of materials: Microscopy or not? Polymer Preprints. 1992, 33, (1): 767. MAMMOGRAPHY/silicon measurement.

Pfleiderer, B., Xu, P., Ackerman, J., and Garrido, L. Study of aging of silicone rubber biomaterials with NMR. Journal of Biomedical Materials Research. 1995 Sep, 29, 1129-1140. SILICONE CHARACTERIZATION.

Phelan, D. L., Mohanakumar, T., McWilliams, J., and et al. Breast implants and autoimmunity: Association with HLA. Human Immunology. 1992, 34, S34. IMMUNE EFFECTS.

Phelps, C. P., Chen, L. T., Poole, L. T., and Menzies, R. A. Variable tissue reactions and endocrine responses to a jugular catheter. Journal of Submicrosc. Cytol. Path. 1995 Jan, 27, (1): 83-89. IMMUNE EFFECTS.

Philippou and et al. Lung fibrosis after inhalation of amorphous silica. Zentralbl Pathol. 1992 Mar, 138, 41-46. SILICA.

Phillips, J. W., de Camara, D. L., Lockwood, M. D., and Grebner, W. C. C. Strength of silicone breast implants. Plast. Reconstr. Surg. 1996 May, 97, (6): 1215-1225. RUPTURE/local complications.

Phua, S. K., Castillo, E., Anderson, J. M., and Hiltner, A. Biodegration of a polyurethane *in vitro*. Journal of Biomedical Materials Research. 1987, 21, 231-246. POLYURETHANE.

Picard, F., Alikacem, N., Guidoin, R., and Auger, M. Multinuclear solid-state NMR spectroscopy of envelopes from virgin and explanted silicone breast prostheses: An exploratory study. Magn Reson Med. 1997, 37, (1): 11-17. SILICONE CHARACTERIZATION/silicon measurement.

Picha, G. J. Mammary implants: Surface modifications and the soft tissue response. Perspectives in Plastic Surgery. 1991, 5, 54. SILICONE CHARACTERIZATION.

Picha, G. J., and Goldstein, J. A. Analysis of the soft-tissue response to components used in the manufacture of breast implants: rat-animal model. Plast. Reconstr. Surg. 1991 Mar, 87, 490-500. SILICONE CHARACTERIZATION/capsule-contracture/local complications.

Picha, G. J., and Goldstein, J. A. Investigation of silicone oil and fumed silica on an adjuvant animal model. Plast. Reconstr. Surg. 197, 100, (3): 643-652. CONNECTIVE TISSUE DISEASE/immune effects.

Picha, G. J., Goldstein, J. A., and Stohr, E. Natural-Y Même polyurethane versus smooth silicone: Analysis of the soft-tissue interaction from 3 days to 1 year in the rat animal model. Plast. Reconstr. Surg. 1990 Jun, 85, (6): 903-916. POLYURETHANE/capsule-contracture/local complications.

Picha, G. J., Goldstein, J., and Stohr, E. Soft tissue response to Même polyurethane covered silicone implants/smooth controls: Three days to one year. Artificial Organs. 1990, 14, (3). POLYURETHANE.

Picha, G. J., and Siedlak, D. J. Ion-beam microtexturing of biomaterials. Medical Device Diagn Ind. 1984, 6, 39. SILICONE CHARACTERIZATION.

Pickrell, K. L., Puckett, C. L., and Given, K. S. Subpectoral augmentation mammaplasty. Plast. Reconstr. Surg. 1977 Sep, 60, (3): 325-336. GENERAL.

Pidutti, R., and Morales, A. Silicone gel-filled testicular prosthesis and systemic disease. Urology. 1993 Aug, 42, (2): 155-157. IMMUNE EFFECTS/connective tissue disease/general.

Piechotta, F. U. Silicone fluid, attractive and dangerous: Collective review and summary of exposure. Aesthetic Plastic Surgery. 1979, 3, 347-351. SILICONE INJECTION.

Pilbrandt, A., and Strindberg, B. Pharmacokinetics of 2,6-cis-diphenylhexamethylcyclotetrasiloxane in man. Acta Pharmacologica et Toxicologica. 1975, 36, (Supplement III): 139-147. TOXICOLOGY.

Pilipshen, S. J., Gerardi, J., Bretsky, S., and Robbins, G. F. The significance of delay in treating patients with potentially curable breast cancer. Breast, Diseases of the Breast. 1984, 10, (3): 16-23. CANCER.

Pinotti, J. A., Costa, M. S., Teixeira, L. C., Keppke, E. M., Baroudi, R., and Gabiatti, J. R. E. Localization of benign breast diseases and proposal of a new approach for aesthetic breast reduction. Breast Dis. 1989, 1, 295-312. GENERAL.

Piscatelli, S. J. Breast capsule contracture: Is fibroblast activity associated with severity? Aesthetic Plast Surg. 1994, 18, (1): 75-79. CAPSULE-CONTRACTURE/local complications.

Pisetsky, D. S. Anti-DNA antibodies in systemic lupus erythematosus. Rheumatic Disease Clinics of North America. 1992 May, 18, (2): 437-454. AI-CTD BACKGROUND.

Pitt, W. G., Park, K., and Cooper, S. L. Sequential protein adsorption and thrombus deposition on polymeric biomaterials. Journal of Colloid and Interface Science. 1986 Jun, 111, (2): 343-362. SILICONE CHARACTERIZATION.

Poblete, J. V. P., Rodgers, J. A., and Wolfort, F. G. Toxic shock syndrome as a complication of breast prostheses. Plast. Reconstr. Surg. 1995 Dec, 96, (7): 1702-1708. INFECTION/local complications.

Pohost, G. M., Blackwell, G. G., and Shellock, F. G. Safety of patients with medical devices during application of magnetic resonance methods. Annals of the New York Academy of Sciences. 1992, 649, 302-312. MAMMOGRAPHY.

Policard, A., and Collet, A. Experimental studies of the pathological reactions to parenteral administrations of submicron amorphous silicas. American Archives of Industrial Health. 1957 Oct, 19. SILICA/toxicology.

Policard, A., and Collet, A. Toxic and fibrosing action of submicroscopic particles of amorphous silica. Industr Hyg Occp Med. 1955, 12, 389-395. TOXICOLOGY/silica.

Pollock, H. Breast capsular contracture: A retrospective study of textured versus smooth silicone implants. Plast. Reconstr. Surg. 1993, 91, (3): 404-407. CAPSULE-CONTRACTURE/local complications.

Polyzois, G. L., Hensten-Pettersen, A., and Kullman, A. An assessment of the physical properties and biocompatibility of three silicone elastomers. The Journal of Prosthetic Dentistry. 1994, 71, (5): 500-504. TOXICOLOGY/general.

Porter, J. F., Kingsland, 3d L. C., Lindberg, D. A., Shah, I., Benge, J. M., Hazelwood, S. E., Kay, D. R., Homma, M., Akizuki, M., Takano, M., and Sharp, G. C. The AI/RHEUM knowledge-based computer consultant system in rheumatology. Arthritis and Rheumatism. 1988, 31, (2): 219-226. AI-CTD BACKGROUND.

Potter, M., Morrison, S., Wiener, F., Zhang, X. K., and Miller, F. W. Induction of plasmacytomas with silicone gel in genetically susceptible strains of mice. Journal of the National Cancer Institute. 1994 Jul 20, 86, (14): 1058-1065. MYELOMA/immune effects.

Press, R. I., Peebles, C. L., Kumagai, Y., Ochs, R. L., and Tan, E. M. Antinuclear autoantibodies in women with silicone breast implants. The Lancet. 1992 Nov 28, 340, 1304-1307. IMMUNE EFFECTS.

Price, J. E., and Barker, D. E. Initial clinical experience with 'low bleed' breast implants. Aesthetic Plastic Surgery. 1983 Jan 1, 7, 255-256. CAPSULE CONTRACTURE/local complications.

Price Jr., J. E. Capsular contraction and deflation associated with inflatable implants. Aesthetic Plastic Surgery. 1983, 7, 257-238. CAPSULE-CONTRACTURE/local complications/rupture/saline.

Price, R., North, C., Wessely, S., and Frasher, V. Estimating the prevalence of chronic fatigue syndrome and associated symptoms in the community. Public Health Reports. 1992, 107, (5): 515-522. AI-CTD BACKGROUND.

Prockop, D. Mutations in collagen genes as a cause of connective-tissue diseases. New England Journal of Medicine. 1992 Feb 20, 326, (8): 540-546. AI-CTD BACKGROUND.

Provost, T. T. R., Watson, K. K., Gaither, and Harley, J. B. The neonatal lupus erythematosus syndrome. J. Rheumatol. 1987, 14, 199-205. CHILDREN'S EFFECTS/breast feeding.

Pryse-Phippils, W., and Murray, T. J. Amyotrophic lateral sclerosis. Essential Neurology. 1992. NEUROLOGIC DISEASE.

Puckett, C. L. Gel bleed and gel migration. Plast. Reconstr. Surg. 1997 Apr, 99, (5): 1410. MIGRATION/local complications/rupture.

Puckett, C. L, Croll, G. H., and Reichel, C. A. A critical look at capsule contracture in subglandular versus subpectoral mammary augmentation. Aesthetic Plast. Surg. 1987, 11, 23. CAPSULE-CONTRACTURE/local complications.

Purohit, A., Ghilchik, M. W., Duncan, L. J., and et al. Aromatase activity and interleukin-6 production by normal and malignant breast tissues. Journal of Clinical Endrocrinology and Metabolism. 1995, 80, 3052-3058. CANCER.

Quinn, S. F., Neubauer, N. M., Sheley, R. C., Demlow, T. A., and Szumowski, J. MR imaging of silicone breast implants: Evaluation of prospective and retrospective interpretations and interobserver agreement. J Magn Reson Imaging. 1996 Jan-1996 Feb 28, 6, (1): 213-218. MAMMOGRAPHY.

Radovan, C. Breast reconstruction after mastectomy using the temporary expander. Plast. Reconstr. Surg. 1982 Feb, 69, (2): 195-206. EXPANDER/reconstruction.

Radovan, C. Reconstruction of the breast after radical mastectomy using temporary expander. Am Soc Plast Reconstr Surg Forum. 1978, 1, 41. EXPANDER/reconstruction.

Radovan, C. Tissue expansion in soft-tissue reconstruction. Plast. Reconstr. Surg. 1984 Oct, 74, (4): 482-490. EXPANDER/local complications.

Rae, V., Pardo, R. J., Blackwelder, P. L., and Falanga, V. Leg ulcers following subcutaneous injection of a liquid silicone preparation. Archives of Dermatology. 1989 May, 125, 5. SILICONE INJECTION.

Rahman, H., and Fagg, P. Silicone granulomatous reactions after first metatarsophalangeal hemiarthroiplasty. Journal of Bone and Joint Surgery. 1993 Jul, 75b, 637-639. GRANULOMAS/local complications/general.

Ramasastry, S. S., Weinstein, L. W., Zerbe, A., Narayanan, K., LaPietra, D., and Futrell, J. W. Regression of local and distant tumor growth by tissue expansion: An experimental study of mammary carcinoma 13762 in rats. Plast. Reconstr. Surg. 1991, 87, (1): 1-7. CANCER.

Ramirez, O. M., and Orlando, J. C. Chest wall deformity during tissue expansion in breast reconstruction. Plastic Surgery Forum. 1986, 9, 148-153. LOCAL COMPLICATIONS/expander.

Randall, T. Antibodies to silicone detected in patients with severe inflammatory reactions. J. Amer. Med. Assoc. 1992 Oct 14, 268, (14): 1821-1822. IMMUNE EFFECTS.

Randall, T. Less maligned, but cut from the same cloth, other silicone implants also have adverse effects. J. Amer. Med. Assoc. 1992 Jul, 268, (1): 12-18. GENERAL.

Ransjö, U., Asplund, O., Gylbert, L., and Jurell, G. Bacteria in the female breast. Scandinavian Journal of Plastic and Reconstructive Surgery. 1985, 19, 87-89. INFECTION.

Rapaport, D. P., Stadelmann, W. K., and Greenwald, D. P. Incidence and natural history of saline-filled breast implant deflations: Comparison of blunt-tipped versus cutting and tapered needles. Plast. Reconstr. Surg. 1997, 100, (4): 1028-1032. SALINE/rupture/local complications.

Rapaport, M. J., Vinnik, C., and Zaren, H. Injectable silicone: Cause of facial nodules, cellulitis, ulceration, and migration. Aesthetic Plastic Surgery. 1996, 20, (3): 267-276. SILICONE INJECTION.

Raposo do Amaral, C. M., Tiziani, V., Cintra, M. L., Amstalden, I., and Palhares, F. B. Local reaction and migration of injected silicone gel: Experimental study. Aesthetic Plastic Surgery. 1993, 17, 335-338. TOXICOLOGY/migration/local complications/silicone injection.

Raso, D. S., Crymes, L. W., and Metcalf, J. S. Histological assessment of fifty breast capsules from smooth and textured augmentation and reconstruction mammoplasty prostheses with emphasis on the role of synovial metaplasia. Modern Pathology. 1994b, 7, (3): 310-316. CAPSULE-CONTRACTURE/local complications.

Raso, D. S., and Greene, W. B. Silicone breast implants: Pathology. Ultrastructural Pathology. 1997, 21, (3): 263-271. CAPSULE-CONTRACTURE/local complications/immune effects/children's effects.

Raso, D. S., and Greene, W. B. Synovial metaplasia of a periprosthetic capsule surrounding a polyurethane foam breast prosthesis. Plast. Reconstr. Surg. 1995 Aug, 35, (2): 201-203. CAPSULE CONTRACTURE.

Raso, D. S., Greene, W. B., Harley, R. A., and Maize, J. C. Silicone deposition in reconstruction scars of women with silicone breast implants. Journal of the American Academy of Dermatology. 1996 Jul, 35, (1): 32-36. CAPSULE-CONTRACTURE/local complications.

Raso, D. S., Greene, W. B., Kalasinsky, V. F., Riopel, M. A., Luke, J. L., Askin, F. B., Silverman, J. F., and Young, V. L. Elemental analysis and clinical implications of calcification deposits associated with silicone breast implants. Annals of Plastic Surgery. 1999 Feb, 42, (2): 117-123. CALCIFICATION/capsule-contracture/mammography.

Raso, D. S., Greene, W. B., and Metcalf, J. Synovial metaplasia of a periprosthetic breast capsule. Archives of Pathology and Laboratory Medicine. 1994a Mar, 118, 249. CAPSULE-CONTRACTURE/local complications.

Raso, D. S., Greene, W. B., Vesely, J. J., and Willingham, M. C. Light microscopy techniques for the demonstration of silicone gel. Archives of Pathology and Laboratory Medicine. 1994b Oct, 118, 984-987. MAMMOGRAPHY/silicon measurement.

Raso, D. S., and Schulte, B. A. Immunolocalization of keratan sulfate, chondroitin-4-sulfate, and chondroitin-6-sulfate in periprosthetic breast capsules exhibiting synovial metaplasia. Plast. Reconstr. Surg. 1996, 98, (1): 78-82. CAPSULE CONTRACTURE/IMMUNE EFFECTS.

Rassaby, J., and Hill, D. Patient's perceptions of breast reconstruction after mastectomy. Medical Journal of Australia. 1983, 2, 173-176. PSYCHOSOCIAL/reconstruction.

Raszewski, R., Guyuron, B., Lash, R. H., McMahon, J. T., and Tuthill, R. J. A severe fibrotic reaction after cosmetic liquid silicone injection. Journal of Cranio-Max Fac Surgery. 1990, 18, 225-228. SILICONE INJECTION.

Ratliff, N. B. Silicone pericarditis. Cleveland Clinical Quarterly. 1984, 51, (1): 185-189. GRANULOMAS/local complications.

Reaby, L. L., and Hort, K. L. Postmastectomy attitudes in women who wear external breast prostheses compared to those who have undergone breast reconstruction. Journal of Behavioral Medicine. 1995, 18, (1): 55-67. PSYCHOSOCIAL/reconstruction.

Reaby, L. L., Hort, L. K., and Vandervord, J. Body image, self-concept, and self-esteem in women who had a mastectomy and either wore an external breast prosthesis or had breast reconstruction and women who had not experienced mastectomy. Health Care for Women International. 1994, 15, (5): 361-375. PSYCHOSOCIAL.

Redelmeier, D. A., Rozin, P., and Kahneman, D. Understanding patients' decisions: Cognitive and emotional perspectives. J. Amer. Med. Assoc. 1993 Jul 7, 270, (1): 72-76. PSYCHOSOCIAL.

Redfern, A. B., and Hoopes, J. E. Subcutaneous mastectomy: A plea for conservatism. Plast. Reconstr. Surg. 1978, 62, (5): 706-707. CANCER.

Redfern, A. B., Ryan, J. J., and Tsugn Su, C. Calcification of the fibrous capsule about mammary implants. Plast. Reconstr. Surg. 1977 Feb, 59, (2): 249-251. CALCIFICATION/capsule-contracture/local complications.

Reed, M. E. Daubert and the breast implant litigation: How is the judiciary addressing the science. Plast. Reconstr. Surg. 1997 Oct, 100, (5): 1322-1326. GENERAL.

Reed, W. A., and Kittle, C. F. Observations on toxicity and use of Antifoam A. AMA Arch Surg. 1959, 78, 220. TOXICOLOGY.

Rees, T. D. The current status of silicone fluid in plastic and reconstructive surgery. Journal of Dermatology and Surgical Oncology. 1976 Mar, 2, (1): 34-38. SILICONE INJECTION.

Rees, T. D., and Ashley, F. L. Treatment of facial atrophy with liquid silicone. American Journal of Surgery. 1966 Apr, 111, 531-535. SILICONE INJECTION.

Rees, T. D., Ashley, F. L., and Delagado, J. P. Silicone fluid injections for facial atrophy —a ten year study. Plast. Reconstr. Surg. 1973a Aug, 52, (2): 118†127. SILICONE INJECTION.

Rees, T. D., Ballantyne, Jr. D. L., and Hawthorne, G. A. Silicone fluid research: A follow-up summary. Plast. Reconstr. Surg. 1970 Jul, 46, (1): 50-56. TOXICOLOGY/silicone injection.

Rees, T. D., Ballantyne, Jr. D. L., Seidman, I., and Hawthorne, G. A. Visceral response to subcutaneous and intraperitoneal injections of silicone in mice. Plast. Reconstr. Surg. 1967 Apr, 39, (4): 402-410. TOXICOLOGY/silicone injection.

Rees, T. D., Ballantyne, Jr. D. L., Seidman, I., and Hawthrone, G. A. Intraperitoneal injections of silicone in mice. Plast. Reconstr. Surg. 1967, 39, 402-410. SILICONE INJECTION.

Rees, T. D., Guy, C. L., and Coburn, R. J. The use of inflatable breast implants. Plast. Reconstr. Surg. 1973b Dec, 52, (6): 609. EXPANDER.

Rees, T. D., Platt, J., and Ballantyne, D. L. An investigation of cutaneous response to dimethylpolysiloxane (silicone liquid) in animals and humans—A preliminary report. Plast. Reconstr. Surg. 1965 Feb, 35, (2): 131-139. CARCINOGENICITY/silicone injection.

Refojo, M. F., Leong, F.-L., Chung, H., Ueno, N., Nemiroff, B., and Tolentino, F. I. Extraction of retinol and cholesterol by intraocular silicone oils. Ophthalmology. 1988 May, 95, (5): 614-618. GENERAL/toxicology.

Regnault, P. Partially submuscular breast augmentation. Plast. Reconstr. Surg. 1977, 59, (1): 72-76. GENERAL.

Regnault, P., Baker, t. J., Gleason, M. C., Gordon, H. L., Grossman, A. R., Lewis, Jr. J. R., Waters, W. R., and Williams, J. E. Clinical trial and evaluation of a proposed new inflatable mammary prosthesis. Plast. Reconstr. Surg. 1972 Sep, 50, (3): 220-226. SALINE/expander.

Reich, J. The surgery of appearance: Psychological and related aspects. The Medical Journal of Australia. 1969 Jul 5: 5-13. PSYCHOSOCIAL.

Reichlin, M. Antibodies to defined antigens in the systemic rheumatic diseases. Bulletin on Rheumatic Diseases. 1993 Dec, 42, (8): 4-6. IMMUNE EFFECTS.

Reichlin, M., and Arnett, Jr. F. C. Multiplicity of antibodies in myositis sera. Arthritis and Rheumatism. 1984 Oct, 27, (10): 1150-1156. IMMUNE EFFECTS/ai-ctd background.

Reiffel, R. S., Rees, T. D., Guy, C. L., and Aston, S. J. A comparison of capsule formation following breast augmentation by saline-filled or gel-filled implants. Aesthetic Plast. Surg. 1983, 7, 113-116. CAPSULE-CONTRACTURE/local complications/saline.

Reimer, G., Rose, K. M., Scheer, U., and Tan, E. M. Autoantibody to RNA polymerase I in scleroderma sera. Journal of Clinical Investigation. 1987 Jan, 79, 65-72. AI-CTD BACKGROUND/immune effects.

Reinberg, Y., Manivel, J. C., and Gonzalez, R. Silicone shedding from artificial urinary sphincter in children. The Journal of Urology. 1993 Aug, 150, 694-696. SILICONE CHARACTERIZATION/local complications.

Reintgen, D., Berman, C., Cox, C., and et al. The anatomy of missed breast cancers. Surg. Oncol. 1993, 2, 65-75. MAMMOGRAPHY.

Renfrew, D. L., Franken, E. A., and Berbaum, K. S. et al. Errors in radiology: classification and lessons in 182 cases presented at a problem case conference. Radiology. 1992, 183, 145-150. MAMMOGRAPHY.

Rennekampff, H.-O., Exner, K., Lemperle, G., and Nemsmann, B. Reduction of capsular formation around silicone breast implants by D-penicillamine in rats. Scandinavian Journal of Plastic and Reconstructive and Hand Surgery. 1992, 26, 253-255. CAPSULE-CONTRACTURE/local complications.

Renneker, R., and Cutler, M. Psychological problems of adjustment to cancer of the breast. J. Amer. Med. Assoc. 1952, 148, (10): 833-838. PSYCHOSOCIAL/cancer.

Renwick, S. B. Silicone breast implants: Implications for society and surgeons. Medical Journal of Australia. 1996, 165, 338-341. GENERAL.

Reyes, H., Ojo-Amaize, E. A., and Peter, J. B. Silicates, silicones and autoimmunity. Israel Journal of Medical Science. 1997 Apr, 33, (4): 239-242. IMMUNE EFFECTS.

Reynolds, H. E., Buckwalter, K. A., Jackson, V. P., Siwy, B. K., and Alexander, S. G. Comparison of mammography, sonography, and magnetic resonance imaging in the detection of silicone-gel breast implant rupture. Annals of Plastic Surgery. 1994 Sep, 33, (3): 247-255. MAMMOGRAPHY/local complications/rupture.

Rheingold, L. M., Yoo, R. P., and Courtiss, E. H. Experience with 326 inflatable breast implants. Plast. Reconstr. Surg. 1994, 93, (1): 118. EXPANDER/local complications/rupture/saline.

Rhie, J. W., Han, S. B., Byeon, J. H., Ahn, S. T., and Kim, H. M. Efficient in vitro model for immunotoxicologic assessment of mammary silicone implants. Plast. Reconstr. Surg. 1998 Jul, 102, (1): 73-77. IMMUNE EFFECTS.

Ricci, J., Alexander, H., Steiner, G. et al. Status of retrieved breast implants and their surrounding tissues. Proc. Soc. Biomater. 1995, 91, 828. EXPLANTATION.

Rice, D. C., Agasthian, T., Clay, R. P., and Deschamps, C. Silicone thorax: A complication of tube thoracostomy in the presence of mammary implants. Annals of Thoracic Surgery. 1995, 60, 1417-1419. RUPTURE/local complications.

Rich, J. D., Shesol, B. F., and Gottlieb, V. Supraclavicular migration of breast injected silicone: Case report. Military Medicine. 1982 May, 147, 404-405. SILICONE INJECTION/migration.

Richards, J. M., Meuzelaar, H. L. C., and Bunger, J. A. Spectrometric and chromatographic methods for the analysis of polymeric explant materials. Journal of Biomedical Materials Research: Applied Biomaterials. 1989, 23, 321-335. SILICON MEASUREMENT/polyurethane.

Richardson, B., and Epstein, W. V. Utility of the fluorescent antinuclear antibody test in a single patient. Annals of Internal Medicine. 1981, 95, (3): 333-338. IMMUNE EFFECTS.

Riddle, L. B. Augmentation mammoplasty. Plast. Reconstr. Surg. March 1986, 11, (3): 30-40. GENERAL.

Riddle, L. B. Expansion exercises: Modifying contracture of the augmented breast. Research in Nursing and Health. 1986, 9, 341-345. CAPSULE-CONTRACTURE/local complications.

Rider, J. A. Intestinal gas and bloating: Treatment with methyl Polysiloxane. Am Pract & Digest Treat. 1960, 11, (1): 52-57. GENERAL.

Ridolfi, R. L., and Hutchins, G. M. Detection of ball variance in prosthetic heart valves by liver biopsy. Hopkins Medical Journal. 1974, 134, 131-140. SILICONE CHARACTERIZATION.

Riefkohl, R., Roberts, T. L., and McCarty, K. S. Lack of adverse effect of silicone implant on sarcoidosis of the breast. Plast. Reconstr. Surg. 1985, 76, (2): 296-298. IMMUNE EFFECTS.

Rigdon, R. H. Local reaction to polyurethane—a comparative study in the mouse, rat, and rabbit. Journal of Biomedical Materials Research. 1973, 7, (1): 79-93. POLYURETHANE.

Ringberg, A. Subcutaneous mastectomy surgical techniques and complications in 176 women. Eur. J. Plast. Surg. 1990, 13, 7-15. GENERAL.

Rintala, A. E., and Svinhufvud, U. M. Effect of augmentation mammaplasty on mammography and thermography. Plast. Reconstr. Surg. 1974 Oct, 54, (4): 390-396. MAMMOGRAPHY.

Rivero, M. A., Schwartz, D. S., and Mies, C. Silicone lymphadenopathy involving intrammary lymph nodes: A new complication of silicone mammaplasty. AJR American Journal of Roentgenology. 1994 May, 162, 1089-1090. LYMPHADENOPATHY/local complications.

Roberts, C., Wells, K. E., and Daniels, S. Outcome study of the psychological changes after silicone breast implant removal. Plast. Reconstr. Surg. 1997, 100, (3): 595-599. PSYCHOSOCIAL/explantation.

Roberts, N., and Williams, P. Silicon measurement in serum and urine by direct current plasma emission spectrometry. Clinical Chemistry. 1990, 36, (6): 970-971. SILICON MEASUREMENT.

Robertson, G., and Braley, S. Toxicologic studies, quality control and efficacy of the Silastic mammary prosthesis. Med Instrum. 1973, 7, (2): 100-103. TOXICOLOGY/general.

Robertson, J. L. A. A complication of transareolar augmentation mammaplasty. Plastic and Reconstructive Surgery. 1973: 263-264. LOCAL COMPLICATIONS/capsule contracture.

Robinson, D. E., Ophir, J., Wilson, L. S., and Chen, C. F. Pulse-echo ultrasound speed measurements: Progress and prospects. Ultrasound in Medicine and Biology. 1991, 17, (6): 633-646. MAMMOGRAPHY.

Robinson, Jr. O. G. et al. Disruption rate of silicone gel prostheses: Report of 200 cases. Aesthetic Plastic Surgery. 1993 Apr. RUPTURE/local complications.

Robinson, Jr. O. G., and Benos, D. J. Spontaneous autoinflation of saline mammary implants. Annals of Plastic Surgery. 1997 Aug, 39, (2): 114-118. SALINE/local complications.

Robinson, Jr. O. G., Bradley, E. L., and Wilson, D. S. Analysis of explanted silicone implants: A report of 300 patients. Annals of Plastic Surgery. 1995 Jan, 34, (1): 1-6. RUPTURE/local complications.

Rockwell, W. B., Casey, H. D., and Cheng, C. A. Breast capsule persistence after breast implant removal. Plast. Reconstr. Surg. 1998, 101, (4): 1085-1088. CAPSULE CONTRACTURE/explantation.

Rodgers, K. Klykken P., Jacobs, J., Frondoza, C., Tomazic, V., and Zelikoff, J. Symposium overview. Immunotoxicity of medical devices. Fundamental and Applied Toxicology. 1997, 36, (1): 1-14. IMMUNE EFFECTS/toxicology.

Rodman, N. F., and Mason, R. G. Compatibility of blood with foreign surfaces. Thrombosis et Diathesis Hemmorrhagica. 1970, 40 (Supplement): 145-155. IMMUNE EFFECTS.

Rodnan, G. P., Benedek, T. G., Medsger, T. A., and Cammarata, R. J. The association of progressive systemic sclerosis (scleroderma) with coal miners' pneumoconiosis and other forms of silicosis. Annals of Internal Medicine. 1967 Feb, 66, (2): 323-334. SILICA.

Rodriguez, M. A., Martinez, M. C., and Lopez-Artiguez, M. et al. Lung embolism with liquid silicone. Journal of Forensic Sciences. 1989 Mar 31, 34, (2): 504-510. SILICONE INJECTION.

Roggendorf, E. J. The biostability of silicone rubbers, a polyamide, and a polyester. J. Biomed. Mater. Res. 1976, 10, 123-143. SILICONE CHARACTERIZATION.

Roggli, V. L., McDonald, J. W., and Shelburne, J. D. The detection of silicone within tissues. Archives of Pathology and Laboratory Medicine. 1994 Oct, 118, 963-964. SILICON MEASUREMENT/local complications.

Rohrich, R. J., Adams, W. P., Beran, S. J., Rathakrishnan, R., Griffin, J., Robinson, J. B., and Kenkel, J. M. An analysis of silicone gel-filled breast implants: diagnosis and failure rates. Plast. Reconstr. Surg. 1998a Dec, 102, (7): 2304-2309. RUPTURE.

Rohrich, R. J., Beran, S. J., Restifo, R. J., and Copit, S. E. Aesthetic management of the breast following explantation: evaluation and mastopexy options. Plast. Reconstr. Surg. 1998b Mar, 101, (3): 827-837. LOCAL COMPLICATIONS/expander.

Rohrich, R. J., Hollier, L. H., and Robinson, Jr. J. B. Determining the safety of the silicone envelope: In search of a silicone antibody. Plast. Reconstr. Surg. 1996 Sep, 98, (4): 455-458. IMMUNE EFFECTS.

Rokeach, L. A., Jannatipour, M., and Hoch, S. O. Heterologous expression and epitope mapping of a human small nuclear ribonucleoprotein-associated Sm-B'/B autoantigen. The Journal of Immunology. 1990 Feb 1, 144, (3): 1015-1022. IMMUNE EFFECTS.

Rolland, C., Guidoin, R., Marceau, D., and Ledoux, R. Nondestructive investigations on ninety-seven surgically excised mammary prostheses. J. Biomed. Mater. Res.: Applied Biomaterials. 1989a, 23, (A3): 285-298. CAPSULE-CONTRACTURE/local complications/explantation.

Rolland, C., Ledoux, R., Guidoin, R., and Marceau, D. First observation of hopeïte and parascholzite in fibrous capsules surrounding silicone breast implants. International Journal of Artificial Organs. 1989b, 12, 180-188. CALCIFICATION/local complications/capsule-contracture.

Rom, W. N., Turner, W. G., Peebles, C., Tan, E. M., and Olsen, D. M. Antinuclear antibodies in Utah coal miners. Chest. 1983 Mar, 83, (3): 515-519. AI-CTD BACKGROUND.

Romano, T. J. Clinical characteristics of silicone breast implant patients. Am J Pain Management. 1996, 6, 13-16. GENERAL/pain.

Roncadin, M., Massarut, S., Perin, T., Arcicasa, M., Canzonieri, V., Rossi, C., and Carbone, A. Breast angiosarcoma after conservation surgery, radiotherapy and prosthesis implant. Acta Oncol. 1998, 37, (2): 209-211. CANCER.

Rosanova, I., Sevastianov, S., and Wan Kim, S. Effect of silicone rubber surface on the calcium balance of human serum. Journal of Biomedical Materials Research. 1991, 25, 459-465. CALCIFICATION/local complications.

Rosato, F. E., and et al. Immediate postmastectomy reconstruction. J Surg Oncol. 1976, 8, 277-280. RECONSTRUCTION.

Rosato, R. M., and Dowden, R. V. Radiation therapy as a cause of capsular contracture. Annals of Plastic Surgery. 1994 Apr, 32, (4): 342-345. CAPSULE-CONTRACTURE/local complications/radiation.

Rosculet, K. A., Ikeda, D. M., Forrest, M. E., Oneal, R. M., Rubin, J. M., Jeffries, D. O., and Helvie, M. A. Ruptured gel-filled silicone breast implants: Sonographic findings in 19 cases. American Journal of Roentgenology. 1992 Oct, 159, 711-716. MAMMOGRAPHY/local complications/rupture.

Rosdy, M., Grisoni, B., and Clauss, L.-C. Proliferation of normal human keratinocytes on silicone substrates. Biomaterials. 1991 Jul, 12, 511-517. IMMUNE EFFECTS/toxicology.

Rose, N. R. The silicone breast implant controversy: The other courtroom. Arthritis and Rheumatism. 1996 Oct, 39, (10): 1615-1618. GENERAL.

Rose, N. R. Silicone breast implants and human disease. Annals of Plastic Surgery. 1992, 28, 499. GENERAL.

Rose, N. R., and Potter, M. The silicone controversy: Towards a resolution. Immunology Today. 1995, 16, (10): 459-460. GENERAL.

Rosen, P. D., Jaba, A. D., Kister, S. J., and et al. Clinical experience with immediate breast reconstruction using tissue expansion or transverse rectus abdominis musculocutaneous flaps. Annals of Plastic Surgery. 1990, 25, 249. RECONSTRUCTION/expander.

Rosen, P. P., and Ernsberger, D. Mammary Fibromatosis. A benign spindle cell tumor with significant risk for local recurrence. Cancer. 1989, 63, 1363-1369. CANCER.

Rosenbaum, J. L., Bernadino, M. E., Thomas, J. L., and Wigley, K. D. Ultrasonic findings in silicone augmented breasts. Southern Medical Journal. 1981 Apr, 74, (4): 455-458. MAMMOGRAPHY.

Rosenbaum, J. T. Lessons from litigation over silicone breast implants: A call for activism by scientists. Science. 1997 Jun 6, 276, 1524-1525. GENERAL.

Rosenberg, C., and Ainen, H. S. Detection of urinary metabolites in toluene diisocyanate exposed rats. J Chromatogr. 1985, 323, 429-433. POLYURETHANE/toxicology.

Rosenberg, M. J. Is there an association between injectable collagen and polymyositis/dermatomyositis? Arthritis and Rheumatism. 1994 May, 37, (5): 747-753. AI-CTD BACKGROUND.

Rosenberg, N. L. The neuromythology of silicone breast implants. Neurology. 1996 Feb, 46, 308-314. NEUROLOGIC DISEASE/connective tissue disease.

Rosenblatt, K., and Thomas, D. WHO collaborative study of neoplasia and steriod contraceptives. International J. Epidemiology. 1993, 22, 192-197. CHILDREN'S EFFECTS/breast feeding.

Rosenbruch, M. Inhalation of amorphous silica: morphological and morphometric evaluation of lung associated lymph nodes in rats. Exp Toxicol Pathol. 1992, 44, 10-14. TOXICOLOGY.

Rosenthal, D. I., Rosenberg, A. E., Schiller, A. L., and Smith, R. J. Destructive arthritis due to silicone: A foreign-body reaction. Radiology. 1983 Oct, 149, 69. LOCAL COMPLICATIONS/general.

Rotatori, D. S., Hathaway, C. L., Steinbach, B. G., and Caffee, H. H. Noninvasive assessment of implant capsules. Plast. Reconstr. Surg. 1991 Apr, 87, (4): 703-707. MAMMOGRAPHY/local complications/capsule-contracture.

Roux, H., Imbert, I., Roudier, J., Quinsat, D., and Catanéo-Fontaine, J. Pathologie autoimmune et chirurgie esthétique. A propos d'un cas. La Revue de Médecine Interne. 1987 Nov-1987 Dec 31, 8, (3): 475-480. CONNECTIVE TISSUE DISEASE.

Rowe, V. K., Spencer, H. C., and Bass, S. L. Toxicological studies on certain commercial silicones and hydrolyzable silane intermediates. Journal of Industrial Hygiene Toxicol. 1948 Nov, 30, (6): 332-352. TOXICOLOGY.

Rowe, V. K., Spencer, H., and Bass, S. Toxicologic studies on certain commercial silicones: Two year dietary feeding study of DC antifoam to rats. Archives of Industrial Hygiene and Occupational Medicine. 1950 May, 1, 539-544. TOXICOLOGY.

Rowland, J. H., Dioso, J., Holland, J. C., Chaglassian, T., and Kinne, D. Breast reconstruction after mastectomy: Who seeks it, who refuses? Plast. Reconstr. Surg. 1995 Apr, 95, (5): 812-822. PSYCHOSOCIAL/reconstruction.

Rowley, M. J. Collagen antibodies in rheumatoid arthritis: Significance of antibodies to denatured collagen and their association with HLA-DR4. Arthritis and Rheumatism. 1986 Feb, 29, (2): 174-184. AI-CTD BACKGROUND.

Rowley, M. J., Cook, A. D., Teuber, S. S., and Gershwin, M. E. Antibodies to collagen: Comparative epitope mapping in women with silicone breast implants, systemic lupus erythematosus, and rheumatoid arthritis. Journal of Autoimmunity. 1994, 7, 775-789. IMMUNE EFFECTS/connective tissue disease.

Rowsell, A. R., Godfrey, A. M., and Richards, M. A. The thinned latissimus dorsi free flap: a case report. Br. J. Plast. Surg. 1986, 39, 210. EXPANDER.

Rudolph, R., and Abraham, J. Tissue effects of new silicone mammary-type implants in rabbits. Annals of Plastic Surgery. 1980 Jan, 4, (1): 14-20. SILICON MEASUREMENT/IMMUNE EFFECTS/capsule contracture/local complications.

Rudolph, R., Abraham, J., Vecchione, T., Guber, S., and Woodword, M. Myofibroblasts and free silicon around breast implants. Plast. Reconstr. Surg. 1978 Aug, 62, (2): 185-196. CAPSULE-CONTRACTURE/saline/local complications.

Rudolph, R., Gruber, S., Suzuki, M., and Woodward, M. The life cycle of the myofibroblast. Surgery, Gynecology and Obstetrics. 1977 Sep, 145, 389-394. CAPSULE-CONTRACTURE/local complications.

Rudolph, R., and Woodward, M. Absence of visible bacteria in capsules around silicone breast implants. Plast. Reconstr. Surg. 1983 Jul, 72, (1): 32-35. INFECTION/local complications/capsule-contracture.

Ruffatti, A., Rossi, L., Calligaro, A., Del Ross, T., Lagni, M., Marson, P., and Todesco, S. Autoantibodies of systemic rheumatic diseases in the healthy elderly. Gerontology. 1990, 36, 104-111. AI-CTD BACKGROUND.

Ruíz-Velasco, M. D. Hyperprolactinemia and mammary prostheses: A report of eight cases. The Journal of Reproductive Medicine. 1986 Apr, 31, (4): 267-270. BREAST FEEDING/local complications.

Russel, I. S., Collins, J. P., Holman, A. D., and Julian, A. S. The use of tissue expansion for immediate breast reconstruction after mastectomy. Med. J. Aust. 1990, 152, 632. RECONSTRUCTION/expander.

Russell, F. E., Simmers, M. H., Hirst, A. E., and Pudenz, R. H. Tumors associated with embedded polymers. Journal of the National Cancer Institute. 1953, 23, 305. CARCINOGENICITY.

Russell, R. C., Pribaz, J., Zook, E. G., Leighton, W. D., Eriksson, E., and Smith, C. J. Functional evaluation of latissimus dorsi donor site. Plast. Reconstr. Surg. 1986 Sep, 78, (3): 336-344. RECONSTRUCTION.

Rustin, M. H. A., Bull, H. A., Ziegler, V., Mehlhorn, J., Haustein, U.-F., Maddison, P. J., James, J., and Dowd, P. M. Silica-associated systemic sclerosis is clinically, serologically and immunologically indistinguishable from idiopathic systemic sclerosis. British Journal of Dermatology. 1990, 123, 725-734. SILICA/connective tissue disease.

Ryan, A. S. The resurgence of breastfeeding in the United States. Pediatrics. 1997, 99, (4): E12. CHILDREN'S EFFECTS/breast feeding.

Ryan, G. B., Cliff, W. J., Gabbiani, G., Irle, C., Montandon, D., Statkov, P. R., and Majno, G. Myofibroblasts in human granulation tissue. Human Pathology. 1974 Jan, 5, (1): 55-67. CAPSULE-CONTRACTURE/local complications.

Ryan, J. J. A lower thoracic advancement flap in breast reconstruction after mastectomy. Plast. Reconstr. Surg. 1982 Apr, 70, (2): 153-158. RECONSTRUCTION.

Rybka, F. J. The experimental value of silicone-sheet, Dacron felt spacers in prevention of capsular contractures. Plast. Reconstr. Surg. 1980, 66, (4): 502-508. CAPSULE-CONTRACTURE/local complications.

Ryu, J., Yahalom, J., Shank, B., Chaglassian, T. A., and McCormick, B. Radiation therapy after breast augmentation or reconstruction in early or recurrent breast cancer. Cancer. 1990 Sep 1, 66, (5): 844-847. CAPSULE-CONTRACTURE/local complications/radiation.

Sabbagh, W. H., Murphy, Jr. R. X., Kucirka, S. J., and Okunski, W. J. Idiosyncratic allergic reaction to textured saline implants. Plast. Reconstr. Surg. 1996 Apr, 97, (4): 820. SALINE/immune effects.

Sahn, E. E., Garen, P. D., Silver, R. M., and Maize, J. C. Scleroderma following augmentation mammoplasty: Report of a case and review of the literature. Archives of Dermatology. 1990 Sep, 126, 1198-1202. CONNECTIVE TISSUE DISEASE.

Salmon, S. E., and Kyle, R. A. Silicone gels, induction of plasma cell tumors, and genetic susceptibility in mice: a call for epidemiologic investigation of women with silicone breast implants. Journal of the National Cancer Institute. 1994 Jul 20, 86, (14): 1040-1041. MYELOMA.

Salomon, J., and Barton, F. E. Augmentation mammaplasty, selected readings. Plast. Reconstr. Surg. 1997, 8, (28): 1-34. GENERAL.

Salthouse, T. N. Some aspects of macrophage behavior at the implant interface. Journal of Biomedical Materials Research. 1984, 18, 395-401. IMMUNE EFFECTS.

Samuels, J. B., Rorhich, R. J., Weatherall, P. T., Ho, A. M. W., and Goldberg, K. L. Radiographic diagnosis of breast implant rupture: Current status and comparison of techniques. Plast. Reconstr. Surg. 1995 Sep, 96, (4): 865-877. MAMMOGRAPHY/local complications/rupture.

Sánchez-Guererro, J., Liang, M. H., Karlson, E. W., Hunter, D. J., and Colditz, G. A. Postmenopausal estrogen therapy and risk of developing systemic lupus erythematosus. Annals of Internal Medicine. 1995b, 122, (6): 430-433. CONNECTIVE TISSUE DISEASE.

Sánchez-Guerrero, J. Autoantibody testing in patients with silicone implants. Clinics in Laboratory Medicine. 1997 Sep, 17, (3): 341-353. IMMUNE EFFECTS.

Sánchez-Guerrero, J., Colditz, G. A., Karlson, E. W., Hunter, D. J., Speizer, F. E., and Liang, M. H. Silicone breast implants and the risk of connective-tissue diseases and symptoms. The New England Journal of Medicine. 1995a Jun 22, 332, (25): 1666-1670. CONNECTIVE TISSUE DISEASE.

Sánchez-Guerrero, J., Schur, P. H., Sargent, J. S., and Liang, M. H. Silicone breast implants and rheumatic disease: Clinical, immunological and epidemiological evidence. Arthritis and Rheumatism. 1994 Feb, 37, (2): 158-168. CONNECTIVE TISSUE DISEASE.

Sánchez-Roman, J., Wichmann, I., Salaberri, J., Varela, J. M., and Nuñez-Roldan, A. Multiple clinical and biological autoimmune manifestations in 50 workers after occupational exposure to silica. Annals of the Rheumatic Diseases. 1993, 52, (7): 534-538. SILICA.

Sanger, J. R., Kolachalam, R., Komorowski, R. A., Yousif, N. J., and Matloub, H. S. Short-term effect of silicone gel on peripheral nerves: A histologic study. Plast. Reconstr. Surg. 1992 May, 89, (5): 931-940. MIGRATION/local complications/neurologic disease.

Sanger, J. R., Komoroswki, R. A., Larson, D. L., Gingrass, R. P., Yousif, N. J., and Matloub, H. S. Tissue humoral response to intact and ruptured silicone gel-filled prostheses. Plast. Reconstr. Surg. 1995 May, 95, (6): 1033-1038. IMMUNE EFFECTS/granulomas/local complications/rupture.

Sanger, J. R., Matloub, H. S. Yousif N. J., and Komorowski, R. Silicone gel infiltration of a peripheral nerve and constrictive neuropathy following rupture of a breast prosthesis. Plast. Reconstr. Surg. 1992 May, 89, (5): 949-952. MIGRATION/local complications/ rupture/neurologic disease.

Sanger, J. R., Sheth, N. K., and Franson, T. R. Adherence of microorganisms to breast prostheses: An in vitro study. Ann. Plast. Surg. 1989, 22, 337. INFECTION.

Sanislow, C., and Zuidema, G. The use of silicone T-tubes in reconstructive biliary surgery in dogs. 1963 Dec. GENERAL.

Sank, A., Chalabian-Baliozian, J., Ertl, D., Sherman, R., Nimini, M., and Tuan, T. L. Cellular responses to silicone and polyurethane prosthetic surfaces. Journal of Surgical Research. 1993, 54, 12-20. POLYURETHANE/capsule-contracture/local complications.

Santerre, J. P., and Labow, R. S. The effect of hard segment size on the hydrolytic stability of polyether-urea-urethanes when exposed to cholesterol esterase. Journal of Biomedical Materials Research. 1997, 36, 223-232. POLYURETHANE.

Santerre, J. P., Labow, R. S., Duguay, D. G., Erfle, D., and Adams, G. A. Biodegradation evaluation of polyether and polyester-urethanes with oxidative and hydrolytic enzymes. Journal of Biomedical Materials Research. 1994, 28, 1187-1199. POLYURETHANE.

Sarwer, D. B., Bartlett, S. P., Bucky, L. P, LaRossa, D., Low, D. W., Pertschuk, M. J., Wadden, T. A., and Whitaker, L. A. Bigger is not always better: body image dissatisfaction in breast reduction and breast augmentation patients. Plast. Reconstr. Surg. 1998a Jun, 101, (7): 1956-1961. PSYCHOSOCIAL.

Sarwer, D. B., Wadden, T. A., Pertschuk, M. J., and Whitaker, L. A. Body image dissatisfaction and body dysmorphic disorder in 100 cosmetic surgery patients. Plast. Reconstr. Surg. 1998b May, 101, (6): 1644-1649. PSYCHOSOCIAL.

Savrin, R. A., Martin, E. W., and Ruberg, R. L. Mass lesion of the breast after augmentation mammaplasty. Archives of Surgery. 1979 Dec, 114, 1423-1424. GRANULOMAS/local complications.

Sazy, J. A., Smith, D. J., Crissman, J. D., Heggers, J. P., and Robson, M. C. Immunogenic potential of carpal implants. Surgical Forum. 606-608. IMMUNE EFFECTS.

Scales, J. T. Discussion on metals and synthetic materials in relation to soft tissue: Tissue reaction to synthetic materials. Proc R Soc Med. 1953, 46, 647-657. TOXICOLOGY.

Schaeberle, M. D., Kalasinsky, V. F., Luke, J. L., Lewis, E. N., Levin, I. W., and Treado, P. J. Raman chemical imaging: Histopathology of inclusions in human breast tissue. Analytical Chemistry. 1996 Jun, 68, (11): 1829-1833. SILICON MEASUREMENT.

Schaefer, C. J., Whalen, J. D., Knapp, T., and Wooley, P. H. The influence of silicone implantation on type II collagen-induced arthritis in mice. Arthritis and Rheumatism. 1997, 40, (6): 1064-1072. IMMUNE EFFECTS/connective tissue disease.

Schafer, A. I., and Miller, J. B. Association of IgA multiple myeloma with pre-existing disease. British Journal of Haematology. 1979, 41, 19-24. MYELOMA.

Schag, C. A., Ganz, P. A., Polinsky, M. L., Fred, C., Hirji, K., and Petersen, L. Characteristics of women at risk for psychosocial distress in the year after breast cancer. Journal of Clinical Oncology. 1993 Apr, 11, (4): 783-793. PSYCHOSOCIAL.

Schain, W. S., Jacobs, E., and Wellisch, D. K. Psychosocial issues in breast reconstruction: Intrapsychic, interpersonal, and practical concerns. Clinics in Plastic Surgery. 1984, 11, 237-251. PSYCHOSOCIAL/reconstruction.

Schain, W. S., Wellisch, D. K., Pasnau, R. O., and Landsverk, J. The sooner the better: A study of psychological factors in women undergoing immediate versus delayed breast reconstruction. American Journal of Psychiatry. 1985, 142, (1): 40-46. PSYCHOSOCIAL.

Schatten, W. E. Reconstruction of breasts following mastectomy with polyurethane-covered gel-filled prostheses. Annals of Plastic Surgery. 1984, 12, 147-156. RECONSTRUCTION/polyurethane.

Scheflan, M., and Kalisman, M. Complications of breast reconstruction. Clinics in Plastic Surgery. 1984 Apr, 11, (2): 343-350. GENERAL/local complications/reconstruction.

Schepers, G., Delahant, A., Bailey, D., Gockeler, E., and Gay, W. The biological action of degussa submicron amorphous silica dust (Dow Corning® silica) v. injection studies. American Archives of Industrial Health. 1957 Dec, 16, (6): 499-513. SILICA/toxicology.

Schiller, V. L., Arndt, R. D., and Brenner, R. J. Aggressive fibromatosis of the chest associated with a silicone breast implant. Chest. 1995 Nov, 108, (5): 1466-1468. LOCAL COMPLICATIONS.

Schirber, S., Thomas, W. O., Finley, J. M., Green, Jr. A. E., and Ferrara, J. J. Breast cancer after mammary augmentation. Southern Medical Journal. 1993, 86, 263-268. MAMMOGRAPHY/cancer.

Schlebusch, L. Negative bodily experience and prevalence of depression in patients with augmentation mammoplasty. S. Afr. Med. J. 1989 Apr 1, 75, 323-326. PSYCHOSOCIAL.

Schlebusch, L Levin A. A psychological profile of women selected for augmentation mammaplasty. S. Afr. Med. J. 1983, 64, 481. PSYCHOSOCIAL.

Schlenker, J. D., Bueno, R. A., Ricketson, G., and Lynch, J. B. Loss of silicone implants after subcutaneous mastectomy and reconstruction. Plast. Reconstr. Surg. 1978 Dec, 62, (6): 853-861. RECONSTRUCTION.

Schlienger, J. L., Haenel, P., and Jaeck, D. Protracted periodic fever and breast prosthesis. Rev Méd Interne. 1994, 15, (8): 557-559. EXPLANTATION/connective tissue disease.

Schluederberg, A., Straus, S., Peterson, P., Blumenthal, S., Komaroff, A. L., Spring, S. B., Landay, A., and Buchwald, D. Chronic fatigue syndrome research: Definition and medical outcome assessment. Annals of Internal Medicine. 1992 Aug 15, 117, (4): 325. AI-CTD BACKGROUND.

Schmidt, G. H. Calcification bonded to saline-filled implants. Plast. Reconstr. Surg. 1993, 92, 1423-1424. CALCIFICATION/local complications.

Schmidt, G. H. Mammary implant shell failure. Annals of Plastic Surgery. 1980 Nov, 5, (5): 369-371. RUPTURE/local complications.

Schneider, E., and Chan, T. W. Selective MR imaging of silicone with the three-point Dixon Technique. Radiology. 1993 Apr, 187, (11): 89-93. MAMMOGRAPHY.

Schnitt, S. J. Tissue Reactions to Mammary Implants: a capsule summary. Adv. Anat. Pathol. 1995, 2, (1): 24-27. CAPSULE-CONTRACTURE.

Schnur, P. L., Weinzweig, J., Harris, J. B., Moyer, T. P., Petty, P. M., Nixon, D., and McConnell, J. P. Silicon analysis of breast and periprosthetic capsular tissue from patients with saline or silicone gel breast implants. Plast. Reconstr. Surg. 1996 Oct, 98, (5): 798-803. SILICON MEASUREMENT/saline/local complications/capsule contracture.

Schnur, P. L., Weinzweig, J., Moyer, T. P., and et al. Silicone analysis of breast and periprosthetic capsular tissue from patients with saline or silicone gel breast implants. Plast Surg Forum. 1994, 17, 200. CAPSULE-CONTRACTURE/local complications/saline/silicon measurement.

Schoen, F. J. Biomaterial-associated infection, neoplasia, and calcification. Trans Am Soc Artif Intern Organs. 1987, 33. INFECTION.

Schottenfeld, D., Burns, C. J., Gillespie, B. W., Laing, T. J., Mayes, M. D., Heeringa, S. G., and Alcser, K. H. The design of a population-based case-control study of systemic sclerosis (scleroderma): commentary on the University of Michigan study. Journal of Clinical Epidemiology. 1995, 48, (4): 583-586. AI-CTD BACKGROUND.

Schover, L. R. The impact of breast cancer on sexuality, body image, and intimate relationships. CA-A Cancer Journal for Clinicians. 1991, 41, (2): 112-120. PSYCHOSOCIAL.

Schubert, M. A., Wiggins, M. J., Schaefer, M. P., Hiltner, A., and Anderson, J. M. Oxidative biodegradation mechanisms of biaxially strained poly(etherurethane urea) elastomers. Journal of Biomedical Materials Research. 1995, 29, 337-347. SILICONE CHARACTERIZATION.

Schuh, M. E., and Radford, D. M. Desmoid tumor of the breast following augmentation mammaplasty. Plast. Reconstr. Surg. 1994 Mar, 93, (3): 603-605. LOCAL COMPLICATIONS.

Schuler, F, Rosato, F, Miller, E, and Horton, C. Silicone protheses and antitumor immunity. An in-vitro rat study. Plast. Reconstr. Surg. 1978 May, 61, (5): 762-766. IMMUNE EFFECTS/cancer.

Schumann, D. Health risks for women with breast implants. Nurse Practitioner. 1994 Jul, 19, (7): 19-30. GENERAL.

Schumann, R., and Taubert, H. D. Long term application of steroids enclosed in dimethylpolysiloxane (Silastic): in vitro and in vivo experiments. Acta Biol. Med. Germ. 1970, 24, 897-920. GENERAL.

Schuster, D. I., and Lavine, D. M. Nine-year experience with subpectoral breast reconstruction after subcutaneous mastectomy in 98 patients utilizing saline-inflatable prostheses. Annals of Plastic Surgery. 1988, 21, 444-451. LOCAL COMPLICATIONS.

Schusterman, M. A., Kroll, S. S., Reece, G. P., Miller, M. J., Ainslie, N., Halabi, S., and Balch, C. M. Incidence of autoimmune disease in patients after breast reconstruction with silicone gel implants versus autogenous tissue: A preliminary report. Annals of Plastic Surgery. 1993 Jul, 31, (1): 1-6. CONNECTIVE TISSUE DISEASE/immune effects.

Schusterman, M. A., Kroll, S. S., and Weldon, M. E. Immediate breast reconstruction: Why the free TRAM over the conventional TRAM flap? Plast. Reconstruct. Surg. 1992 Aug, 90, (2): 255-261. RECONSTRUCTION.

Schwartz, G. F. Benign neoplasms and inflammation of the breast. Clinical Obstetrics and Gynecology. 1982 Jun, 25, (2): 373-385. CANCER.

Schwartz, G. F., Feig, S. A., and Patchefsky, A. S. Clinicopathologic correlations and significance of clinically occult mammary lesions. Cancer. 1978 Mar, 41, (3): 1147-1153. MAMMOGRAPHY/cancer.

Scott, I. R., Muller, N., Fitzpatrick, D., and Burhenne, L. Ruptured breast implant: Computed tomographic and mammographic findings. J. Can. Assoc. Radiol. 1988, 39, 152-154. RUPTURE/local complications/mammography.

Scully, S. J. Augmentation mammaplasty without contracture. Annals of Plastic Surgery. 1981, 6, 262-269. CAPSULE-CONTRACTURE/local complications.

Seckel, B. R., and Costas, P. D. Total versus partial musculofascial coverage for steroid-containing double-lumen breast implants in augmentation mammaplasty, with discussion by Tebbetts, J.B. Annals of Plastic Surgery. 1993 Apr, 30, (4): 296-301. STEROIDS/local complications.

Seckel, B. R., and Hyland, W. T. Soft-tissue expander for delayed and immediate breast reconstruction. Surg Clin North Am. 1985, 65, 383. EXPANDER/reconstruction.

Segall, M., and Bach, F. H. HLA and disease: The perils of simplifications. The New England Journal of Medicine. 1990, 322, (26): 1879-1880. IMMUNE EFFECTS.

Segreti, J., and Levin, S. The role of prophylactic antibiotics in the prevention of prosthetic device infection. Infectious Disease Clinics of North America. 1989 Jun, 3, (2): 357-370. INFECTION/local complications.

Seleznick, M. J., Martinez-Osuna, P., Espinoza, L. R., and Vasey, F. B. Is silicone associated with connective tissue disease? J Fla Med Assoc. 1991 Feb, 78, (2): 85-87. CONNECTIVE TISSUE DISEASE.

Selmanowitz, V. J., and Orentreich, N. Medical-grade fluid silicone. J. Dermatol. Surg. Oncol. 1977, 3, (6): 597-611. SILICONE INJECTION.

Semple, J. L., Lugowski, S. J., Baines, C. J., Smith D. C., and McHugh, A. Breast milk contamination and silicone implants: Preliminary results using silicon as a proxy measurement for silicone. Plast. Reconstr. Surg. 1998 Aug, 102, (2): 528-33. SILICON MEASUREMENT/breast feeding/children's effects.

Sepai, O., Henschler, D., Czech, S., Eckert, P., and Sabbioni, G. Exposure to toluenediamines from polyurethane-covered breast implants. Toxicol. Lett. 1995, 77, 371-378. TOXICOLOGY/polyurethane.

Sergott, T. J., Limoli, J. P., Baldwin, C. M., and Laub, D. R. Human adjuvant disease, possible autoimmune disease after silicone implantation: A review of the literature, case studies, and speculation for the future. Plast. Reconstr. Surg. 1986 Jul, 78, (1): 104-110. IMMUNE EFFECTS/connective tissue disease.

Serletti, J. M., and Moran, S. L. The combined used of the TRAM and expanders/implants in breast reconstruction. Plast. Reconstr. Surg. 1988 May, 40, (5): 510-514. RECONSTRUCTION/expander.

Sevastianov, V. I., and Tseytlina, E. A. The activation of the complement system by polymer materials and their blood compatibility. Journal of Biomedical Materials Research. 1984, 18, 969-978. IMMUNE EFFECTS.

Sevastjanova, N. A., Mansurova, L. A., Dombrovska, L. E., and Slutskii, L. I. Biochemical characterization of connective tissue reaction to synthetic polymer implants. Biomaterials. 1987 Jul, 8, 242-247. CAPSULE-CONTRACTURE/local complications.

Sever, C. E., Leith, C. P., Appenzeller, J., and Foucar, K. Kikuchi's histiocytic necrotizing lymphadenitis associated with ruptured silicone breast implant. Archives of Pathology and Laboratory Medicine. 1996 Apr, 120, (4): 380-385. IMMUNE EFFECTS.

Shack, R. B. Is silicone safe? Let science decide. Southern Medical Journal. 1996 Feb, 89, (2): 251-252. GENERAL.

Shah, Z., Lehman, J. A., and Stevenson, G. Capsular contracture around silicone implants: The role of intraluminal antibiotics. Plast. Reconstr. Surg. 1982 May, 69, (5): 809-812. INFECTION/local complications.

Shah, Z., Lehman, J. A., and Tan, J. Does infection play a role in breast capsular contracture. Plast. Reconstr. Surg. 1981 Jul, 68, (1): 34. CAPSULE-CONTRACTURE/local complications/infection.

Shainkin-Kestenbaum, R., Adler, A. J., and Berlyne, G.M. Inhibition of superoxide dismutase activity by silicon. Journal of Trace Elements and Electrolytes in Health and Disease. 1990 Mar, 4, 97. SILICONE CHARACTERIZATION/toxicology.

Shanklin, D. R., and Smalley, D. L. Quantitative aspects of cellular responses to silicone. International Journal of Occupational Medicine and Toxicology. 1995 Nov, 4, (1): 99-111. IMMUNE EFFECTS/granulomas.

Shapiro, M. A. Smooth vs. rough: An 8-year survey of mammary prostheses. Plast. Reconstr. Surg. 1989 Sep, 84, (3): 449-457. POLYURETHANE/capsule-contracture/local complications.

Sharma, R. K., and Jackson, I. T. Breast reconstruction following removal of silicone implants: A new technique. Aesthetic Plastic Surgery. 1995, 19, 247-250. GENERAL/reconstruction/explantation.

Sharp, G. C., Irvin, W. S., May, C. M., Holman, H. R., McDuffie, F. C., Hess, E. V., and Schmid, F. R. Association of antibodies to ribonucleoprotein and Sm antigens with mixed connnective tissue disease, system lupus erythematosus and other rheumatic diseases. The New England Journal of Medicine. 1976 Nov 18, 295, (21): 1149-1154. IMMUNE EFFECTS/connective tissue disease/ai-ctd background.

Shaw, W. W. Microvascular free flap breast reconstruction. Clinics in Plastic Surgery. 1984 Apr, 11, (2): 333-341. RECONSTRUCTION.

Sheard, C. Contact dermatitis from platinum and related metals. A.M.A. Archives of Dermatology. 1955, 71, 357-360. PLATINUM/toxicology.

Shedbalkar, A. R., Devata, A., and Padanilam, T. A study of effects of radiation on silicone prosthesis. Plast. Reconstr. Surg. 1980 Jun, 65, (6): 805-810. RADIATION/local complications.

Shen, G., Ojo-Amaize, E. A., Agopian, M. S., and Peter, J. B. Silicate antibodies in women with silicone breast implants: Development of an assay for detection of humoral immunity. Clinical and Diagnostic Laboratory Immunology. 1996 Mar, 3, (2): 162-166. IMMUNE EFFECTS/silica.

Shepard, R. J., Rhind, S., and Shek, P. N. Exercise and the immune system. Natural killer cells, interleukins, and related response. Sports Med. 1994, 18, 340-369. AI-CTD BACKGROUND.

Shermis, R. B., Adler, D. D., Smith, D. J., and Hall, J. D. Intraductal silicone secondary to breast implant rupture. Breast Dis. 1990, 3, 17-20. LOCAL COMPLICATIONS/rupture/migration.

Sherrer, Y. R. Current status of silicone breast implants [editorial]. Cleveland Clinic Journal of Medicine. 1992 Sep-1992 Oct 31, 59, (5): 539-541. GENERAL.

Shestak, K. C., Ganott, M. A., Harris, K. M., and Losken, H. W. Breast masses in the augmentation mammaplasty patient: the role of ultrasound. Plast. Reconstr. Surg. 1993 Aug, 92, (2): 209-216. MAMMOGRAPHY/cancer.

Shields, C., and Eagle, Jr. R. Pseudo-Schnabel's cavernous degeneration of the optic nerve secondary to intraocular silicone oil. Archives of Ophthalmology. 1989 May, 107, 714-717. SILICONE CHARACTERIZATION/local complications/general.

Shields, H. C., Fleischer, D. M., and Weschler, C. J. Comparisons among VOC's measured in three types of commercial buildings with different occupant densities. Indoor Air. 1996, 6, 2-17. TOXICOLOGY.

Shiokawa, Y., Kumagai, Y., Nishino, N., and Abe, C. Postmammoplasty connective tissue disease (human adjuvant disease). Rev Int Rheumatol. 1978, 7, 225. CONNECTIVE TISSUE DISEASE.

Shipley, R. H., O'Donnell, J., and Bader, K. Personality characteristics of women seeking breast augmentation: Comparison to small-busted and average-busted controls. Plast. Reconstr. Surg. 1977 Sep, 60, (3): 369-376. PSYCHOSOCIAL.

Shons, A. R., and Schubert, W. Silicone breast implants and immune disease. Annals of Plastic Surgery. 1992 May, 28, (5): 491-497. GENERAL/immune effects/connective tissue disease.

Shousha, S., Schoenfeld, A., Moss, J., Shore, I., and Sinnett, H. D. Light and electron microscopic study of an invasive cribriform carcinoma with extensive microcalcification developing in a breast with silicone augmentation. Ultrastructural Pathology. 1994, 18, 519-523. CANCER.

Sibbitt, W. L. Jr., and Bankhurst, A. D. Natural killer cells in connective tissue disorders. Clin. Rheum. 1985, 11, 507-521. AI-CTD BACKGROUND.

Sichere, P., Faudot-Bel, X., Pellerin, M., and Bieder, L. Shoulder pain as the inaugural manifestation of silicone breast implant intolerance. Rev Rheum Engl Ed. 1995, 62, 151-152. PAIN/local complications.

Sickles, E. A., Filly, R. A., and Callen, P. W. Breast cancer detection with sonography and mammography: Comparison using state-of-the-art equipment. AJR American Journal of Roentgenology. 1983, 140, 843-845. MAMMOGRAPHY/cancer.

Sickles, E. A., and Herzog, K. Intramammary scar tissue: A mimic of the mammographic appearance of carcinoma. American Journal of Roentgenology. 1980 Aug, 135, 349-352. MAMMOGRAPHY.

Sickles, E. A., Ominsky, S. H., Soluto, R. A., Galvin, H. B., and Monticciolo, D. L. Medical audit of a rapid-throughput mammography screening practice: methodology and results of 27,114 examinations. Radiology. 1990, 175, 323-327. MAMMOGRAPHY.

Siddiqui, W. H., and Hobbs, E. J. Subchronic dermal toxicity of trifluoropropylmethylcyclotrisiloxane in rabbits. Drug and Chemical Toxicology. 1982, 5, (4): 415-426. TOXICOLOGY.

Siddiqui, W. H., and Schardein, J. L. One generation reproduction study of silicone gel and Silastic II mammary envelope implants in rats. Toxicologist. 1993, 13, (75): 193. TOXICOLOGY.

Siddiqui, W. H., Schardein, J., Cassidy, S. L., and Meeks, R. Reproductive and developmental toxicity studies of silicone elastomer q7-2423/q7-2551 in rats and rabbits. Fundamental and Applied Toxicology. 1994b, 23, 377-381. TOXICOLOGY.

Siddiqui, W. H., Schardein, J., Cassidy, S. L., and Meeks, R. Reproductive and developmental toxicity studies of silicone gel Q7-2159A in rats and rabbits. Fundamental and Applied Toxicology. 1994a, 23, 370-376. TOXICOLOGY.

Signorini, M., Grisotti, A., Ponzielli, G., Pajardi, G., and Gilardino, P. Self-expanding prostheses complicating augmentation mammoplasties. Aesthetic Plastic Surgery. 1994, 18, (2): 195-199. EXPANDER.

Sihm, F., Jagd, M., and Pers, M. Psychological assessment before and after augmentation mammaplasty. Scandinavian Journal of Plastic and Reconstructive and Hand Surgery. 1978, 12, (3): 295-298. PSYCHOSOCIAL.

Silicosis and Silicate Disease Committee (Craighead, J. E., Lemerman, J., and Abraham, J. L.) Diseases associated with exposure to silica and nonfibrous silicate minerals. Archives of Pathology and Laboratory Medicine. 1988 Jul, 112, 673-720. GENERAL/ silica.

Silman, A. J. Epidemiology of scleroderma. Annals of Rheumatic Disease. 1991, 50, 846-853. AI-CTD BACKGROUND.

Silman, A. J. Epidemiology of systemic sclerosis. Current Opinions in Rheumatology. 1996, 8, (6): 585-589. AI-CTD BACKGROUND.

Silman, A. J., and Hochberg, M. C. Occupational and environmental influences on scleroderma. Rheumatic Disease Clinics of North America. 1996 Nov, 22, (4): 737-749. AI-CTD BACKGROUND.

Silman, A. J., and Jones. S. What is the contribution of occupational environmental factors to the occurrence of scleroderma in men? Annals of the Rheumatic Diseases. 1992, 51, 1322-1324. AI-CTD BACKGROUND.

Silver, H. Reduction of capsular contracture. Plast. Reconstr. Surg. 1982, 69, (5): 802-808. CAPSULE CONTRACTURE/local complications.

Silver, R. M., Sahn, E. E., Allen, J. A., Sahn, S., Greene, W., and Maize, J. C. Demonstration of silicon in sites of connective-tissue disease in patients with silicone-gel breast implants. Archives of Dermatology. 1993 Jan, 129, 63-68. CONNECTIVE TISSUE DISEASE/local complications/migration.

Silverman, B. G., Brown, S. L., Bright, R. A., Kaczmarek, R. G., Arrowsmith Lowe, J. B., and Kessler, D. A. Reported complications of silicone gel breast implants: An epidemiologic review. Annals of Internal Medicine. 1996 Apr 15, 24, (8): 744-756. GENERAL/ connective tissue disease/cancer/local complications.

Silverman, S., Gluck, O., Silver, D., Tessar, J., Wallace, D., Neumann, K., Metzger, A., and Morris, R. Incidence of autoantibodies in symptomatic patients and asymptomatic patients with breast implants. Abstracts of Immunology. 1995 Mar 13. IMMUNE EFFECTS.

Silverstein, J. J., Murphy, G. P., Bostwick, J., Byrd, B. F., Snyderman, R. K., and Weber, W. E. Breast reconstruction: State-of-the-art for 1990. Cancer. 1991, 68, 5 (Supplement): 1180-1181. GENERAL/reconstruction.

Silverstein, M. J., Gamagami, P., Colburn, W. J., and et al. Nonpalpable breast lesions: Diagnosis with slightly overpenetrated scteen-film mammography and hook wire—directed biopsy in 1014 cases. Radiology. 1989, 171, 633-638. MAMMOGRAPHY.

Silverstein, M. J., Gamagami, P., and Handel, N. Missed breast cancer in an augmented woman using implant displacement mammography. Annals of Plastic Surgery. 1990c Sep, 25, (3): 210-213. CANCER/mammography.

Silverstein, M. J., Gierson, E. D., Gamagami, P., Handel, N., and Waisman, J. R. Breast cancer diagnosis and prognosis in women augmented with silicone gel-filled prostheses. Cancer. 1990b, 66, 97-101. MAMMOGRAPHY/cancer.

Silverstein, M. J., Handel, N., Gamagami, P., Gierson, E. D., Furmanski, M., and Collins, A. R. Breast cancer diagnosis and prognosis in women following augmentation with silicone gel-filled prostheses. European Journal of Cancer. 1992, 28, 635-640. MAMMOGRAPHY/cancer.

Silverstein, M. J., Handel, N., Gamagami, P., Waisman, J. R., Gierson, E. D., Rosser, R. J., Steyskal, R., and Colburn, W. Breast cancer in women after augmentation mammoplasty. Archives of Surgery. 1988 Jun, 123, (5): 681-685. MAMMOGRAPHY/cancer.

Silverstein, M. J., Handel, N., and Gamagani, P. The effect of silicone-gel-gilled implants on mammography. Cancer. 1991 Sep 1, 68, (Supplement): 1159-1163. MAMMOGRAPHY.

Silverstein, M. K., Handel, N., Gamagami, P., Waisman, E., and Gierson, E. D. Mammographic measurements before and after augmentation mammoplasty. Plast. Reconstr. Surg. 1990a Dec, 86, (6): 1126-1130. MAMMOGRAPHY.

Simeonova, P. P., and Luster, M. I. Iron and reactive oxygen species in the asbestos-induced tumor necrosis factor—a response to alveolar macrophages. American Journal of Respir. Cell. Mol. Biol. 1995 Jun, 12, (6): 676-683. IMMUNE EFFECTS.

Sinclair, A., and Hallam, T. R. The determination of dimethylpolysiloxane in beer and yeast. Analyst. 1971 Feb, 96, 149-154. SILICON MEASUREMENT.

Sinclair, T. M., Kerrigan, C. L., and Buntic, R. Biodegradation of the polyurethane foam covering of breast implants. Plast. Reconstr. Surg. 1993 Nov, 92, (6): 1003-1013. POLYURETHANE/toxicology.

Singletary, S. E. Skin-sparing mastectomy with immediate breast reconstruction: Is it safe? Breast Diseases. 1995, 6, (3): 259-260. RECONSTRUCTION.

Sinha, S., Gorczyca, D. P., Debruhl, N. D., Shellock, F. G., Gausche, V. R., and Bassett, L. W. MR imaging of silicone breast implants: Comparison of different coil arrays. Radiology. 1993 Apr, 187, (1): 284-286. MAMMOGRAPHY.

Sinow, J. D., and Cunningham, B. L. Intraluminal lidocaine for analgesia after tissue expansion: A double-blind prospective trial in breast reconstruction. Annals of Plastic Surgery. 1992 Apr, 28, (4): 320-325. PAIN/local complications/expander.

Sinow, J. D., Halvorsen, Jr. R. A., Matts, J. P., Schubert, W., Letourneau, J. G., and Cunningham, B. L. Chest-wall deformity after tissue expansion for breast reconstruction. Plast. Reconstr. Surg. 1991 Dec, 88, (6): 998-1004. EXPANDER/local complications/reconstruction.

Skolnick, A. A. Ultrasound may help detect breast implant leaks. J. Amer. Med. Assoc. 1992 Feb 12, 267, (6): 786. MAMMOGRAPHY/local complications/rupture.

Slade, C. L. Subcutaneous mastectomy: Acute complications and long-term follow-up. Plast. Reconstr. Surg. 1984 Jan, 73, (1): 84-90. RECONSTRUCTION/local complications.

Slade, C. L., and Peterson, H. D. Disappearance of polyurethane cover of the Ashley Natural Y prosthesis. Plast. Reconstr. Surg. 1982 Sep, 70, (5): 379-382. POLYURETHANE.

Slater, C. A., Davis, R. B., and Shmerling, R. H. Antinuclear antibody testing. A study of clinical utility. Archives of Internal Medicine. 1996, 156, (13): 1421-1425. AI-CTD BACKGROUND/immune effects.

Slavin, S. A., and Colen, S. R. Sixty consecutive breast reconstructions with the inflatable expander: A critical appraisal. Plast. Reconstr. Surg. 1990, 86, (5): 910-919. RECONSTRUCTION/expander.

Slavin, S. A., and Goldwyn, R. M. Silicone gel implant explantation: Reasons, results, and admonitions. Plast. Reconstr. Surg. 1995 Jan, 95, (1): 63-69. EXPLANTATION/psychosocial/rupture/capsule-contracture/local complications.

Slavin, S. A., Schnitt, S. J., Duda, R. B., Houlihan, M. J., Koufman, C. N., Morris, D. J., Troyan, S. L., and Goldwyn, R. M. Skin-sparing mastectomy and immediate reconstruction: oncologic risks and aesthetic results in patients with early-stage breast cancer. Plast Reconstr Surg. 1998 Jul, 102, (1): 49-62. RECONSTRUCTION/local complications.

Sluis-Cremer, G. K., Hessel, P. A., Nizdo, E. H., Churchill, A. R., and Zeiss, E. A. Silica silicosis and progressive systemic sclerosis. British Journal of Industrial Medicine. 1985, 42, 838-843. SILICA.

Sluis-Cremer, G. K., Hessell, P. A., Hnizdo, E., and Churchill, A. R. Relationship between silicosis and rheumatoid arthritis. Thorax. 1986, 41, 596-601. SILICA.

Smahel, J. Fibrous reactions in the tissues which surround silicone breast prostheses. British Journal of Plastic Surgery. 1978b Jan, 31, 250-253. CAPSULE-CONTRACTURE/local complications.

Smahel, J. Foreign material in the capsules around breast prostheses and the cellular reaction to it. British Journal of Plastic Surgery. 1979, 32, 35-42. CAPSULE CONTRACTURE/local complications/silicon measurement.

Smahel, J. Histology of the capsules causing constructive fibrosis around breast implants. British Journal of Plastic Surgery. 1977, 30, 324-329. CAPSULE-CONTRACTURE/local complications.

Smahel, J. Tissue reactions to breast implants coated with polyurethane. Plast. Reconstr. Surg. 1978a, 61, (1): 80-85. POLYURETHANE/capsule contracture/local complications.

Smahel, J., Hurwitz, P. J., and Hurwitz, N. Soft tissue response to textured silicone implants in an animal experiment. Plast. Reconstr. Surg. 1993 Sep, 92, (3): 474-479. CAPSULE-CONTRACTURE/local complications.

Smahel, J., Schneider, K., and Donski, P. Bizarre implants for augmentation mammaplasty: long term human reaction to polyethylene strips. Br J Plast Surg. 1977 Oct, 30, 287-290. GENERAL.

Smalley, D. L., Levine, J. J., Shanklin, D. R., Hall, M. F., and Stevens, M. V. Lymphocyte response to silica among offspring of silicone breast implant recipients. Immunobiology. 1996a, 196, (5): 567-574. IMMUNE EFFECTS/children's effects/silica.

Smalley, D. L., Shanklin, D. R., Hall, M. F., and Stevens, M. V. Detection of lymphocyte stimulation by silicon dioxide. International Journal of Occupational Medicine and Toxicology. 1995a Jan, 4, (1): 63-70. IMMUNE EFFECTS/silica.

Smalley, D. L., Shanklin, D. R., Hall, M. F., Stevens, M. V., and Hanissian, A. Immunologic stimulation of T lymphocytes by silica after use of silicone mammary implants. FASEB Journal. 1995b Mar, 9, 424-427. SILICA/immune effects.

Smalley, D., Hall, M. F., Shanklin, D. R., and Stevens, M. Immunologic markers in silicone breast implant recipients. International Journal of Occupational Medicine and Toxicology. 1995c, 4, (1): 147-153. IMMUNE EFFECTS.

Smart, C. R., Hendrick, R. E., Rutledge, J. H., and Smith R.A. Benefit of mammography screening in women ages 50 to 49 years. Cancer. 1995, 75, 1619-1626. MAMMOGRAPHY.

Smedley, H., Datrak, M., Sikora, K., and Wheeler, T. Neurological effects of recombinant human interferon. British Medical Journal. 1993 Jan 22, 286, 262-264. NEUROLOGIC DISEASE.

Smith, D. S. False-positive radiographic diagnosis of breast implant rupture: Report of two cases. Annals of Plastic Surgery. 1985, 14, 166-167. MAMMOGRAPHY/rupture/local complications.

Smith, H. R. Review. Do silicone breast implants cause autoimmune rheumatic disease. J. Biomater. Sci. Polymer Edn. 1995, 7, (2): 115-121. GENERAL.

Smith Jr., D. J., Sazy, J. A., Crissman, J. D., Niu, X.-T., Robson, M. C., and Heggers, J. P. Immunogenic potential of carpal implants. Journal of Surgical Research. 1990 Jan, 48, 13-20. IMMUNE EFFECTS/general.

Smith, L.F., Smith, T.T., Yeary, E., McGee, J.M., and Malnar, K. Squamous cell carcinoma of the breast following silicone injection of the breasts. J. Okla. State Med. Assoc. 1999, 92, (3): 126-130. CANCER.

Snow, J., Harasaki, H., Kasick, J., Whalen, r., Kiraly, R., and Nosé, Y. Promising results with a new textured surface intrathoracic variable volume device for LVAS. Transactions—American Society for Artificial Internal Organs. 1981, 27, 485-489. CAPSULE-CONTRACTURE/local complications.

Snow, R. B., and Kossovsky, N. Hypersensitivity reaction associated with sterile ventriculoperitoneal shunt malfunction. Surg Neurol. 1989, 31, 209-214. IMMUNE EFFECTS/local complications.

Snyder, J. W. Silicone breast implants. Can emerging medical, legal, and scientific concepts be reconciled? The Journal of Legal Medicine. 1997, 18, (2): 133-220. GENERAL.

Snyder, R. C., and Breder, C. V. High-performance liquid chromatographic determinations of 2,4- and 2,6-toluenediamine in aqueous extracts. Journal of Chromatography. 1982, 236, 429-440. TOXICOLOGY/polyurethane.

Snyder, R. E. Xeromammography—a reason for using saline-filter in breast prostheses. Plast. Reconstr. Surg. 1978, 61, 107. MAMMOGRAPHY/saline.

Snyderman, R. K., and Lizardo, J. G. Statistical study of malignancies found before, during, or after routine breast plastic operations. Plastic and Reconstructive Surgery. 1960 Mar, 25, (3): 253-256. CANCER/reconstruction.

Söderholm, K.-J. M., and Shang, S.-W. Molecular orientation of silane at the surface of colloidal silica. Journal of Dental Researchives. 1993 Jun, 72, (6): 1050-1054. SILICONE CHARACTERIZATION/silica.

Soderquist, M. E., and Walton, A. G. Structural changes in proteins adsorbed in polymer surfaces. Journal of Colloid and Interface Science. 1980, 75, (2): 386-397. TOXICOLOGY.

Solomon, G. A clinical and laboratory profile of symptomatic women with silicone breast implants. Seminars in Arthritis and Rheumatism. 1994a Aug, 24, (1 (Supplement 1)): 29-37. CONNECTIVE TISSUE DISEASE/immune effects.

Solomons, E. T., and Jones, J. K. The determination of polydimethylsiloxane (silicone oil) in biological materials: A case report. Journal of Forensic Sciences. 1975, 20, 191-199. SILICONE INJECTION/silicon measurement.

Sontag, J. M. Carcinogenicity of substituted-benzenediamines (phyenylenediamines) in rats and mice. JNCI. 1981 Mar, 66, (3): 591-602. CARCINOGENICITY.

Soo, M. S., Kornguth, P. J., Georgiade, G. S., and Sullivan, D. C. Seromas in residual fibrous capsules after explantation: Mammographic and sonographic appearances. Radiology. 1995, 194, 863-862. MAMMOGRAPHY/local complications/explantation.

Soo, M. S., Kornguth, P. J., Walsh, R., Elenberger, C. D., and Georgiade, G. S. Complex radial folds versus subtle signs of intracapsular rupture of breast implants: MR findings with surgical correlation. American Journal of Roentgenology. 1996 Jun, 166, 1421-1427. MAMMOGRAPHY/rupture/local complications.

Soo, M. S., Kornguth, P. J., Walsh, R., Elenberger, C., Georgiade, G. S., DeLong, D., and Spritzer, C. E. Intracapsular implant rupture: MR findings of incomplete shell collapse. Journal of Magnetic Resonance Imaging. 1997, 7, (4): 724-730. MAMMOGRAPHY/rupture/local complications.

Sorahan, T., and Pope, D. Mortality and cancer morbidity of production workers in the United Kingdom flexible polyurethane foam industry. British Journal of Industrial Medicine. 1993, 50, 528-536. TOXICOLOGY/polyurethane/cancer.

Spagnolo, F., and Malone, W. M. Quantitative determination of small amounts of toluene diisocyanate monomer in urethane adhesives by gel permeation chromatography. Journal of Chromatographic Science. 1976 Feb, 14, 52-56. TOXICOLOGY/polyurethane.

Spear, S. L., and Baker, Jr. J. L. Classification of capsular contracture after prosthetic breast reconstruction. Plast. Reconstr. Surg. 1995 Oct, 96, (5): 1119-1123. CAPSULE-CONTRACTURE/local complications/reconstruction.

Spear, S. L., and Majidian, A. Immediate breast reconstruction in two stages using textured, integrated-valve tissue expanders and breast implants: A retrospective review of 171 consecutive breast reconstructions from 1989 to 1996. Plast. Reconstr. Surg. 1998 Jan, 101, (1): 53-63. EXPANDER/reconstruction.

Spear, S. L., Matsuba, H., Romm, S., and Little, J. W. Methyl prednisolone in double-lumen gel-saline submuscular mammary prostheses: A double-blind, prospective, controlled clinical trial. Plast. Reconstr. Surg. 1991 Mar, 87, (3): 483-487. CAPSULE-CONTRACTURE/local complications/steroids.

Speirs, A. L., and Blocksman, R. New implantable silicone rubbers: An experimental evaluation of tissue response. Plast. Reconstr. Surg. 1963 Feb, 31, (2): 166-175. GENERAL/toxicology.

Spielvogel, D. E., and Hannenman, L. E. 2,6-cis-diphenylhexamethylcyclotetrasiloxane: Physicochemical properties and analytical methods. Acta Pharmacologica et Toxicologica. 1975, 36, (Supplement III): 25-32. TOXICOLOGY/silicone characterization.

Spiera, H., and Kerr, L. D. Scleroderma following silicone implantation: A cumulative experience of 11 cases. J. Rheumatol. 1993, 20, (6): 958-961. CONNECTIVE TISSUE DISEASE.

Spiera, H., and Spiera, R. F. Silicone breast implants and connective tissue disease: An overview. The Mount Sinai Journal of Medicine. 1997 Nov, 64, (6): 363-371. CONNECTIVE TISSUE DISEASE.

Spiera, R. F., Gibofsky, A., and Speira, H. Silicone gel filled breast implants and connective tissue disease: An overview. J. Rheumatol. 1994, 21, (2): 239-245. GENERAL/connective tissue disease.

Spiera, R., Gibofsky, A., and Spiera, H. Immunological reactions to silicone implants: Risk and management. Clinical Immunotherapy. 1994 Jun, 1, (6): 406-411. IMMUNE EFFECTS.

Spiers, E. M., Grotting, J. C., and Omura, E. F. An epidermal proliferative reaction associated with a silicone gel breast implant. The American Journal of Dermatopathology. 1994, 16, (3): 315-319. LOCAL COMPLICATIONS/polyurethane.

Spilizewski, K. L., Marchant, R. E., Anderson, J. M., and Hiltner, A. *In vivo* leucocyte interactions with the NHLBI-DTB primary reference materials: Polyethylene and silica-free polymethylsiloxane. Biomaterials. 1987 Jan, 8, 12-17. IMMUNE EFFECTS.

Spitalny, H. H. Reconstruction of the breast. Chir. Plast. 1981, 6, 87. RECONSTRUCTION/infection.

Spitzer, W. O., Harth, M., Goldsmith, C. H., Norman, G. R., Dickie, G. L., Bass, M. J., and Newell, J. P. The arthritic complaint in primary care: Prevalence, related disability, and costs. The Journal of Rheumatology. 1976, 3, (1): 88-99. AI-CTD BACKGROUND.

Srivastava, M. D., Rossi, T. M., and Lebenthal, E. Serum soluble interleukin-2 receptor, soluble CD8 and soluble intercellular adhesion molecule-1 levels in Crohn's disease, celiac disease, and systemic lupus erythematosus. Research Communications in Molecular Pathology and Pharmacology. 1995 Jan, 87, (1): 21-26. AI-CTD BACKGROUND/immune effects.

Stabile, R. J., Santoro, E., Dispaltro, F., and Sanfilippo, L. J. Reconstructive breast surgery following mastectomy and adjunctive radiation therapy. Cancer. 1980 Jun 1, 45, (11): 2738-2743. RADIATION/reconstruction.

Stafford, H. A., Anderson, C. J., and Reichlin, M. Unmasking of anti-ribosomal P autoantibodies in healthy individuals. J. Immunol. 1995, 155, 2754-2761. CHILDREN'S EFFECTS/breast feeding.

Stanford, J. L, Weiss, N. S., Voigt, L. F., Daling, J. R., Habel, L. A., and Rossing, M. A. Combined estrogen and progestin hormone replacement therapy in relation to risk of breast cancer in women. J. Amer. Med. Assoc. 1995, 274, (2): 137-142. CANCER.

Stanislawski, L., Serne, H., Stanislawski, M., and Jozefowicz, M. Conformational changes of fibronectin induced by polystyrene derivatives with a heparin-like function. Journal of Biomedical Materials Research. 1993, 27, 619-626. SILICONE CHARACTERIZATION/general.

Stark, B., Göbel, M., and Jaeger, K. Intraluminal cyclosporine A reduces capsular thickness around silicone implants in rats. Annals of Plastic Surgery. 1990 Feb, 24, 156-161. LOCAL COMPLICATIONS/capsule contracture.

Stark, G. B., and et al. Intraluminal cyclosporine A. Annals of Plastic Surgery. 1990, 24, (15): 6-61. CAPSULE CONTRACTURE.

Steen, V. D., Conte, C., Santoro, D., Casterline, G. L. Z., Oddis, C. V., and Medsger, T. A. Twenty-year incidence survey of systemic sclerosis. Arthritis and Rheumatism. 1997 Mar, 40, (3): 441-445. CONNECTIVE TISSUE DISEASE/ai-ctd background.

Steen, V. D., and Medsger, T. A. Epidemiology and natural history of systemic sclerosis. Rheumatic Disease Clinics of North America. 1990 Feb, 16, (1): 10. AI-CTD BACKGROUND.

Steen, V. D., Powell, D. I., and Medsger, Jr. T. A. Clinical correlations and prognosis based on serum autoantibodies in patients with systemic sclerosis. Arthritis and Rheumatism. 1988, 31, 196-203. CONNECTIVE TISSUE DISEASE.

Steenland, K., and Brown, D. Mortality study of gold miners exposed to silica and nonasbestiform amphibole minerals: An update with 14 more years of follow-up. American Journal of Industrial Medicine. 1995 Feb, 27, (2): 217-229. SILICA.

Steenland, K., and Goldsmith, D. F. Silica exposure and autoimmune diseases. American Journal of Industrial Medicine. 1995, 28, 603-608. SILICA.

Stefanek, M. E., Helzlsouer, K. J., Wilcox, P. M., and Houn, F. Predictors of and satisfaction with bilateral prophylactic mastectomy. Preventive Medicine. 1995, 24, 412-419. PSYCHOSOCIAL.

Stein, J., Lewis L. N. et al. In situ determination of the active catalyst in hydrosilylation reactions using highly reactive Pt(0) catalyst precursors. J. Amer. Chem. Soc. 1999, 121, 3693. SILICONE CHEMISTRY/toxicology.

Stein, Z. A. Silicone breast implants: epidemiological evidence of sequelae. American Journal of Public Health. 1999 Apr, 89, (4): 484-486. CONNECTIVE TISSUE DISEASE.

Steinbach, B. G., Hardt, N. S., Abbitt, P. L., Lanier, L., and Caffee, H. H. Breast implants, common complications and concurrent breast disease. Radiographics. 1993, 13, 95-118. GENERAL/local complications.

Stern, K., Doyon, D., and Racine, R. Preoccupation with the shape of the breast as a psychiatric symptom in women. Canadian Psychiatric Association Journal. 1959 Oct, 4, (4): 243-254. PSYCHOSOCIAL.

Sternberg, E. M. Pathogenesis-Environmental. Systemic Sclerosis. p. 203-228. TOXICOLOGY.

Sternberg, T. R., Ashley, F. L., Winer, H. H., and Lehman, R. Tissue reactions to injected silicone liquids. Der Hautarzt. 1964, 15, 281. SILICONE INJECTION.

Stevens, L, McGrath, M, Druss, R, and et al. The psychological impact of immediate breast reconstruction for women with early breast cancer. Plast. Reconstr. Surg. 1984 Apr, 73, (4): 619-626. PSYCHOSOCIAL/reconstruction.

Stevens, P. E., Dibble, S. L., and Miaskowski, C. Prevalence, characteristics, and impact of postmastectomy pain syndrome: An investigation of women's experiences. Pain. 1995, 61, 61-68. PAIN/local complications.

Stewart, N. R., Monsees, B. S., Destouet, J. M., and Rudloff, M. A. Mammographic appearance following implant removal. Radiology. 1992, 185, (1): 83-85. MAMMOGRAPHY/explantation.

Stocks, M. R., Williams, D. G., and Maini, R. N. Analysis of a positive feedback mechanism in the anti-Sm autoantibody reponse in MRL/MPJ-lpr/lpr mice. Eur. J. Immunol. 1991, 21, 267-272. CHILDREN'S EFFECTS/breast feeding.

Stocks, M. R., Williams, D. G., and Maini, R. N. Differential induction of lupus associated antinuclear antibodies in MRL mice by monoclonal anti-Sm antibodies. Clin. Exp. Immunol. 1987, 67, 492-499. CHILDREN'S EFFECTS/breast feeding.

Stokes, K. B. Polyether polyurethanes: Biostable or not. Journal of Biomaterials Applications. 1988 Oct, 3, 228-259. POLYURETHANE.

Stombler, R. E. Breast implants and the FDA: Past, present, and future. ACS Bull. 1993, 78 (6), 11-15. GENERAL.

Stomper, P., Kopans, D., Sadowsky, N. L., Sonnenfeld, M. R., Swann, C. A., Gelman, R. S., Meyer, J. E., Jochelson, M. S., Hunt, M. S., and Allen, P. D. Is mammography painful? A multicenter patient survey. Archives of Internal Medicine. 1988 Mar, 148, 521-524. MAMMOGRAPHY/pain.

Stone, J., and Dowden, R. V. Breast implant endoscopy: Detecting leaks in silicone-gel breast implants. AORN Journal. 1994 May, 59, (5): 1007-1015. LOCAL COMPLICATIONS/rupture.

Stone, Jr. W. Alloplasty in the surgery of the eye. The New England Journal of Medicine. 1958 Mar 6, 258, (10): 486-490. GENERAL.

Stratton, K. R., Howe, C. J., and Johnston, R. B. Causality and evidence in adverse events associated with childhood vaccines: evidence bearing on causality. Washington, DC: National Academy Press, 1994. GENERAL.

Strickland, R. W., Tesar, J. T., Berne, B. H., Hobbs, B. R., and Lewis, D. M. The frequency of sicca syndrome in an elderly female population. J. Rheumatol. 1987, 14, (4): 766-771. AI-CTD BACKGROUND.

Strom, B. L., Reidenberg, M. M., Freundlich, B., and Schinnar, R. Breast silicone implants and risk of systemic lupus erythematosis. Journal of Clinical Epidemiology. 1994, 47, (10): 1211-1214. CONNECTIVE TISSUE DISEASE.

Strom, S. S., Baldwin, B. J., Sigurdson, A. J., and Schusterman, M. A. Cosmetic saline breast implants: A survey of satisfaction, breast-feeding experience, cancer screening, and health. Plast. Reconstr. Surg. 1997, 100, (6): 1553-1557. PSYCHOSOCIAL/breast feeding/children's effects /saline.

Stroman, P. W., Rolland, C., Dufour, M., Grondin, P., and Guidoin, R. G. Appearance of low signal intensity lines in MRI of silicone breast implants. Biomaterials. 1996 May, 17, (10): 983-988. MAMMOGRAPHY/capsule-contracture/local complications/rupture.

Struyf, N. J., Snoeck, H. W., Bridts, C. H., and et al. Natural killer cell activity in Sjogren's syndrome and systemic lupus erythematosus: stimulation with interferons and interleukin-2 and correlation with immune complexes. Ann. Rheum. Dis. 1990, 49, 690-693. AI-CTD BACKGROUND.

Stuart, R., Littlewood, A., Maddison, P., and Hall, N. Elevated serum interleukin-6 levels associated with active disease in systemic connective tissue disorders. Clinical and Experimental Rheumatology. 1995, 13, 17-22. IMMUNE EFFECTS/AI-CTD BACKGROUND.

Su, C. W., Dreyfuss, D. A., Krizek, T. J., and Leoni, K. J. Silicone implants and the inhibition of cancer. Plast. Reconstr. Surg. 1995 Sep, 96, (3): 513-518. CARCINOGENICITY/polyurethane.

Sultan, M. R., Smith, M. L., Estabrook, A., Schnabel, F., and Singh, D. Immediate breast reconstruction in patients with locally advanced disease. Annals of Plastic Surgery. 1997 Apr, 38, (4): 345-349. CANCER/reconstruction.

Sundaram, K., and Kincl, F. A. Sustained release hormonal preparations. 2. Factors controlling the diffusion of steroids through dimethylpolysiloxane membranes. Steroids. 1968, 12, (4): 517-524. STEROIDS.

Suster, S., Phillips, M., Wallack, M., and Robinson, M. J. Carcinoma of the breast arising at the site of liquid silicone injection. South. Med. J. 1987, 80, 57. SILICONE INJECTION/cancer.

Sutherland, K., Mahoney, J. R. II, Coury, A. J., and Eaton, J. W. Degradation of biomaterials by phagocyte-derived oxidants. Journal of Clinical Investigation. 1993, 92, 2360-2367. POLYURETHANE/toxicology.

Svahn, J. K., Vastine, V. L., Landon, B. N., and Dobke, M. K. Outcome of mammary prostheses explantation: A patient perspective. Annals of Plastic Surgery. 1996 Jun, 36, (6): 594-600. PSYCHOSOCIAL/explantation.

Swan, S. Disease occurrence in silicone breast implanted women: Estimates from the sample of domestic claimants. Journal of Womens Health. 1995 Oct 1. CONNECTIVE TISSUE DISEASE.

Swan, S. H. Epidemiology of silicone-related disease. Seminars in Arthritis and Rheumatism. 1994, 24, (1 (Supplement 1)): 38-43. CONNECTIVE TISSUE DISEASE.

Swanson, A. B. Durability of silicone implants—An in vivo study. Orthopedic Clinics of North America. 1973 Oct, 4, (4): 1097-1112. SILICONE CHARACTERIZATION/general.

Swanson, A. B., Nalbandian, R. M., Zmugg, T. J., Williams, D., Jaeger, S., Maupin, B. K., and Swanson, G. G. Silicone implants in dogs. Clinical Orthopaedics and Related Research. 1984 Apr, 184, 293-301. TOXICOLOGY.

Swanson J.W., and Lebeau, J. E. The effect of implantation on the physical properties of silicone rubber. Journal of Biomedical Materials. 1974 Jan, 8, 357-367. SILICONE CHARACTERIZATION.

Symmers, W. St. C. Silicone mastitis in topless waitresses and some other varieties for foreign-body mastitis. British Medical Journal. 1968, 3, 19-22. SILICONE INJECTION.

Szycher, M., Lee, S. J., and Siciliano, A. A. Breast prostheses: A critical review. Journal of Biomaterials Applications. 1991 Apr, 5, 256-281. POLYURETHANE/general.

Szycher, M., and Poirer, V. L. Polyurethanes in implantable devices. Medical Devices and Diagnostic Industry. 1984 May, 6, (5): 44-49. POLYURETHANE.

Szycher, M., and Siciliano, A. A. Polyurethane-covered mammary prostheses: A nine-year follow-up assessment. Journal of Biomaterials Applications. 1991b, 5, 282-322. POLYURETHANE/local complications.

Szycher, M., and Siciliano, A. A. An assessment of 2,4-TDA formation from Surgitek polyurethane foam under simulated physiological conditions. Journal of Biomaterials Applications. 1991a Apr, 5, 323-336. TOXICOLOGY/polyurethane.

Tabari, K. Augmentation mammaplasty with simaplast implant. Plast. Reconstr. Surg. 1969 Nov, 44, (5): 468-470. GENERAL/saline.

Tabatowski, K., Elson, C. E., and Johnston, W. W. Silicone lymphadenopathy in a patient with a mammary prosthesis. Acta Cytologica. 1990 Jan-1990 Feb 28, 34, (1): 10-14. LYMPHADENOPATHY/granulomas/local complications.

Taggart, I., and Bantick, G. L. Mammography and breast implants. British Journal of Plastic Surgery. 1995, 48, 49-52. MAMMOGRAPHY.

Talmor, M., Rothaus, K. O., Shannahan, E., Cortese, A. F., and Hoffman, L. A. Sqamous cell carcinoma of the breast after augmentation with liquid silicone injection. Annals of Plastic Surgery. 1995 Jun, 34, (6): 619-623. CANCER/silicone injection.

Tan, E. M. Antinuclear antibodies: Diagnostic markers for autoimmune diseases and probes for cell biology. Advances in Immunology. 1989, 44, 93-151. IMMUNE EFFECTS.

Tan, E. M. Immunologic changes in women with silicone breast implants. Today In Medicine/Obstetrics & Gynecology. 1993 Jan 1: 21-22. IMMUNE EFFECTS.

Tan, E. M., Feltkamp, T. E. W., Smolen, J. S., Butcher, B., Dawkins, R., Fritzler, M. J., Gordon, T., Hardin, J. A., Kalden, J. R., Lahita, R. G., Maini, R. N., McDougal, J. S., Rothfield, N. F., Smeenk, R. J., Takasaki, Y., Wiik, A., Wilson, M. R., and Koziol, J. A. Range of antinuclear antibodies in healthy individuals. Arthritis and Rheumatism. 1997 Sep, 40, (9): 1601-1611. AI-CTD BACKGROUND/immune effects.

Tan, E. M., Rodnan, G. P., Garcia, I., Moroi, T., Fritzier, M. J., and Peebles, C. Diversity of antinuclear antibodies in progressive systemic sclerosis: Anti-centromere antibody and its relationship to CREST syndrome. Arthritis and Rheumatism. 1980 Jun, 23, (6): 615-617. AI-CTD BACKGROUND/immune effects.

Tanaka, K., Wakabayashi, M., Tanaka, M., Ohno, T., and Hoshi, E. A case of human adjuvant disease with polyneuropathy. Clinical Neurology. 1985 Sep 1, 25, (9): 1075-1080. NEUROLOGIC DISEASE/connective tissue disease.

Tanaka, T., Maeda, T., Hayashi, Y., Imai, S., Funakawa, K., and Nose, T. Silicon concentrations in maternal serum and breast milk in the postpartum period. Jpn. J. Hyg. 1990, 45, 919-925. BREAST FEEDING/silicon measurement.

Tang, L., and Eaton, J. W. Fibrin(ogen) mediates acute inflammatory responses to biomaterials. J Exp Med. 1993, 178, 2147-2156. IMMUNE EFFECTS.

Tang, L., and Eaton, J. W. Inflammatory responses to biomaterials. American Journal of Clinical Pathology. 1995, 103, (4): 466-471. IMMUNE EFFECTS/polyurethane.

Tang, P. M., Petrelli, M., and Robecheck, P. J. Stromal sarcoma of the breast. Cancer. 1979, 43, 209-217. CANCER.

Tansini, I. Sopra il mio nuovo processo di amputazione della mamella. Gaz. Med. Ital. 1906, 57, 141. RECONSTRUCTION.

Tarpila, E., Ghassemifar, R., Fagrell, D., and Berggren, A. Capsular contracture with textured versus smooth saline-filled implants for breast augmentation: A prospective clinical study. Plast. Reconstr. Surg. 1997 Jun, 99, (7): 1934-1939. CAPSULE-CONTRACTURE/local complications.

Taupmann, R. E., and Adler, S. Silicone pleural effusion due to iatrogenic breast implant rupture. Southern Medical Journal. 1993 May, 86, (5): 570-571. MIGRATION/local complications/rupture.

Taylor, S. R., and Gibbons, D. F. Effect of surface texture on the soft tissue response to polymer implants. Journal of Biomedical Materials Research. 1983, 17, 205-227. CAPSULE-CONTRACTURE/local complications.

Tebbetts, J. B. Transaxillary subpectoral augmentation mammoplasty: Long term follow up and refinements. Plast. Reconstr. Surg. 1984 Nov, 74, (5): 636-647. CAPSULE-CONTRACTURE/local complications.

Tebbetts, J. B. What is adequate fill? Implications in breast implant surgery. Plast. Reconstr. Surg. 1996 Jun, 97, (7): 1451-1454. RUPTURE/local complications.

Tebbetts, J. B., and Barton, F. E. Augmentation mammaplasty. Selected Readings in Plastic Surgery. 1987, 4, (29): 1-18. GENERAL.

Teimourian, B., and Adham, M. N. Survey of patients' response to breast reconstruction. Annals of Plastic Surgery. 1982, 9, (4): 321-325. PSYCHOSOCIAL.

Temple, W. J., Lindsay, R. L., Magi, E., and Urbanski, S. J. Technical considerations for prophylactic mastectomy in patients at high risk for breast cancer. The American Journal of Surgery. 1991 Apr, 161, 413-415. CANCER.

Tenenbaum, S. A., Rice, J. C., Espinoza, L. R., Cuellar, M. L., Plymale, D. R., Sander, D. M. Williamson L. L., Haislip, A. M., Gluck, O. S., Tesser, J. R. P., Nogy, L., Stribrny, K. M., Bevan, J. A., and Garry, R. F. Use of antipolymer antibody assay in recipients of silicone breast implants. The Lancet. 1997a Feb 15, 349, 449-454. IMMUNE EFFECTS.

Terry, M. B., Skovron, M. L., Garbers, S., Sonnenschein, E., and Toniolo, P. The estimated frequency of cosmetic breast augmentation among U.S. women, 1963 through 1988. American Journal of Public Health. 1995 Aug, 85, (8): 1122-1124. PREVALENCE.

Teuber, S. S., and Gershwin, M. E. Autoantibodies and clinical rheumatic complaints in two children of women with silicone gel breast implants. International Archives of Allergy and Immunology. 1994, 103, 105-108. CONNECTIVE TISSUE DISEASE/children's effects.

Teuber, S.S., Howell, L. P., Yoshida, S. H., and Gershwin, M. E. Remission of sarcoidosis following removal of silicone gel breast implants. International Archives of Allergy and Immunology. 1994, 105, 404-407. IMMUNE EFFECTS.

Teuber, S.S., Ito, L. K., Anderson, M., and Gershwin, M. E. Silicone breast implant - Associated scarring dystrophy of the arm. Archives of Dermatology. 1995b Jan, 131, 54-56. MIGRATION/local complications.

Teuber, S.S., Reilly, D.A., Howell, L., Oide, C., and Gershwin, M.E. Severe migratory granulomatous reactions to silicone gel in 3 patients. Rheumatol. 1999, 26, (3): 699-704. LOCAL COMPLICATIONS.

Teuber, S.S., Rowley, M. J., Yoshida, S. H., Ansari, A. A., and Gershwin, M. E. Anti-collagen autoantibodies are found in women with silicone breast implants. Journal of Autoimmunity. 1993 Jan, 6, 367-377. IMMUNE EFFECTS.

Teuber, S.S., Saunders, R. L., Halpern, G. M., Brucker, R. F., Conte, V., Goldman, B. D., Winder, E. E., Wood, W. G., and Gershwin, M. E. Elevated serum silicon levels in women with silicone gel breast implants. Biological Trace Element Research. 1995a May, 48, 121-130. SILICON MEASUREMENT.

Teuber, S.S., Yoshida, S. H., and Gershwin, M. E. Immunopathic effects of silicone breast implants. Western Journal of Medicine. 1995c May, 162, (5): 418-425. IMMUNE EFFECTS.

Theophelis, L. G., and Stevenson, T. R. Radiographic evidence of breast implant rupture. Plast. Reconstr. Surg. 1986 Nov, 78, (5): 673-675. MAMMOGRAPHY/rupture/local complications.

Thomas, 3rd W. O., Harper, L. L., Wong, S. W., Michalski, J. P., Harris, C. N., Moore, J. T., and Rodning, C. B. Explantation of silicone breast implants. The American Surgeon. 1997 May, 63, (5): 421-429. EXPLANTATION.

Thomas, C., and Robinson, J. A. The antinuclear antibody list. When is a positive result clinically relevant? Postgrad. Med. 1993, 94, 55-58. AI-CTD BACKGROUND.

Thomas, P. R. S., Ford, H. T., and Gazet, J. Use of silicone implants after wide local excision of the breast. British Journal of Surgery. 1993, 80, (7): 868-870. RADIATION/capsule-contracture/local complications.

Thomsen, J. L., Christensen, L., Nielsen, M., Brandt, B., Breiting, V. B., Felby, S., and Nielsen, E. Histologic changes and silicone concentrations in human breast tissue surrounding silicone breast prostheses. Plast. Reconstr. Surg. 1990 Jan, 85, (1): 38-41. SILICON MEASUREMENT.

Thomson, H. G. The fate of the pseudosheath pocket around silicone implants. Plast. Reconstr. Surg. 1973 Jun, 51, (6): 667-671. CAPSULE-CONTRACTURE/local complications.

Thornton, J. W., Argenta, L. C., McClatchey, K. D., and Marks, M. W. Studies on the endogenous flora of the human breast. Ann. Plast. Surg. 1988, 20, (1): 39-42. INFECTION.

Thuesen, B., Siim, E., Christensen, L., and Schroder, M. Capsular contracture after breast reconstruction with the tissue expansion technique. A comparison of smooth and textured silicone breast prostheses. Scandinavian Journal of Plastic and Reconstructive Surgery and Hand Surgery. 1995, 29, (1): 9-13. CAPSULE-CONTRACTURE/expander/local complications.

Timberlake, G. A., and Looney, G. R. Adenocarcinoma of the breast associated with silicone injections. Journal of Surgical Oncology. 1986, 32, 79-81. SILICONE INJECTION/cancer.

Tinkler, J. Breast implants: Is there an association with connective tissue disease? Health Trends. 1994, 26, (1): 25-26. GENERAL.

Tirelli, U., Marotta, G., Improta, S., and Pinto, A. Immunological abnormalities in patients with chronic fatigue syndrome. Scandinavian Journal of Immunol. 1994, 40, 601-608. IMMUNE EFFECTS/CONNECTIVE TISSUE DISEASE.

Tiziani, V., Cintra, M. L., Raposo do Amaral, C. M., Sabbatini, R. M. E., and Lima, R. P. R. Lack of lymph-node reaction to subcutaneously injected silicone gel—histological and computer-aided morphometric study in rats. Scandanavian Journal of Plastic and Reconstructive Surgery and Hand Surgery. 1995, 29, (4): 303-311. TOXICOLOGY/lymphadenopathy.

Tobin, G., Shaw, R. C., and Goodpasture, H. C. Toxic shock syndrome following breast and nasal surgery. Plast. Reconstr. Surg. 1987 Jul, 80, (1): 1111-1114. INFECTION/local complications.

Tobin, H. A. Incidence of capsular contracture in polyurethane versus smooth implants. American Journal of Cosmetic Surgery. 1989, 6, 177. POLYURETHANE/capsule-contracture/local complications.

Tobin, H. R., and Middleton, W. G. Revision mammoplasty using the Replicon implant. The American Journal of Cosmetic Surgery. 1987, 4, (3): 201-204. CAPSULE-CONTRACTURE/polyurethane/local complications.

Todhunter, J. A., and Farrow, M. G. Current scientific considerations in regard to defining a "silicone syndrome" disease and the formation of silica from silicone. International Journal of Toxicology. 1998, 17, 449-463. CONNECTIVE TISSUE DISEASE/silica.

Toennissen, J., Schrudde, J., and Niermann, W. Experience with 250 cases of subcutaneous breast implants. British Journal of Plastic Surgery. 1982, 35, 458-465. LOCAL COMPLICATIONS/reconstruction.

Tolhurst, D. E. Nutcracker technique for compression rupture of capsules around breast implants. Plast. Reconstr. Surg. 1978 Nov, 62, (5): 795. RUPTURE/capsule-contracture/local complications/closed capsulotomy.

Tollefson, D. F., Bandyk, D. F., Kaebnick, H. W., and et al. Surface biofilm disruption: Enhanced recovery of microorganisms from vascular prostheses. Archives of Surgery. 1987 Jan, 122, 38-43. INFECTION.

Tomazic, V. J., Withrow, T. J., and Hitchines, V. M. Adverse reactions associated with medical device implants. Periodicum Biologorum. 1991, 93, 547-554. GENERAL.

Touchette, N. Silicone implants and autoimmune disease: Studies fail to gel. The Journal of NIH Research. 1992 May, 4, 49-52. GENERAL/connective tissue disease.

Trabulsy, P. P., Anthony, J. P., and Mathes, S. J. Changing trends in postmastectomy breast reconstruction: A 13-year experience. Plast. Reconstr. Surg. 1994 Jun, 93 (7), 1418-1427. RECONSTRUCTION.

Travis, W. D., Balogh, K., and Abraham, J. L. Silicone granulomas: Report of three cases and review of the literature. Human Pathology. 1985 Jan, 16, 19-27. GRANULOMAS/local complications.

Trichopoulos, D., and Lipman, R. D. Mammary gland mass and breast cancer risk. Epidemiology. 1992, 3, 523-526. CANCER.

Troilius, C. Total muscle coverage of a breast implant is possible through the transaxillary approach. Plast. Reconstr. Surg. 1995 Mar, 95, (3): 509-512. GENERAL.

Trolius, C. Correction of implant ptosis after a transaxillary subpectoral breast augmentation. Plast. Reconstr. Surg. 1996 Oct, 98, (5): 889-895. GENERAL.

Truong, L. D., Cartwright, J., Goodman, M. D., and Woznicki, D. Silicone lymphadenopathy associated with augmentation mammaplasty: Morphologic features of nine cases. The American Journal of Surgical Pathology. 1988, 12, (6): 484. LYMPHADENOPATHY/local complications.

Truppman, E. S., Ellenby, J. D., and Schwartz, B. M. Fungi in and around implants after augmentation mammaplasty. Plast. Reconstr. Surg. 1979 Dec, 64, (6): 804-806. INFECTION/local complications.

Tsang, W. Y. W., Chan, J. K. C., and Ng, C. S. Kikuchi's lymphadenitis: A morphologic analysis of 75 cases with special reference to unusual features. The American Journal of Surgical Pathology. 1994, 18, (3): 219-231. LYMPHADENOPATHY.

Tsuchiya, T., Hata, H., and Nakamura, A. Studies on the tumor-promoting activity of biomaterials: Inhibition of metabolic cooperation by polyurethane and silicone. Journal of Biomedical Materials Researchives. 1995 Jan, 29, (1): 113-119. CANCER.

Turnbull, A. R., Turner, D. T., Fraser, J. D., Lloyd, R. S., Lang, C. J., and Wright, R. Autoantibodies in early breast cancer: a stage related phenomenon. Br. J. Cancer. 1978, 38, 461-463. AI-CTD BACKGROUND.

Turner, F. C. Sarcoma at sites of subcutaneously implanted Bakelite discs in rats. Journal of the National Cancer Institute. 1941, 2, 81-83. CARCINOGENICITY.

Tytherleigh, M., Koshy, C. E., and Evans, J. Phantom Breast Pain. Plast. Reconstr. Surg. 1998, 102, (3): 921. PAIN.

Uchida, K., Fukami, A., Hori, M., and et al. Breast cancers following a breast implant. Rinshou-Geka. 1981, 36, 129-132. CANCER.

Ueki, A., Yamaguchi, M., Ueki, H., Watanabe, Y., Ohsawa, G., Kinugawa, K., Kawakami, Y., and Hyodoh, F. Polyclonal human t-cell activation by silicate in vitro. Immunology. 1994, 82, 332-335. IMMUNE EFFECTS/silica.

Umansky, C., and Wilkinson, T. S. Infection associated with polyurethane-coated implants. Plast. Reconstr. Surg. 1985, 75, (6): 925-926. INFECTION/local complications/polyurethane.

Umeda, M. Production of rat sarcoma by injections of propylene glycol solution of M-Toluylenediamine (Plates XXIII and XXIV). GANN. 1955, 46, 597-603. POLYURETHANE/cancer.

Unger, P. D., and Friedman, M. A. High-performance liquid chromatography of 2,6- and 2,4-diaminotoluene, and its application to the determination of 2,4-diaminotoluene in urine and plasma. Journal of Chromatography. 1979, 174, 379-384. TOXICOLOGY/polyurethane.

Unzeitig, G. W., Frankl, G., Ackerman, M., and O'Connell, T. X. Analysis of the prognosis of minimal and occult breast cancers. Archives of Surgery. 1983 Dec, 118, 1403-1404. CANCER/mammography.

Uretsky, B. F., O'Brien, J. J., Courtiss, E. H., and Becker, M. D. Augmentation mammoplasty associated with a severe systemic illness. Annals of Plastic Surgery. 1979 Nov, 3, (5): 445-447. IMMUNE EFFECTS.

Utell, M. J., Gelein, R., and Yu, C. P. et al. Quantitative exposure of humans to an octamethylcyclotetrasiloxane (D4) vapor. Toxicological Sciences. 1998, 44, 206-213. TOXICOLOGY.

Valaoras, V. G., MacMalom, B., Trichopoulos, D., and Polychronopoulou, A. Lactation and reproductive histories of breast cancer patients in greater Athens, 1965-1967. International Journal of Cancer. 1969, 4, 350-363. CANCER/breast feeding.

Van Dam, F. S. A. M., and Bergman, R. B. Psychosocial and surgical aspects of breast reconstruction. European Journal of Surgical Oncology. 1988, 14, 141-149. PSYCHOSOCIAL/reconstruction.

Van Heerden, J. A., Jackson, I. T., Martin, J. K., and Fisher, J. Surgical technique and pitfalls of breast reconstruction immediately after mastectomy for carcinoma: Initial experience. Mayo Clinic Proceedings. 1987 Mar, 62, 185-191. RECONSTRUCTION/expander.

Van Ierssel, G. J., Mieremet-Ooms, M. A., van der Zon, A. M., and et al. Effect of cortisol and ACTH on corticosteroid-suppressed peripheral blood natural killer cells from healthy volunteers and patients with Crohn's disease. Immunopharmacology. 1996, 34, 97-104. AI-CTD BACKGROUND.

Van Kooten, T. G., Whitesides, J. F., and von Recum, A. F. Influence of silicone (PDMS) surface texture on human skin fibroblast proliferation as determined by cell cycle analysis. J. Biomed. Mat. Res. 1998, 43, 1-14. CAPSULE CONTRACTURE/toxicology.

Van Natta, B. W., Thurston, J. B., and Moore, T. S. Silicone breast implants—Is there cause for concern? Indiana Med. 1990 Mar, 83, 184-185. GENERAL.

Van Nunen, S. A., Gatenby, P. A., and Basten, A. Post-mammoplasty connective tissue disease. Arthritis and Rheumatism. 1982 Jun, 25, (6): 694-697. CONNECTIVE TISSUE DISEASE.

Van Oss, C. J., Singer, J. M., and Gillman, C. F. The influence of particulate carriers and of mineral oil in adjuvants on the antibody response in rabbits to human gamma globulin. Immunological Communications. 1976, 5, (3): 181-188. IMMUNE EFFECTS.

Van Rappard, J. H., Sonneveld, G. J., van Twisk, R., and Borghouts, J. M. Pressure resistance of breast implants as a function of implantation time. Annals of Plastic Surgery. 1988, 21, 566-569. RUPTURE/local complications.

Van Venrooij, W. J., Charles, P., and Maini, R. N. The consensus workshops for the detection of autoantibodies to intracellular antigens in rheumatic diseases. Journal of Immunological Methods. 1991, 140, 181-189. IMMUNE EFFECTS/connective tissue disease.

Van Wingerden, J. J., and van Staden, M. M. Ultrasound mammography in prosthesis-related breast augmentation complications. Annals of Plastic Surgery. 1989 Jan, 22, (1): 32-35. MAMMOGRAPHY.

Vanderford, M. L., Smith, D. H., and Olive, T. The image of plastic surgeons in news media coverage of the silicone breast implant controversy. Plast. Reconstr. Surg. 1995 Sep, 96, (3): 521-538. PSYCHOSOCIAL.

Vanderhoof, J. A., Rapoport, P. J., and Paxson, C. L. Manometric diagnosis of lower esophageal sphincter incompetence in infants: Use of a small, single-lumen perfused catheter. Pediatrics. 1978, 62, (5): 805-808. CHILDREN'S EFFECTS/breast feeding.

Vanderwilde, R., Morrey, B., Melberg, M. W., and vinh, T. N. Inflammatory arthritis after failure of silicone rubber replacement of the radial head. The Journal of Bone and Joint Surgery. 1994 Jan, 76-B, (1): 78-81. GENERAL/local complications.

Vann, R. D., Riefkohl, R., Georgiade, G. S., and Georgiade, N. G. Mammary implants, diving, and altitude exposure. Plast. Reconstr. Surg. 1988 Feb, 81, (2): 200-203. LOCAL COMPLICATIONS.

Vanore, J., O'Keefe, R., and Pikscher, I. Complications of silicone implants in foot surgery. Clinics in Podiatry. 1984 Apr, 1, (1): 175-196. GENERAL/local complications.

Varaprath, S., Frye, C. L., and Hamelink, J. Aqueous solubility of permethylsiloxanes (silicones). Environ Toxicol and Chem. 1996(8): 1263-1265. SILICONE CHARACTERIZATION.

Varga, J., and Jimenez, S. A. Augmentation mammoplasty and scleroderma: Is there an association? Archives of Dermatology. 1990 Sep, 126, (9): 1220-1223. CONNECTIVE TISSUE DISEASE.

Varga, J., Schumacher, R., and Jimenez, S. A. Systemic sclerosis after augmentation mammoplasty with silicone implants. Annals of Internal Medicine. 1989 Sep, 111, (5): 377-383. CONNECTIVE TISSUE DISEASE.

Vargas, A. Shedding of silicone particles from inflated breast implants. Plast. Reconstr. Surg. 1979 Aug, 64, (2): 252-253. LOCAL COMPLICATIONS/silicon measurement.

Vasconez, L. O., Psillakis, J., and Johnson-Giebeik, R. Breast reconstruction with contralateral rectus abdominis myocutaneous flap. Plast. Reconstr. Surg. 1983 May, 71, (5): 668-675. RECONSTRUCTION.

Vasey, F. B. A rheumatologist's view of silicone. International Journal of Occupational Medicine and Toxicology. 1995, 4, (1): 203-209. GENERAL.

Vasey, F. B., Havice, D. L., and Bocanegra, T. S. Clinical findings in symptomatic women with silicone breast implants. Seminars in Arthritis and Rheumatism. 1994 Aug, 24, (1 (Supplement 1)): 22-28. CONNECTIVE TISSUE DISEASE/explantation.

Vasquez, B., Given, K. S., and Houston, G. C. Breast augmentation: A review of subglandular and submuscular implantation. Aesthetic Plastic Surgery. 1987, 11, 101-105. STEROIDS/saline/local complications.

Vaughan, G. T., and Florence, T. M. Platinum in the human diet, blood, hair and excreta. The Science of the Total Environment. 1992, 111, (1): 47-58. PLATINUM.

Vayssairat, M., Mimoun, M., Houot, B., Abuaf, N., Rouquette, A. M., and Chaouat, M. Hashimoto's thyroiditis and silicone breast implants: 2 cases [abstract]. Journal des Maladies Vasculaires. 1997 Jul, 22, (3): 198-199. IMMUNE EFFECTS.

Venta, L. A., Salomon, C. G., Flisak, M. E., Venta, E. R., Izquierdo, R., and Angelats, J. Sonographic signs of breast implant rupture. American Journal of Roentgenology. 1996 Jun, 166, (6): 1413-1419. RUPTURE/mammography/local complications.

Verneuil. Memoires de Chirurgie, Paris. 1887. RECONSTRUCTION.

Vesterberg, O., Alessio, L., Brune, D., and et al. International project for producing reference values for concentrations of trace elements in human blood and urine - TRACY. Scandinavian Journal of Work and Environmental Health. 1993, 19 , ((Suppl 1)): 19-26. TOXICOLOGY.

Vial, T., and Descotes, J. Clinical toxicity of cytokines used as haemopoietic growth factors. Drug Safety. 1995, 13, (6): 371-406. AI-CTD BACKGROUND/immune effects.

Victor, S. J., Brown, D. M., Horwitz, E. M., Martinez, A. A., Kini, V. R., Pettinga, J. E., Shaheen, K. W., Benitez, P., Chen, P. Y., and Vicini, F. A. Treatment outcome with radiation therapy after breast augmentation or reconstruction in patients with primary breast carcinoma. Cancer. 1998 Apr 1, 82, (7): 1303-1309. RADIATION/reconstruction.

Villota, R., and Hawkes, J. Food applications and the toxicological and nutritional implications of amorphous silicon dioxide. Clinical Reviews In Food, Science and Nutrition. 1986, 23, (4): 289-322. SILICA.

Vimalasiri, P. A. D. T., Burford, R. P., and Haken, J. K. Chromatographic analysis of elastomeric polyurethanes. Rubber Chemistry and Technology. 60, 555-577. POLYURETHANE.

Vinnik, C. A. Spherical contracture of fibrous capsules around breast implants: Prevention and treatment. Plast. Reconstr. Surg. 1976b Nov, 58, (5): 555-560. CAPSULE-CONTRACTURE/local complications.

Vinton, A. L., Traverso, W., and Zehring, D. Immediate breast reconstruction following mastectomy is as safe as mastectomy alone. Archives of Surgery. 1990 Oct, 125, 1303-1308. RECONSTRUCTION.

Virden, C. P., Dobke, M. K., Stein, P., Parsons, C. L., and Frank, D. H. Subclinical infection of the silicone breast implant surface as a possible cause of capsular contracture. Aesthetic Plastic Surgery. 1992, 16, 173-179. CAPSULE-CONTRACTURE/infection.

Vistnes, L. M., Bentley, J. W., and Fogarty, D. C. Experimental study of tissue response to ruptured gel-filled mammary prostheses. Plast. Reconstr. Surg. 1977 Jan, 59, 31-34. RUPTURE/local complications.

Vistnes, L. M., Ksander, G. A., Isaacs, G., and Rozner, L. Elevated glycosaminoglycans and chondroitin 4-sulfate, and other properties of contracted human prosthesis capsules. Annals of Plastic Surgery. 1981, 7, 195-203. CAPSULE-CONTRACTURE.

Vistnes, L. M., Ksander, G. A., and Kosek, J. Effects of local instillation of tramcinolone on the capsules around silicone bag-gel prostheses in animals. Plast. Reconstr. Surg. 1978 Nov, 62, (5): 739-750. STEROIDS/local complications/capsule-contracture.

Vistnes, L. M., Ksander, G. A., and Kosek, J. Study of encapsulation of silicone rubber implants in animals: A foreign body reaction. Plast. Reconstr. Surg. 1978 Oct, 62, (4): 580-588. CAPSULE-CONTRACTURE/local complications.

Vogt, P. A., Seider, H. A., Moufarrege, R., Leikensohn, J. R., Ersek, R. A., Eisenberg, H. V., and Armstrong, D. P. Surface-patterned silicone implants decrease contracture for soft breast prostheses. Contemporary Surgery. 1990 Sep, 37, 25-29. CAPSULE-CONTRACTURE/local complications.

Vojdani, A. Highlights of the recent Immunology of Silicone Workshop, National Cancer Institute, March 13-14, 1995. Intl. J. Occup. Med. Toxicol. 1995, 4(1), 197-201. IMMUNE EFFECTS/local complications/migration/connective tissue disease.

Vojdani, A. Neuroimmunologic evaluation of patients with silicone implants. International Journal of Occupational Medicine and Toxicology. 1995a Jan 1, 4, (1): 25-62. IMMUNE EFFECTS/neurologic disease.

Vojdani, A., Brautbar, N., and Campbell, A. Immunologic and biologic markers for silicone. Journal of Toxicology and Industrial Health. 1994a, 10, (1/2): 25-41. IMMUNE EFFECTS.

Vojdani, A., Brautbar, N., and Campbell, A. W. Antibody to silicone and native macromolecules in women with silicone breast implants. Immunopharmacology and Immunotoxicology. 1994b, 16, (4): 497-523. IMMUNE EFFECTS.

Vojdani, A., Campbell, A., and Brautbar, N. Immune functional impairment in patients with clinical abnormalities and silicone breast implants. Toxicology and Industrial Health. 1992b, 8, (6): 415-429. IMMUNE EFFECTS.

Vojdani, A., Ghoneum, M., and Brautbar, N. Immune alteration associated with exposure to toxic chemicals. Toxicol. Ind. Hlth. 1992a, 8, (5): 239-254. IMMUNE EFFECTS.

Von Frey, H.-P., Lemperle, G., and Exner, K. Siliconomas and rheumatoid symptoms—A known and a questionable complication of silicone implants. Hanchir Mikrochir Plast Chir. 1992, 24, 171-177. GRANULOMAS/local complications/connective tissue disease.

Von Heimburg, D., Exner, K., Kruft, S., and Lemperle, G. The tuberous breast deformity: classification and treatment. Brit. J. Plast. Surg. 1996, 49, (6): 339-345. RECONSTRUCTION.

Von Mikecz, A., Konstantinov, K., Buchwald, D. S., Gerace, L., and Tan, E. M. High frequency of autoantibodies to insoluble cellular antigens in patients with chronic fatigue syndrome. Arthritis and Rheumatism. 1997 Feb, 40, (2): 295-305. AI-CTD BACKGROUND/immune effects.

Von Smitten, K., and Sundell, B. The impact of adjuvant radiotherapy and cytotoxic chemotherapy on the outcome of immediate breast reconstruction by tissue expansion after mastectomy for breast cancer. European Journal of Surgical Oncology. 1992, 18, 119-123. EXPANDER/radiation/reconstruction/infection/local complications.

Vondracek, P., and Gent, A. N. Slow decomposition of silicone rubber. Journal of Applied Polymer Science. 1982, 27, 4517-4523. SILICONE CHARACTERIZATION.

Vuursteen, P. J. The Krakatau syndrome, a late complication of retroglandular mammary augmentation. British Journal of Plastic Surgery. 1992, 45, 34-37. CAPSULE CONTRACTURE/local complications/calcification.

Wagner, H., Beller F.K., and Pfautsch, M. Electron and light microscopy examination of capsules around breast implants. Plast. Reconstr. Surg. 1977 Jul, 60, (1): 49-55. CAPSULE CONTRACTURE/polyurethane.

Wagner, S. K. Breast implant imaging homes in on tiny leaks. Diagn Imaging. 1996, 3, 51-57. MAMMOGRAPHY.

Wakabayashi, G., Gelfand, J. A., Jung, W. K., Connolly, R. J., Burke, J. F., and Dinarello, C. A. *Staphylococcus epidermidis* induces complement activation, tumor necrosis factor and interleukin 1: A shock-like state and tissue injury in rabbits without endotoxemia. Comparison to *Escherichia coli*. Journal of Clinical Investigation. 1991 Jun, 87, 1925. INFECTION.

Walden, K. J., Thompson, J. K., and Wells, K. E. Body image and psychological sequelae of silicone breast explantation: Preliminary findings. Plast. Reconstr. Surg. 1997 Oct, 100, (5): 1299-1306. PSYCHOSOCIAL.

Walker, J., Walker, S., and Grace, A. Topographic quantitative evoked response to pattern-reversal visual stimuli patients with siliconosis following breast implantation: objective evidence for involvement of the central nervous system as a common complication. Intl. J. Occup. Med. Immun. Toxicol. 1996, 5, (1): 25-28. NEUROLOGIC DISEASE.

Walker, L. E., Breiner, M. J., and Goodman, C. M. Toxic shock syndrome after explantation of breast implants: a case report and review of the literature. Plast. Reconstr. Surg. 1997 Mar, 99, (3): 875-879. INFECTION.

Walker, Q. J., and Langlands, A. O. The misuse of mammography in the management of breast cancer. The Medical Journal of Australia. 1986 Sep, 145, (2): 185-187. MAMMOGRAPHY.

Wallace, D. J., Basbug, E., Schwartz, E., Clements, P., Metzger, A. L., Furst, D. E., and Klinenberg, J. R. A comparison of systemic lupus erythemotosus and scleroderma patients with and without silicone breast implants. Journal of Clinical Rheumatology. 1996 Oct, 2, (5): 257-261. CONNECTIVE TISSUE DISEASE.

Wallace, J. R. Foreign body reaction to dimethylpolysiloxane (silastic): Report of case. Journal of the American Dental Association. 1967 Jul 1, 75, (1): 172-173. GENERAL/local complications.

Wallace, M. S., Wallace, A. M., Lee, J., and Dobke, M. K. Pain after breast surgery: A survey of 282 women. Pain. 1996, 66, 195-205. PAIN/local complications.

Walsh, F. W., Solomon, D. A., Espinoza, L. R., Adams, G. D., and Whitelocke, H. E. Human adjuvant disease: A new cause of chylous effusions. Archives of Internal Medicine. 1989 May, 149, 1194-1196. CONNECTIVE TISSUE DISEASE.

Walsh, L. G., and Greene, W. B. Electron probe microanalysis of silicone: Problems in quantitation. Bull Southeastern Electron Microscopy Soc. 1992, 24, 28. SILICON MEASUREMENT.

Wang, G. B., Santerre, J. P., and Labow, R. S. High-performance liquid chromatographic separation and tandem mass spectrometric identification of breakdown products associated with the biological hydrolysis of a biomedical polyurethane. Journal of Chromatography. 1997 Sep, 698, (2): 69-80. POLYURETHANE/toxicology.

Ward, C. M. Cosmetic and reconstructive surgery of the breast. British Journal of Medicine. 1985, 290, 1337-1339. GENERAL.

Ward, J., Cohen, I. K., and Brown, P. W. Immediate breast reconstruction with tissue expansion. Plast. Reconstr. Surg. 1987 Oct, 80, (4): 559-566. CAPSULE-CONTRACTURE/local complications/expander/reconstruction.

Warheit, D. B., McHugh, T. A., and Hartsky, M. A. Differential pulmonary responses in rats inhaling crystalline, colloidal or amorphous silica dusts. Scandinavian Journal of Work and Environmental Health. 1995, 21, (2): 19-21. SILICA.

Warner, E., Lipa, M., Pearson, D., and Weizel, H. A. Silicone mastopathy mimicking malignant disease of the breast in Southeast Asian patients. Canadian Medical Association Journal. 1991, 144, (5): 569-571. SILICONE INJECTION.

Wasicek, C. A., and Reichlin M. Clinical and serological differences between systemic lupus erythematosus patients with antibodies to Ro versus patients with antibodies to Ro and La. J Clin Invest. 1982 Apr, 69, (4): 835-843. AI-CTD BACKGROUND.

Watanabe, N., Yasuda, Y., Kato, K., and Nakamura, T. Determination of trace amounts of siloxanes in water, sediments and fish tissues by inductively coupled plasma emission spectrometry. The Science of the Total Environment. 1984, 34, 169-176. SILICON MEASUREMENT.

Watkins, L. R., Wiertelak, E. P., Goehler, L. E., Smith, K. P., Martin, D., and Maier, S. F. Characterization of cytokene-induced hyperalgesia. Brain Research. 1994, 654, 15-26. AI-CTD BACKGROUND.

Watson, J. Some observations on breast augmentation procedures over the past two decades. Aesthetic Plastic Surgery. 1976, 1, 89-97. GENERAL.

Watson, J. Some observations on free fat grafts: with reference to their use in mammaplasty. Brit. J. Plast. Surg. 1959, 3, 263-274. RECONSTRUCTION.

Webster, D. J., Mansel, R. E., and Hughes, L. E. Immediate reconstruction of the breast after mastectomy: Is it safe? Cancer. 1984, 53, (6): 1416-1419. RECONSTRUCTION.

Webster, R. C. Injectable silicone for small augmentations: Twenty year experience in humans. American Journal of Cosmetic Surgery. 1984, 1, (4): 1-10. SILICONE INJECTION.

Weightman, B., Simon, S., Rose, R., Paul, I., and Radin, E. Environmental fatigue testing of silastic finger joint prostheses. J. Biomed. Mat. Res. Symposium. 1972, 3, 15-24. SILICONE CHEMISTRY/silicone characterization.

Weiner, D. L., Aiache, A. E., and Silver, L. A new soft, round, silicone gel breast implant. Plast. Reconstr. Surg. 1974, 53, (2): 174-178. GENERAL.

Weiner, S. R., and Paulus, H. E. Chronic arthropathy occurring after augmentation mammoplasty. Plast. Reconstr. Surg. 1986 Feb, 77, (2): 185-192. CONNECTIVE TISSUE DISEASE.

Weinreb, J. C., and Newstead, G. MR imaging of the breast. Radiology. 1995 Sep, 196, 593-610. MAMMOGRAPHY.

Weinzweig, J., Schnur, P. L., McConnell, J. P., Harris, J. B., Petty, P. M., Moyer, T. P., and Nixon, D. Silicon analysis of breast and capsular tissue from patients with saline or silicone gel breast implants: II. Correlation with connective-tissue disease. Plastic and Reconstructive Surgery. 1998 Jun, 101, (7): 1836-1841. SILICON MEASUREMENT.

Weisman, M. H., Vecchione, T. R., Albert, D., Moore, L. T., and Mueller, M. R. Connective-tissue disease following breast augmentation: A preliminary test of the human adjuvant disease hypothesis. Plast. Reconstr. Surg. 1988 Oct, 82, (4): 626-630. CONNECTIVE TISSUE DISEASE.

Weizer, G., Malone, R. S., Netscher, D. T., Walker, L. E., and Thornby, J. Utility of magnetic resonance imaging and ultrasonography in diagnosing breast implant rupture. Annals of Plastic Surgery. 1995 Apr, 34, (4): 352-361. RUPTURE/local complications/mammography.

Wellisch, D. K., Schain, W. S., Noone, R. B., and Little, J. W. III. The psychological contribution of nipple addition in breast reconstruction. Plastic and Reconstructive Surgery. 1987 Nov, 80, (5): 699-704. PSYCHOSOCIAL/reconstruction.

Wellisch, D. K., Schain, WS., Noone, R. B., and Little, J. W. Psychosocial corelates of immediate versus delayed reconstruction of the breast. Plastic and Reconstructive Surgery. 1985 Nov, 76, (5): 713-717. PSYCHOSOCIAL/reconstruction.

Wells, A. F., Daniels, S., Gunasekaran, S., and Wells, K. E. Local increase in hyaluronic acid and interleukin-2 in the capsules surrounding silicone breast implants. Annals of Plastic Surgery. 1994 Jul, 33, (1): 1-5. IMMUNE EFFECTS/capsule contracture.

Wells, K. E., Cruse, C. W., Baker, Jr. J. L., Daniels, S. M., Stern, R. A., Newman, C., Seleznich, M. J., Vasey, F. B., Brozena, S., Albers, S. E., and Fenske, N. The health status of women following cosmetic surgery. Plast. Reconstr. Surg. 1994 Apr, 93, (5): 907-912. CONNECTIVE TISSUE DISEASE.

Wells, K. E., Roberts, C., Daniels, S. M., Hann, D., Clement, V., Reintgen, D., and Cox, C. E. Comparison of psychological symptoms of women requesting removal of breast implants with those of breast cancer patients and healthy controls. Plast. Reconstr. Surg. 1997 Mar, 99, (3): 680-685. PSYCHOSOCIAL/explantation.

Wells, K. E., Roberts, C., Daniels, S., Kearney, R. E., and Cox, C. E. Psychological and rheumatic symptoms of women requesting silicone breast implant removal. Annals of Plastic Surgery. 1995 Jun, 34, (6): 572-577. PSYCHOSOCIAL/explantation.

Wells, R. L. Experience with polyurethane-covered silicone-gel implants. Plast. Reconstr. Surg. 1988 Jul, 82, (1): 193. POLYURETHANE.

Wengle, H-P. The psychology of cosmetic surgery: A critical overview of the literature 1960-1982, part I. Annals of Plastic Surgery. 1986, 16, (5): 435-443. PSYCHOSOCIAL.

West, J. K. Thoeretical analysis of hydrolysis of polydimethylsiloxane (PDMS). Journal of Biomedical Materials Research. 1997, 35, (4): 505-511. SILICON MEASUREMENT/silicone characterization.

Wey, P. D., Highstein, J. B., and Borah, G. L. Immediate breast reconstruction in the high-risk adjuvant setting. Annals of Plastic Surgery. 1997 Apr, 38, (4): 342-344. CANCER/reconstruction.

Whalen, R. L. Improved textured surfaces for implantable prostheses. Transactions of the American Society of Artificial Internal Organs. 1988, 34, 887-892. POLYURETHANE/capsule-contracture/local complications.

Whalen, R. L., Bowen, M. A., Fukumura, F., Fukamachi, K., Muramoto, K., Higgins, P., Brown, J., and Harasaki, H. The effects of radiation therapy on the tissue capsule of soft tissue implants. ASAIO J. 1994, 3403, M365-M370. RADIATION/expander/capsule-contracture/local complications.

Whidden, P. G. Observations and conclusions from 20 years' experience with the single-lumen inflatable breast implant with 3500 patients. Canadian Journal of Plastic Surgery. 1993, 1, 39. SALINE.

White, B., Bauer, E. A., Goldsmith, L. A., Hochberg, M. C., Katz, L. M., Korn, J. H., Lachenbruch, P. A., LeRoy, E. C., Miltrane, M. P., Paulus, H. E., Postlethwaite, A. E., and Steen, B. Guidelines for clinical trials and systemic sclerosis (scleroderma). Arthritis and Rheumatism. 1995 Mar, 38, (3): 351-360. AI-CTD BACKGROUND.

White, E, Malone, K., Weiss, N., and Daling, J. Breast cancer among young US women in relation to oral contraceptive use. Journal of the National Cancer Institute. 1994 Apr 6, 86, (7): 505-514. CANCER.

White, Jr. KL and Klykken, PC. The non-specific binding of immunoglobulins to silicone implant materials: the lack of a detectable silicone specific antibody. Immunological Investigations. 1998, 27, (4&5): 221-235. IMMUNE EFFECTS.

White, K. L. Use of brown Norway rat and the NZBxW mouse models of SLE to assess effect of silicone gel, metals, and other xenobiotics on autoimmune disease. The Toxicologist. 1996, 42, 403. TOXICOLOGY/connective tissue disease.

Whitehouse, M. W., Orr, K. J., Beck, F. W. J., and Pearson, C. M. Freund's adjuvants: Relationship of arthritogenicity and adjuvanticity in rats to vehicle composition. Immunology. 1974, 27, 311-330. IMMUNE EFFECTS.

Whiteside, T. L., and Friberg, D. Natural killer cells and natural killer cell activity in chronic fatigue syndrome. The American Journal of Medicine. 1998 Sep 28, 105, (3A): 247S-34S. AI-CTD BACKGROUND.

Whorton, D., and Wong, O. Scleroderma and silicone breast implants. Western Journal of Medicine. 1997 Sep, 167, (3): 159-165. CONNECTIVE TISSUE DISEASE.

Wichems, D. N., Calloway, C. P. Jr., Fernando, R., Jones, B. T., and Morykwas, M. J. Determination of silicone in breast tissue by graphite furnace continuum source atomic absorption spectometry. Applied Spectroscopy. 1993 Oct, 47, 1577-1579. MIGRATION/silicon measurement.

Wickham, M. G., Rudolph, R., and Abraham, J. Silicon identification in prostheses-associated fibrous capsules. Science 199:437. 1978 Jan, 199, 437. SILICON MEASUREMENT/capsule contracture/local complications.

Wickman, M. Breast reconstruction: past achievements, current status, and future goals. Scand. J. Plast. Reconstr. Hand. Surg. 1995, 29, 81-100. RECONSTRUCTION.

Wickman, M., Johansson, O., and Forslind, B. Dimensions of capsular collagen fibrils: Image analysis of rapid compared with slow tissue expansion for breast reconstruction. Scandinavian Journal of Plastic and Reconstructive and Hand Surgery. 1992, 26, 281-285. EXPANDER/capsule-contracture/local complications.

Wickman, M., Johansson, O., Olenius, M., and Forslind, B. A comparison of the capsules around smooth and textured silicone prostheses used for breast reconstruction. Scandinavian Journal of Plastic and Reconstructive and Hand Surgery. 1993, 27, (1): 15-22. CAPSULE-CONTRACTURE/local complications/expander/reconstruction.

Wickman, M., and Jurell, G. Low capsular contraction rate after primary and secondary breast reconstruction with a textured expander prosthesis. Plast. Reconstr. Surg. 1997 Mar, 99, (3): 692-697. EXPANDER/capsule-contracture/reconstruction/local complications.

Wigren, R., Elwing, H., Erlandsson, R., Welin, S., and Lundstöm, I. Structure of adsorbed fibrinogen obtained by scanning force microscopy. Federation of European Biomedical Societies. 1991 Mar, 280, (2): 225-228. IMMUNE EFFECTS/general.

Wilflingseder, P., Hoinkes, G., Hussl, H., Papp, C., Mikuz, G., and Propst, A. Silicone radiation measurements around mammary type implants: Animal model for evaluation of materials and implantation sites. Chir Plast. 1982, 6, 189. SILICON MEASUREMENT.

Wilflingseder, P., Hoinkes, G., and Mikuz, G. Tissue reactions from silicone implant in augmentation mammaplasties. Congresso Nazionale di Chirurgia Plastica. 1983, 38, 877-880. CAPSULE CONTRACTURE/local complications.

Wilflingseder, P., Propst, A., and Mikuz, G. Constrictive fibrosis following silicone implants in mammary augmentation. Chir. Plast. 1974 Jul, 2, 251. CAPSULE-CONTRACTURE/local complications.

Wilkie, T. F. Late development of granuloma after liquid silicone injections. Plast. Reconstr. Surg. 1977 Aug, 60, (2): 179-188. SILICONE INJECTION.

Wilkinson, T. S. Polyurethane coated implants. Plast. Reconstr. Surg. 1985, 75, 925. POLYURETHANE.

Williams, C. W. Silicone gel granuloma following compressive mammography. Aesthetic Plastic Surgery. 1991, 15, 49-51. MAMMOGRAPHY/rupture/local complications/granulomas.

Williams, C. W., Aston, S., and Rees, T. D. The effect of hematoma on the thickness of pseudosheaths around silicone implants. Plast. Reconstr. Surg. 1975 Aug, 56, (2): 194-198. CAPSULE-CONTRACTURE/local complications/hematomas.

Williams, G. H., and Silman, A. J. Review of U.K. data on the rheumatic diseases: 9-Scleroderma. British Journal of Rheumatology. 1991, 30, 365-367. AI-CTD BACKGROUND.

Williams, H. J., Alarcon, G. S., and Neuner, R. Early undifferentiated connective tissue disease. V. An inception cohort five years later: disease remissions and changes in diagnoses in well established and undifferentiated connective tissue disease. The Journal of Rheumatology. 1998, 25, 261-268. AI-CTD BACKGROUND.

Williams, H. J., Weisman, M. H., and Berry, C. C. Breast implants in patients with differentiated and undifferentiated connective tissue disease. Arthritis and Rheumatism. 1997, 40, (3): 437-440. CONNECTIVE TISSUE DISEASE.

Williams, J. E. Experiences with a large series of Silastic breast implants. Plast. Reconstr. Surg. 1972 Mar, 49, (3): 253-258. EXPANDER/hematomas/capsule-contracture/pain/local complications.

Williams, K., Walton, R., and Bunkis, J. Aspergillus colonization association with bilateral silicone mammary implants. Plast. Reconstr. Surg. 1982. INFECTION/local complications.

Williford, M. E. Mammography: evaluation following breast augmentation. NCMJ. 1991 Oct, 52, (10): 515-519. MAMMOGRAPHY.

Wilsnack, R. E., and Bernadyn, S. A. Blood compatibility of medical device materials as measured by lymphocyte function. Biomaterials Medical Devices and Artifical Organs. 1979, 7, 527. IMMUNE EFFECTS/general.

Wilson, R. B., Gluck, O. S., Tesser, J. R. P., Rice, J. C., Meyer, A., and Bridges, A. J. Anti-polymer antibody reactivity in a subset of patients with fibromyalgia correlates with severity. J. Rheumatol. 1999, 26, 402-407. IMMUNE EFFECTS.

Winder, A. E., and Winder, B. D. Patient counseling: Clarifying a woman's choice for breast reconstruction. Patient Education and Counseling. 1985, 7, 65-75. PSYCHOSOCIAL.

Winding, O., Christensen, L., Thomsen, J. L., Nielsen, M., Breiting, V., and Brandt, B. Silicon in human breast tissue surrounding silicone gel prostheses—a scanning electron microsopy and energy dispersive X-ray investigation of normal, fibrocystic and periprosthetic breast tissue. Scand J Plast Reconstr Surg Hand Surg. 1988, 22, 127-130. CAPSULE CONTRACTURE.

Winer, E. P., Fee-Fulkerson, C. C., Fulkerson, G. G., Catoe, K. E., Conaway, M., Brunatti, C., Holmes, V., and Rimer, B. K. Silicone controversy: A survey of women with breast cancer and silicone implants. Journal of the National Cancer Institute. 1993 Sep 1, 85, (17): 1407-1411. CANCER/psychosocial.

Winer, L. H., Sternberg, T. H., Lehman, R., and Ashley, F. L. Tissue reactions to injected silicone liquids. Archives of Dermatology. 1964 Dec, 90, 588-598. SILICONE INJECTION.

Winther, J. F., Bach, F. W., Friis, S., Blot, W. J., Mellemkjær, L., Kjøller, K., Høgsted, C., McLaughlin, J. K., and Olsen, J. H. Neurologic disease among women with breast implants. Neurology. 1998 Apr, 50, 951-955. NEUROLOGIC DISEASE.

Wintsch, W., Smahel, J., and Clodius, L. Local and regional lymph node response to ruptured gel-filled mammary prosthesis. British Journal of Plastic Surgery. 1978, 349, 31. POLYURETHANE/local complications/rupture/lymphadenopathy.

Wise, R. J. A new inflatable implant for breast augmentation. Plast. Reconstr. Surg. 1974a Mar, 53, (3): 360-363. GENERAL/expander.

Wolf, L. E., Lappé, M., Peterson, R. D., and Ezrailson, E. G. Human immune response to polydimethylsiloxane (silicone): screening studies in a breast implant population. FASEB. 1993 Oct, 7, 1265-1268. IMMUNE EFFECTS.

Wolfe, F. Fibromyalgia. Epidemiology of Rheumatic Disease. 1990 Aug, 16, (3): 681-698. AI-CTD BACKGROUND.

Wolfe, F., Ross, K., Anderson, J., Russell, I. J., and Hebert, L. The prevalence and characteristics of fibromyalgia in the general population. Arthritis and Rheumatism. 1995b, 38, (1): 19-28. AI-CTD BACKGROUND.

Wolfe, F., Smythe, H. A., Yunus, M. B., Bennett, R. M., Bombardier, C., Goldenberg, D. L., Tugwell, P., Campbell, S. M., Abeles, M., Clark, P., Fam, A. G., Farber, S. J., Fiechtner, J. J., Franklin, C. M., Gatter, R. A., Hamaty, D., Lessard, J., Lichtbround, A. S., Masi, A. T., McCain, G. A., Reynolds, W. J., Romano, T. J., Russell, I. J., and Sheon, R. P. The American College of Rheumatology 1990 criteria for the classification of fibromyalgia. Arthritis and Rheumatism. 1990 Feb, 33, (2): 160-172. AI-CTD BACKGROUND.

Wong, J. H., Jackson, C. F., Swanson, J. S., Palmquist, M. A., Oyama, A. A., Miller, S. H., and Fletcher, W. S. Analysis of the risk reduction of prophylactic partial mastectomy in Sprague-Dawley rats with 7,12 dimethylbenzanthracine-induced breast cancer. Surgery. 1986, 99, 67-91. GENERAL/cancer.

Wong, O. A critical assessment of the relationship between silicone breast implants and connective tissue disease. Regulatory Toxicology and Pharmacology. 1996, 23, 74-85. CONNECTIVE TISSUE DISEASE.

Woods, J. E., Irons, Jr. G. B., and Arnold, P. G. The case for submuscular implantation of prostheses in reconstructive breast surgery. Annals of Plastic Surgery. 1980, 5, 115-122. CAPSULE-CONTRACTURE/local complications/reconstruction.

Woods, J. E., and Mangan, M. A. Breast reconstruction with tissue expanders: Obtaining an optimal result. Annals of Plastic Surgery. 1992 Apr, 28, (4): 390-396. EXPANDER/reconstruction/saline.

Worden, J. W., and Weisman, A. D. The fallacy in postmastectomy depression. The American Journal of the Medical Sciences. 1977 Mar-1977 Apr 30, 273, (2): 169-175. PSYCHOSOCIAL/cancer.

Worseg, A., Kuzbari, R., Tairych, G., Korak, K., and Holle, J. Long term results of inflatable mammary implants. British Journal of Plastic Surgery. 1995, 48, (4): 183-188. EXPANDER/local complications/capsule-contracture/rupture.

Worsing, R. A., Engber, W. D., and Lange, T. A. Reactive synovitis from particulate silastic. J Bone Joint Surg. 1982, 64A, 581-585. TOXICOLOGY.

Worton, E. W., Seifert, L. N., and Sherwoor, R. Late leakage of inflatable silicone breast prostheses. Plast. Reconstr. Surg. 1980 Mar, 65, (3): 302-306. EXPANDER/saline/local complications/rupture.

Wustrack, K. O., and Zarem, H. A. Surgical management of silicone mastitis. Plast. Reconstr. Surg. 1979 Feb, 63, (2): 224-229. SILICONE INJECTION.

Wyatt, L. E., Sinow, J. D., Wollmna, J. S., Sami, D. A., and Miller, T. A. The influence of time on human breast capsule histology: smooth and textured silicone-surfaced implants. Plast. Reconstr. Surg. 1998 Nov, 102, (6): 1922-1931. CAPSULE-CONTRACTURE.

Xavier, R. M., Yamauchi, Y., Nakamura, M., Tanigawa, Y., Ishikura, H., Tsunematsu, T., and Kobayashi, S. Antinuclear antibodies in healthy aging people: a prospective study. Mech. Aging Dev. 1995, 78, 145-154. AI-CTD BACKGROUND.

Xiao, K., and Appleby, A. J. Physical and bioelectrochemical behavior of polydimethylsiloxanes in physiologic electrolytes. J. Clean Technol. Environ. Toxicol. Occup. Med. 1995, 5, (3): 249-257. SILICONE CHARACTERIZATION.

Yadin, O., Sarov, B., Naggan, S., Slhor, H., and Shoenfeld, Y. Natural autoantibodies in the serum of healthy women—A five year follow-up. Clin Exp Immunol. 1989, 75, 402-406. AI-CTD BACKGROUND/immune effects.

Yager, J. S., and Chaglassian, T. Polyester as a bioimplantable material. Annals of Plastic Surgery. 1998 May, 40, (5): 502-505. GENERAL.

Yamazaki, T., Kinjo, T., and et al. Experience with mammography of the augmentation mammoplasty in relation to breast cancer detection. Jpn J Clin Radiol. 1977, 22, 861. MAMMOGRAPHY/cancer.

Yeoh, G., Russell, P., and Jenkins, E. Spectrum of histological changes reactive to prosthetic breast implants: A clinopathological study of 84 patients. Pathology. 1996 Aug, 28, (3): 232-235. CAPSULE-CONTRACTURE/calcification/local complications.

Yoshida, S. H., Chang, C. C., Teuber, S. S., and Gershwin, M. E. Silicon and silicone: Theoretical and clinical implications of breast implants. Regulatory Toxicology and Pharmacology. 1993, 17, 3-18. GENERAL.

Yoshida, S. H., and Gershwin, M. E. Autoimmunity and selected environmental factors of disease induction. Seminars in Arthritis and Rheumatism. 1993 Jun, 22, (6): 339. IMMUNE EFFECTS.

Yoshida, S. H., Swan, S., Teuber, S. S., and Gershwin, M. E. Silicone breast implants: Immunotoxic and epidemiologic issues. Life Sciences. 1995, 56, (16): 1299-1310. IMMUNE EFFECTS/connective tissue disease.

Yoshida, S. H., Teuber, S. S., German, J. B., and Gershwin, M. E. Immunotoxicity of silicone: Implications of oxidant balance towards adjuvant activity. Fd Chem Toxic. 1994 Jun, 32, (11): 1089-1100. IMMUNE EFFECTS/toxicology.

Yoshida, T., Tanaka, M., Okamoto, K., and Hirai, S. Neurosarcoidosis following augmentation mammoplasty with silicone. Neurological Research. 1996 Aug, 18, (4): 319-320. SILICONE INJECTION/connective tissue disease/neurologic disease.

Yoshikawa, M., Sakamoto, T., Mitoro, A., Mochi, T., Tsujii, H., and et al. Autoimmunity during alpha-interferon therapy for chronic hepatitis. C. Gastroenterologia Japonica 28:109. 1993 May. IMMUNE EFFECTS.

Yoshino, S. Silicone-induced arthritis in rats and possible role for T cells. Immunobiology. 1994, 192, 40-47. IMMUNE EFFECTS/connective tissue disease.

Yoshino, S., Quattrocchi, E., and Weiner, H. L. Suppression of antigen-induced arthritis in Lewis rats by oral administration of type II collagen. Arthritis and Rheumatism. 1995 Aug, 38, (8): 1092-1096. IMMUNE EFFECTS.

Young, V. L. Guidelines and indications for breast implant capsulectomy. Plast. Reconstr. Surg. 1998 Sep, 102, (3): 884-894. CAPSULE CONTRACTURE/general.

Young, V. L. Overview of the Development and Testing of Trilucent Breast Implants. Perspectives in Plastic Surgery. 1997, 10, (2): 1-48. TOXICOLOGY/local complications/mammography/general.

Young, V. L., Bartell, T., Destouet, J. M., Monsees, B., and Logan, S. E. Calcification of breast implant capsule. Southern Medical Journal. 1989 Sep, 82, (9): 1171-1173. CALCIFICATION/capsule-contracture/local complications/mammography.

Young, V. L., Diehl, G. J., Eichling, J., Monsees, B. S., and Destouet, J. The relative radiolucencies of breast implant filler materials. Plast. Reconstr. Surg. 1993a May, 91, (6): 1066-1072. MAMMOGRAPHY/saline/general.

Young, V. L., Hertl, M. C., Murray, P. R., Jensen, J., Witt, H., and Schorr, M. W. Microbial growth inside saline-filled breast implants. Plast. Reconstr. Surg. 1997 Jul, 100, (1): 182-196. INFECTION/local complications/saline.

Young, V. L., Hertl, M. C., Murray, P., and Lambros, V. S. *Paecilomyces variotii* contamination in the lumen of a saline-filled breast implant. Plast. Reconstr. Surg. 1995a Nov, 96, (6): 1430-1434. INFECTION/local complications/saline.

Young, V. L., Lund, H., Destouet, J., Pidgeon, L., and Ueda, K. Biocompatibility of radiolucent breast implants. Plast. Reconstr. Surg. 1991b Sep, 88, (3): 462-474. MAMMOGRAPHY/general.

Young, V. L., Lund, H., Destouet, J., Pidgeon, L., and Ueda, K. Effect of breast implants on mammography. Southern Medical Journal. 1991a Jun, 84, (6): 707-714. MAMMOGRAPHY/polyurethane.

Young, V. L., Lund, H., Ueda, K., Pidgeon, L., Schorr, M. W., and Kreeger, J. Bleed of and biologic response to triglyceride filler used in radiolucent breast implants. Plast. Reconstr. Surg. 1996b May, 97, (6): 1179-1193. MAMMOGRAPHY/local complications/general.

Young, V. L., and Nemecek, A. R. How safe are silicone breast implants? South Med J. 1993, 86, 932-944. GENERAL.

Young, V. L., Nemecek, J. R., Gilliam, C., Schwartz, B. D., and Wick, M. Immunohistochemical analysis of periprosthetic capsular tissue from breast implant patients. Plastic Surgery Forum. 1993b. CAPSULE-CONTRACTURE/local complications.

Young, V. L., Nemecek, J. R., and Nemecek, D. A. The efficacy of breast augmentation: Breast size increase, patient satisfaction, and psychological effects. Plast. Reconstr. Surg. 1994 Dec, 94, (7): 958-969. PSYCHOSOCIAL.

Young, V. L., Nemecek, J. R., Schwartz, B. D., Phelan, D. L., and Schorr, M. W. HLA typing in women with breast implants. Plast. Reconstr. Surg. 1995b Dec, 96, 1497-1519. CONNECTIVE TISSUE DISEASE/immune effects.

Youngjohn, J., Spector, J., and Mapou, R. Neuropsychological findings in silicone breast implant complainants: Brain damage, somatization, or compensation neuroses. Clinical Neuropsychologist. 1996. NEUROLOGIC DISEASE/psychosocial.

Yu, L. T., Latorre, G., Marotta, J., Batich, C., and Hardt, N. S. In vitro measurement of silicone bleed from breast implants. Plastic and Reconstructive Surgery. 1996 Apr, 97, (4): 756-764. SILICON MEASUREMENT/local complications.

Yule, G. J., Concannon, M. J., Croll, G., and Puckett, C. L. Is there liability with chemotherapy following immediate breast construction? Plast. Reconstr. Surg. 1996 Apr, 97, (5): 969-973. CANCER/reconstruction.

Yunus, M. B. Towards a model of pathophysiology of fibromyalgia. J. Rheumatol. 1992, 19, 846. AI-CTD BACKGROUND.

Yunus, M. B., Hussey, F. X., and Aldag, J. C. Antinuclear antibodies and connective tissue disease features in fibromyalgia syndrome: A controlled study. J. Rheumatol. 1993, 20, (9): 1157-1560. AI-CTD BACKGROUND.

Yunus, M., Masi, A. T., Calabro, J. J., Miller, K. A., and Feigenbaum, S. L. Primary fibromyalgia (fibrositis): Clinical study of 50 patients with matched normal controls. Seminars in Arthritis and Rheumatism. 1981 Aug, 11, (1): 151-171. AI-CTD BACKGROUND.

Zachariae, H. Silicone breast implants and connective tissue diseases. Ugeskr Laeger. 1997, 159, (28): 4410-4411. CONNECTIVE TISSUE DISEASE.

Zapka, J., Stoddard, A., Costanza, M., and Greene, H. Breast cancer screening by mammography: Utilization and associated factors. American Journal of Public Health. 1989, 79, (11): 1499-1502. MAMMOGRAPHY/cancer.

Zazgornik, J., Piza, H., Kaiser, W., Bettelheim, P., Steiner, G., Smolen, J., Biesenbach, G., and Maschek, W. Autoimmune reactions in patients with silicone breast implants. Wien Klin Wochenschr. 1996, 108, (24): 781-787. IMMUNE EFFECTS.

Zeigler, J. M. The function, chemistry, and form of platinum in breast implants [letter to Dr. Herdman]. Rio Rancho, NM: Silchemy, 1998 Aug. TOXICOLOGY.

Zhang, W., and Reichlin, M. Some autoantibodies to Ro/SS-A and La/SS-B are antiidiotypes to anti-double-stranded DNA. Arthritis Rheum. 1996, 39, 522-531. CHILDREN'S EFFECTS/breast feeding.

Zhang, Y. Z. Tissue response to commercial silicone and polyurethane elastomers after different sterilization procedures. Biomaterials. 1996, 98, (7): 1324-1325. SILICONE CHARACTERIZATION/polyurethane.

Ziats, N. P., Miller, K. M., and Anderson, J. M. *In vitro* and *in vivo* interactions of cells with biomaterials. Biomaterials. 1988 Jan, 9, 5-13. CAPSULE-CONTRACTURE/local complications/general.

Zide, B. Complications of closed capsulotomy after augmentation. Plast. Reconstr. Surg. 1981, 67, (5): 697. CLOSED CAPSULOTOMY/capsule contracture/local complications/rupture.

Ziegler, L. D., and Kroll, S. S. Primary breast cancer after prophylactic mastectomy. American Journal of Clinical Oncology. 1991, 14, (5): 451-454. CANCER.

Ziegler, V. V., Haustein, U.-F., Mehlhorn, J., Münzberger, H., and Rennau, H. Silica induced scleroderma: Scleroderma-like syndrome or progressive systemic sclerosis? Dermatol. Mon. schr. 1986 Jan, 172, 86-90. SILICA/connective tissue disease.

Zimman, O. A., Robles, J. M., and Lee, J. C. The fibrous capsule around mammary implants—an investigation. Aesthetic Plastic Surgery. 1978, 2, 217-234. CAPSULE-CONTRACTURE/local complications.

Zimmerli, W., Lew, P. D., and Waldvogel, F. A. Pathogenesis of foreign body infection. Evidence of local granulocyte defect. Journal of Clinical Investigation. 1984 Apr, 73, 1191-1200. INFECTION.

Zollman, W., Chavis, D. D., Wentland, M. J., and Lai, K. D. Breast augmentation mammoplasty using a saline filled prosthesis: An eighteen-year survey. Prepublication communication. 1996. SALINE.

Zones, J. S. The political and social context of silicone breast implant use in the United States. J. Long-Term Effects Med. Implants. 1992, 1, (3): 225-241. GENERAL/prevalence.

Zweiman, B. Immunologic aspects of neurological and neuromuscular diseases. J. Amer. Med. Assoc. 1992 Nov 25, 268, (20): 2918-2922. NEUROLOGIC DISEASE /ai-ctd background.

OTHER REFERENCES

Abeles, M., Manu, P., Lane, T., and Matthews, D. Evaluation of musculoskeletal complaints in patients with the chronic fatigue syndrome [abstract]. Arthritis and Rheumatism. 1992, 24, (Supplement): S212. AI CTD BACKGROUND.

Abeles, M., and Waterman, J. An evaluation of silicone breast implant patients for silicone associated disease [abstract]. Arthritis and Rheumatism. 1995 Sep, 38, (9 (Supplement)): S325. CONNECTIVE TISSUE DISEASE/immune effects.

Abeles, M., and Waterman, J. The relation of depression and symptoms of women with silicone breast implants [abstract]. American College of Rheumatism Abstract, Regional Meeting, 1995 Feb. PSYCHOSOCIAL.

Abraham, J. L. Breast implants and connective tissue diseases [letter]. The New England Journal of Medicine. 1995 Nov 23, 333, (21): 1424. CONNECTIVE TISSUE DISEASE/letter.

Acha-Orbea, H. Bacterial and viral superantigens: Roles in autoimmunity? Annals of Rheumatic Disease. 1993, 52, S6-S16. AI-CTD BACKGROUND.

Adamson, A. W., and Gast, A. P. Physical Chemistry of Surfaces. 6th Edition ed. New York: John Wiley & Sons, Inc, 1997. SILICONE CHARACTERIZATION.

Agence Nationale pour le Développement de l'Évaluation Médicale. Silicone gel-filled breast implants. France: ANDEM, 1996 May. GENERAL.

Agency for Toxic Substances and Disease Registry. Toxicological Profile for Tin and Compounds. U.S.Public Health Service, ATSDR, Atlanta, GA., TP-91/27, 1992 Sep. TOXICOLOGY.

Agnew, J. R. Silicone gel breast implants [letter]. J. Amer Med Assoc. 1994 Jul 27, 272, (4): 271. GENERAL/letter.

Ahn, C. Y. Ruptured breast implant [letter-reply]. Plast. Reconstr. Surg. 1995 Jul, 96, (1): 234. RUPTURE/local complications/letter.

Alasia, S. T., and Ambroggia, G. P. Autoimmune connective tissue disease and silicone implants. Presented at International Breast Implant RS, Berlin Congress, 1993, Berlin. CONNECTIVE TISSUE DISEASE.

American Academy of Pediatrics, Committee on Drugs. Transfer of drugs and other chemicals into human milk. Elk Grove Village, IL: AAP, 1989. BREAST FEEDING.

American College of Rheumatology. Statement on Silicone Breast Implants [position paper]. [http://www.rheumatology.org/position/implant1.html]: American College of Rheumatology, 1995 Oct 22. GENERAL.

American Conference of Governmental Industrial Hygienists. Threshold Limit Values and Biological Exposure Indices. 1998. TOXICOLOGY.

American Society for Testing and Materials. Standard Classification for Silicone Elastomers Used in Medical Applications—Standard F 604-78, Annual Book of Standards Vol. 13.01: Medical Devices. Philadelphia: American Society for Testing and Materials, 1983b. SILICONE CHARACTERIZATION.

American Society for Testing and Materials. Standard Specifications for Implantable Breast Prostheses. 1983a. SILICONE CHARACTERIZATION.

American Society of Plastic and Reconstructive Surgeons (ASPRS). Indications for Explantation of Breast Implants. 1992. EXPLANTATION.

American Society of Plastic and Reconstructive Surgeons (ASPRS). First National Survey Asks Women How They Feel about Breast Implants. Chicago: American Society of Plastic and Reconstructive Surgeons, 1990 Nov 19. PSYCHOSOCIAL.

American Society of Plastic and Reconstructive Surgeons (ASPRS). Reoperation on women with breast implants [position paper]. Arlington Heights, Ill.: ASPRS, 1994 Jun. GENERAL.

American Society of Plastic and Reconstructive Surgeons (ASPRS). National Clearinghouse of Plastic Surgery Statistics [Internet]. http:www.plasticsurgery.org/mediactr/stats.html. 1992, 1996, 1997. PREVALENCE.

American Thoracic Society. Adverse effects of crystalline silica exposure. Am. J. Respir. Crit. Care. Med. 1997, 155, 761-765. SILICA.

Anderson, J. M. Analysis of the surface morphology of recovered silicone mammary prostheses [discussion]. Plast. Reconstr. Surg. 1983 Jun, 71, (6): 803-804. SILICONE CHARACTERIZATION.

Anderson, J. M., and Miller, K. Biomaterial biocompatibility and the macrophage. Biomaterials. 1984 Jan, 5, 5-10. CAPSULE CONTRACTURE.

Angell, M. Antipolymer antibodies, silicone breast implants, and fibromyalgia. The Lancet. 1997, 349, (9059): 1171-1172. GENERAL/connective tissue disease/immune effects.

Angell, M. Breast implants—protection or paternalism? (Editorial). The New England Journal of Medicine. 1992 Jun 18, 326, (25): 1695-1696. GENERAL.

Angell, M. Do breast implants cause systemic disease? [editorial]. The New England Journal of Medicine. 1994 Jun 16, 330, (24): 1748-1749. GENERAL/connective tissue disease.

Angell, M. Science in the courtroom [letter-reply]. The New England Journal of Medicine. 1994, 331, (16): 1099. GENERAL.

Angell, M. Science on Trial. The clash of medical evidence and the law in the breast implant case. W.W. Norton and Company, 1996. GENERAL.

Angelotti, N. C. Analysis of polymers, mixtures, and compositions. Smith, A. L., ed. The Analytical Chemistry of Silicones. John Wiley & Sons, Inc., 1991, pp. 47-69. SILICONE CHARACTERIZATION.

Annelin, R. B., and Isquith, A. J. Trace analysis of organosilicon in human urine and milk by the ASFT technique [abstract]. Midland, Mich.: Dow Corning Corporation, 1980 May 29. SILICON MEASUREMENT/toxicology/breast feeding.

Archer, R. R. Breast implants [letter]. Plast. Reconstr. Surg. 1997 Aug, 100, (2): 555. GENERAL.

Arkfeld, D., and Lau, C. Deficiency of insulin-like growth factor-1 in silicone breast implant patients with fibromyalgia. Arthritis and Rheumatism. 1994 Sep, 37, (9 (Supplement)): 270. IMMUNE EFFECTS/connective tissue disease.

Arkfeld, D., and Liston, S. Detection of silicone-gel breast implant leakage by magnetic resonance imaging [abstract]. Arthritis and Rheumatism. 1993 Sep, 36, (9 (Supplement)): S71. MAMMOGRAPHY/rupture.

Asaadi, M. *Salmonella* infection following breast reconstruction [letter]. Plast. Reconstr. Surg. 1995 Dec, 96, (7): 1749-1750. INFECTION/local complications/capsule-contracture.

Ashbell, T. S. Outpatient breast surgery under intercostal block anesthesia [discussion]. Plast. Reconstr. Surg. 1980 Feb: 239-240. PAIN.

Ashbell, T. S. Re: Analysis of explanted silicone implants: A report of 300 patients and reply [letter]. Annals of Plastic Surgery. 1995 Jun, 34, (6): 671. EXPLANTATION/closed capsulotomy/letter.

Atherton, J. C. Risk of connective tissue disease among women with breast implants: Authors should have made better use of matched control group [letter]. British Medical Journal. 1998 Aug 15, 317, 470-471. CONNECTIVE TISSUE DISEASE/letter.

Autian, J. Toxicology of Plastics in Cassarett, L. J., and Doull, J. D. Editors. Toxicology, first edition. 1975b. TOXICOLOGY.

Azavedo, E., and Bone, B. Imaging breasts with silicone implants. Eur. Radiol. 1999, 9, (2): 349-355. MAMMOGRAPHY.

Aziz, N. M., Vasey, F. B., Leaverton, P. E., Wolff, P. A., and Felber, E. Comparison of Clinical Status among Women Retaining or Removing Gel Breast Implants. Bethesda, Md.: National Cancer Institute, 1998. EXPLANTATION/connective tissue disease.

Bachman, J. J. Boyle's law and breast implants [letter]. The New England Journal of Medicine. 1994 Aug 18, 331, (7): 483-484. LOCAL COMPLICATIONS.

Baines, C. J. A Selected Overview of Current Evidence on the Health Effects of Silicone Gel-Filled Breast Implants. Toronto, Ont.: 1998 Mar 27. GENERAL.

Baines, C. J. A. Silicone gel breast implants [letter]. J. Amer. Med. Assoc. 1994 Jul 27, 272, (4): 272. GENERAL.

Baker, Jr. J. L. Augmentation mammaplasty. Symposium on aesthetic surgery of the breast. St. Louis: The C.V. Mosby Company, 1978, pp. 256-263. CAPSULE CONTRACTURE/ steroids/local complications.

Baker, Jr. J. L. Augmentation Mammaplasty. in: Peck, G. C. Ed. Complications and Problems in Aesthetic Plastic Surgery. New York: Gower Medical Publishing, 1992. GENERAL.

Baker, Jr. J. L. Classification of spherical contractures. Paper presented at the Aesthetic Breast Symposium. Scottsdale, AZ: Aestheetic Breast Symposium, 1975. CAPSULE-CONTRACTURE/local complications.

Baker, Jr. J. L. On closed compression to rupture capsules around breast implants [letter-reply]. Plast. Reconstr. Surg. 1977 Jun, 59, (6): 841. CLOSED CAPSULOTOMY/rupture/local complications/letter.

Baker, Jr. J. L., Chandler, M., and Levier, R. R. Occurrence and activity of myofibroblasts in human capsular tissue surrounding mammary implants [discussion]. Plast. Reconstr. Surg. 1981 Dec, 68, (6): 913-914. CAPSULE-CONTRACTURE/local complications/ saline.

Baker, M. F. Treatment of silicone implant associated symptoms [abstract]. Arthritis and Rheumatism. 1996, 39, (9 (Supplement)): S51. CONNECTIVE TISSUE DISEASE.

Ballester, O. F., Garland, L. L., and Vasey, F. Multiple myeloma (MM) and monoclonal gammopathies (MG) in women with silicone breast implants. Blood. 1994, 84, (10): 643a. MYELOMA.

Bar-Meir, E., Teuber, S. S., Lin, H.-C., Alosachie, I., Borka, N., Shen, B., Peter, J. B., Gershwin, M. E., and Shoefeld, Y. Autoantibody profile of women with silicone breast implants [abstract]. Arthritis and Rheumatism. 1994 Sep, 37, (9 (Supplement)): S422. IMMUNE EFFECTS.

Barbuto, J. P. Breast implants and autoimmunity [letter]. Western Journal of Medicine. 1994 Jul, 161, (1): 90-91. IMMUNE EFFECTS.

Barnes, R. E. Long-term results with polyurethane-covered breast implants [letter]. Plast. Reconstr. Surg. 1992 May, 89, (5): 994-995. POLYURETHANE/capsule-contracture/ local complications/letter.

Barr, S. G., Martin, L. M., and Edworthy, S. M. Do breast implant recipients report a unique cluster of symptoms? Arthritis & Rheumatism. 1998 Sep, 41, (9). CONNECTIVE TISSUE DISEASE.

Barrer, R. Chapters IX And X. Diffusion in and through solids. The University Press: New York, 1941 Jan 1, p. 382-453. GENERAL/local complications.

Bartel, D. R. Sclerodermalike esophageal disease in children of mothers with silicone breast implants [letter]. J. Amer. Med. Assoc. 1994 Sep 14, 272, (10): 767. CHILDREN'S EFFECTS/breast feeding.

Barthel, H. R., Barraza, O., and Meier, L. G. Evaluating the health risks of breast implants [letter-reply]. The New England Journal of Medicine. 1996, 335, (15): 1155. GENERAL.

Bartlett, S. P. Saline made viscous with polyethylene glycol: A new alternate breast implant filler material [discussion]. Plast. Reconstr. Surg. 1996 Dec, 98, (7): 1214-1215. GENERAL.

Barton Jr., F. E., and Burns, A. J. Immunologic responses to breast implants: A prospective study. Plastic Surgery Scientific Abstracts. 1993 Apr. IMMUNE EFFECTS.

Basbug, E., Schwartz, E., Wallace, D. J., Nessim, S., and Klinenberg, J. R. Clinical and laboratory features of 30 patients with systemic lupus erythematosus and silicone breast implants [abstract]. Arthritis and Rheumatism. 1995 Sep, 38, (9 (Supplement)): S265. IMMUNE EFFECTS/connective tissue disease.

Baselt, R. C., and Cravey, R. H. Disposition of Toxic Drugs and Chemicals in Man. 3rd ed. Chicago: Year Book Medical Publishers, 1989. PLATINUM.

Bassett, L. W., and Brenner, R. J. Considerations when imaging women with breast implants [commentary]. American Journal of Roentgenology. 1992 Nov, 159, 979-981. MAMMOGRAPHY.

Bassett, L. W., Hendrick, R. E., Bassford, T. L., Butler, P. F., Carter, D., and DeBor, M. Quality Determinants of Mammography. clinical practice guideline no. 13. AHCPR publication no. 95-0632 ed. Rockville, Md.: U.S. Department of Health and Human Services, Public Health Service, Agency for Health Care Policy and Research, 1994. MAMMOGRAPHY.

Bates, D. W., Buchwald, D., Lee, J., and et al. Clinical laboratory findings of systemic rheumatic disorders in "symptomatic" woman with silicone breast implants [abstract]. Arthritis and Rheumatism. 1992, 35, (9 (Supplement)): S12. CONNECTIVE TISSUE DISEASE.

Bates, H. K., Cunny, H. C., and LaBorde, J. B. Developmental toxicity evaluation of polydimethylsiloxane injection in the Sprague-Dawley rat. in. Silicone in Medical Devices, Proceedings of a Conference, 1991: DHHS: pp 127-137. TOXICOLOGY/children's effects.

Bates, H. K., Filler, R., and Kimmel, C. Developmental toxicity study of polydimethylsiloxane injection in the rat [abstract]. Teratology. 1985, 31, (3): 50. TOXICOLOGY.

Bayer, R. Editor's note: science, justice, and breast implants. American Journal of Public Health. 1999 Apr, 89, (4): 483. GENERAL.

Bayer, Goldschmidt, Wacker-Chemie, and Haus der Technik. Silicones: Chemistry and Technology. Germany: CRC Press, 1991. SILICONE CHARACTERIZATION.

Beasley, M. E. Eighty-four consecutive breast reconstructions using a textured silicone tissue expander [discussion]. Plast. Reconstr. Surg. 1992 Jun, 89, (6): 1035-1036. POLYURETHANE/expander/reconstruction/capsule-contracture/local complications.

Becker, H. Capsulectomy—medically or legally indicated? [letter]. Plast. Reconstr. Surg. 1992 Oct, 90, (4): 731. LOCAL COMPLICATIONS/general /letter.

Bell, M. L. Inflatable breast implants [letter]. Plast. Reconstr. Surg. 1983 Feb, 71, (2): 281-282. SALINE/letter/local complications.

Bellia, J. P., Birchall, J. D., and Roberts, N. B. Beer: A dietary source of silicon [letter]. The Lancet. 1994, 343, 235. SILICON MEASUREMENT/letter.

Benmeir, P., Lusthaus, S., and Baruchin, A. Laparoscopic breast augmentation [letter]. Plast. Reconstr. Surg. 1994 Jul, 94, (1): 215. LOCAL COMPLICATIONS/letter.

Bennett, R. M. The fibromyalgia syndrome: Myofascial pain and the chronic fatigue syndrome. Textbook of Rheumatology. 1993, p. 471. AI-CTD BACKGROUND.

Beraka, G. J. Rupture of implants following mammography [letter]. Plast. Reconstr. Surg. 1995 Apr, 95, (5): 936-937. MAMMOGRAPHY/rupture/local complications.

Berg, W. A., Caskey, C. I., Kuhlman, J. E., Hamper, U. M., Chang, B. W., Anderson, N. D., and et al. Comparative evaluation of MR imaging and US in determining breast implant failure [abstract]. Radiology. 1994 Nov, 193, (P (Supplement)): 318. MAMMOGRAPHY.

Berkel, H. Breast augmentation and the risk of subsequent breast cancer [letter-reply]. The New England Journal of Medicine. 1993 Mar 4, 328, (9): 663. CANCER.

Berlin Jr., C. M. Silicone breast implants and breastfeeding. Breastfeeding Abstracts. 1996 Feb, 15, (3): 17-18. BREAST FEEDING/children's effects.

Bernet, V. J., and Finger, D. R. Graves disease following silicone breast implantation [letter]. J. Rheumatol. 1994, 21, (11): 2169. CONNECTIVE TISSUE DISEASE/letter.

Bernstein, S. A. Axillary lymphadenopathies due to silicone implants [letter-reply]. J. Rheumatol. 1994, 21, (5): 965-966. LYMPHADENOPATHY/local complications/granulomas/letter.

Bertolin, S. M., Gonzalez, R., and Amorrurtu, J. Leakage of silicone gel through a cutaneous fistula [letter]. Plast. Reconstr. Surg. 1994 Jun, 93, (7): 1531-1532. RUPTURE/local complications/letter.

Bestler, J. M. Ruptured breast implant [letter]. Plast. Reconstr. Surg. 1995 Jul, 96, (1): 234. IMMUNE EFFECTS/rupture/letter.

Bignall, J. Silicones and connective tissue disease [letter]. The Lancet. 1993 Apr 17, 341, 1019. LETTER/capsule contracture.

Bischoff, F., and Bryson, G. Carcinogenesis through solid state surfaces. Progress in Experimental Tumor Research. New York: Nafner Publishing Company, Inc., 1964, p. 85-133. CARCINOGENICITY.

Black, C. M., Impose, S., and Stevens, W. M. R. Augmentation mammoplasty and connective tissue disease. Arthritis and Rheumatism. 1989, 32, 578. CONNECTIVE TISSUE DISEASE.

Black, O. Vestibular and auditory function abnormalities in silicone breast implant patients [abstract]. Presented at Combined Otolaryngological Spring Meetings, 1997 May. NEUROLOGIC DISEASE.

Blackburn Jr., W. D., Grotting, J., and Everson, M. P. Lack of findings of systemic rheumatic disorders in symptomatic women with silicone breast implants [abstract]. Arthritis and Rheumatism. 1992 Oct, 35 , (9 (Supplement)): S212. CONNECTIVE TISSUE DISEASE.

Blais, P. Problems with Saline-Filled Implants: A 10-Year Retrospective. Presented to the IOM Committee on the Safety of Silicone Breast Implants, 1998 Jul 24, Washington, D.C. SALINE/infection/local complications.

Bleiweiss, I. J., and Copeland, M. Capsular synovial metaplasia and breast implants, with reply by Raso, et al. [letter]. Archives of Pathology and Laboratory Medicine. 1995 Feb, 119, (2): 115. CAPSULE-CONTRACTURE/local complications/saline/letter.

Blocksma, R., and Braley, S. Implantation Materials. in. Plastic Surgery: A Concise Guide to Clinical Practice. 1968. GENERAL.

Boley, W. F., and LeVier, R. R. Immunological Enhancing Activities of Organosilicon Compounds and Non-functional Fluids. Midland, Mich.: Dow Corning Corporation, 1974 Oct 2. IMMUNE EFFECTS/toxicology.

Bommer, J., Ritz, E., Waldherr, R., and Gastner, M. Silicone cell inclusions causing multiorgan foreign body reaction in dialysed patients [letter]. The Lancet. 1981 Jun 13: 1314. SILICON MEASUREMENT/local complications/letter.

Borenstein, D. Clinical manifestations of 100 consecutive women with silicone breast implants [abstract]. Arthritis and Rheumatism. 1993 Sep, 36, (9 (Supplement)): S117. CONNECTIVE TISSUE DISEASE.

Borenstein, D. Operational Criteria for Systemic Silicone Related Disease (SSRD), Executive Committee of the Silicone Related Disease Research Group. in Tugwell, P., 1998. 1994a. CONNECTIVE TISSUE DISEASE.

Borenstein, D. Siliconosis: A spectrum of illness. Seminars in Arthritis and Rheumatism. 1994b Aug, 24, (1 (Supplement 1)): 1-7. CONNECTIVE TISSUE DISEASE.

Borzelleca, J. History of Toxicology. in: Hayes. Principles and Methods of Toxicology. 3rd edition ed. New York: Raven Press, 1994.

Bostwick III, J. Plastic and Reconstructive Breast Surgery. St. Louis, Mo.: Quality Medical Publishing, 1990. GENERAL.

Botti, G., Villedieu, R., and Garibaldi, V. Postoperative self-expansion in augmentation mammaplasty [letter]. Plast. Reconstr. Surg. 1994 May, 93, (6): 1310. LOCAL COMPLICATIONS.

Bowlin, S. J., Perkins, L. L., and Duel, L. A (Dow Corning Corp.). Clinical Evaluation of Dow Corning Silicone Breast Implants. in. Amer. Soc. Plast. Reconstr. Surg. Nurses, 1998 Oct 3-1998 Oct 8, Boston, MA. 1998. RUPTURE/capsule-contracture/local complications.

Braley, S. The present status of mammary implant materials. In: Masters, F. W., and Lewis, Jr. J. R., Eds. Symposium on Aesthetic Surgery of the Face, Eyelid, and Breast. St. Louis: C.V. Mosby, 1972, p. 149-151. GENERAL.

Braley, S. Silicone fluids with added adulterants [letter]. Plast. Reconstr. Surg. 1970, 45, (3): 288. SILICONE INJECTION.

Brand, K. G. Polyurethane-coated silicone implants and the question of capsular contracture [letter]. Plast. Reconstr. Surg. 1984 Mar, 73, (3): 498. POLYURETHANE/capsule-contracture/letter.

Brandon, H. J., Wolf, C., Jerina, K., and Young, L. Mechanical, Chemical, and Physical Analyses of Explanted Silicone Gel Breast Implants. 1998a Mar. RUPTURE.

Brandon, H. J., Young, L., Jerina, K., and Wolf, C. Effect of Implantation on Breast Implant Material Properties. 1997d Oct. RUPTURE.

Brandon, H. J., Young, L., Jerina, K., and Wolf, C. Long Term Aging of Silastic II Silicone Gel Breast Implants. 1998d May. RUPTURE.

Brandon, H. J., Young, L., Jerina, K., and Wolf, C. Variability in the Properties of Silicone Gel Breast Implants. 1998c Apr. RUPTURE.

Brandon, H. J., Young, L., Jerina, K., Wolf, C., and Schorr, M. A. Diagnosis of Ruptured Breast Implants Using Scanning Electron Microscopy. 1997a Oct. RUPTURE.

Brandon, H. J., Young, L., Jerina, K., Wolf, C., and Schorr, M. W. Comparison of Breast Implant Shell Strengths and Rupture Rates. 1998f Oct. RUPTURE.

Brandon, H. J., Young, V. L., Jerina, K. L., and Wolf, C. J. Assessment of Long Term Aging of Silicone Gel Breast Implants. 1998b Apr. SILICONE CHARACTERIZATION.

Brandon, H. J., Young, V. L., Jerina, K. L., and Wolf, C. J. Tear Strength of Explanted Silicone Gel Breast Implants. 1998e Sep. RUPTURE.

Brandon, H. J., Young V.L., Jerina, K. L., Wolf, C. J., and Schorr, M. W. Case Studies of Breast Implant Failure Using Scanning Electron Microscopy. 1997b Oct. RUPTURE.

Brandon, H. J., Young, V. L., Wolf, C. J., and Jerina, K. L. Long-Term Material Stability of Explanted Breast Implants. 1997c Sep. RUPTURE.

Brautbar, N., and Vojdani, A. Immunologic and clinical aspects of silicone in women with breast implants. in: Gorczyca, D. P., and Brenner, R. J., eds. The Augmented Breast: Radiologic and Clinical Perspectives. New York and Stuttgart: Thieme, 1997, p. 189-205. IMMUNE EFFECTS/connective tissue disease.

Brautbar, N., Vojdani, A., and Campbell, A. W. Silicone implants and systemic immunological disease: Review of the literature and preliminary results [editorial]. Toxicology and Industrial Health. 1992, 8, (5): 231-237. GENERAL/CONNECTIVE TISSUE DISEASE.

Brawer, A. E. (Monmouth Medical Center). Bones, Groans, and Silicone: Beauty and the Beast. Arthritis and Rheumatism: Abstracts of Scientific Presentations, 1994 Jun: p. 365. IMMUNE EFFECTS/CONNECTIVE TISSUE DISEASE.

Brawer, A. E. Silicon and matrix macromolecules: New research opportunities for old diseases from analysis of potential mechanisms of breast implant toxicity. (unpublished). 1998 Jun. GENERAL.

Brent, J. (University of Colorado Health Sciences Center). The Medical Toxicology of Silicone Breast Implants. transcript of IOM Committee on the Safety of Silicone Breast Implants, 1998 Jul 24, Washington, D.C. TOXICOLOGY.

Bridges, A. J. Silicone implant controversy continues [letter]. The Lancet. 1994 Nov 26, 344, 1451-1452. GENERAL/letter.

Bridges, A. J., Anderson, J. D., Burns, D. E., Kemple, K., Kaplan, J. D., and Lorden, T. Autoantibodies in patients with silicone implants. Current Topics in Microbiology and Immunolgoy, Immunology of Silicones. 1996, 210, 277-282. IMMUNE EFFECTS.

Bridges, A. J., Conley, C., Wang, G., Burns, D., and Vasey, F. A clinical and immunologic evaluation of women with SBI and symptoms of rheumatic disease. American College of Rheumatism Meeting. 1993b Nov: Abstract #184. CONNECTIVE TISSUE DISEASE/immune effects.

Bridges, A. J., and Lorden, T. Sicca syndrome in women with silicone implants: Absence of serum autoantibodies [abstract]. Arthritis and Rheumatism. 1993 Sep, 36, (9 (Supplement)): S70. CONNECTIVE TISSUE DISEASE/immune effects.

Bright, R. A., and Moore, Jr. R. M. Estimating the prevalence of women with breast implants [letter]. American Journal of Public Health. 1996 Jun, 86, (6): 891-892. PREVALENCE/letter.

Brody, G. S. The effect of breast implants on the radiographic detection of microcalcification and soft-tissue masses [discussion]. Plast. Reconstr. Surg. 1989, 84, (5): 779-780. MAMMOGRAPHY/local complications/calcification.

Brody, G. S. Knowledge, concern, and satisfaction among augmentation mammaplasty patients [discussion]. Annals of Plastic Surgery. 1993 Jan, 30, (1): 20-22. PSYCHOSOCIAL.

Brody, G. S. Lactation after augmentation mammaplasty [letter]. Obstetrics and Gynecology. 1996 Jun, 87, (6): 1062-1063. BREAST FEEDING/letter.

Brody, G. S. The Même implant [discussion]. Plast. Reconstr. Surg. 1984, 73, 420. POLYURETHANE.

Brody, G. S. Reconstruction of the breast using polyurethane-coated prostheses [discussion]. Plast. Reconstr. Surg. 1984 Mar, 73, (3): 420-421. POLYURETHANE/capsule-contracture/local complications/reconstruction.

Brody, G. S. Scleroderma after silicone augmentation mammoplasty [letter]. J. Amer. Med. Assoc. 1988 Nov 25, 260, (20): 236-238. CONNECTIVE TISSUE DISEASE.

Brody, G. S. Scleroderma-like esophageal disease in children of mothers with silicone breast implants [letter]. J. Amer. Med. Assoc. 1994a Sep 14, 272, (10): 770. CHILDREN'S EFFECTS/breast feeding/letter.

Brody, G. S. Silicone breast implant safety: Physical, chemical, and biologic problems [letter-reply]. Plast. Reconstr. Surg. 1997 Jan, 99, (1): 260-261. CAPSULE-CONTRACTURE/local complications/migration/rupture/letter.

Brody, G. S. Silicone gel breast implants [letter]. J. Amer. Med. Assoc. 1994 Jul 27, 272, (4): 271. GENERAL/letter.

Brody, G. S., and Deapen, D. M. Breast cancer diagnosis in the augmented patient [letter]. Archives of Surgery. 1989 Feb, 124, 256-257. MAMMOGRAPHY.

Brooks, P. M. Silicone breast implantation: Doubts about the fears [editorial]. Medical Journal of Australia. 1995 Apr 17, 162, 432-434. GENERAL.

Broughton, A., and Thrasher, J. D. Autoantibodies associated with silicone breast implants [abstract]. Clinical Chemistry. 1993, 39, (6): 1139. IMMUNE EFFECTS.

Brown, S. L., Mann, J., Merner, M. L., and Woo, E. Toxic Shock Syndrome: Post-Surgical Infection in Women after Mammoplasty. Unpublished FDA report: 1997a Oct 6. INFECTION/local complications.

Brown, S. L., and Silverman, B. G. Silicone Gel Breast Implants: A Regulatory Perspective and Report On Published Epidemiologic Studies (Abstract No. T64). 1996 Annual Conference of ISEE, 1996 Jul. CONNECTIVE TISSUE DISEASE.

Brown, S., Patten, B. M., Cooke, N., Ostermeyer-Shoaib, B., and Jhingran, S. C. Silicone breast implants: Association with abnormal SPECT scans and memory defects [abstract]. Canadian Journal of Neurological Sciences. 1993(Supplement 4): S177. NEUROLOGIC DISEASE.

Brownstein, M. L., and Owsley, Jr. J. Q. Augmentation mammaplasty: A survey of the major complications. in: Owsley, J. Q., and Peterson, R. A., eds. Symposium on Aesthetic Surgery of the Breast. St. Louis: Mosby, 1978, p. 267. INFECTION/steroids/capsule-contracture/local complications.

Brucker, R. Bleed of a biologic response to triglyceride filler used in radiolucent breast implants [letter]. Plast. Reconstr. Surg. 197 Jun, 99, (7): 2107-2108. GENERAL.

Bryant, H. H. Project BBL 722: X3-0294-70D (RP) Radiopaque Silicone Rubber, X3-0146-50D (RP) Radiopaque Silicone Rubber. Midland, Mich.: Dow Corning Corporation, 1982 Aug 23. TOXICOLOGY.

Bryant, H., Brasher, P. M. A., van de Sande, J. H., and Turc, J-M. Review of methods in breast augmentation: A risk factor for breast cancer [letter]. The New England Journal of Medicine. 1994, 330, (4): 293. CANCER/letter.

Bui, H. X., Del Rosario, A. D., Ballouk, F., and et al. Reaction to silicone breast implants: Morphologic, immunofluorescent, and electron probe x-ray microanalytic (EPXMA) findings. Modern Pathology. 1993, 6, 12A. immune effects.

Bulpitt, K., Weiner, S. R., and Paulus, H. E. Comparison of the systemic manifestations associated with polyurethane-coated and non-coated silicone breast implants [abstract]. Arthritis and Rheumatism. 1992 Sep, 35, (9 (Supplement)): S161. POLYURETHANE/connective tissue disease/local complications.

Burkhardt, B. R. 1985 supplement to augmentation mammaplasty and capsular contracture. An annotated review and guide to the literature. Privately published, Tucson Arizona. 1985. GENERAL.

Burkhardt, B. R. Absence of visible bacteria in capsules around silicone breast implants [discussion]. Plast. Reconstr. Surg. 1983 Jul, 72, (1): 32-35. INFECTION/local complications/capsule-contracture.

Burkhardt, B. R. Are the polyurethane-covered implants really as good as they're cracked up to be? If so, why haven't I switched? [expert commentary]. Perspectives in Plastic Surgery. 1988, 2, (1): 165-167. POLYURETHANE/capsule-contracture/local complications.

Burkhardt, B. R. Breast implants: A brief history of their development, characteristics, and problems. Grant, Vasconez, and Williams, Eds. Postmastectomy Reconstruction. 2 ed. 1988, pp. 68-83. GENERAL.

Burkhardt, B. R. Comparing contracture rates: Probability theory and the unilateral contracture [editorial]. Plast. Reconstr. Surg. 1984 Oct, 74, (4): 527-529. CAPSULE-CONTRACTURE/local complications.

Burns, C. G. The Epidemiology of Systemic Sclerosis: A Population-Based Case-Control Study [doctoral dissertation]. Ann Arbor, Mich.: University of Michigan, 1994. AI-CTD BACKGROUND.

Busch, H. Silicone toxicology. Seminars in Arthritis and Rheumatism. 1994 Aug, 24, (1 (Supplement 1)): 11-17. GENERAL/toxicology.

Butler, J. E., Lu, E. P., Navarro, P., and Christiansen, B. The adsorption of proteins on a polydimethylsiloxane elastomer (pep) and their antigenic behavior. Current Topics in Immunology and Microbiology: Immunology of Silicones. 1996, 210, 75-84. IMMUNE EFFECTS/silicone characterization.

Cabot Corporation. Cab-O-Sil, properties and functions. Tuseola Ill.: 1990. SILICA.

Cadier, M. A., and Hobby, J. A. Silicone breast implants and drug-induced arthralgia [letter]. Plast. Reconstr. Surg. 1997 Apr, 99, (5): 1464. CONNECTIVE TISSUE DISEASE.

Caffee, H. H. The biophysical and histologic properties of capsules formed by smooth and textured silicone implants in the rabbit [discussion]. Plast. Reconstr. Surg. 1992b Jun, 89, (6): 1043-1044. CAPSULE-CONTRACTURE/local complications.

Caffee, H. H. Capsular contracture: A prospective study of the effect of local antibacterial agents [discussion]. Plast. Reconstr. Surg. 1986 Jun, 77, (6): 919-932. CAPSULE-CONTRACTURE/local complications/infection.

Caffee, H. H. Capsule thickness and breast firmness [letter]. Plast. Reconstr. Surg. 1992c Feb, 89, (2): 380. CAPSULE-CONTRACTURE/local complications.

Caffee, H. H. Classification of capsular contracture after prosthetic breast reconstruction [discussion]. Plast. Reconstr. Surg. 1995 Oct, 96, (5): 1124. CAPSULE-CONTRACTURE/local complications.

Caffee, H. H. The conventional and low-bleed implants for augmentation mammoplasty. Plast. Reconstr. Surg. 1992a, 90, (2): 343. BLEED-LEAKAGE/letter.

Caffee, H. H. Could tight breast capsules squeeze a significant amount of silicone gel out of an implant? [letter-reply]. Plast. Reconstr. Surg. 1993a Sep, 92, (3): 558. CAPSULE-CONTRACTURE/local complications.

Caffee, H. H. The effect of siltex texturing and povidone-iodine irrigation on capsular contracture around saline inflatable breast implants [discussion]. Plast. Reconstr. Surg. 1994 Jan, 93, (1): 123-128. CAPSULE-CONTRACTURE/local complications.

Caffee, H. H. The effects of hematomas on implant capsular contracture. Ann. Plast. Surg. 1986b, 16, 102. HEMATOMA.

Caffee, H. H. Intraductal migration of silicone from intact gel breast prostheses [discussion]. Plast. Reconstr. Surg. 1995 Mar, 95, (3): 563-566. LOCAL COMPLICATIONS.

Caffee, H. H. Life span of silicone gel-filled mammary prostheses [discussion]. Plast. Reconstr. Surg. 1997 Dec, 100, (7): 1727-1728. CAPSULE-CONTRACTURE/local complications/infection/rupture/pain.

Caffee, H. H. Methyl prednisolone in double-lumen gel-saline submuscular mammary prostheses: A double-blind, prospective, controlled clinical trial [discussion]. Plast. Reconstr. Surg. 1991 Mar, 87, (3): 488-489. CAPSULE-CONTRACTURE/local complications/steroids.

Caffee, H. H. Rupture and aging of silicone gel breast implants [discussion]. Plastic and Reconstructive Surgery. 1993b Apr, 91, (5): 835-836. RUPTURE.

Caffee, H. H. Short-term effect of silicone gel on peripheral nerves: A histologic study [discussion]. Plast. Reconstr. Surg. 1992d May, 89, (5): 941-942. NEUROLOGIC DISEASE.

Caldwell, J. R. Silicone and silliness. Probabilistic prevarication in the legal arena [editorial]. Journal of the Florida Medical Association. 1994, 81, (9): 596-598. GENERAL.

Campbell, A. W. List of Symptoms Frequently Caused by Silicone Implants [Web Page]. Accessed 1997 Nov 6. Available at: http://wee.geocities.com/HotSprings/8689/symptoms.html. SILICONE CHARACTERIZATION.

Cantoch, S., and Fairclough, P. Breast augmentation and the risk of subsequent breast cancer [letter]. The New England Journal of Medicine. 1993 Mar 4, 329, (9): 662. CANCER.

Capozzi, A. Polyurethane-covered gel mammary implants [letter]. Plastic Reconstructive Surgery. 1982 May, 69, 904. POLYURETHANE/letter.

Carlisle, E. M. Silicon as an essential trace element in animal nutrition. Evered, D., and O'Connor, M., eds. Silicon Biochemistry: CIBA Foundation Symposium 121. New York: Wiley, 1986, p. 123-129. GENERAL.

Carlström, D., and Falkenberg, G. The crystal and molecular structure of 2,6-*cis*-diphenylhexamethylcyclotetrasiloxane. Acta Pharmacologica et Toxicologica. 1975 Jan 1, 36 (Supp. III), 17-24 ,Chapter II. SILICONE CHARACTERIZATION.

Carter, D. Tissue reaction to breast implants [editorial]. American Journal of Clinical Pathology. 1994 Nov, 102, (5): 565-566. CAPSULE-CONTRACTURE/local complications.

Carver, J. F., inventor. Cast gel implantable prosthesis. 4,470,160. 1984 Sep 11. GENERAL.

Casarett, L. J. Chapter 1. in: Cassarett, L. J., and Doull, J. D. Eds. Toxicology. first edition ed. McMillan, 1975. TOXICOLOGY.

Cash, T. F., Winstead, B. A., and Janda, L. H. The great American shape up. Psychology Today. 1986 Apr: 30-37. GENERAL.

Cederna, J. P. Hematoma as a late complication in breast reconstruction with silicone gel prostheses [letter]. Plast. Reconstr. Surg. 1995 Jul, 96, (1): 235-236. HEMATOMA/local complications/letter.

Cederna, J. P. Partial deflation of a saline breast implant [letter]. Plastic and Reconstructive Surgery. 1996 Mar, 97, (3): 684. SALINE/local complications/rupture.

Celli, B. R., and Kovnat, D. M. Acute pneumonitis after subcutaneous injections of silicone [letter]. The New England Journal of Medicine. 1983 Oct 6, 309, (14): 856-857. SILICONE INJECTION.

Centeno, J. A., Luke, J. L., Kalasinskyi, V. F., and Mullick. Biophysical Characterization of Silicone Breast Explants by Laser Raman Microprobe and Infrared Microspectroscopy. American Chemical Society Aug. 21-26: 1994. SILICONE MEASUREMENT/silicone characterization.

Centeno, J. A., Ramos, M. S., Mullick, F. G., Offiah, O. O., Rastogi, T., and Panos, R. G. Biophysical findings associated with silicone-gel breast implants: Determination of silicon, calcium, and magnesium levels in capsular tissues. in. Metal Ions in Biology and Medicine. Paris: Eurotext, 1998, p. 362-366. SILICON MEASUREMENT/capsule-contracture/local complications/saline/calcification.

Centers for Disease Control (CDC). Diagnostic tests for silicone breast disease. MMWR Morbidity and Mortality Weekly Report. 1996, 45, 111-112. GENERAL.

Chan, E. K. L., and Pollard, K. M. Autoantibodies to ribonucleoprotein particles by immunoblotting. Rose, N. R., Friedman, H., and Fahey, J. L., eds. Manual of Clinical Laboratory Immunology. 4th ed. ed. Washington, D.C.: American Society for Microbiology, 1992, p. 755-761. IMMUNE EFFECTS.

Chandler Jr., P. J. Re: Connective tissue disease and other rheumatic conditions following breast implants in Denmark [letter]. Annals of Plastic Surgery. 1998 Jan, 40, (1): 103-104. CONNECTIVE TISSUE DISEASE.

Chang, Y. Pathogenesis of adjuvant arthritis in rats. Arthritis and Rheumatism. 1978 Jan-1978 Feb 28, 21, (1): 169-170. AI-CTD BACKGROUND.

Chantelau, E. Silicone oil released from disposable insulin syringes. Diabetes Care. 1986 Nov-1986 Dec 31, 9, (6): 672-673. TOXICOLOGY/letter.

Chantelau, E. A., and Berger, M. Pollution of insulin with silicone oil, a hazard of disposable plastic syringes. The Lancet. 1985 Jun 22, 1, (8443): 1459. GENERAL/letter.

Chase, D. R., Mallot, R. L., Weeks, D. A., Oberg, K. C., and Chase, R. L. Correspondence re: J.A. Emory, S.S. Spanier, G. Kasnic, Jr., N.S. Hardt. The Synovial Structure of Breast-Implant-Associated Bursae. Modern Pathology 7:728, 1994. [letter]. Modern Pathology. 1996, 9, (2): 157-158. CAPSULE-CONTRACTURE/local complications/letter.

Chase, D. R., Obert, K. C., Chase, R. L., Mallot, R. L., and Weeks, D. A. Silicone breakdown and capsular synovial metaplasia in textured-wall saline breast implants [letter]. Plast. Reconstr. Surg. 1996 Jan, 97, (1): 249. CAPSULE-CONTRACTURE/local complications.

Chastre, J., Basset, F., and Gilbert, C. Acute pneumonitis after subcutaneous injections of silicone [letter-reply]. The New England Journal of Medicine. 1983b Oct 6, 310, (14): 856-857. SILICONE INJECTION/letter.

Chawla, A., and Hinberg, I. Laboratory evaluation of explanted gel filled silicone breast implants. Fifth World Biomaterials Congress, Toronto, Canada. 1996 Jun. EXPLANTATION/rupture.

Chilcote, W. A., Dowden, R. V., Paushter, D. M., Hale, J. C., Desberg, A. L., Singer, A. A., and et al. Detection with US of silicone gel breast implant leaks: A prospective analysis [abstract]. Radiology. 1993 Nov, 189, (P): 155. MAMMOGRAPHY/rupture/local complications.

Chin, H. P., Harrison, E. C. Blankenhorn D. H., and Moacanin, J. Lipids in silicone rubber valve prosthesis after human implantation. Circulation. 1971, 43, ((Supplement 1)): I-51-I-56. SILICONE CHARACTERIZATION.

Chow, H. Y., Calabrese, L. H., Wilke, W. S., and Cash, J. M. Is silicone associated illness really chronic fatigue syndrome? [abstract]. Arthritis and Rheumatism. 1995 Sep, 38, (9 (Supplement)): 264. IMMUNE EFFECTS/connective tissue disease.

Chow, H. Y., Cash, J. M., Calabrese, L. H., and Wilke, W. S. Patients with chronic fatigue syndrome (CFS) and silicone-associated illness (SAI) are similarly disabled [abstract]. Arthritis and Rheumatism. 1996 Sep, 39, (9 (Supplement)): S52. CONNECTIVE TISSUE DISEASE.

Claman, H. N. Autoimmunity after silicone breast implants [letter, with response by Ellis, T.M., Hardt, N.S., and Atkinson, M.A.]. Annals of Allergy, Asthma, and Immunology. 1997 Aug, 79, (2): 89-90. IMMUNE EFFECTS.

Claman, H. N. Breast implants and autoimmunity [letter-reply]. Western Journal of Medicine. 1994 Jul, 161, (1): 91-92. IMMUNE EFFECTS.

Claman, H. N., and Giorno, R. C. Silicone and antinuclear antibodies [abstract]. J Allergy Clin Immunol. 1993, 92, 212. CONNECTIVE TISSUE DISEASE/IMMUNE EFFECTS.

Claman, H. N., and Robertson, A. D. Antinuclear antibodies in apparently healthy women with breast implants. Current Topics in Microbiology and Immunology: Immunology of Silicones. 1996, p. 265-268. IMMUNE EFFECTS.

Clarson, S. J., and Semlyen, J. A. Siloxane Polymers. Englewood Cliffs, N.J.: PTR Prentice Hall, 1993. SILICONE CHARACTERIZATION.

Clayton, G. D., and Clayton, F. E. 33, Tin. in. Patty's Industrial Hygiene and Toxicology. 4th ed. John Wiley and Sons, Inc., 1994. TOXICOLOGY.

Coble, Jr. Y. D. Silicone gel breast implants [letter]. J. Amer. Med. Assoc. 1994 Jul 27, 272, (4): 273. GENERAL/letter.

Coccaro, S. F. Dealing with the ruptured silicone gel breast implant [letter]. Plast. Reconstr. Surg. 1993 Sep, 92, (3): 557. RUPTURE/local complications/letter.

Cocke, W. M. "Nutcracker" technique for compression rupture of capsules around breast implants. Plast. Reconstr. Surg. 1978 Nov, 62, (5): 772-773. CLOSED CAPSULOTOMY/rupture.

Cohen, F. J. Identification and location of extravasated silicone gel using magnetic resonance imaging [letter]. Plast. Reconstr. Surg. 1993 Jun, 91, (7): 1371. MAMMOGRAPHY.

Cohen, I. K. Antibiotics in the tissue expander to decrease the rate of infection [letter-reply]. Plast. Reconstr. Surg. 1988 Jan, 81, (1): 138. PAIN/infection/local complications/expander.

Cohen, I. K. The effectiveness of alpha-tocopherol (vitamin E) in reducing the incidence of spherical contracture around breast implants [discussion]. Plast. Reconstr. Surg. 1981 Nov, 68, (5): 699. CAPSULE-CONTRACTURE/local complications.

Cohen, I. K. Impact of the FDA ban on silicone breast implants [editorial]. Journal of Surgical Oncology. 1994, 56, (1): 1. GENERAL.

Cohen, I. K. Leakage of Breast Prostheses. Arch Surg. 1984 May, 119, 615. RUPTURE/deflation.

Cohen, I. K. On mammography in the presence of breast implants [letter]. Plast. Reconstr. Surg. 1978b Aug, 62, (2): 287. MAMMOGRAPHY/letter.

Cohen, I. K. On the use of soluble steroids within inflatable breast prostheses [letter]. Plast. Reconstr. Surg. 1978a Jul, 62, (1): 105-106. STEROIDS/local complications/capsule-contracture.

Cohen, I. K., and Roberts, C. Lidocaine relieves pain with tissue expansion of the breast [letter]. Plast. Reconstr. Surg. 1987 Mar, 79, (3): 489. PAIN/local complications/expander/letter.

Cohen, I. K., and Scheflan, M. The value of xeromammography for ruptured breast implants [letter]. Plast. Reconstr. Surg. 1982 May, 69, (5): 898-890. MAMMOGRAPHY/letter.

Cohen, J. J. T-cell response in women with silicone breast implants [letter]. Clinical and Diagnostic Laboratory Immunology. 1995 Mar, 2, (2): 253. IMMUNE EFFECTS/letter.

Collier, F. C., and Dawson, A. D. Insulin syringes and silicone oil. Lancet. 1985 Sep 14. TOXICOLOGY.

Collis, N., Dhoo, C. T. K., and Sharpe, D. T. Media are too eager to link silicone to disease [letter]. British Medical Journal. 1998 Feb, 316, (7129): 477. GENERAL/letter.

Cook, R. R. Sclerodermalike esophageal disease in children of mothers with silicone breast implants [letter]. J. Amer. Med. Assoc. 1994 Sep 14, 272, (10): 767-768. CHILDREN'S EFFECTS/letter.

Cook, R. R., Curtis, J. M., and Perkins, L. L. Rupture of silicone-gel breast implants. The Lancet. 1998, 351, 520-521. RUPTURE/letter.

Cook, R. R., Delongchamp, R. R., Woodbury, M., and et al. Breast Implant Prevalence. Midland, Mich.: Dow Corning Corporation, 1993 Mar 17. PREVALENCE.

Cook, R. R., Hoshaw, S. J., and Perkins, L. L. Failure of silicone gel breast implants: Analysis of literature data for 1652 explanted prostheses [letter]. Plast. Reconstr. Surg. 1998 Apr, 101, (4): 1162. RUPTURE/letter/local complications.

Cook, R. R., and Perkins, L. L. The prevalence of breast implants among women in the United States. Current Topics in Microbiology and Immunology: Immunology of Silicones. 1996, p. 419-425. PREVALENCE.

Cooper, C., and Dennison, E. Do silicone breast implants cause connective tissue disease: There is still no clear evidence that they do [editorial]. British Medical Journal. 1998 Feb, 316, 403-404. GENERAL/connective tissue disease.

Copeland, M. Capsular synovial metaplasia as a common response to both textured and smooth implants [discussion]. Plastic and Reconstructive Surgery. 1996 Jun, 97, (7): 1434-1435. CAPSULE CONTRACTURE.

Corrin, B. Silicone lymphadenopathy [letter]. Journal of Clinical Pathology. 1982, 35, (8): 901-902. LYMPHADENOPATHY/local complications/letter.

Courtiss, E. Inflatable breast implants [letter-reply]. Plast. Reconstr. Surg. 1995 Mar, 95, (3): 600. EXPANDER/rupture/local complications/capsule-contracture/letter.

Crase, B. L. (La Leche League International, Center for Breast Feeding Information). Letter To: Dear Friend [La Leche position paper]. Schaumburg, Ill., 1996 May. BREAST FEEDING/children's effects.

Crofoot, S. D., and Plotzke, K. P. A Pilot Study for the Determination of 14C-Octamethylcyclotetrasiloxane (D4) Pharmacokinetics in Fischer 344 Rats Following a Single Nose-Only Vapor Inhalation Exposure to 700 ppm 14D-D4. Midland, Mich.: Dow Corning Corporation, 1996 Jun 25. TOXICOLOGY.

Cronin, T. D. One-stage reconstruction of a projecting nipple: The quadrapod flap [discussion]. Plast. Reconstr. Surg. 1983b Jan, 71, (1): 133. RECONSTRUCTION.

Cronin, T. D. Silicone breast implant. Rubin, L. R., Ed. Biomaterials In Reconstructive Surgery. St. Louis: The C.V. Mosby Company, 1983a. GENERAL.

Cronin, T. D., and Gerow, F. J. Augmentation mammoplasty: A new "natural feel" prosthesis. Transactions of the Third International Congress of Plastic Surgery, Oct. 13-18, 1963. Excerpta Medica Foundation. 1963: 41-49. GENERAL.

Cruz-Korchin, N. Re: Effectiveness of silicone sheets in the prevention of hypertrophic breast scars [letter-reply]. Annals of Plastic Surgery. 1997 May, 38, (5): 547. LOCAL COMPLICATIONS/letter.

Cuéllar, M. L., Citera, G., Scopelitis, E., Sandifer, M., Cabrera, G., Gutierrez, M., Silveira, L. H., and Espinoza, L. R. High prevalence of serum antinuclear antibodies in women with silicone breast implants [abstract]. Arthritis and Rheumatism. 1993 Sep, 36, (9 (Supplement)): S219. IMMUNE EFFECTS.

Cuéllar, M. L., and Espinoza, L. R. Chest pain and breast implants [letter]. Southern Medical Journal. 1996 Jan, 89, (1): 97. PAIN/local complications/letter.

Cuéllar, M. L., and Espinoza, L. R. Silicone breast implants and connective tissue disease [letter]. J. Rheumatol. 1994, 21, (10): 1979. CONNECTIVE TISSUE DISEASE/immune effects/letter.

Cuéllar, M. L., Espinoza, L. R., Ochs, R., and Tan, E. M. Clinical outcome of silicone breast implant (SBI) women following implant removal [abstract]. Arthritis and Rheumatism. 1995 Sep, 38, (9 (Supplement)): S264. IMMUNE EFFECTS/connective tissue disease/explantation.

Cuéllar, M. L., Gutiérrez, M., Cabrera, G., Gharavi, A., and Espinoza, L. R. Soluble intercellular adhesion molecule I (sICAM-1) and other acute phase reactants such as ESR and CRP are not elevated in silicone breast implant patients [abstract]. Arthritis and Rheumatism. 1993 Sep, 36, (9 (Supplement)): S219. CONNECTIVE TISSUE DISEASE/immune effects.

Cuéllar, M. L., Scopelitis, E., Citera, G., Gutiérrez, M., Silveira, L. H., and Espinoza, L. R. A prospective clinical evaluation of 300 women with silicone breast implants [abstract]. Arthritis and Rheumatism. 1993 Sep, 36, (9 (Supplement)): S219. CONNECTIVE TISSUE DISEASE.

Cuéllar, M. L., Stein, Jr. T. W., Espinoza, L. R., Tan, E. M., and Ochs, R. L. Immunoblot analysis of sera from women with silicone breast implants (SBI) [abstract]. Arthritis and Rheumatism. 1994 Sep, 37, (9 (Supplement)): S422. IMMUNE EFFECTS.

Cuéllar, M. L., Stein, T., Espinoza, L. R., Tan, E. M., and Ochs, R. L. Prevalence of antinuclear antibodies (ANAs) in women with silicone breast implants (SBI): Clinical associations [abstract]. Arthritis and Rheumatism. 1994 Sep, 37, (9 (Supplement)): S270. IMMUNE EFFECTS.

Cunningham, B. L. Distribution of organosilicon polymers in augmentation mammaplasties at autopsy [discussion]. Plast. Reconstr. Surg. 1997 Jul, 100, (1): 204-205. SILICON MEASUREMENT.

Cunningham, B. L. Enhanced activity of lysosomal ß-galactosidase after silicone implantation: An experimental study in rats [editorial]. J Lab Clin Med. 1993, 121, 734-736. IMMUNE EFFECTS.

Curtis, J. M. Non-Regulated Study: Determination of low levels of silicones in human breast milk by aqueous silanol functionality test: Amendment to Report No. 1991-I0000-36332. Midland, Mich.: Dow Corning Corporation, 1997. BREAST FEEDING/children's effects.

Curtis, J. M., Bejarano, M. A., and Zimmer, M. A. Determination of low levels of silicones in human breast milk by aqueous silanol functionality test. Midland, Mich.: Dow Corning Corporation, 1991. CHILDREN'S EFFECTS/breast feeding/silicon measurement.

Curtis, J. M., and Hoshaw, S. J. Mechanical (Tensile) Test Data of Explanted Silastic Breast Implants Demonstrate Elastomer Stability *In Vivo*. Midland, MI: Dow Corning Corporation, 1998 Mar. RUPTURE.

Cutting, W. C. Toxicity of silicones. Stanford Medical Bulletin. 1952 Feb, 10, (1): 23-26. TOXICOLOGY.

Davis, G. S. Immunologic Aspects of Pneumoconioses in Asbestosis and Silicosis. Lynch, J. P., and DeRemee, R. A., Eds. Immunologically Mediated Pulmonary Disease. 1991, p. 111-155. SILICA.

Davis, J., Campagna, J., Perrillo, R., and Criswell, L. Clinical Characteristics of 343 Patients With Breast Implants. J. Rheumatol. 1995 Oct: S263. CONNECTIVE TISSUE DISEASE/expander/rupture/local complications.

Davis, P. Augmentation mammoplasty: Beauty or beast? [editorial]. J. Rheumatol. 1993, 20, (6): 927-928. GENERAL/local complications/connective tissue disease.

De Camara, D. L., and Sheridan, J. M. Leaking gel implants [letter-reply]. Plast. Reconstr. Surg. 1993 Dec, 92, (7): 1411. RUPTURE/local complications/letter.

De Jong, W. H., Spiekstra, S. W., and van Loveren, H. Detection of antipolymer antibodies (APA) in serum of women with silicone breast implants. Introduction and performance of the assay in the RIVM. The Netherlands: Ministry of Health, Welfare and Sports, Public Health Supervisory Service, Inspectorate of Health Care, 1998 Oct. IMMUNE EFFECTS.

De Lange, E. E., Bosworth, J. E., DeAngelis, G. A., and Morgan, R. F. MR imaging of breast implants [abstract]. Radiology. 1992, 185, 378. MAMMOGRAPHY.

De Vries, C. P., and Siddiqui, W. H. Acute Oral Toxicity of a Platinum Catalyst. Midland, Mich.: Dow Corning Corporation, 1982 Aug 18. PLATINUM/toxicology.

de Waal, J. C., Vaillant, W., Baltzer, J., and Zander, J. Carcinoma of the breast behind a breast prosthesis [letter]. Computerized Radiology. 1987, 11, (4): 207. MAMMOGRAPHY/cancer/letter.

Deapen, D. M., and Brody, G. Re: Induction of plasmacytomas with silicone gel in genetically susceptible strains of mice [letter]. Journal of the National Cancer Institute. 1995 Feb 15, 87, (4): 315. MYELOMA.

Deapen, D. M., and Brody, G. S. Breast augmentation and the risk of subsequent breast cancer [letter]. The New England Journal of Medicine. 1993 Mar 4, 328, (9): 662-663. CANCER.

DeGussa Corp., Ridgefield Park N. J. Aerosil Fumed Silica. SILICA.

DETector Engineering and Technology, Inc. Selective detection of cyclic silicon compounds extracted from silicone breast implants. DET Report No. 22. Walnut Creek, Calif.: DETector Engineering and Technology, Inc., 1992 Mar. TOXICOLOGY.

Digby, J. M., and Wells, A. L. Malignant lymphoma with intranodal refractile particles after insertion of silicone prostheses [letter]. The Lancet. 1981 Sep 12, 2, (8246): 580. CANCER.

Dobbie, J. W., and Smith, M. J. B. Urinary and serum silicon in normal and uremic individuals. Evered, D., and O'Connor, M., eds. Silicon Biochemistry: CIBA Foundation Symposium 121. New York: Wiley, 1986, p. 194-213. SILICON MEASUREMENT.

Dolsky, R. L. Infection after augmentation mammaplasty [letter-reply]. Plast. Reconstr. Surg. 1986 Sep, 78, (3): 425. INFECTION/polyurethane/letter/local complications.

Dolsky, R. L. Polyurethane-coated implants [letter]. Plastic and Reconstructive Surgery. 1985 Dec, 76, (6): 974-975. POLYURETHANE/capsule-contracture/local complications/infection/letter.

Donis, R. K. Breast implants and contracture, with replies by Biggs, T.M., and Gylbert, L. [letter]. Plast. Reconstr. Surg. 1990 Oct, 86, (4): 809-810. CAPSULE-CONTRACTURE/local complications/letter.

Dow Corning Corporation. A 28-day Oral Gavage Study of Octamthylcyclotetrasiloxane in Male and Female Rats with Attachments and Cover Letter Dated 04/08/88. Washington, D.C.: OPPT, U.S. Environmental Protection Agency, 1988. TOXICOLOGY.

Dow Corning Corporation. Acute Toxicity and Industrial Handling Hazards of Dow Corning® Platinum No. 1 and Dow Corning® Platinum No. 2. 1973 Sep 10. PLATINUM/TOXICOLOGY.

Dow Corning Corporation. Acute Toxicologic Properties and Industrial Handling Hazards of Dow Corning® X-2-7018. 1973 Sep 10. TOXICOLOGY.

Dow Corning Corporation. Comparative eye irritation of specially prepared Dow Corning 200 fluids with cover letter. Washington, D.C.: OPPT, U.S. Environmental Protection Agency, 1985. CANCER.

Dow Corning Corporation. Comparison of the Primary Skin Irritation Potential and the Effects of Repeated Prolonged Skin Exposures to Various Volatile Experimental Cosmetics Fluids with SD Alcohol 40. Washington, D.C.: OPPT, U.S. Environmental Protection Agency, 1986. TOXICOLOGY.

Dow Corning Corporation. Dermal absorption of Dow Corning F-218 Fluid in the Adult Male Rat, Primate, and Human. Washington, D.C.: OPPT, U.S. Environmental Protection Agency, 1989. TOXICOLOGY.

Dow Corning Corporation. Dimethypolysiloxane fluid - C14 (Dow Corning® 360 medical fluid C14) distribution and disposition in rats following subcutaneous injection. Midland, Mich.: Dow Corning Corporation, 1972 Apr 7. TOXICOLOGY.

Dow Corning Corporation. Evaluation of the dermal irritation potential of 13 personal care fluids. TSCA 8d submission 87-8215092, microfiche number OTS-0206762. Washington, D.C.: OPPT, U.S. Environmental Protection Agency, 1985. TOXICOLOGY.

Dow Corning Corporation. Gel Silicone Mammary Implant Rupture Complaint History. Dallas, Tex.: Jim Curtis, 1996 Nov 9. RUPTURE.

Dow Corning Corporation. Implant Information Booklet: Silicone Breast, Chin and Testicular Implants. Midland, Mich.: Dow Corning Corporation, 1998 Sep. GENERAL.

Dow Corning Corporation. Inhalation Studies and Industrial Hygiene Survey for Octamethylcyclotetrasiloxane (D4). Washington, D.C.: OPPT, U.S. Environmental Protection Agency, 1989. TOXICOLOGY.

Dow Corning Corporation. Mammary implant material formulations, MDF-077, and Q7-2423. Surgery Device Panel, U. S. Food and Drug Administation. Silicone Breast Implant Team Leaders' Report. Washington, D.C.: U.S. Food and Drug Administration, 1968, pp. 42, 51. GENERAL.

Dow Corning Corporation. Medtox Project—Analysis of internal safety studies relevant to health care materials and products. Midland, Mich.: Dow Corning Corporation, 1987 Feb 23. TOXICOLOGY.

Dow Corning Corporation. Metabolism of Octamethylcyclotetrasiloxane in the Monkey. Washington, D.C.: OPPT, U.S. Environmental Protection Agency, 1988. TOXICOLOGY.

Dow Corning Corporation. Platinum. Midland, Mich.: Dow Corning Corporation, 1995. PLATINUM/toxicology.

Dow Corning Corporation. Range Finding Eye Irritation Test on Hexamethyldisiloane (DC 200 Fluid). Washington, D.C.: OPPT, U.S. Environmental Protection Agency, 1986. TOXICOLOGY.

Dow Corning Corporation. Results of range finding toxicological tests on dimethyl cyclic tetramer. Washington, D.C.: OPPT, U.S. Environmental Protection Agency, 1985. TOXICOLOGY.

Dow Corning Corporation. Results of range finding toxicological tests on octamethylcyclotetrasiloxane. Washington, D.C.: OPPT, U.S. Environmental Protection Agency, 1985. TOXICOLOGY.

Dow Corning Corporation. Silastic II Mammary Implant, H. P., and Silastic MSI Mammary Implant, H. P., Premarket Approval Application. Midland, Mich.: Dow Corning Corporation, 1991. SILICONE CHARACTERIZATION.

Dow Corning Corporation. Then-octanol/Water Partition Coefficient of octamethylcyclotetrasiloxane). Washington, D.C.: OPPT, U.S. Environmental Protection Agency, 1987. TOXICOLOGY.

Dow Corning Corporation. Toxicity studies on hexamthyldisiloxane (DC 200 fluid). Washington, D.C.: OPPT, U.S. Environmental Protection Agency, 1986. TOXICOLOGY.

Dow Corning Corporation. Toxicity studies on TX-135A. Washington, D.C.: OPPT, U.S. Environmental Protection Agency, 1986. TOXICOLOGY.

Dow Corning Corporation. Two-Year Implant Studies with Silastic Materials in Dogs. Midland, Mich.: Dow Corning Corporation, 1970 Apr 14. TOXICOLOGY.

Dow Corning Corporation. U.S., and International Studies of Breast Implants and Rupture. 1997 Dec. RUPTURE.

Dowden, R. V. Definition of terms for describing loss of gel from breast implants [letter]. American Journal of Roentgenology. 1993 Jun, 160, 1360. RUPTURE.

Dowden, R. V. Proper terminology for status of breast implants [letter]. Plast. Reconstr. Surg. 1993 May, 91, (6): 1174. RUPTURE/letter.

Dowden, R. V., and Anain, S. Leaking gel implants [letter]. Plast. Reconstr. Surg. 1993 Dec, 92, (7): 1411. RUPTURE/local complications/letter.

Dowden, R. V., Young, V. L., and Colon, G. A. Failed implant versus silicone bleed [letter]. Plast. Reconstr. Surg. 1996 Dec, 98, (7): 1323. LOCAL COMPLICATIONS/rupture/letter.

Dugowson, C. E., Daling, J., Koepsell, T. D., Voigt, L., and Nelson, J. L. Silicone breast implants and risk for rheumatoid arthritis [abstract]. Arthritis and Rheumatism. 1992 Sep, 35, 9 (Supplement): 66. CONNECTIVE TISSUE DISEASE.

Duvic, M. Sézary syndrome in association with silicone breast implant [letter-reply]. Journal of the American Academy of Dermatology. 1995 Dec, 33, (6): 1060-1061. IMMUNE EFFECTS/ connective tissue disease/cancer/letter.

Eaborn, C. Reactions of silicon-carbon bonds. Organosilicon Compounds. London: Butterworths Scientific Publications, 1960, p. 122-505, Chapters 4-17. SILICONE CHARACTERIZATION.

Edelman, D. A., Grant, S., and van Os, W. A. A. Breast cancer and silicone breast implants. International Journal of Gynecology & Obstetrics. 1994, 47, 295-296. CANCER/letter.

Edelman, D. A., Grant, S., and Van Os, W. A. A. Breast cancer and silicone breast implants. International Journal of Gyn Obstetrics. 1994 Dec, 47, (3): 295-296. CANCER/letter.

Edison, R. B. Capsular contracture: A new concept for an old problem [letter]. Plast. Reconstr. Surg. 1991 Jan, 87, (1): 198. POLYURETHANE/capsule-contracture/local complications/letter.

Edlavitch, S. Antipolymer antibodies, silicone breast implants, and fibromyalgia [letter]. The Lancet. 1997 Apr 19, 349, (9059): 1170. IMMUNE EFFECTS/connective tissue disease/letter.

Edminston, Jr. C. E., and Sanger, J. R. Re: Fibroblast behavior in vitro is unaltered by products of staphylococci cultured from silicone implants [letter]. Annals of Plastic Surgery. 1994 Jun, 32, (6): 650-653. INFECTION/local complications/letter.

Edmond, J., and Versaci, A. D. Late complication of closed capsulotomy of the breast. Plastic and Reconstructive Surgery. 1980 Sep. RUPTURE/closed capsulotomy/local complications/letter.

Edworthy, S. M., and Martin, L. Local connective tissue effects of saline and silicone breast implants: The Alberta experience. Arthritis and Rheumatism. 1995 Sep, 38, (9 (Supplement)): S325. CAPSULE CONTRACTURE/local complications/immune effects/connective tissue disease/saline.

Edworthy, S. M., Martin, L., and Talavera, R. Symptoms reported by breast implant patients: rheumatic disease or not? Arthritis and Rheumatism. 1993 Sep, 36, (9 (Supplement)): S118. CONNECTIVE TISSUE DISEASE/immune effects.

Egilman, D. S., and Stubbs, C. Evaluating the health risks of breast implants [letter-reply]. The New England Journal of Medicine. 1996 Oct 10, 335, (15): 1154-1155. GENERAL/letter.

Ehrlich, G. E. Regarding silicone implants and rheumatic disorders [letter]. Arthritis and Rheumatism. 1995 May, 38, (5): 721-722. GENERAL/letter.

Eisenbaum, A. M. The safety of silicone for ophthalmic use [letter]. Plast. Reconstr. Surg. 1994 Nov, 94, (6): 895. GENERAL/letter.

Eklund, G. W. Collapse of a breast implant after mammography [letter-reply]. AJR American Journal of Roentgentology. 1990 Jun, 154, 1345-1346. CAPSULE-CONTRACTURE/local complications/rupture/mammography/letter.

Elbaz, J. S., and Ohana, J., Prostheses mammaires. Medicine et Sciences Internatinales, Paris. 1982. GENERAL.

Ellenberg, A. H. Steroids in breast implants [letter]. Plast. Reconstr. Surg. 1983 Feb, 71, (2): 282-283. STEROIDS/local complications/letter.

Engel, A., and Lamm, S. H. Risk of sarcomas of the breast among women with breast augmentation [letter]. Plast. Reconstr. Surg. 1992 Mar, 89, 571-572. CANCER/letter.

Englert, M., Morris, D., and March, L. Silicone? Silica? Scleroderma. A need to look further? [letter]. Australia New Zealand Journal of Medicine. 1996, 26, (6): 858. GENERAL/connective tissue disease/silica/letter.

Environ Corporation. Evaluation of the safety of silicone gel-filled breast prostheses: issues related to human health. Arlington, VA : Environ Corporation, 1991 Jul 3. LOCAL COMPLICATIONS.

Epstein, W. A. Sclerodermalike esophageal disease in children of mothers with silicone breast implants [letter]. J. Amer. Med. Assoc. 1994 Sep 14, 272, (10): 768. CHILDREN'S EFFECTS/breast feeding/letter.

Epstein, W. A. Silicone breast implants and breast feeding [letter]. J. Rheumatol. 1997, 24, (5): 1013. BREAST FEEDING/children's effects.

Epstein, W. A. Silicone breast implants and sclerodermalike esophageal disease in breast-fed infants [letter]. J. Amer. Med. Assoc. 1996 Jan 17, 275, (3): 184. CHILDREN'S EFFECTS/breast feeding/letter.

Erlank, J. D. Ultrasound for diagnosis of ruptured breast implant [letter]. Plast. Reconstr. Surg. 1992 May, 89, (5): 995. MAMMOGRAPHY/rupture/local complications/letter.

Ersek, R. A. Capsule thickness and breat firmness [letter-reply]. Plast. Reconstr. Surg. 1992 Feb, 89, (2): 380. CAPSULE-CONTRACTURE/local complications/letter.

Ersek, R. A. Textured silicone breast implants [letter]. Plast. Reconstr. Surg. 1995 Apr, 95, (4): 771-772. POLYURETHANE/letter.

Ersek, R. A. Total implant tracking system [letter]. Plast. Reconstr. Surg. 1990 Oct, 86, (4): 808-809. GENERAL/letter.

Eschbach, C. S., and Schulz, C. O. Chemical characterization of silicone gel-filled breast prosthesis materials, redacted. McGhan Medical Corporation, 1994 Jan 19. TOXICOLOGY.

European Committee on Quality Assurance and Medical Devices in Plastic Surgery. Consensus Declaration EQUAM—June 28, 1996 [position paper]. Regensburg: EQUAM, 1996 Jun. GENERAL.

European Committee on Quality Assurance and Medical Devices in Plastic Surgery. Consensus Declaration on Breast Implants-July 4, 1998. Regensburg: EQUAM, 1998 Jul. GENERAL.

Evans, G. R. D. Silicone tissue assays [letter-reply]. Plast. Reconstr. Surg. 1995 Apr, 95, (4): 770-771. SILICON MEASUREMENT/letter.

Everson, M. P. Silicone immunology [letter]. Science and Medicine. 1997 Jan-1997 Feb 28, 4, (1): 3. IMMUNE EFFECTS/letter.

Everson, M. P., and Blackburn Jr., W. D. Antipolymer antibodies, silicone breast implants and fibromyalgia [letter]. The Lancet. 1997 Apr 19, 349, (9059): 1171. IMMUNE EFFECTS/connective tissue disease/letter.

Everson, M. P., Bradley, Jr. E. L., and Blackburn, Jr. W. D. Silicone gel and hypersensitivity [letter]. Plast. Reconstr. Surg. 1996 Dec, 98, (7): 1324-1325. IMMUNE EFFECTS/letter.

Everson, M. P., Koopman, W. J., and Blackburn, Jr. W. D. Elevated expression of soluble intercellular adhesion molecule-1 (sICAM-1) in rheumatoid arthritis (RA) and systemic lupus erythematosus [abstract]. Arthritis and Rheumatol. 1992, 35, (Supplement): S48. IMMUNE EFFECTS.

Felix, K., Janz, S., Pitha, J., Williams, J. A., Mushinski, E. B., Bornkamm, G. W., and Potter, M. Cytotoxicity and membrane damage in vitro by inclusion complexes between gamma-cyclodextrin and siloxanes. Potter, M., and Rose, N., eds. Current Topics In Microbiology and Immunology: Immunology of Silicones. Heidelberg: Springer-Verlag, 1996, pp. 93-99. TOXICOLOGY.

Fenske, N. A., and Vasey, F. B. Silicone associated connective-tissue disease: The debate rages [editorial]. Archives of Dermatology. 1993 Jan, 129, (1): 97-98. CONNECTIVE TISSUE DISEASE.

Ferdinandi, E. S., and Beattie, G. Method Development for the Determination of 14C-Octamethylcyclotetrasiloxane (D4) Pharmacokinetics in the Rat Following Single Nose-Only Vapor Inhalation Exposure to 14C-D4. Midland, Mich.: Dow Corning Corporation, 1996a Jul 31. TOXICOLOGY.

Ferdinandi, E. S., and Beattie, G. Pharmacokinetics of 14C-octamethylcyclotetrasiloxane (D4) in the Rat Following 14 Repeat Daily Nose-Only Vapor Inhalation Exposures to Unlabeled D4 and a Single Exposure (Day 15) to 14C-D4 at Two Dose Levels. Midland, Mich.: Dow Corning Corporation, 1997 Aug 25. TOXICOLOGY.

Ferdinandi, E. S., and Beattie, G. Pharmacokinetics of 14C-Octamethylcyclotetrasiloxane (D4) in the Rat Following Single Nose-Only Vapor Inhalation Exposure to 14C-D4 at Three Dose Levels. Midland, Mich.: Dow Corning Corporation, 1996b Sep 27. TOXICOLOGY.

Field, T., and Bridges, A. J. Clinical and laboratory features of patients with scleroderma and silicone implants. Current Topics in Microbiology and Immunology: Immunology of Silicones. 1996, p. 419-425. CONNECTIVE TISSUE DISEASE.

Findlay, J., and Krueger, J. F. Skin sensitization study of Dow Corning® 2-0707 Intermediate (platinum #4) using the guinea pig maximization test (GPMT). Chicago, Ill.: IIT Research Institute, 1996b Oct 30. PLATINUM/toxicology.

Findlay, J., and Krueger, J. F. Skin sensitization study of Dow Corning® 3-8015 Intermediate (platinum #2) using the guinea pig maximization test (GPMT). Chicago, Ill.: IIT Research Institute, 1996a Oct 30. PLATINUM/toxicology.

Finegold, I. Silicone gel breast implants [letter]. J. Amer. Med. Assoc. 1994 Jul 27, 272, (4): 271-272. GENERAL/letter.

Fisher, J. C. Analysis of explanted silicone implants: A report of 300 patients [invited discussion]. Annals of Plastic Surgery. 1995 Jan, 34, (1): 6-7. RUPTURE/local complications.

Fisher, J. C. The silicone controversy—when will science prevail? [commentary]. The New England Journal of Medicine. 1992 Jun 18, 326, (25): 1696-1698. GENERAL.

Fivenson, D., Saed, G., and Ladin, D. T-cell response profile in silicone gel breast implant capsules. Joint Meeting of the Central Society for Clinical Research, Midwest Section American Federation for Clinical Research, Midwest Society for Pediatric Research and the Central Region Society for Investigative Dermatology. Clin Res. 1992, 40, 709A. IMMUNE EFFECTS.

Flaningam, O. L., and Langley, N. R. Physical properties and polymer structure. Smith, A. L., ed. The analytical chemistry of silicones. John Wiley & Sons, Inc., 1991, pp. 135-173. SILICONE CHARACTERIZATION.

Flick, J. A. Sclerodermalike esophageal disease in children of mothers with silicone breast implants [letter]. J. Amer. Med. Assoc. 1994 Sep 14, 272, (10): 770. CHILDREN'S EFFECTS/breast feeding.

Florke, O., W., Martin, B., and Bendo, L. et al. Silica. in: Elvers, B., Hawkins, S., Russy, W., and Schulz, G. Eds. Ullmann's Encyclopedia of Industrial Chemistry, Vol A23. New York: VCH Publishers, 1993. SILICA.

Fodor, P. B. Breast reconstruction in patients after chest-wall irradiation [letter]. Plast. Reconstr. Surg. 1997 Jan, 99, (2): 274. RECONSTRUCTION/expander/letter.

Food and Drug Administration. 144 Guidance for gel-filled breast prostheses—1992 [Web Page]. 1992. Available at: www.fda.gov/cdrh/ode/107.html. GENERAL.

Food and Drug Administration. Background information on the possible health risks of silicone breast implants. Rockville, MD: U.S. Food and Drug Administration, 1988. GENERAL.

Food and Drug Administration. Breast Implants: An information update. 1997 Jul. GENERAL/polyurethane.

Food and Drug Administration. Chronology of FDA Activities. Rockville, Md: Department of Health and Human Services, 1998. GENERAL.

Food and Drug Administration. General and plastic surgery devices, effective data of requirement for premarket approval of silicone inflatable breast prosthesis. Federal Register. 1993 Jan 8, Part X, (21 CFR Part 878): 3436-3443. GENERAL.

Food and Drug Administration. General and plastic surgery devices, effective data of requirement for premarket approval of silicone gel-filled breast prosthesis, final rule. Federal Register. 1991 Apr 10, Part V, (21 CFR Part 878): 14620-14627. GENERAL.

Food and Drug Administration. General and plastic surgery devices, effective date of requirement for premarket approval of silicone gelfilled breast prosthesis. Federal Register. 1990 May 17, 55, (96): 20568-20577. GENERAL.

Food and Drug Administration U.S. Food and Drug Administration. General and Plastic Surgery Devices Panel Meeting Transcript. Washington, D.C., 1988 Nov 22. GENERAL.

Food and Drug Administration. U.S. Food and Drug Administration. General and Plastic Surgery Devices Panel Meeting Transcript. Washington, D.C., 1989 Jan 26. GENERAL.

Food and Drug Administration. General and Plastic Surgery Devices Panel Meeting Transcript. Washington, D.C., 1992a Feb 18. GENERAL.

Food and Drug Administration. Hearing before the Human Resources and Intergovernmental Relations Subcommittee of the Committee on Government Operations, House of Representatives, 1990 Dec 18, Washington, D.C. Washington, D.C.: U.S. Government Printing Office, 1991a. GENERAL.

Food and Drug Administration. Important Information on Breast Implants. Food and Drug Administration, 1991b Sep. POLYURETHANE/general.

Food and Drug Administration. Medical devices, device tracking, final rules and request for comments. Federal Register. 1993 Aug 16, Part IV, (21 CFR Part 821): 43442-43455. GENERAL.

Food and Drug Administration. An Overview of the Final Regulations Implementing the Mammography Quality Standards Act of 1992. Rockville, MD: U.S. Department of Health and Human Services, 1997 Oct. MAMMOGRAPHY/general.

Food and Drug Administration. Quality Mammography Standards, Final Rule. Federal Register. 1997 Oct 28, 21 CFR Parts 16 and 900, 55853-55994. MAMMOGRAPHY/general.

Food and Drug Administration. Stratemeyer, M. E., Project Officer. Silicone in Medical Devices: Conference Proceedings, 1991 Feb, Baltimore, Md. Rockville, Md.: U.S. Department of Health and Human Services, 1991 Dec. GENERAL.

Food and Drug Administration. Study of children breast fed by women with breast implants. Rockville, Md.: U.S. Department of Health and Human Services, 1994 Jan. BREAST FEEDING/general.

Food and Drug Administration. Update: Study of TDA Released from Polyurethane Foam-Covered Breast Implants. Rockville, Md.: U.S. Department of Health and Human Services, 1995 Jun 27. POLYURETHANE/toxicology/general.

Food and Drug Administration, Office of Science and Technology. The effect of fold flaws in breast implant shells' failure characteristics. Annual report, Fiscal year 1998. Rockville, Md.: U.S. Department of Health and Human Services, 1998a RUPTURE/local complications.

Food and Drug Administration. Collagen and Liquid Silicone Injections. Rockville, Md.: U.S. Department of Health and Human Services, 1991 Aug. SILICONE INJECTION/general.

Forsythe, R. L. Silicone gel implant failure [letter]. Plast. Reconstr. Surg. 1992 Oct, 90, (4): 729-730. RUPTURE/local complications/migration/letter.

Foster, M. T., and et al. Mycobacterial infections associated with augmentation mammoplasty—Florida, North Carolina, Texas. MMWR. 1978: 513. INFECTION/local complications.

Fourie, L. R., and Lamont, A. Silicone-gel-filled breast implants [editorial]. South African Medical Journal. 1991 Sep 21, 80, 307-308. GENERAL.

Francel, T. J. Silcone-gel implant longevity (abstract). San Diego: American Society for Plastic and Reconstructive Surgery, 1998. RUPTURE/local complications.

Frank, G. I. Science in the courtroom [letter]. New England Journal of Medicine. 1994, 331, (16): 1099. GENERAL/letter.

Frechette, C. N. Subcutaneous Mastectomy [letter]. Plast. Reconstr. Surg. 1990, 86, (1): 166. POLYURETHANE/letter.

Freeman, B. S. On the implantation of free silicone gel [letter]. Plast. Reconstr. Surg. 1977, 60, (5): 780. SILICONE INJECTION/letter.

Freeman, H. A., and Durall, R. L. Microscopical characterization. Smith, A. L. The Analytical Chemistry of Silicones. John Wiley & Sons, Inc., 1991, pp. 219-253. SILICONE CHARACTERIZATION.

Freundlich, B., Sandorfi, N., Altman, C., and Tomaszewski, J. Monocyte/macrophage infiltrates in the salivary glands of women with silicone breast implants. Current Topics in Microbiology and Immunology: Immunology of Silicones. 1996, p. 419-425. IMMUNE EFFECTS/CONNECTIVE TISSUE DISEASE.

Freundlich, B., Tomaszewski, J., and Callegari, P. A Sjögren's-like syndrome in women with silicone-gel breast implants [abstract]. Arthritis and Rheumatism. 1992, 35 (Supplement), S67. IMMUNE EFFECTS/connective tissue disease.

Frisch, E. E. Invited discussion on spontaneous autoinflation of saline mammary implants [reply]. Annals of Plastic Surgery. 1998, 40, (1): 101-103. SALINE/letter/rupture.

Frisch, E. E. Silicone breast implant. Rubin, L. R., Ed. Biomaterials In Reconstructive Surgery. St. Louis: The C.V. Mosby Company, 1983. GENERAL.

Frisch, E. E. Silicone chemistry and pharmacokinetics. in. Silicone in medical devices, Proceeding of a Conference, 1991: DHHS, 1991. SILICONE CHEMISTRY/silicone characterization.

Frisch, E. E. Spontaneous autoinflation of saline mammary implants [discussion]. Annals of Plastic Surgery. 1997 Aug, 39, (2): 118-121. SALINE.

Frisch, E. E., and Langley, N. R. Biodurability evaluation of medical-grade high performance silicone elastomer. In: Fraker, A. C., and Griffith, C. D., Eds. Corrosion and Degradation of Implant Materials: Second Symposium, ASTM Special Technical Publication 859. Philadelphia: American Society for Testing and Materials, 1985, p. 67. RUPTURE/local complications.

Fritzler, M. J. Immunofluorescent antinuclear antibody tests. In: Rose, N. R., Friedman, H., and Fahey, J. L. Manual of Clinical Laboratory Immunology. Third ed. Washington, D.C.: American Society for Microbiology, 1986, p. 733-739. IMMUNE EFFECTS/ai-ctd background.

Fuchs, H., Johnson, J. S., and Sergent, J. S. Still more on breast implants and connective tissue diseases [letter]. The New England Journal of Medicine. 1995 Aug 24, 333, (5): 526. CONNECTIVE TISSUE DISEASE.

Furst, A., and Rading, S. B. Platinum (Pt). in: Wexler, P. Ed. Encyclopedia of Toxicology. Academic Press, 1998. TOXICOLOGY.

Gabriel, S. E., Melton, L. J., Woods, J. E., O'Fallon, W. M., and Kurtland, L. T. Silicone-containing breast implants and connective tissue diseases: A population-based retrospective cohort study [abstract]. Arthritis and Rheumatism. 1993, 36 (Supplement), S70. CONNECTIVE TISSUE DISEASE.

Gabriel, S. E., O'Fallon, W. M., and Kurland, L. T. Breast implants and connective-tissue diseases [letter-reply]. The New England Journal of Medicine. 1994 Nov 3, 331, (18): 1233-1234. CONNECTIVE TISSUE DISEASE/letter.

Gabriel, S. E., O'Fallon, W. M., Kurland, L. T., and Melton, L. J. Letters to the Editor [letter]. Life Sciences. 1995, 57, (19): 1737-1740. CONNECTIVE TISSUE DISEASE/letter.

Galbraith, T. W., Duwe R.L., and Malczewski, R. M. Development of a Positive Control for the Primary Popliteal Lymph Node Assay in Mice Using Ammonium Hexachloroplatinate. Midland, Mich.: Dow Corning Corporation, 1993 Jul 21. PLATINUM/toxicology.

Gallagher, H. S., Leis, H. P., Snyderman, R. V., and Urban, J. A. The Breast [book review by Clifford C. Snyder]. St. Louis: C.V. Mosby Co., 1978. GENERAL.

Garland, L. L., Ballester, O. F., Vasey, F. B., Benson, K., Moscinski, L. C., Farmelo, M. J., Rodriguez, M. J., and Rapaport, D. P. Multiple myeloma in women with silicone breast implants. Serum immunoglobulin and interleukin-6-studies in women at risk. Curr Top Microbiol Immunol. 1996, 210, 361-366. MYELOMA.

Garrido, L., and Ackerman, J. L. Re: Do patients with silicone-gel breast implants have elevated levels of blood silicon compared with control patients? [letter]. Annals of Plastic Surgery. 1995 Oct, 35, (4): 441-442. SILICON MEASUREMENT/letter.

Garrido, L., Bogdanova, A., Cheng, L. L., Pfleiderer, B., Tokareva, E., Ackerman, J. L., and Brady, T. J. Detection of silicone migration and biodegradation with NMR. Current Topics in Microbiology and Immunology. 1996, 210, 49-58. MIGRATION/mammography.

Garrido, L., Pfleiderer, B., and Jenkins, B. G. et al. Erratum. Mag. Res. Med. 1998, 40, (5): 689. SILICON MEASUREMENT.

Geary, R. S., Dammann, M., and Mason, R. A Qualification Study of the Methods for Measuring Extractable Platinum Content in Dow Corning Silicone Gel-Filled Mammary Implant Devices: Draft Final Report Prepared for Dow Corning Corporation. San Antonio, Tex.: Southwest Research Institute, 1994 Oct. PLATINUM/toxicology.

Georgiade, N. G. The role of the rectus abdominis myocutaneous flap in breast reconstruction [discussion]. Plast. Reconstr. Surg. 1982 Feb, 69, (2): 215. RECONSTRUCTION.

German Government. Answer of the Federal Government to a request of the SPD. 1998 Nov 5. GENERAL.

Gerow, F. J. Breast implants. in: Georgiade, N. G., ed. Reconstructive Breast Surgery. St. Louis, Mo.: The C.V. Mosby Company, 1976, p. 31-49. GENERAL.

Glasser, J. W., Lee, N. C., and Wingo, P. A. Does Breast Augmentation Increase the Risk of Breast Cancer? In: Proceedings of Epidemiologic Intelligence Service, 38th Annual Conference, 1989 Apr 3-1989 Apr 8, Atlanta. Centers for Disease Control, 1989. CANCER.

Gluck, O. S., Tessar, J. R. P., Tenenbaum, S. A., and et al. Development of a laboratory marker for fibromyalgia [abstract]. Arthritis and Rheumatism. 1996, 39, 590. AI-CTD BACKGROUND.

Goin, M. K. The psychological impact of immediate breast reconstruction for women with early breast cancer [discussion]. Plast. Reconstr. Surg. 1984 Apr, 73, (4): 627-628. PSYCHOSOCIAL/reconstruction.

Gold, A. H. Mammary prostheses: Size and shape relationships. in: Rubin, L. R., Ed. Biomaterials in Reconstructive Surgery. St. Louis: The C.V. Mosby Company, 1983. GENERAL.

Goldberg, E. P. Evaluating the health risks of breast implants [letter]. The New England Journal of Medicine. 1996 Oct 10, 335, (15): 1154. GENERAL/letter.

Goldberg, E. P. Silicone breast implant safety: Physical, chemical, and biologic problems [letter]. Plast. Reconstr. Surg. 1997 Jan, 99, (1): 258-260. RUPTURE/capsule-contracture/migration/local complications/letter.

Goldberg, E. P., and Widenhouse, C. Failure of silicone gel breast implants: Analysis of literature data for 1652 explanted prostheses [letter-reply]. Plast. Reconstr. Surg. 1998, 101, (4): 1163-1164. RUPTURE/letter/local complications.

Goldberg, E. P., Widenhouse, C., Marotta, J., and Martin, P. Failure of silicone gel breast implants: Analysis of literature data for 1652 explanted prostheses [letter]. Plast. Reconstr. Surg. 1997 Jul, 100, (1): 281-284. RUPTURE/local complications/letter.

Goldblum, R. M., Pyron, D., and Shenoy, M. Modulation of IgG binding to silicone by human serum albumin [abstract]. FASEB J. 1995, 9, A1029 (abstr 5967). IMMUNE EFFECTS.

Goldman, J. A. Silicone augmentation mammoplasty (SAM): A specific musculoskeletal spectrum due to these implants? Arthritis and Rheumatism. 1991, 34, R35. CONNECTIVE TISSUE DISEASE.

Goldman, J. A., Lamm, S. H., Cooper, W., and Cooper, L. Breast implants are not associated with an excess of connective tissue disease (CTD). Arthritis and Rheumatism. 1992, 35 Suppl, S65 (Abstr.). CONNECTIVE TISSUE DISEASE.

Goldsmith, Silverman, and Solomon. Methodology for Estimating Sensitivity and Specificity for Systemic Silicone-Related Disorders (Ssrd) (Abstract T128). 1996 Annual Conference of ISEE, 1996, 1996 Jul. CONNECTIVE TISSUE DISEASE.

Gordon, P. B. Malignant breast masses detected only with US [abstract]. Radiology. 1994, 193, 177. MAMMOGRAPHY.

Gott, D. M., and Tinkler, J. J. B., editors. Silicone Implants and Connective Tissue Disease. London: UK Medical Devices Agency, 1994 Dec. GENERAL.

Gottlieb, L. J., and Greenwald, D. P. Quantitative analysis of lidocaine HCI delivery by diffusion across tissue expander membranes [discussion]. Plast. Reconstr. Surg. 1992, 89, (5): 900-907. PAIN/general.

Grasso, P., Golberg, L., and Fairweather, F. A. Injection of silicones in mice [letter]. The Lancet. 1964 Jul 11, 2, 96. TOXICOLOGY/silicone injection/letter.

Grazer, F. M., and Heinrichs, H. L. Augmentation Mammaplasty: survey of 200 consecutive implants. Symposium on Aesthetic Surgery of the Breast. St Louis, Mo.: Mosby, 1978. GENERAL.

Greco, D. Silicone modification: A chemical and bacteriological study. Proceedings of the X Congress of the International Confederation for Plastic and Reconstructive Surgeons, June 28-July 3, 1992. vol. 3 ed. Madrid, Spain: International Confederation for Plastic and Reconstructive Surgeons, 1992. GENERAL.

Greene, W. B. Silicon in rat knee joints after subcutaneous injection of dimethylpolysiloxane gel breast implant material. 52nd annual meeting of the Microscopy Society of America and the 29th annual meeting of the Microbeam Analysis Society, 1994: pp 182-183. SILICON MEASUREMENT/local complications.

Greene, W. B., and Walsh, L. G. Silicone in remote tissues after breast augmentation mammoplasty. Bull. Southeast Electron Microscopy Society. 1992, 24, 27A. MIGRATION/local complications.

Greenwald, D. P., Randol.ph, M., and May, Jr. J. W. Mechanical analysis of explanted silicone breast implants (letter). Plast. Reconstr. Surg. 1997, 99, (7): 2117. RUPTURE/local complications/letter.

Groh, C. L. Acute Toxicity and Industrial Handling Hazards of Dow Corning® Platinum No. 1 and Dow Corning® Platinum No. 2. Midland, Mich.: Dow Corning Corporation, 1973 Sep 10. PLATINUM/toxicology.

Groh, C. L. Acute Toxicologic Properties and Industrial Handling Hazards of Dow Corning® X-2-7018. Midland, Mich.: Dow Corning Corporation, 1972 Nov 10. PLATINUM/toxicology.

Groth, D., Kommineni, C., Morman, W., Stettler, L., and Wagner, W. Pathologic effects of inhaled amorphous silicas in animals. Presented at ASTM International Symposium on Health Effects, 1979 Nov 6. SILICA.

Guidoin, R., Rolland, C., King, M., Roy, P., and Therrien, M. Morphological analysis of 269 surgically excised mammary prostheses. In: Food and Drug Administration. Silicone in Medical Devices, 1991 Feb, Baltimore, Md. Rockville, Md.: U.S. Department of Health and Human Services, 1991 Feb 1, c1991. RUPTURE/expander/local complications.

Guidoin, R., Rolland, C., Roy, P. E., Marois, M., and Blais, P. Foam Separation in Polyurethane-Covered Breast Prostheses. In: High Performance Biomaterials, Szycher, M. Ed. Lancaster, Pa.: Technomic Publishing Co. 1991a, pp. 191-206. POLYURETHANE.

Gurdin, M. Augmentation Mammaplasty. in: Goldwyn, R. M. The Unfavorable Result in Plastic Surgery. Boston, Mass.: Little, Brown and Company, 1972, p. 353-385. GENERAL.

Guthrie, R. H., and Podolsky, D. The truth about breast implants. New York: John Wiley and Sons, 1994.

Hall, F. M. Breast augmentation and the risk of subsequent breast cancer [letter]. The New England Journal of Medicine. 1993 Mar 4, 329, (9): 661. CANCER/letter.

Hall, F. M., Homer, M. J., D'Orsi, C. J., and Eklund, G. W. Mammography of the augmented breast [letter]. American Journal of Roentgenology. 1989 Nov, 153, 1098-1099. MAMMOGRAPHY/letter.

Handel, N. Does irradiation to the augmented breast produce scar contracture? [letter-reply]. Plast. Reconstr. Surg. 1992 Feb, 89, (2): 381. RADIATION/capsule-contracture/local complications/letter.

Handel, N. Health risks of failed silicone gel breast implants, with reply by Duffy, M.J. [letter]. Plast. Reconstr. Surg. 1995 May, 95, (6): 1129-1131. GENERAL/local complications/rupture/letter.

Harris, K. M., Ganott, M. A., and Skolnich, M. L. US appearance of ruptured silicone breast implants [letter-reply]. Radiology. 1994, 190, 584. MAMMOGRAPHY/local complications/rupture.

Hawes, D. R. Collapse of a breast implant after mammography [letter]. American Journal of Roentgentology. 1990 Jun, 154, 1345. RUPTURE/mammography/letter.

Hayes Jr., H. Could tight breast capsules squeeze a significant amount of silicone gel out of an implant? [letter-reply]. Plast. Reconstr. Surg. 1993 Sep, 92, (3): 558. CAPSULE-CONTRACTURE/local complications.

Hazleton Washington. Combined chronic toxicity and oncongenicity study in rats. Vienna, VA: Hazleton Washington, Inc., 1992. TOXICOLOGY/carcinogenicity.

Heaney, P. J. Structure and chemistry of the low-pressure silica polymorphs. Heaney, P. J., Prewitt, C. T., and Gibbs, G. V., Eds. Silica, Physical Behavior, Geochemistry and Materials Application. Washington, D.C.: Mineralogical Society of America, 1994, p. 41-49. SILICA.

Heaney, P. J., Prewitt, C. T., and Gibbs, G. V. Silica physical behavior, geochemistry and materials applications. in. Reviews in Mineralogy. Washington, D.C.: Mineralogical Society of America, 1994. SILICA.

Hedges, L. K and Ioriani, P. MRI diagnosis of leaking silicone implants using a silicone saturation technique. Works In Progress: 10th Annual Meeting of Society of Magnetic Resonance In Medicine, 1991 Aug 10. MAMMOGRAPHY/rupture/local complications.

Heinlein and Bassett, L. W. Positioning. in: Bassett, L. W. et al. Diagnosis of Diseases of the Breast. W. B. Saunders, 1997. MAMMOGRAPHY.

Hemley, P. J. High-pressure behavior of silica. Heaney, P. J., Prewitt, C. T., and Gibbs, G. V., Eds. Silica: Physical Behavior, Geochemistry and Materials Application. Washington, D.C.: Mineralogical Society of America, 1994, p. 1-40. SILICA.

Hennekens, C. H. Lee I-Min, Cook, N. R., Hebert, P. R., Karlson, E. W., LaMotte, F., Manson, J. E., and Buring, J. E. Breast implants and connective-tissue disease [letter-reply]. J. Amer. Med. Assoc. 1996 Jul 10, 276, (2): 103. CONNECTIVE TISSUE DISEASE/letter.

Hepburn, C. Polyurethane elastomers. Applied Science. New York, 1982, p. Chapter 11. POLYURETHANE.

Herman, S. Infection surrounding Meme implants (letter). Plast. Reconstr. Surg. 1985, 75, (6): 926. INFECTION/local complications/letter.

Herrinton, L. J. The epidemiology of monoclonal gammopathy of unknown significance: A review. In: Current Topics in Microbiology and Immunology: Immunology of Silicones. 1996, p. 389-395. MYELOMA.

Hersemann, S. Health Outcomes in Women With Silicone Breast Implants: Analysis of The 1988 NHIS Data [abstract]. Presented at Sept. 1995 Meeting of American College of Epidemiology, 1995 Sep. CONNECTIVE TISSUE DISEASE.

Herzog, P. Silicone granuloma detection by ultrasonography [letter]. Plast. Reconstr. Surg. 1989 Nov, 84, (5): 856-857. MAMMOGRAPHY/granulomas/local complications/letter.

Herzog, P. M., Exner, K., Holtermueller, K. H., Quayson, J., and Lemperle, G. Detection with US of implant rupture and siliconomas [abstract]. Radiology. 1993, 189, 155. MAMMOGRAPHY/local complications/rupture/granulomas.

Hess, E. V. Environmental lupus syndromes [editorial]. British Journal of Rheumatology. 1995, 34, (7): 597-599. AI-CTD BACKGROUND.

Hester, Jr. T. R., and Bostwick, F. Implants and Expanders. in. Plastic and Reconstructive Breast Surgery, Bostwick, III, J., Ed., Vol I. St. Louis, Mo.: Quality Medical Publishing, Inc., 1990. EXPANDER.

Heywang, S. H., and Lissner, J. Carcinoma of the breast behind a breast prosthesis: Choice of imaging modality [letter]. Computerized Radiology. 1987, 11, (4): 209-211. MAMMOGRAPHY/cancer/letter.

Hill, A. B. The environment and disease: association or causation? Proceedings of the Royal Society of Medicine. 1965, 58, 295-300. GENERAL.

Hill, S. L., Landavere, M. G., and Rose, N. R. The adjuvant effect of silicone gel and silicone elastomer particles in rats. Current Topics in Microbiology and Immunology. 1996, 210, 123-137. IMMUNE EFFECTS.

Ho, L. C. Y. Endoscopic-assisted augmentation mammaplasty [letter]. British Journal of Plastic Surgery. 1996, 49, (8): 576-577. LOCAL COMPLICATIONS/rupture/capsule-contracture/local complications/saline/letter.

Ho, W. C. Radiographic evidence of breast implant rupture [letter]. Plast. Reconstr. Surg. 1987 Jun, 79, (6): 1009-1010. LOCAL COMPLICATIONS/rupture/mammography.

Hochberg, M. C. Silicone breast implants and rheumatic disease [editorial]. British Journal of Rheumatology. 1994, 33, (7): 601-602. CONNECTIVE TISSUE DISEASE.

Hochberg, M. C., and Perlmutter, D. L. The association of augmentation mammoplasty with connective tissue disease, including systematic sclerosis (scleroderma): A meta-analysis. Current Topics in Microbiology and Immunology: Immunology of Silicones. 1996, p. 411-417. CONNECTIVE TISSUE DISEASE.

Hochberg M.C., Perlmutter, D. L., White, B., Steen, V., Medsger, T. A., Weisman, M., and Wigley, F. M. The association of augmentation mammoplasty with systemic sclerosis: Results from a multi-centered case-control study [abstract]. Arthritis And Rheumatism. 1994, 37, (9 (Supplement)): S369. CONNECTIVE TISSUE DISEASE.

Hochberg, M. C., Schein, O. D., Munoz, B., Anhalt, G., Provost, T. T., and West, S. The prevalence of dry eye, dry mouth, autoimmunity and primary Sjögren's syndrome in the general population [abstract]. Arthritis and Rheumatism. 1996 Sep, 39, (9 (Supplement)): S66. AI-CTD BACKGROUND.

Hochberg, M. C., White, B., Medsger, T. A., Weisman, M., and Wigley, F. M. The association of augmentation mammoplasty with systemic sclerosis: preliminary results from a case-control study [abstract]. Arthritis and Rheumatism. 1993, 36, (9 (Supplement)): S71. CONNECTIVE TISSUE DISEASE.

Hodgkinson, D. J. Silicone breast implants: Implications for society and surgeons [letter]. Medical Journal of Australia. 1997 Jun 2, 166, (11): 615-616. GENERAL.

Hoffman, S. Breast augmentation with autologous tissue: An alternative to implants [discussion]. Plast. Reconstr. Surg. 1995 Aug, 96, (2): 385. GENERAL.

Hoffman, S. The dilemma of capsular contracture [letter]. Plast. Reconstr. Surg. 1980, 66, (3): 477. CAPSULE-CONTRACTURE/local complications/letter.

Hollingsworth, P. N., Pummer, S. C., and Dawkins, R. L. Antinuclear antibodies. Peter, J. B., and Shoenfeld, Y., Eds. Autoantibodies. Amsterdam: Elsevier, 1996. AI-CTD BACKGROUND.

Holten, I. W. R. Intraductal migration of silicone [letter]. Plast. Reconstr. Surg. 1996 Oct, 98, (5): 903. MIGRATION/local complications/letter.

Hoshaw, S. J., Klykken, P. C., and Abbott, J. P. Silicone breast implants and breast feeding [letter]. J. Rheumatol. 1997, 24, (5): 1014. BREAST FEEDING/letter/children's effects.

Howell, B. F. Low molecular weight leachables from medical grade polymers. Final Report, U.S. Department of Commerce, et al., Prepared For FDA and the Center For Medical Devices: U.S. Department of Commerce, 1982 Apr. SILICONE CHARACTERIZATION.

Hulka, B. Epidemiological analysis of silcone breast implants and connective tissue disease in silicone breast implants in relation to connective tissue disease. National Science Panel, 1998 Nov 17. TISSUE DISEASE.

Hunter, C. A. Silastic® MDX4-4210 Medical Elastomer Extraction Study. Midland, Mich.: Dow Corning Corporation, 1988 Jun 2. PLATINUM/toxicology.

Hurst, N. M. Lactation after augmentation mammoplasty/letter reply. Obstetrics and Gynecology. 1996a Jun, 87, (6): 1063. BREAST FEEDING/letter.

Iler, R. K. The occurrence, dissolution and deposition of silica. Chemistry of Silica. 1979a, pp. 3-104. SILICA.

Iler, R. K. The surface chemistry of amorphous synthetic silica interaction with organic molecules in an aqueous medium. In: Dunnom, D. D., Ed. Health Effects of Synthetic Silica Particulates, ASTM STP 732. Philadelphia: American Society for Testing and Materials, 1981, p. 3. SILICA.

Iler, R. K. The surface chemistry of silica. Chemistry of Silica. 1979b, pp. 622-714. SILICA.

Independent Advisory Committee on Silicone-Gel-Filled Breast Implants. Summary of the report on silicone-gel-filled breast implants. Can. Med. Assoc. J. 1992, 147, (8): 1141-1146. GENERAL.

Independent Review Group. Silicone Gel Breast Implants: The Report of the Independent Review Group. Cambridge, England: Jill Rogers Associates, 1998 Jul. GENERAL.

IOM Scientific Workshop. Transcripts of invited participants' presentations. National Academy of Sciences, Public Access Office, 1998 Jul 22. GENERAL.

Isquith, A. J. Salmonella/Mammalian—Microsome Plate Incorporation Mutagenicity Assay (AMES Test) and Eschericia Coli WP2 uvrA Reverse Mutation Assay with a Confirmatory Assay of Dow Corning® 7-9172 Part A. Midland, Mich.: Dow Corning Corporation, 1992 Dec 9. TOXICOLOGY.

Isquith, A. J., Galbraith, T. W., Duwe, R. L., and Klykken, P. C. A Sub-Chronic Distribution Study of 14C-Labeled Silicone Gel (Laboratory Preparation of Dow Corning® Q7-2159A) in the Mouse Following Subcutaneous Implantation [abstract]. Midland, Mich.: Dow Corning Corporation, 1991. TOXICOLOGY.

Isquith, A. J., and Miller, B. J. Mutagenicity Evaluation of Platinum II Concentrate in the Ames Bacterial Assay. Midland, Mich.: Dow Corning Corporation, 1981 Oct 8. PLATINUM/toxicology.

Israelachvili, J. N. Some therodynamic aspects of intermolecular forces. Intermolecular and Surface Forces. Orlando, Fla.: Academic Press, Inc., 1985, p. 12-23. IMMUNE EFFECTS.

Iverson, R. E. Breast implants and patient satisfaction [letter-reply]. Plast. Reconstr. Surg. 1992 May, 89, (5): 996. PSYCHOSOCIAL/letter.

Iverson, R. E. Patient Survey Commissioned by the American Society of Plastic and Reconstructive Surgeons 1990. Arlington Heights, Ill.: American Society of Plastic and Reconstructive Surgeons, 1990. PSYCHOSOCIAL.

Jackson, A. Tissue culture testing of platinum complexes for MDF-0185 elastomers (letter to Talcott, T). Dow Corning Corp, Midland, Mich. 1972 Jun 6. PLATINUM/toxicology.

Jackson, L. W., and Dennis, G. J. Blood silicon determination in patients with silicone breast implants [abstract]. Arthritis and Rheumatism. 1997 (Supplement). SILICON MEASUREMENT.

Jackson, LW., Dennis, G. J., and Centeno, J. A. Analytical determination of blood silicon in patients with silicone breast implants. In: Metal Ions in Biology and Medicine. 5 ed. Paris, 1998, p. 33-38. SILICON MEASUREMENT.

Jacobs, J. C., and Fimundo, L. F. Silicone implants and autoimmune disease [letter]. The Lancet. 1994 Feb 5, 343, 354-355. CONNECTIVE TISSUE DISEASE/letter.

Jacobs, J. C., Hensle, T. W., Imundo, L. F., and D'Agati, V. Do silicone testicular implants increase the risk of systemic lupus erythematosus (SLE) in children? Micro-vascular immune complexes may be demonstrated in the fibro-muscular tissue around silicone implants [abstract]. Arthritis and Rheumatism. 1994 Sep, 37, (9 (Supplement)): S271. IMMUNE EFFECTS/connective tissue disease.

Jacobs, J. C., Imundo, L., and Chander, P. Do silicone implants increase the risk of systemic lupus erthematosus (SLE) in children? [abstract]. Arthritis and Rheumatism. 1994 Jun, 37 , (6 (Supplement)): R42. CONNECTIVE TISSUE DISEASE.

Jahr, J. Possible health hazards from different types of amorphous silicas. Health Effects of Synthetic Silica Particulates. ASTM Special Technical Publication ed. pp. 199-210. SILICA.

Jankauskas, S. Scleroderma after silicone augmentation mammaplasty: Is there a causative relationship? [letter]. Plast. Reconstr. Surg. 1989 Jan, 83, (1): 198. CONNECTIVE TISSUE DISEASE/letter.

Jeng, L. Summary Report of the Dow Corning 1985-1987 Silicone Implant Study. Memorandum report to Melvin Stratmeyer, Chief of the Health Sciences Branch, Food and Drug Administration. Washington, D.C.: Food and Drug Administration, 1988 Aug 3. CANCER.

Jenny, H. A Re-Evaluation of the External Rupturing of the Mammary Pseudocapsule [unpublished manuscript]. Palm Springs, Calif.: 1980 Mar. CAPSULE-CONTRACTURE/ rupture/local complications.

Jenny, H. A. Silcone-gate: exposing the breast implant scandal. Siloam Springs, AR: Silicongate, 1994. GENERAL.

Jin, Y., Fan, Z., and Tang, Y. Clinical applications of China-made saline-filled breast implants: A report of 62 cases [abstract]. Chung Hua Cheng Hsing Shao Shang Wai Ko Tsa Chih. 1996 Jul, 12, (4): 257-259. SALINE.

Jobe, R. P. Effect of implants on chest wall [letter]. Plast. Reconstr. Surg. 1983 Dec, 72, (6): 919-920. LOCAL COMPLICATIONS/letter.

Jobe, R. P. in. Symposium on Aesthetic Surgery of the Breast. St Louis, Mo.: C. V. Mosby, Co., 1978. GENERAL.

Jordan, M. E., and Blum, R. W. M. Should breast-feeding by women with silicone implants be recommended? Archives of Pediatric and Adolescent Medicine. 1996, 150, (8): 880-881. BREAST FEEDING/letter.

Kaminski, N. Scientific evaluation of Dow Corning studies designed to determine potential effects on host defense and immunogenicity of silicone fluid, gel and elastomer. 1995 Jan 5. TOXICOLOGY/immune effects.

Karns, M. E., and Cullison, C. A. Breast implants and connective-tissue disease [letter]. J. Amer. Med. Assoc. 1996 Jul 10, 276, (2): 101-102. CONNECTIVE TISSUE DISEASE/ letter.

Karstedt, B. D., inventor. Platinum Complexes of Unsaturated Siloxanes and Platinum Containing Organopolysiloxanes. General Electric Company, assignee. US 3,775,452. 1973 Nov 27. PLATINUM.

Karstedt, B. D., inventor. Platinum Complexes of Unsaturated Siloxanes and Platinum Containing Organopolysiloxanes. General Electric Company, assignee. US 3,814,730. 1974 Jun 4. PLATINUM.

Karstedt, B. D., inventor. Platinum-Vinylsiloxanes [Hydrosilation Catalysts]. General Electric Company, assignee. US 3,715,334. 1973 Feb 6. PLATINUM.

Kasper, C. S. Pathology of breast implant capsules. Seminars in Breast Diseases. 1998, 1, (4): 168-175. MAMMOGRAPHY.

Kasukawa, R., Tojo, T., Miyawaki, S., Yoshida, H., Tanimoto, K., Nobunaga, M., Suzuki, T., Takasaki, Y., and Tamura, T. Preliminary diagnostic criteria for classification of mixed connective tissue disease. Kasukawa, R., and Sharp, G. C., eds. Mixed Connective Tissue Disease and Anti-Nuclear Antibodies. Japan: Elsevier Science Publishers, B.V. (Biomedical Division), Japan Intractable Diseases Research Foundation, 1987, p. 41-47. AI-CTD BACKGROUND.

Katzin, W. E., and Feng, L. J. Phenotype of lymphocytes associated with the inflammatory reaction to silicone-gel breast implants [abstract]. Mod Pathol. 1994, 7, 17A. IMMUNE EFFECTS.

Kaye, B. L. Augmentation mammaplasty: A critical review of 200 patients. in: Owsley, J. Q., and Peterson, R. A., eds. Symposium on Aesthetic Surgery of the Breast. St. Louis: Mosby, 1978, p. 267. INFECTION/steroids/capsule-contracture/granulomas/local complications.

Kayler, L. K., and Goodman, P. H. Breast implants increase the risk of arthralgia: An epidemiological meta-analysis [abstract]. Journal of Investigative Medicine. 1995 Feb, 43, (1): 129a. CONNECTIVE TISSUE DISEASE.

Keech, Jr. M. A. Anaplastic T-cell lymphoma in proximity to a saline-filled breast implant [letter]. Plastic and Reconstructive Surgery. 1997 Aug, 100, (2): 554-555. SALINE/cancer.

Kemple, K. L., Black, F. O., and Pesznecker, S. C. Disturbances in Vestibular Function in Women With Silicone Breast Implants. Abstract from the Am. Coll. Rheum. Meeting: October 22-26, 1995, San Franciso. 1995 Oct 22-1995 Oct 26. NEUROLOGIC DISEASE.

Kemple, K. L., and Pestronk, A. Antiglycolipid antibodies in symptomatic women with silicone breast implants [abstract]. Arthritis and Rheumatism. 1995 Sep, 38, (9 (Supplement)): S264. IMMUNE EFFECTS.

Kent, B. D. Silicone gel breast implants [letter]. J. Amer. Med. Assoc. 1994 Jul 27, 272, (4): 272. GENERAL.

Kerkvlliet, N. I. Review of animal studies relevant to silicone toxicology. In: Silicone breast implants in relation to connective tissue diseases and immunologic dysfunction. National Science Panel, 1998 Nov 17. TOXICOLOGY.

Kerr, L., and Speira, H. Graves disease following silicone breast implantation [letter-reply]. J. Rheumatol. 1994, 21, (11): 2169. GENERAL/letter.

Kessler, D. A., Merkatz, R. B., and Schapiro, R. A call for higher standards for breast implants [commentary]. J. Amer. Med. Assoc. 1993 Dec 1, 270, (21): 2607-2608. GENERAL.

Kessler, D. A., Merkatz, R. B., and Schapiro, R. Silicone gel breast implants [letter-reply]. J. Amer. Med. Assoc. 1994 Jul 27, 272, (4): 273-274. GENERAL/letter.

Keystone, E., Peters, W., Snow, K., Rubin. L., and Smith, D. Frequency of autoantibody detection in patients with silicone-gel implants [abstract]. Arthritis and Rheumatism. 1993 Sep, 36, (9 (Supplement)): S71. IMMUNE EFFECTS.

Kim, D. C., and Buinewicz, B. R. Removal of silicone from breast implants [letter]. Plast. Reconstr. Surg. 1995 Nov, 96, (6): 1486. GENERAL.

Kirk, J. F., Marotta, J. S., Widenhouse, C. W., and Goldberg, E. P. (University of Florida, Gainesville). A Novel Method for Characterizing Silicone Breast Implant "Gel" Flow Properties. In: 23rd Annual Meeting of the Society for Biomaterials, 1997 Apr 4, New Orleans, La. Society for Biomaterials, c1997. SILICONE CHARACTERIZATION.

Kirwan, L. Two cases of apparent silicone allergy [letter]. Plast. Reconstr. Surg. 1995 Jul, 96, (1): 236-237. LOCAL COMPLICATIONS/immune effects /letter.

Klykken, P. C. A Life-time Implant Study with Dow Corning® Q7-2159A in Rats. Midland, Mich.: Dow Corning Corporation, 1998 Jun 30. TOXICOLOGY.

Klykken, P. C., Duew, R., Galbraith, T., and Isquith, A. Absence of an immunological reaction to Dow Corning® Q7-2159A gel, 36321. Midland, Mich.: Dow Corning Corporation, 1991a Jun 6. IMMUNE EFFECTS/toxicology.

Klykken, P. C., Duwe, R. L., Galbraith, T. W., and Isquith, A. J. Absence of an Immunological Reaction to Dow Corning® Q7-2423 H.P. Elastomer [abstract] 36323. Midland, Mich.: Dow Corning Corporation, 1991b. IMMUNE EFFECTS/toxicology.

Klykken, P. C., Duwe, R. L., Galbraith, T. W., and Isquith, A. J. Absence of an Immunological Reaction to Dow Corning® Q7-2870 PDMS Fluid [abstract] 36322. Midland, Mich.: Dow Corning Corporation, 1991c. IMMUNE EFFECTS/toxicology.

Klykken, P. C., Duwe, R. L., Galbraith, T. W., and Isquith, A. J. Host Resistance to Listeria Monocytogenes: Absence of an Immunomodulatory Effect by Q7-2159A Silicone Gel [abstract]. Midland, Mich.: Dow Corning Corporation, 1991d. IMMUNE EFFECTS/ toxicology.

Klykken, P. C., Duwe, R. L., Galbraith, T. W., and Isquith, A. J. Host Resistance to Listeria Monocytogenes: Absence of an Immunomodulatory Effect by Q7-2423 H.P. Elastomer [abstract]. Midland, Mich.: Dow Corning Corporation, 1991e. IMMUNE EFFECTS/ toxicology.

Klykken, P. C., Galbraith, T. W., and Kolesar, G. B. A Subchronic Toxicology Evaluation and Splenic Antibody Forming Cell Response to Sheep Erythrocytes following a 28-day Whole Body Inhalation Exposure with Octamethylcyclotetrasiloxane (D4) in Rats. Midland, Mich.: Dow Corning Corporation, 1997 Sep 30. TOXICOLOGY.

Klykken, P. C., Galbraith, T. W., and Woolhiser, M. R. A Humoral Adjuvancy Study of Octamethylcyclotetrasiloxane (D4), Mammary Gel Bleed and the Following Dow Corning® Mammary Implant Components after Intramuscular Injection in the Rat: Q7-2159A Gel, 7-2317 Int Fluid (1000 CS), SFD-119 fluid, Q1-0043 Int, 4-2776 Fluid, and 3-8015 Int (Platinum II). Midland, Mich.: Dow Corning Corporation, 1994 Mar 29. IMMUNE EFFECTS/platinum/toxicology.

Klykken, P. C., Galbraith, T. W., Woolhiser, M. R., and et al. A Humoral Adjuvancy Study of Dow Corning® Silicone Fluids Alone (360 fluid, 20 CS, 7-2317, 1000 CS) and Dow Corning® 360 fluid, 20 CS, Mixed with Dow Corning® Mammary Gel (Q7-2159A) or McGhan Mammary Gel in the Rat. Midland, Mich.: Dow Corning, 1993. IMMUNE EFFECTS/toxicology.

Klykken, P. C., Levier, R. R., and Mast, R. W. Immunological investigations of silicone gel in mice and rats [abstract]. Toxicolgist. 1994 Mar, 14, 20. TOXICOLOGY/immune effects.

Klykken, P. C., and White, K. The adjuvancy of silicones: Dependency on compartmentalization. Current Topics in Microbiology and Immunology: Immunology of Silicones. Midland, Mich.: Dow Corning Corporation, 1996, pp. 113-121. IMMUNE EFFECTS.

Klykken, P. C., Woolhyiser, N., Nelson, S., Goodman, D., and Mast, R. A lifetime implant study of silicone mammary gel in female Sprague Dawley rats (Dow Corning, annual meeting) [abstract]. Society of Toxicology. 1995 Mar: Abstract # 1066. TOXICOLOGY.

Koeger, A-C and Nguyen, J-M. Epidemiology of scleroderma among women: Assessment of risk from exposure to silicone and silica [letter]. The Journal of Rheumatology. 1997, 24, (9): 1853. CONNECTIVE TISSUE DISEASE/silica /letter.

Koeger, A. C., Rozenberg, S., Chaibi, P., Gutmann, L., and Bourgeois, P. Connective tissue disease associated with silicone alveolitis due to silicone spray. A prospective series [abstract]. Arthritis and Rheumatism. 1995 Sep, 38, (9 (Supplement)): S342. CONNECTIVE TISSUE DISEASE.

Koeger, C., Alcaix, D., Rozenberg, S., Arnaud, J., Camns, J.-P., and Bourgeois, P. Silica-induced connective tissue diseases do still occur [abstract]. Arthritis and Rheumatism. 1992, 35 (Supplement), S67. SILICA/connective tissue disease.

Kolesar, G. B. 1 Month repeated dose inhalation study with decamethylchclopentasiloxane in rats. 1995c: Dow Corning Corp, Midland, Mich., 1995c. TOXICOLOGY.

Kolesar, G. B. 1-Month repeated dose inhalation toxicity study with octamethylcyclotetrasiloxane in rats. Midland, Mich.: Dow Corning Corporation, Health and Environmental Sciences, 1995a Mar 14. TOXICOLOGY.

Kolesar, G. B. 3 month repeated dose inhalation study with decamethylcyclopentasiloxane in rats. Dow Corning Corp., Midland, Mich., 1995d. TOXICOLOGY.

Kolesar, G. B. 3-Month repeated dose inhalation toxicity study with octamethylcyclotetrasiloxane in rats with 1-month recovery period. Midland, Mich.: Dow Corning Corporation, Health and Environmental Sciences, 1995b Mar 6. TOXICOLOGY.

Kolesar, G. B. An acute whole body vapor inhalation toxicity study with hexamethyldisiloxane in albino rats. Midland, Mich.: Dow Corning Corporation, Health and Environmental Sciences, 1997 Jan 17. TOXICOLOGY.

Koons, C. R. Breast implants and autoimmunity [letter]. Western Journal of Medicine. 1994 Jul, 161, (1): 91. IMMUNE EFFECTS/connective tissue disease/letter.

Korn, J. H. Antipolymer antibodies, silicone breast implants and fibromyalgia [letter]. The Lancet. 1997 Apr 19, 349, (9059): 1171. IMMUNE EFFECTS/connective tissue disease/ letter.

Kossovsky, N. Death of the "non-specific foreign body reaction" [editorial]. Trends in Polymer Science. 1, (7): 190-191. GENERAL.

Kossovsky, N. Pathophysiological basis of silicone bioreactivity. in: Stratmeyer, M. E., Project Officer. Silicone in Medical Devices, 1991 Feb, Baltimore, Md. Rockville, Md.: U.S. Department of Health and Human Services, 1991 Dec. IMMUNE EFFECTS.

Kossovsky, N., Conway, D., Kossovsky, R., and Petrovich, D. Novel anti-silicone surface-associated antigen antibodies (anti-SSA(x)) may help differentiate symptomatic patients with silicone breast implants from patients with classical rheumatological disease. Current Topics in Microbiology and Immunology. 1996, 210, 327-336. IMMUNE EFFECTS.

Kossovsky, N., Gelman, A., Hnatyszyn, H. J., Rajguru, S., Mena, E. A., Crowder, J., Torres, M., and Zemanovich, G. Adjuvant effect of silicone on the formation of anti-insulin and anti-fibronectin antibodies [abstract]. Arthrtis and Rheumatism. 1994 Sep, 37, (9 (Supplement)): S271. IMMUNE EFFECTS.

Kossovsky, N., Heggers, J. P., Parsons, R. W., and Robson, M. C. Analysis of the surface morphology of recovered silicone mammary prostheses [discussion]. Plast. Reconstr. Surg. 1983 Jun, 71, (6): 803-804. INFECTION/capsule contracture.

Kossovsky, N., Heggers, J. P., and Robson, M. C. The bioreactivity of silicone. Williams, D. F., ed. CRC Critical Reviews in Biocompatibility. Boca Raton: CRC Press, 1987, p. 53-85. GENERAL/immune effects.

Kovarsky, J. Science in the courtroom [letter]. The New England Journal of Medicine. 1994, 331, (16): 1099. GENERAL/letter.

Krech, J. A. Jr. Anaplastic T-cell lymphoma in proximity to a saline-filled breast implant [letter]. Plast. Reconstr. Surg. 1997, 100, 554-555. CANCER.

Kruggell, J. L. MRI for diagnosis of breast implant rupture [letter]. Plast. Reconstr. Surg. 1994 Oct, 94, (5): 741-742. MAMMOGRAPHY/local complications/rupture/letter.

Kulig, K., Brent, J., and Phillips, S. Chest pain and breast implants [letter]. Southern Medical Journal. 1996 Jan, 89, (1): 98-99. PAIN/local complications/letter.

Kurland L.T. Lack of association of multiple sclerosis and silicone breast implants, World Federation of Neurology. World Federation of Neurology Meeting, 1995 May, University of Washington. 1995. NEUROLOGIC DISEASE.

Kurland, L. T., and Homburger, H. A. Epidemiology of autoimmune and immunological diseases in association with silicone implants: is there an excess of clinical disease or antibody response in population-based or other controlled studies? Current Topics in Microbiology and Immunology. 1996, 210, 427-430. CONNECTIVE TISSUE DISEASE.

Kvistad, K. A., Smenes, E., Thuomas, K. A., Gribbestad, I. S., and Samdal, F. Magnetic tomography in diagnosis of breast implant rupture [abstract]. Tidsskr Nor Laegeforen. 1997 Sep 20, 117, (22): 3226-3228. MAMMOGRAPHY.

Kyle, R. A. Monoclonal Gammopathy of Undetermined Significance. Current Topics in Microbiol Immunology. 1996, 210, 375-383. MYELOMA.

Lacey, J. V. Jr. The epidemiology of undifferentiated connective tissue disease in women: assessment of risks of reproductive history and exogenous estrogens, medical devices, and environmental chemicals. Ann Arbor, Mich.: University of Michigan, 1998, c1998. CONNECTIVE TISSUE DISEASE.

Lacey, Jr. J. V., Laing, T. J., Gillespie, B. W., and Schottenfeld, D. Epidemiology of scleroderma among women: Assessment of risk from exposure to silicone and silica [letter-reply]. The Journal of Rheumatology. 1997, 24, (9): 1854-1855. CONNECTIVE TISSUE DISEASE/letter.

Laing, T. J., Gillespie, B. W., and Lacey, Jr. J. V. et al. The association between silicone exposure and undifferentiated connective tissue disease and women in Michigan and Ohio (abstract). Arthritis and Rheumatism. 1996, 39, S150. CONNECTIVE TISSUE DISEASE/immune effects.

Laing, T., Gillespie, B., Burns, C., Garabrant, D., Heeringa, S., Alcser, K., and Schottenfeld, D. Risk factors for scleroderma among Michigan women [abstract]. Arthritis and Rheumatism. 1995, 38, (9 (Supplement)): S341. AI-CTD BACKGROUND.

Lake, R. S., and Radonovich, M. F. Action of Polydimethylsiloxanes on the Reticuloendothelial System of Mice: Basic Cellular Interactions and Structure-Activity Relationships. Midland, Mich.: Dow Corning Corporation, Bioscience Research Laboratory, 1975 Oct 30. IMMUNE EFFECTS/toxicology.

Lake, R. S., Radonovich, M. F., and Boley, W. F. Potentiation of Endotoxin Induced Interferon in Mice Treated with Octamethyleyclotetrasiloxane. Presentation [Abstract]. Midland, Mich.: Dow Corning Corporation, 1975. IMMUNE EFFECTS/toxicology.

Lambing, C. A. A 28-day Inhalation Toxicity and Splenic Antibody Formation Study of Decamethylcyclopentasiloxane. Midland, Mich.: Dow Corning Corporation, 1996 Dec 4. TOXICOLOGY.

Lamm, S. H. Antipolymer antibodies, silicone breast implants, and fibromyalgia [letter]. The Lancet. 1997 Apr 19, 349, (9059): 1170-1171. IMMUNE EFFECTS /connective tissue disease/letter.

Landfield, H. Sterilization of medical devices based on polymer selection and stabilization techniques. in: Szycher, M., Editor. Biocompatible polymers, metals, and composites. Lancaster, PA: Technomic Publishing Co, Inc., 1983. RADIATION.

Lane, T. H., and Burns, S. A. Silica, silicon and silicone, unraveling the mystery. p.c.: Dow Corning Corp. Midland, Mich., 1998. SILICA/silicone chemistry.

Lane, T. H., Curtis, J. M., and Klykken, P. C. Silicone Breast Implants: Composition & Information. Midland, Mich.: Dow Corning Corporation, 1998 Mar 18. TOXICOLOGY/silicone characterization.

Lane, T. H., and Kenan, J. J. Comments on Process Aids used in the Manufacture of Breast Implants. Midland, Mich.: Dow Corning Corporation, 1998 Aug 28. TOXICOLOGY.

Lane, T. H., and Kennan, J. J. "Low Molecular Weight Silicones Are Widely Distributed after a Single Subcutaneous Injection in Mice" Kala, Lykissa, Neely and Lieberman, *Am J. Pathol*,1998, 152(3), 645-649. Midland, Mich.: Dow Corning Corporation, 1998 Aug 28. TOXICOLOGY.

Lane, T. H., and Kennan, J. J. Reponse to Lykiss' comments on July 22nd at the IOM meeting. Midland, Mich.: Dow Corning Corporation, 1998 Aug 28. TOXICOLOGY.

Lane, T. H., and Kennan, J. J. Response to IOM Committee Questions (4/21/98): Process Aids, Cure Temperature, Environmental Platinum, Breast Milk, and "Bleed" Information. Midland, Mich.: Dow Corning Corporation, 1998 Apr 28. TOXICOLOGY/platinum/breast feeding.

Lane, T. H., and Kennan, J. J. Response to Questions Related to Platinum from the July 22nd IOM Meeting on the Safety of Silicone Breast Implants. Midland, Mich.: Dow Corning Corporation, 1998 Aug 28. PLATINUM/toxicology.

Lane, T. H., and Kennan, J. J. Response to the Statements made by Tom Talcott at the July 22nd IOM Meeting. Midland, Mich.: Dow Corning Corporation, 1998 Aug 28. TOXICOLOGY.

Lane, T. H., and Kennan, J. J. Rupture Etiology. Midland, Mich.: Dow Corning Corporation. RUPTURE/local complications.

Langer, A. M., and Nolan, R. P. Physiochemical properties of quartz controlling biological activity. Silica, Silicosis and Cancer—Surface Properties. pp. 125-135. SILICA.

Langley, N. R., and Swanson, J. W. Effects of Subcutaneous Implantation, Through Two Years, on the Physical Properties of Medical Grade Tough Rubber (MDF-0198) [abstract]. Midland, Mich.: Dow Corning Corporation, 1976 May. SILICONE CHARACTERIZATION.

Lappe, M. A. Chemical Deception: the toxic threat to health and the environment. Sierra Club Books. 1992 Nov. TOXICOLOGY.

Laub, D. R., and Lebovic, G. S. Oncologic aspects of augmentation mammaplasty [letter]. Plast. Reconstr. Surg. 1995, 95, (7): 1145-1149. MAMMOGRAPHY/letter/cancer.

Laurencin, C. T., and Elgendy, H. M.. The biocompatibility and toxicity of degradable polymeric materials: Implications for drug delivery. Domb/A.J., ed. Polymeric Site-Specific Pharmacotherapy. 1994, p. 27-46. TOXICOLOGY.

Lazar, A. P., and Lazar, P. Localized morphea after silicone gel breast implantation: More evidence for a cause-and-effect relationship [letter]. Archives of Dermatology. 1991 Feb, 127, (2): 263. CONNECTIVE TISSUE DISEASE/letter.

Le, U. L., and Munson, A. E. Differential effects of octamethylcyclotetrasiloxane (D4) on $CD4^-$ and CD8+ -T cell functions in B63CF1 mice [abstract]. SOT 1997 Annual Meeting. 1997: 265. IMMUNE EFFECTS/toxicology.

LeBeau, J. E. Evaluation of Dow Corning gel strip as to its ability to produce asensitization phenomena upon guinea pig skin. 1967 Nov 1. TOXICOLOGY.

LeBeau, J. E., and Gorzinski, S. J. Dimethylpolysiloxane fluid-14C (Dow Corning 360 medical fluid-14C) distribution and diposition in rats following subcutaneous injection. Midland, Mich.: Dow Corning Corporation, 1972 Apr 7. TOXICOLOGY.

Leibman, A. J. Microscopic demonstration of intraductal extension of silicone from a ruptured breast implant [letter-reply]. Plast. Reconstr. Surg. 1993 Jul, 92, (1): 176. MIGRATION/rupture/local complications/letter.

Leininger, R. I., and Bigg, D. M. Polymers. Von Recum and American, ed. Handbook of Biomaterials Evaluation, Scientific, Technical and Clinical Testing of Implant Materials. New York: Macmillan, 1986. SILICONE CHARACTERIZATION.

Lelah, M. D., and Cooper, S. L. Polyurethanes in Medicine. Boca Raton, Fla.: CRC Press, Inc., 1986. POLYURETHANE.

Lemen, J. K. Rat Teratology Study via Surgical Implant. Vienna, Va.: 1991 May 1. TOXICOLOGY/polyurethane.

Lemen, J. K., and Wolfe, G. W. Combined Chronic Toxicity and Oncogenicity Study in Rats. Vienna, Va.: 1993 Jan 13. CARCINOGENICITY/toxicology/polyurethane.

Lemperle, G. Invited commentary on Santos Heredero and Mayoral Semper. European Journal of Plastic Surgery. 1992, 15, 3-4. SALINE/connective tissue disease/immune effects.

LeRoy, E. C. HLA typing in women with breast implants [discussion]. Plast. Reconstr. Surg. 1995, 96, 1520. IMMUNE EFFECTS.

LeRoy, E. C., Black, C., Fleischmajer, R., Jablonska, S., Krieg, T., Medsger, Jr. T. A., Rowell, N., and Wollheim, F. Scleroderma (systemic sclerosis) classification, subsets and pathogenesis [editorial]. J. Rheumatol. 1988, 15, (2(?)): 202-205. AI-CTD BACKGROUND.

Letterman, G., and Schurter, M. History of augmentation mammaplasty. in: Owsley Jr., JQ and Peterson, RA, Editors. Symposium on Aesthetic Surgery of the Breast : proceedings of the symposium of the Educational Foundation of the American Society of Plastic and Reconstructive Surgeons, inc., and the American Society for Aesthetic Plastic Surgery, inc., held at Scottsdale, Arizona, November 23-26, 1975. St. Louis, MO: C.V. Mosby Co., 1978. GENERAL.

LeVier, R. R. Could tight breast capsules squeeze a significant amount of silicone gel out of an implant? [letter-reply]. Plast. Reconstr. Surg. 1993 Sep, 92, (3): 557-558. CAPSULE-CONTRACTURE/local complications/letter.

LeVier, R. R. Preparation techniques for silicone gel in the evaluation of its in vivo effects [letter-reply]. Plast. Reconstr. Surg. 1993 Oct, 92, (5): 979. TOXICOLOGY/letter.

LeVier, R. R., Chandler, M., and Wendel, S. The pharmacology of silanes and siloxanes. Bendz and Lindquist, eds. Biochemistry of Silicon and Related Problems. Plenum Publishing , 1977 Aug 23. SILICONE CHARACTERIZATION.

Levin, M. Breast augmentation and the risk of subsequent breast cancer [letter]. The New England Journal of Medicine. 1993 Mar 4, 328, (9): 661. CANCER/letter.

Levine, A. M. Breast implants and connective-tissue diseases [letter]. The New England Journal of Medicine. 1994 Nov 3, 331, (18): 1233. CONNECTIVE TISSUE DISEASE/letter.

Levine, J. J., and Illowite, N. T. Silicone breast implants and sclerodermalike esophageal disease in breast-fed infants [letter-reply]. Journal of American Medical Association. 1996 Jan 17, 275, (3): 184-185. CHILDREN'S EFFECTS/breast feeding/letter.

Levine, J. J., and Llowite, N. T. Sclerodermalike esophageal disease in children of mothers with silicone breast implants [letter-reply]. J. Amer. Med. Assoc. 1994 Sep 14, 272, (10): 769-770. CHILDREN'S EFFECTS/breast feeding/letter.

Levine, J. L., Ilowite, N. T., Pettei, M. J., and Trachtman, H. Silicone breast implants and breast feeding [letter-reply]. J. Rheumatol. 1997, 24, (5): 1014-1015. BREAST FEEDING/children's effects.

Levine, M. D. Sclerodermalike esophageal disease in children of mothers with silicone breast implants [letter]. Journal of the American Medical Association. 1994 Sep 14, 272, (10): 769. CHILDREN'S EFFECTS.

Levine, R. A. Ultrasound for diagnosis of ruptured breast implant [letter-reply]. Plast. Reconstr. Surg. 1992 May, 89, (5): 995. MAMMOGRAPHY/rupture/local complications/letter.

Levinson, J. Breast reconstruction: A patient's view [letter]. Plast. Reconstr. Surg. 1984 Apr, 73, (4): 703. PSYCHOSOCIAL/reconstruction/letter.

Lewy, R. I. Antinuclear antibodies, Lipid disturbances and central nervous system imaging abnormalities in silicone breast implant users (abstract). J. Invest. Med. 1995, 43, 333A. IMMUNE EFFECTS/neurologic disease.

Lewy, R. I. Breast implant controversy deserves more study [letter-reply]. Texas Medicine. 1994 Feb, 90, (2): 7-8. GENERAL/letter.

Lewy, R. I. Outcomes of breast implant court-ordered disease classification at a clinic in Houston, Texas. 1996 Aug. GENERAL.

Lewy, R. I., and Ezrailson, E. Laboratory studies in breast implant patients: ANA positivity, gammaglobulin levels, and other autoantibodies. Current Topics in Microbiology and Immunology: Immunology of Silicones. 1996, p. 419-425. IMMUNE EFFECTS.

Liang, M. H. Silicone breast implants and systemic rheumatic disease. Some smoke but little fire to date [editorial]. Scandinavian Journal of Rheumatology. 1997, 26, (6): 409-411. CONNECTIVE TISSUE DISEASE.

Liang, M. H., Karlson, E., and Sánchez-Guerrero, J. Breast implants and connective tissue diseases [letter-reply]. The New England Journal of Medicine. 1995 Nov 23, 333, (21): 1424. CONNECTIVE TISSUE DISEASE/letter.

Liau, M., Ito, S., and Koren, G. Sclerodermalike esophageal disease in children of mothers with silicone breast implants [letter]. J. Amer. Med. Assoc. 1994 Sep 14, 272, (10): 769. CHILDREN'S EFFECTS/breast feeding/connective tissue disease/letter.

Lightfoote, M. M., Bushar, G., Greenfield, W., and Langone, J. J. Animal models for predicting autoimmune response to biomaterials [abstract]. J Allergy Clin Immunol. 99, (1 (Part 2)): S195. IMMUNE EFFECTS.

Little, III J. W. The use of intradermal tattoo to enhance the final result of nipple-areola reconstruction [discussion]. Plast. Reconstr. Surg. 1986 Apr, 77, (4): 676. RECONSTRUCTION.

Litvak, J. Breast implants and connective-tissue disease [letter]. J. Amer. Med. Assoc. 1996 Jul 10, 276, (2): 102-103. CONNECTIVE TISSUE DISEASE/letter.

Lockhorn, N., Lacy, S., and Lucas, L. Biocompatibility evaluations of medical grade silicone elastomers. Fifth World Biomaterials Congress, Toronto, Canada. 1996 Jun. TOXICOLOGY.

Looney, R. J., and et al. Immunological effects of respiratory exposure to siloxane in humans [abstract]. Fundamental and Applied Toxicology (Supplement: The Toxicologist). 1996 Mar 10, 30 (Part 2), (16): 85. IMMUNE EFFECTS/toxicology.

Lorentzen, R. J. Human epidemiology data on silicone breast implants. FDA Letter. 1988 Sep 22. PREVALENCE/general.

Love, L. A., Weiner, S. R., Vasey, F. B., Crofford, L. T., Oddis, C. V., Starr, M. R., Bridges, A. J., Targoff, I. N., Gurley, R. C., and Miller, F. W. Clinical and immunogenic features of women who develop myositis after silicone implants [abstract]. Arthritis and Rheumatism. 1992, 25, (9 (Supplement)): S46. IMMUNE EFFECTS/connective tissue disease.

Love, S. M. Patient selection for prophylactic mastectomy: Who is at high risk? [discussion]. Plast. Reconstr. Surg. 1983 Sep, 72, (3): 332-333. CANCER.

Lu, E. P. Protein antigens adsorbed on silicone are poorly recognized compared to when absorbed on polystyrene [abstract]. FASEB Journal. 1995 Mar 10, 9, (4): A1030. IMMUNE EFFECTS.

Lu, L. B., Patten, B. M., and Shoaib, B. O. Noncardiac chest pain in silicone breast implants: A pseudo-heart attack syndrome? [abstract]. Arthritis and Rheumatism. 1993 Sep, 36, (9): S219. PAIN/local complications.

Luce, E. A. Breast implants and connective-tissue diseases [letter-reply]. The New England Journal of Medicine. 1994 Nov 3, 331, (18): 1233-1234. CONNECTIVE TISSUE DISEASE/letter.

Lugowski, S., Smith, D. C., Semple, J., Peters, W., and McHugh, A. Silicon levels in blood, breast milk and breast capsules of patients with silicone breast implants and controls. Fifth World Biomaterials Congress, Toronto, Canada. 1996 Jun. SILICON MEASUREMENT/breast feeding/capsule-contracture/local complications/children's effects.

Lundberg, G. D. The breast implant controversy: A clash of ethics and law [editorial]. J. Amer. Med. Assoc. 1993 Dec, 270, (21): 2608. GENERAL.

Luster, M. I., Munson, A. E., White, K. L., and McCay, J. A. Immunotoxicity of Silicone in Female B6C3F1 mice—180 Day Exposure. Richmond, VA: Medical College of Virginia, Virginia Commonwealth University, 1993. TOXICOLOGY/immune effects.

Luu, H. M. D. Silicone, An Update Review. GENERAL.

Lynch, W. The Handbook of Silicone Rubber Fabrication. New York: Van Nostrand Reinhold Company, 1978. SILICONE CHEMISTRY.

MacDonald, P. M. Letter to the Editor. Mangetic Resonance in Medicine. 1999, in press. SILICON MEASUREMENT/migration/letter.

Macklin, R. Ethics, epidemiology, and law: the case of silicone breast implants. American Journal of Public Health. 1999 Apr, 89, (4): 487-489. GENERAL.

Malata, C. M., Naylor, I. L., Nutbrown, M., and Timmons, M. J. Modulation of experimental capsular contracture around silicone gel-filled breast prostheses in a rodent model. Eur J Sur Res. 1994b, 26, (SA): 57. CAPSULE-CONTRACTURE/local complications.

Malata, C. M., Naylor, I. L., and Timmonds, M. J. Smooth versus textured breast implants: A rodent study [abstract]. British Journal of Surgery. 1993, 80, ((Supplement)): 512. CAPSULE-CONTRACTURE/local complications.

Malczewski, R. M. A comparative histology study of cellular responses to commonly used implant materials. Society of Biomaterials. 1994: Abstract. IMMUNE EFFECTS/toxicology.

Malczewski, R. M. Ninety-day implant study of Dow Corning Q7-2167/68-gel (Q7-2159 A). Midland, Mich.: Dow Corning Corporation, 1985a Oct 3. TOXICOLOGY.

Malczewski, R. M. Skin sensitization study of Dow Corning q7-2146/50 gel. Dowcorning Tox. File No. 2332-3 ed. 1985b Oct 7. TOXICOLOGY.

Malczewski, R. M. Skin sensitization study of Dow Corning q7-2167/68 gel. Dowcorning Tox. File No. 2476-12 ed. 1985c Feb 25. TOXICOLOGY.

Malczewski, R. M., Varaprath, S., and Bolger, C. An assessment of the MeSIO 3/2 content of feces and urine obtained 24 hours after the oral administration of D4 to rats. Midland, MI: Dow Corning Corporation, 1988 Aug 17. TOXICOLOGY.

Malczewski, R. M., Woolhiser, M. R., and Mudgett, S. L. A Humoral Adjuvancy Study in the Rat of Dow Corning® Silicone Gel (Q7-2159A) Preparations and Mammary Gel Bleed [abstract]. Midland, Mich.: Dow Corning Corporation, 1993. IMMUNE EFFECTS/toxicology.

Maldonado-Cocco, J. A. Axillary lymphadenopathies due to silicone implants [letter]. The Journal of Rheumatology. 1994, 21, (5): 965-966. LYMPHADENOPATHY/local complications/granulomas/letter.

Malone, K. E., Stanford, J. L., Daling, J. R., and Voigt, L. F. Implants and Breast Cancer. The Lancet. 1992, 339, (May 30): 1365. CANCER/letter.

Malone, R. S., Schwartz, Jr L. A., Lamki, N., and Watson, Jr. A. B. Pitfalls in US evaluation of patients with silicone gel breast implants [abstract]. Radiology. 1994, 193, 177. MAMMOGRAPHY.

Mann, R. D. Breast implants: The tyranny of the anecdote [editorial]. Journal of Clinical Epidemiology. 1995, 48, (4): 504-506. GENERAL.

Manresa, J. M., and Manresa, F. Silicone pneumonitis [letter]. The Lancet. 1983 Dec 10, 2, 1373. GENERAL/letter.

Manson, J. M., and Kang, Y. J. Chapter 28. in: Hayes, A. W. Ed. Principles and Methods of Toxicology. New York: Raven Press, 1994. TOXICOLOGY.

Marion, R. B. Polyurethane-covered breast implant [letter]. Plast. Reconstr. Surg. 1984 Nov, 74, (5): 728-729. POLYURETHANE/infection/local complications/letter.

Marion, R. B. Silicone tissue assays [letter]. Plast. Reconstr. Surg. 1995 Apr, 95, (4): 770. SILICON MEASUREMENT/saline/letter.

Mark, J. E. Silicon-containing polymers. In: Ziegler, J. M., and Fearon, F. W. G., eds. Silicon-Based Polymer Science: A Comprehensive Resource. Washington, D.C.: American Chemical Society, 1990, p. 47-70. SILICONE CHARACTERIZATION.

Markman, B. S., Colletti, M., and Miller, S. M. Silicone Mastopathy and Autoimmune Disease [abstract]. Silicone Mastopathy and Autoimmune Disease, 1993. IMMUNE EFFECTS/CONNECTIVE TISSUE DISEASE.

Marotta, J. S., Amery, D. P., Widenhouse, C. W., Martin, P. J., and Goldberg, E. P. (University of Florida, Gainesville). Degradation of Physical Properties of Silicone Gel Breast Implants and the High Rate of Implant Failures. In: 24th Anntial Meeting of the Society for Biomaterials, 1998 Apr, San Diego, Calif. Society for Biomaterials, c1998. SILICONE CHARACTERIZATION/local complications/explantation.

Marotta, J. S., and Goldberg, E. P. (University of Florida, Gainesville). Extraction Studies with Breast Implant Silicone Elastomer shells and "Gels" Indicate very High Concentrations of Soluble Uncross-Linked Silicones. In: 23rd Annual Meeting of the Society for Biomaterials, 1997 Apr 4, New Orleans, La. Society for Biomaterials, c1997. SILICONE CHARACTERIZATION.

Marotta, J., Latoore, G., Batich, C., Hardt, N., and Yu, L. Measurement of silicon in tissue sites both adjacent to and distant from ruptured and intact silicone breast implants. Fifth World Biomaterials Congress, Toronto, Canada, 1996 May 29-1996 Jun 2, Toronto, Canada. 1996b May 29. SILICON MEASUREMENT/rupture/local complications.

Marotta, J., Latorre, G., Batich, C., Hardt, S., and Yu, L. Measurement of gel bleed from silicone breast implants. Fifth World Biomaterials Congress, Toronto, Canada. 1996a May. SILICON MEASUREMENT/rupture/local complications.

Martellock, A. The hydrolytic degradation of silicone polymers. Waterford, NY: General Electric Company, 1966 Mar 24. SILICONE CHEMISTRY.

Martin, J. E. The effect of breast implants on the radiographic detection of microcalcification and soft tissue masses [discussion]. Plastic and Reconstructive Surgery. 1989 Nov, 84, (5): 781-782. MAMMOGRAPHY/calcification.

Martin, L. Silicone breast implants and connective tissue diseases: An ongoing controversy [editorial]. The Journal of Rheumatology. 1995, 22, (2): 198-200. GENERAL/connective tissue disease.

Martin, L., Edworthy, S. M., Barr, S., Wall, W., and Fritzler, M. J. Autoantibody profiles in patients with breast implants: The Alberta experience [abstract]. Arthritis and Rheumatism. 1995 Sep, 38, (9 (Supplement)): S264. IMMUNE EFFECTS.

Martin, L., Edworthy, S. M., and Fritzler, M. J. Autoantibodies in patients with saline and silicone gel filled breast implants [abstract]. Arthritis and Rheumatism. 1993 Sep, 36, (9 (Supplement)): S117. SALINE/immune effects.

Martínez-Osuna, P., Espinoza, L. R., Gresh, J. P., Seleznik, M., Germain, B., and Vasey, F. B. Silicone-associated connective tissue disease (CTD) following mammoplasty: Clinical course after implant removal [abstract]. Arthritis and Rheumatism. 1990, 33, (9 (Supplement)): S156. CONNECTIVE TISSUE DISEASE/explantation.

Mathes, S. J. Breast implantation—The quest for safety and quality [editorial]. The New England Journal of Medicine. 1997 Mar 6, 336, (10): 718-719. GENERAL.

Mathias, J., Burns, D., Verm, R., Clench, M., and Loftin, C. Enteric neuropathy by antro-duodenal manometry in patients with silicone breast disease (SBD) [abstract]. Annual Meeting of American Gastroenterological Association and American Association for Study of Liver Disease, 1996 May. NEUROLOGIC DISEASE.

Maxwell, G. P. Breast reconstruction utilizing subcutaneous tissue expansion followed by polyurethane-covered silicone implants: A six-year experience [discussion]. Plast. Reconstr. Surg. 1991 Oct, 88, (4): 640-641. EXPANDER/polyurethane/reconstruction.

Maxwell, G. P. Hyaluronic acid-filled mammary implants: An experimental study [discussion]. Plast. Reconstr. Surg. 1994 Aug, 94, (2): 316-317. GENERAL.

Maxwell, G. P., and Falcone, P. A. Eighty-four consecutive breast reconstructions using a textured silicone tissue expander. Plast. Reconstr. Surg. 1992 Jun, 89, (6): 1022-1034. POLYURETHANE/expander/reconstruction.

Maxwell, G. P., and Hammond, D. C. Breast implants: Smooth vs. textured. In: Habal, M. B., ed. Advances in Plastic and Reconstructive Surgery. St. Louis: Mosby-Year Book, 1993, p. 209-220. POLYURETHANE/capsule contracture/local complications.

Maxwell, G. P., McGibbon, B. M., and Hoopes, J. E. Vascular considerations in the use of a latissimus dorsi myocutaneous flap after mastectomy with an axillary dissection. Plast. Reconstr. Surg. 1979, 64, (6): 771-780. RECONSTRUCTION.

Maxwell, G. P., and Perry, L. The capsule in various types of breast implants [letter]. Plast. Reconstr. Surg. 1995 Apr, 95, (5): 937. CAPSULE CONTRACTURE/local complications/saline/polyurethane.

May, D. S., and Stroup, N. E. The incidence of sarcomas of the breast among women in the United States, 1973-1986 [letter]. Plastic Reconstructive Surgery. 1991 Jan, 87, (1): 193-194. CANCER/letter.

McCarty, G. A., Valencia, D. W., and Fritzler, M. J. Antinuclear antibodies: contemporary techniques and clinical applications to connective tissue diseases. New York: Oxford University Press, 1984. AI-CTD BACKGROUND.

McDonald, A. H., Schneider, M. M., Gudenkauf, L., and Sanger, J. R. Silicone gel enhances autoimmunity in nzb mice but fails to induce disease in balb/c mice [abstract]. Journal of Allergy and Clinical Immunology. 99, (1 (Part 2)): S195. IMMUNE EFFECTS/toxicology.

McDonald, A. H., Weir, K., and Sanger, J. R. Silicone-induced T cell proliferation in mice. Current Topics in Microbiology and Immunology: Immunology of Silicones. 1996, p. 189-198. IMMUNE EFFECTS/toxicology.

McGhan Medical Corporation. Large Simple Trial (LST) PMA#P940038 Final Report. McGhan Medical Corporation, (undated). LOCAL COMPLICATIONS/capsule-contracture/deflation/rupture/infection.

McGhan Medical Corporation. Mammary Implants for Augmentation and Reconstruction of the Breast (AR90 Clinical Study). Preliminary Report: Silicone-Filled Implants at Five Years. McGhan Medical Corporation, 1998. RUPTURE/local complications/capsule-contracture.

McGrath, M. Listeria infection of silicone breast implant [discussion]. Plast. Reconstr. Surg. 1994 Sep. INFECTION/local complications.

McGrath, M. Reduced capsule formation around soft silicone rubber prostheses coated with solid collagen [invited comment]. Annals of Plastic Surgery. 1985, 14, 359-360. CAPSULE-CONTRACTURE/local complications.

McGrath, M. H. Capsular contracure in the augmented breast. Rudolph, R., Editor. Problems in aesthetic surgery: biological causes and clinical solutions. St. Louis, MO: C.V. Mosby Company, 1986, pp. 405-422. CAPSULE CONTRACTURE/local complications.

McGrath, M. H. The fibrous capsules around static and dynamic implants: their biochemical, histological, and ultrastructural characteristics [invited comment]. Annals of Plastic Surgery. 1987, 19, (3): 208-214. CAPSULE-CONTRACTURE/local complications/ expander.

McKim, Jr. J. M. Effects of Decamethylcyclopentasiloxane (D5) on Hepatic Cytochrome P450, UDP-Glucuronosyltransferase, and epoxide Hydrolase in the Female Fischer 344 Rat. Midland, Mich.: Dow Corning Corporation, 1997 Sep 22. TOXICOLOGY.

McKim, Jr. J. M. Effects of Octamethylcyclotetrasiloxane on Liver Size and Enzyme Induction: A Pilot Feasibility Study. Midland, Mich.: Dow Corning Corporation, 1996a Sep 26. TOXICOLOGY.

McKim, Jr. J. M. Effects of Octamethylcyclotetrasiloxane on Liver Size and Enzyme Induction: A Pilot Feasibility Study II. Midland, Mich.: Dow Corning Corporation, 1996b Dec 17. TOXICOLOGY.

McKinney, P. Silicone implants [letter]. Plast. Reconstr. Surg. 1992 Oct, 90, (4): 730. GENERAL/letter.

McKissock, P. K. Evaluating breast parenchymal maldistribution with regard to mastopexy and augmentation mammaplasty [discussion]. Plast. Reconstr. Surg. 1990 Oct, 86, (4): 720-721. LOCAL COMPLICATIONS.

McLaughlin, J. K., Fraumeni, J. F., Olsen, J., and Mellemkjaer, L. Re: Breast implants, cancer, and systemic sclerosis [letter]. Journal of the National Cancer Institute. 1994 Sep 21, 86, (18): 1424. CONNECTIVE TISSUE DISEASE/cancer/letter.

McLaughlin, J. K, Fraumeni, Jr. J. F., and Nyren, O. Silicone breast implants and risk of cancer? J. Amer. Med. Assoc. 1995a Jan 11, 273, (2): 116. CANCER/letter.

McLaughlin, J. K., Olsen, J. H., Friis, S., Mellemkjaer, L., and Fraumeni, J. F. Re: Breast implants, cancer, and systemic sclerosis. Journal of the National Cancer Institute. 1995b, 87, 1415-1416. CONNECTIVE TISSUE DISEASE/cancer/letter.

Mease, P. J., Overman, S. S., and Green, D. J. Clinical symptoms/signs and laboratory features in symptomatic patients with silicone breast implants. Arthritis and Rheumatism. 1995, 38, (9 (Supplement)): S324. CONNECTIVE TISSUE DISEASE.

Medical Devices Agency. Silicone Gel Breast Implants: Summary of the Current Situation. London, United Kingdom: Medical Devices Agency, 1997 Feb. GENERAL.

Medical Engineering Corporation. Final report on the pilot study of urine and serum samples from women with Meme and Replicon breast implants. Protocol OT114-001 ed. Department of Human Pharmacology, Bristol-Myers Squibb Pharmaceutical Research Institute, 1995 Jul 14. SILICON MEASUREMENT/carcinogenicity/toxicology/ polyurethane.

Medina, F., Vero, O., Miranda, J. M., and Fraga, A. Elevated prolactin levels in women with Silicone gel breast implants and with mineral mixed oil injections (abstract). Arthritis & Rheumatism. 1995, 38, (9 Supplement): s324. IMMUNE EFFECTS/breast feeding/ local complications.

Medtox. Analysis of internal safety studies relevant to health care materials and products. 1987 Feb 23. TOXICOLOGY.

Mellon Institute of Industrial Research. The single dose and sub-acute toxicity of stabilizer d-2. EPA/OTS Doc. No. 878213501, NTIS/OTS Doc. No. 0205839: University of Pittsburgh, 1994. TOXICOLOGY.

Melmed, E. P. Breast capsular contracture [letter-reply]. Plast. Reconstr. Surg. 1997 Nov, 100, (6): 1619-1620. CAPSULE CONTRACTURE/local complications/letter.

Melmed, E. P. Breast implants [letter-reply]. Plast. Reconstr. Surg. 1997 Aug, 100, (2): 555. GENERAL/letter.

Mentor H/S. Siltex® and Smooth-Surface Low-Bleed Gel-Filled Mammary Prostheses (Reconstruction Adjunct Study). 1992. GENERAL.

Microbiological Associates, Inc. Salmonella/Mammalian—Microsome Plate Incorporation Mutagenicity Assay (AMES Test) and Eschericia Coli WP2 uvrA Reverse Mutation Assay with a Confirmatory Assay of Dow Corning® 7-9172 Part A. Midland, Mich.: Dow Corning Corporation, 1994 Aug 24. TOXICOLOGY.

Middleton, G., McFarlin, J., and Lipsky, P. Fibromyalgia in systemic lupus erythematosus [abstract]. Arthritis and Rheumatism. 1994, 37, (9 (Supplement)): S223. AI-CTD BACKGROUND.

Middleton, M. S. Breast Implant Classification. in: Gorczyca, D. P., and Brenner, R. J., eds. The Augmented Breast. New York-Stuttgart: Thieme, 1997, p. 28-44. GENERAL.

Middleton, M. S. Mammary Implant Product List: 1962-1998. Unpublished document. 1998a. GENERAL.

Middleton, M. S. Pitfalls in breast implant MR imaging. Scientific Exhibit Abstract (submitted for 1995 RSNA). 1995 Jan 1. MAMMOGRAPHY.

Middleton, M. S., Huang, J. S., Mattrey, R., Hesselink, J. R., Dobke, M., Freeman, W. R., and Udkoff, R. In-vitro and in-vivo MR evaluation of silicone implants currently in use. Presentation for Association of University Radiologists, 1996 Apr 22. MAMMOGRAPHY.

Miller, S. H. Does irradiation to the augmented breast produce scar contracture? [letter]. Plast. Reconstr. Surg. 1992 Feb, 89, (2): 380-381. CAPSULE-CONTRACTURE/local complications/radiation/letter.

Miller, S. H. Silicone breast implants and antipolymer antibodies [letter]. The Lancet. 1997 Sep 6, 350, (9079): 740. IMMUNE EFFECTS/letter.

Mladick, R. A. Inflatable breast implants [letter]. Plast. Reconstr. Surg. 1995, 95, (3): 600. EXPANDER.

Modan, B. Breast augmentation and the risk of subsequent breast cancer [letter]. The New England Journal of Medicine. 1993 Mar 4, 328, (9): 661. CANCER/letter.

Mogelvang, L. C. Breast implants [letter]. Plast. Reconstr. Surg. 1995 Jul, 96, (1): 236. GENERAL/letter.

Mogelvang, L. C. Chest pain and breast implants [letter]. Southern Medical Journal. 1996 Jan, 89, (1): 97-98. PAIN/local complications/letter.

Mogelvang, L. C. Oncologic aspects of augmentation mammaplasty [letter]. Plast. Reconstr. Surg. 1995 Apr, 95, (5): 935-936. MAMMOGRAPHY/cancer/letter.

Molenaar, A. Breast implants and patient satisfaction [letter]. Plast. Reconstr. Surg. 1992 May, 89, (5): 995-996. PSYCHOSOCIAL/letter.

Mongey, A.-B., and Hess, V. E. The role of environment in systemic lupus erythematosus and associated disorders. Wallace, Hahn (eds.). Dubois Lupus Erythematosus. 1997, p. Chapter 3:31-47. AI-CTD BACKGROUND.

Montandon, D. Myofibroblasts and free silicon around breast implants [letter]. Plast. Reconstr. Surg. 1979, 63, (5): 719-720. CAPSULE-CONTRACTURE/local complications/letter.

Morain, W. D. The role of iodine-releasing silicone implants in prevention of spherical contracture in mice (discussion). Plast. Reconstr. Surg. 1982, 69, (6): 960-961. INFECTION/local complications.

Morey, S. D., and North, J. A. Final Report on Low Bleed Mammary Implants. Technical Report to Dow Corning Wright from Battelle Columbus Division. Columbus, Oh.: Battelle, 1986 Jul 2. TOXICOLOGY/local complications.

Morgan, E. Capsular contracture [letter]. Plast. Reconstr. Surg. 1983 Feb, 71, (2): 281. CAPSULE-CONTRACTURE/local complications/letter.

Morgan, R. F., and Rodeheaver, G. T. Measurement of capsular contracture: The conventional breast implant and the Pittsburgh implant [discussion]. Plast. Reconstr. Surg. 1989 Dec, 84, (6): 902. CAPSULE-CONTRACTURE/local complications.

Morse, J. H., and Spiera, H. Autoimmune diseases, immunoglobulin isotypes and lymphocyte subsets in 30 females with breast augmentation mammoplasty [abstract]. Arthritis and Rheumatism. 1992, 35 (Supplement), S65. IMMUNE EFFECTS.

Morse, J. H., Spiera, H., Zhang, Y., and Fotino, M. Autoimmune diseases and HLA typing in 60 females with silicone breast implants [abstract]. Arthritis and Rheumatism. 1993, 36 (Supplement), S132. IMMUNE EFFECTS.

Morse, J. H., Spiera, H., Zhang, Y., and Fotino, M. Scleroderma (SSc) in women with silicone implants exhibits the same association of an amino acid sequence in the HLA-DQB1 first domain found in idiopathic SSc [abstract]. Arthritis and Rheumatism. 1994 Sep, 37, (9 (Supplement)): S421. IMMUNE EFFECTS/connective tissue disease.

Moss, A. J., Hamburger, S., Moore, R., Jeng, L. L., and Howie, L. J. Use of selected medical device implants in the United States, 1988. Advance data from vital and health statistics, no. 191. Hyattsville, Md.: National Center for Health Statistics, 1991 Feb 26. PREVALENCE.

Moss-Morris, R., Petrie, K. J., Large, R. G., and Kydd, R. R. Neuropsychological deficits in chronic fatigue syndrome—artifact or reality? [editorial]. Journal of Neurology, Neurosurgery, and Psychiatry. 1996, 60, 474-477. NEUROLOGIC DISEASE/AI-CTD BACKGROUND.

Muhanna, A., Rubin, L, Keystone, E., Peters, W., Ayer, L, and Fritzler, M. Silicone breast implants and rheumatic disease—clinical and immunological investigations [abstract]. Arthritis and Rheumatism. 1992 Sep, 35, (9 (Supplement)): S65. CONNECTIVE TISSUE DISEASE/immune effects.

Munson, A. E., McCay, J. A., Brown, R. D., Musgrove, D. L., Butterworth, L. F., White, K. L. Jr., Lane, T. H., and Klykken, P. C. The immune status of Fischer 334 rats administered octamethylcyclotetrasiloxane (D4) by oral gavage [abstract]. SOT 1997 Annual Meeting. 1997: 265. IMMUNE EFFECTS/toxicology.

Munson, A. E., White, K. L. Jr., Mccay, J. A., Musgrove, D., Brown, R., Stern, M. L., and Luster, M. I. Immunotoxicology of silicone in female b6c3f1 mice—10 day exposure, studies at immunotoxicology program, Med. Col. of Va. 1992. TOXICOLOGY/immune effects.

Munten, J., Hunter, C., and Veresh, L. Biological Safety Evaluation of Dow Corning® Q7-2245 Medical Grade Elastomer. Midland, Mich.: Dow Corning Corporation, 1985 Sep 10. TOXICOLOGY.

Murray, J. E. Factors for safety in use of silicone [editorial]. Plast. Reconstr. Surg. 1967 Apr, 39, (4): 427. GENERAL.

Naim, J. O., Ippolito, K. M., Lanzafame, R. J., and van Oss, C. J. Induction of type II collagen arthritis in the DA rat using silicone gel as adjuvant. Current Topics in Microbiology and Immunology. 1996, 210, 103-111. IMMUNE EFFECTS/toxicology.

Naim, J. O., Lanzafame, R. J., and van Oss, C. J. Breast implants and connective-tissue diseases [letter]. The New England Journal of Medicine. 1994 Nov 3, 331, (18): 1232. CONNECTIVE TISSUE DISEASE/letter.

Naim, J. O., Satoh, M., Ippolito, K. M. L., and Reeves. The effect of silicone gels and oils on anti-nuclear antibody formation in BALB/c mice [abstract]. J Allergy Clin Immunol. 1997b, 99, (1 (Part 2)): S195. IMMUNE EFFECTS.

Nardella, F. A. Oral and ocular sicca syndrome in women with silicone breast implants [abstract]. Arthritis and Rheumatism. 1995 Sep, 38, (9 (Supplement)): S264. IMMUNE EFFECTS/connective tissue disease.

National Cancer Institute. Bioassay of 2,4-Diaminotoluene for Possible Carcinogenicity. Technical Report Series No. 162. Bethesda, Md.: U.S. Department of Health, Education, and Welfare, Public Health Service, National Institutes of Health, 1978. CARCINOGENICITY/toxicology/polyurethane.

National Cancer Institute. Bioassay of Dibutyltin Diacetate for Possible Carcinogenicity. Washington, D.C.: Carcinogenesis Program. TOXICOLOGY.

National Institute for Occupational Safety and Health (NIOSH). Bulletin 53. Toluene diisocyanate (TDI) and toluenediamine (TDA). Evidence of carcinogenicity. Cincinnati, Ohio: NIOSH, 1989. CARCINOGENICITY/toxicology/polyurethane.

National Institute of Arthritis and Musculoskeletal and Skin Diseases, National Institute of Health. Scientific Workshop Summary: Summary of the Atypical Rheumatic Disease and Silicone Breat Implants Workshop. Washington, D.C.: 1997 Apr 17. CONNECTIVE TISSUE DISEASE.

National Institute of Arthritis and Musculoskeletal and Skin Diseases, NIH. Scientific Workshop Summary: The Neuroscience and Endocrinology of Fibromyalgia. Washington, D.C.: National Institutes of Health, 1996 Dec. AI-CTD BACKGROUND.

National Institutes of Health, National Cancer Institute. Cancer Statistics Review 1973-1989. Miller, B. A., Ries, L. A. G., Hankey, B. F., Kosary, C. L., and Edwards, B. K., eds. Bethesda, Md.: National Cancer Institute, 1992. CANCER.

National Library of Medicine. Hazardous Substances Data Bank. Micromedix, Inc. Denver, Colo. TOXICOLOGY.

National Toxicology Program (NTP). TR-162, Bioassay of 2, 4-Diaminotoluene for Possible Carcinogenicity (CAS No. 95-80-7). National Toxicology Program, NIH, 1978. POLYURETHANE, toxicology.

Netscher, D. T. Positive cultures around breast prostheses [letter-reply]. Plast. Reconstr. Surg. 1996 Jul, 98, (1): 186. INFECTION/local complications/letter.

Niazi, Z. B. M. Positive cultures around breast prostheses [letter]. Plast. Reconstr. Surg. 1996 Jul, 98, (1): 186. INFECTION/local complications/letter.

Nickoloff, B. J. The cytokine network in psoriasis [editorial]. Archives of Dermatology. 1991 Jun, 127, 871-884. GENERAL.

Niessen, F. B. Re: Effectiveness of silicone sheets in the prevention of hypertrophic breast scars [letter]. Annals of Plastic Surgery. 1997 May, 38, (5): 547. LOCAL COMPLICATIONS.

Nightingale, S. L. From the Food and Drug Administration: Moratorium on silicone gel breast implants. J. Amer. Med. Assoc. 1992 Feb 12, 267, (6): 787. GENERAL.

Nightingale, S. L. From the Food and Drug Administration: Silicone breast implant decision. J. Amer. Med. Assoc. 1992 Jun 24, 267, (24): 3262. GENERAL.

[No authors listed]. No link between disease and breast implants. South African Medical Journal. July 1994, 84, (7): 15-17. GENERAL.

Noone, R. B. A review of the possible health implications of silicone breast implants. Cancer. 1997 May 1, 79, (9): 1747-1756. GENERAL/cancer/connective tissue disease/local complications/mammography.

Noone, R. B., Sigal, R. K., Naama, H., and Daly, J. M. Silicone increases murine macrophage cytotoxicity. 1994 International Symposium on Plastic Surgery, Florence, Italy, 1994b May 23. IMMUNE EFFECTS.

Nordström, R. E. A. Antibiotics in the tissue expander to decrease the rate of infection [letter]. Plast. Reconstr. Surg. 1988 Jan, 81, (1): 137-138. PAIN/infection/local complications/expander/letter.

Nuttall, K. L., Gordon, W. H., and Ash, K. O. Breast implants and urinary platinum [letter]. Clinical Chemistry. 1994, 40, (9): 1787. PLATINUM/toxicology/local complications/letter.

Nyrén, O., McLaughlin, J. K., Blot, W. J., Boice Jr., J. D., Engquist, M., and Hakelius, L. Risk of connective tissue disease among women with breast implants: Authors' reply [letter-reply]. British Medical Journal. 1998b. CONNECTIVE TISSUE DISEASE/letter.

Nyrén, O., McLaughlin, J. K., Blot, W. J., Boice Jr., J. D., Engquist, M., and Hakelius, L. Risk of connective tissue disease among women with breast implants: Authors' reply [letter-reply]. British Medical Journal. 1998b. CONNECTIVE TISSUE DISEASE/letter.

O'Hanlon, T. P., Okada, S., Love, L. A., Dick, G., Young, V. L., and Miller, F. W. Immunohistopathology and T-cell receptor gene expression in capsules surrounding silicone breast implants. Current Topics in Microbiology and Immunology: Immunology of Silicones. 1996, p. 419-425. IMMUNE EFFECTS.

O'Looney, P. A. Chapter Executive Directors. New York: 1992 Feb 19. NEUROLOGIC DISEASE.

Ojo-Amaze, E. A., Lin, H.-C., Agopian, M. S., Peter, J. B., Conte, V., and Brucker, R. F. T-cell response in women with silicone breast implants [letter-reply]. Clinical and Diagnostic Laboratory Immunology. 1995 Mar, 2, (2): 253-254. IMMUNE EFFECTS/letter.

Olbourne, N. A. Re: Factors affecting the rupture of silicone-gel breast implants [letter]. Annals of Plastic Surgery. 1994 Oct, 33, (4): 462-463. RUPTURE/local complications/letter.

Oneal, R. M., and Argenta, L. C. Steroids in breast implants [letter-reply]. Plast. Reconstr. Surg. 1983 Feb, 71, (2): 283. STEROIDS/local complications/letter.

Onken, H. D. The impact of the media on women with breast implants [letter]. Plast. Reconstr. Surg. 1994 May, 93, (6): 1312-1313. GENERAL/psychosocial/letter.

Orel, S. G., Schnall, M. D., Hochman, M. G., Powell, C. M., Torosian, M. H., and Rosato, E. F. Impact of MR imaging and MR-guided biopsy on detection and staging of breast cancer [abstract]. Radiology. 1994 Nov, 193, (P (Supplement)): 318. MAMMOGRAPHY/cancer.

Ory, H. W., and Schlesselman, J. J. Breast Implants and Connective Tissue Disease: A Review of the Epidemiologic Literature. Transcript of thc IOM Committee on the Safety of Silicone Breast Implants, 1998 Jul 24, Washington, D.C. CONNECTIVE TISSUE DISEASE.

Osborn, T. G., Ghosh, S., Hanna, V. E., Wilson, V. K., and Moore, T. L. Treatment of women with silicone gel breast implants [abstract]. Arthritis and Rheumatism. 1993, 36, (9 (Supplement)): S71. CONNECTIVE TISSUE DISEASE.

Osborn, T. G., Lawrence, J. M., Madson, K. L., Ghosh, S., and Moore, T. L. Silicone gel breast implants: Spectrum of rheumatologic complaints. Arthritis and Rheumatism. 1992, 35, (9 (Supplement)): S162. CONNECTIVE TISSUE DISEASE.

Osborn, T. G., Nesher, G., and Moore, T. L. Effect of silicone injection on skin thickness and antinuclear antibody in the tight-skin mouse [abstract]. Arthritis and Rheumatism. 1994 Sep, 37, (9 (Supplement)): S27. IMMUNE EFFECTS/toxicology.

Osborn, T. G, Wilson, V. G., Hanna, V. E., Ghosh, S., and Moore, T. L. Laboratory evaluation of rheumatologic patients with silicone gel breast implants [abstract]. Arthritis and Rheumatism. 1993 Sep, 36, (9 (Supplement)): S118. IMMUNE EFFECTS/connective tissue disease.

Osborn, T., Moore, T., and McMurtry, P. Effect of polydimethylsiloxane on autoimmune parameters in C57BL-B6 lpr/lpr mice [abstract]. Arthritis and Rheumatism. 1995 Sep, 38, (9 (Supplement)): S325. IMMUNE EFFECTS.

Ostermeyer-Shoaib, B., and Patten, B. M. Chest pain and breast implants [letter-reply]. Southern Medical Journal. 1996b, 89, (1): 99-100. PAIN/local complications.

Ostermeyer-Shoaib, B., and Patten, B. M. A high incidence of breast implant failure in women with neurologic and rheumatic symptoms [abstract]. Canadian Journal of Neurological Science. 1993b Sep, 20, (Supplement 4): S79. NEUROLOGIC DISEASE/connective tissue disease.

Ostermeyer-Shoaib, B., and Patten, B. M. A motor neuron disease syndrome occurring in women with silicone breast implant failure [abstract]. Canadian Journal of Neurological Science. 1993c Sep, 20, (Supplement 4): S110. NEUROLOGIC DISEASE.

Ostermeyer-Shoaib, B., and Patten, B. M. A multiple sclerosis-like syndrome in women with breast implants or silicone fluid injections into breasts [abstract]. Neurology. 1994, 44, (Supplement 2): A158. NEUROLOGIC DISEASE.

Ostermeyer-Shoaib, B., and Patten, B. M. Multiple sclerosis-like syndrome in women with silicone breast implants: A novel neurological disease with rheumatological symptoms [abstract]. Arthritis and Rheumatism. 1995 Sep, 38, (9 (Supplement)): S264. NEUROLOGIC DISEASE.

Ostermeyer-Shoaib, B., and Patten, B. M. Rheumatologic and neurologic findings in silicone adjuvant breast disease. Arthritis and Rheumatism. 1992c Nov, 35 , (9 (Supplement)): S66. CONNECTIVE TISSUE DISEASE/neurologic disease.

Ostermeyer-Shoaib, B., and Patten, B. M. Silicone adjuvant breast disease: More neurological cases [abstract]. Annals of Neurology. 1992b, 32, (2): 254. NEUROLOGIC DISEASE.

Ostermeyer-Shoaib, B., and Patten, B. M. Silicone breast implants or silicone injections associated with the development of autoimmune diseases [abstract]. The 7th Congress European Section Berlin-Germany June 2-6, 1993, International Confederation for Plastic and Reconstructive Surgery. 1993. NEUROLOGIC DISEASE/CONNECTIVE TISSUE DISEASE/silicone injection.

Ostermeyer-Shoaib, B., and Patten, B. M. Systemic disease in women following the insertion of saline breast implants [abstract]. Southern Medical Journal. 1993, 86, 118. CONNECTIVE TISSUE DISEASE/saline.

Ostermeyer-Shoaib, B., Patten, B. M., and Ashizawa, T. Motor neuron disease after silicone breast implants and silicone injections into the face [abstract]. Annals of Neurology. 1992c Aug, 32, (2): 254. NEUROLOGIC DISEASE/silicone injection.

Owen, M. J. Silixane surface activity. in: Zeigler, J. M., and Fearon, F. W. G., eds. Silicon-Based Polymer Science—A Comprehensive Resource, Advances In Chemistry Series. 1990, p. 705-739. SILICONE CHARACTERIZATION/silicone chemistry.

Owsley, Jr. J. Q., and Peterson, R. A. Symposium on Aesthetic Surgery of the Breast: proceedings of the symposium of the Educational Foundation of the American Society of Plastic and Reconstructive Surgeons, Inc., and the American Society for Aesthetic Plastic Surgery, Inc., held at Scottsdale, Arizona, Nov. 23-26, 1975. St Louis, Mo.: C. V. Mosby, Co. 1978. GENERAL.

Palmon, L. U., Foshager, M. C., Everson, L. I., and Cunningham, B. L. Use of ruptured breast implants: Sensitivity of snowstorm appearance [abstract]. Radiology. 1994, 193, 177. MAMMOGRAPHY/rupture/local complications.

Pandeya, N. K. Transumbilical insertion of saline-filled breast implants [letter]. Plast. Reconstr. Surg. 1997 Apr, 99, (4): 1198. SALINE/letter.

Pangman, W. J., inventor. Compound prothesis. Pangman, W. J., assignee. U.S. 3,559,214. 1971 Feb 2. POLYURETHANE.

Pappas, M. A., Schmidt, C. C., Shanbhag, A. S., Whiteside, T. A., Rubash, H. E., and Herndon, J. H. Biological response to particulate debris from nonmetallic orthopedic implants. Wise, D. L., and et al., eds. Human Biomaterials Applications. Totowa, N.J.: Humana Press Inc., 1996: 115. GRANULOMAS/local complications/general.

Pardue, A. M. Systemic illness and augmentation mammaplasty [letter]. Annals of Plastic Surgery. 1980 May, 4, (5): 436. CONNECTIVE TISSUE DISEASE/letter.

Parsons, R. W., Kossovsky, N., Heggers, J. P., and Robson, M. C. Observation of cellular immune phenomena provoked by silicone. In: International Confederation for Plastic and Reconstructive Surgery. The VIII International Congress of Plastic Surgery, June 26-July 1, 1983. Montreal: International Confederation for Plastic and Reconstructive Surgery, 1983, p. 18-19. IMMUNE EFFECTS.

Pasteris, J. D., Wopenka, B., Freeman, J. J., Young, V. L., and Brandon, H. J. Detection of silica in breast implant capsules [abstract]. 1998. SILICA.

Peled, I. J. Capsular contracture in a diabetic patient [letter]. Plast. Reconstr. Surg. 1983 Feb, 71, (2): 281. CAPSULE-CONTRACTURE/local complications/letter.

Pennisi, V. R. On mammography in the presence of breast implants [letter-reply]. Plast. Reconstr. Surg. 1978 Aug, 62, (2): 287-288. MAMMOGRAPHY/saline/letter.

Perrin, E. R. On the use of soluble steroids within inflatable breast prostheses [letter-reply]. Plast. Reconstr. Surg. 1978 Jul, 62, (1): 106. STEROIDS/local complications/capsule-contracture/letter.

Persoff, M. M. Problems with the use of soluble steroids within inflatable breast prostheses containing soluble steroids [letter]. Plast. Reconstr. Surg. 1978, 62, (1): 106. STEROIDS/local complications/capsule-contracture/letter.

Peters, W. J. An outcome analysis of 100 women. Plast. Reconstr. Surg. 1998, 40, 105. CAPSULE CONTRACTURE/letter-reply.

Peters, W. J. Re: Factors affecting the rupture of silicone-gel breast implants [letter-reply]. Annals of Plastic Surgery. 1994 Oct, 33, (4): 624-628. RUPTURE/local complications/letter.

Peters, W. J. Silicone gel as an adjuvant [letter]. Plast. Reconstr. Surg. 1995 Feb, 95, (2): 417-418. IMMUNE EFFECTS/letter.

Peters, W. J., Keystone, E., Lee, P., Pugash, R., Rubin, L., and Smith, D. Silicone gel breast implants and connective tissue disease: An analysis of 500 consecutive patients. New Orleans: Plastic Surgical Forum, Annual Scientific Meeting, 1993 Sep 18. CONNECTIVE TISSUE DISEASE.

Peters, W. J., Smith, D., and Lugowski, S. Re: Do patients with silicone-gel breast implants have elevated levels of blood silicon compared with control patients? [letter-reply]. Annals of Plastic Surgery. 1995c Oct, 35, (4): 442-443. SILICON MEASUREMENT/letter.

Peters, W. J., Smith, D., and Lugowski, S. Silicon capsule assays with low-bleed silicone gel implants [letter]. Plast. Reconstr. Surg. 1996 May, 97, (6): 1311-1312. SILICON MEASUREMENT.

Peters, W. J., Smith, D., Lugowski, S., Mchugh, A., Macdonald, P., and Baines, C. Silicon and silicone levels in patients with silicone implants. Potter, M., and Rose, N., eds. Current Topics In Microbiology and Immunology: Immunology of Silicones. Heidelberg: Springer-Verlag, 1996, pp. 39-48. SILICON MEASUREMENT.

Petit, J. Y., Lê, M., and Mouriesse, H. Breast augmentation and the risk of subsequent breast cancer [letter]. The New England Journal of Medicine. 1993 Mar 4, 328, (9): 661-662. CANCER/letter.

Petrek, J. A. Cystosarcoma phyllodes. Harris, Jr., Hellman, S., Henderson, I. G., and Kinne, D. W., eds. Breast Disease. J.B. Lippincott Co., 1987a, pp. 583-589. CANCER.

Petrek, J. A. Other cancers in the breast. Harris, Jr., Hellman, S., Henderson, I. G., and Kinne, D. W., eds. Breast Diseases. Philadelphia: J.B. Lippincott Co., 1987b, pp. 712-717. CANCER.

Pfister, W. R. Permeation kinetics of c q7-2167/2168 silicone gel through silastic, silastic II and silastic MSI mammary envelopes. Dow Corning, 1990 Mar 27. TOXICOLOGY.

Pfleiderer, B. Evaluation of exposure to silicone in the liver of women with breast implants by h-mrs. Annual Meeting of The Society of Magneticresonance , 1995: 209. MIGRATION/local complications/silicon measurement.

Piccoli, C. W. Imaging modalities for breast implants [invited discussion]. Annals of Plastic Surgery. 1994 Sep, 33, (3): 256-257. MAMMOGRAPHY.

Piccoli, C. W. Imaging of the patient with silicone gel breast implants. Seminars in Breast Disease. 1968, 1, (4): 176-189. MAMMOGRAPHY.

Pickford, M. A., and Webster, M. H. C. Implant rupture by mammography [letter]. British Journal of Plastic Surgery. 1994, 47, 512. MAMMOGRAPHY/local complications/rupture.

Pincus, T., and Callahan, L. Self report of morning stiffness and rheumatic diseases: Similarities in patients with rheumatoid arthritis and fibromyalgia [abstract]. Arthritis and Rheumatism. 1995. AI-CTD BACKGROUND.

Placik, O. J. Scleroderma-like esophageal disease in children of mothers with silicone breast implants [letter]. J. Amer. Med. Assoc. 1994 Sep 14, 272, (10): 768-769. CHILDREN'S EFFECTS/breast feeding/connective tissue disease/letter.

Plotzke, K. P., and McMahon, J. M. *In Vitro* Percutaneous Absorption of 14C-Decamethylcyclopentasiloxane (D5) in Rat Skin. Midland, Mich.: Dow Corning Corporation, 1996 Aug 14. TOXICOLOGY.

Plotzke, K. P., McMahon, J. M., and Hubbell, B. G. *In Vivo* Percutaneous Absorption of 14C-Decamethylcyclopentasiloxane (D5) in the Rat. Midland, Mich.: Dow Corning Corporation, 1996 Sep 30. TOXICOLOGY.

Plotzke, K. P., McMahon, J. M., Hubbell, B. G., Neeks, R. G., and Mast, R. W. Dermal absorption and disposition of 14C-decamethylcyclopentasiloxane D5 in rats [abstract]. Toxicologist. 1994 Mar, 14, 1720. TOXICOLOGY.

Plotzke, K. P., and Salyers, K. L. A Pilot Study to Determine if Classical Inducing Agents Alter the Metabolic Profile of a Single Dose of 14C-Octamethylcyclotetrasiloxane (D4) in Rats. Midland, Mich.: Dow Corning Corporation, 1997 Oct 3. TOXICOLOGY.

Pollock, H. Breast capsular contracture [letter]. Plast. Reconstr. Surg. 1997 Nov, 100, (6): 1619-1620. CAPSULE-CONTRACTURE/local complications/letter.

Pollock, H. Polyurethane-covered breast implant [letter]. Plast. Reconstr. Surg. 1984 Nov, 74, (5): 729. POLYURETHANE/infection/local complications/letter.

Poppi, V. Capsular contracture after augmentation mammaplasty [letter]. Plast. Reconstr. Surg. 1985 Mar, 75, (3): 442. CAPSULE-CONTRACTURE/local complications/letter.

Potter, M., and Morrison, S. Plasmacytoma development in mice injected with silicone gels. Current Topics in Microbiology and Immunology: Immunology of Silicones. 1996, pp. 397-407. IMMUNE EFFECTS/myeloma.

Praet, S. F. E., van Blomberg, MK., and Mulder, J. W. et al. Anti-polymeric antibodies, rheumatic complaints and silicone leakage of breast implants. 14th European League Against Rheumatism Congress. 1999 Jun 6-1999 Jun 11, Poster Presentation, abstract. IMMUNE EFFECTS.

Pramod, N. K. Breast implant rupture due to gunshot injury [letter]. Plast. Reconstr. Surg. 1994 Nov, 94, (6): 893-894. RUPTURE/local complications/letter.

Price, R. I. M. Failure of steroid instillation to prevent capsular contracture after augmentation mammaplasty [letter]. Plast. Reconstr. Surg. 1976 Mar, 57, (3): 371. STEROIDS/local complications/capsule-contracture.

Pruzinsky, T. What influences public perceptions of silicone breast implants? [discussion]. Plast. Reconstr. Surg. 1994 Aug, 94, (2): 326-327. PSYCHOSOCIAL.

Puckett, C. L. Mammograms of the reconstructed breast [editorial]. Plast. Reconstr. Surg. 1991 Sep, 88, (3): 482-483. MAMMOGRAPHY/reconstruction.

Rabkin, C. S., Silverman, S., Tricot, G., Garland, L. L., Ballester, O., and Potter, M. The National Cancer Institute Silicone Implant/Multiple Myeloma Registry. Current Topics in Microbiology and Immunology: Immunology of Silicones. 1996, p. 385-387. MYELOMA.

Radiation Sterilization Working Group. Draft TIR on radiation sterilization material qualification. 1996 Aug 23. RADIATION.

Rajan, S. S., Clauw, D. J., Grossman, L. W., Myers, K. J., and Patt, R. H. Breath-hold mrs for the detection of silicone migration to the liver [abstract]. Proceedings of Society of Magnetic Resonance and European Society For Magnetic Resonance In Medicine and Biology. August 19-25, 1995, Nice, France., 1995 Aug. MIGRATION/local complications.

Ramon, I., Ullmann, Y., and Peled, I. J. Re: Infection following breast reconstruction [letter]. Annals of Plastic Surgery. 1991, 27, 179-180. INFECTION/local complications/letter.

Raso, D. S. Alternative light microscopy techniques for the demonstration of silicone. Annual Meeting of the U.S. and Canadian Academy of Pathology, 1994 Mar, San Francisco. Abst #101. SILICON MEASUREMENT.

Raso, D. S. Breast prostheses, the immune response, and B- and T-lymphocytes [letter]. Plast. Reconstr. Surg. 1994 Mar, 93, (3): 649-650. IMMUNE EFFECTS/letter.

Raso, D. S. Microscopic demonstration of intraductal extension of silicone from a ruptured breast implant [letter]. Plast. Reconstr. Surg. 1993 Jul, 92, (1): 176. MAMMOGRAPHY/rupture/local complications/migration/letter.

Raso, D. S., and Crymes, L. W. Synovial metaplasia of periprosthetic breast capsules. Modern Pathology. 1993, 6, 19A. CAPSULE-CONTRACTURE.

Raso, D. S., Greene, W. B., Greene, A. S., and McGown, S. T. The absence of esophageal lesions in maternal progeny of silicone-injected rats [letter]. Plast. Reconstr. Surg. 1997 May, 99, (6): 1784-1785. BREAST FEEDING/children's effects/connective tissue disease/letter.

Raso, D. S., Greene, W. B., and Metcalf, J. S. Capsular synovial metaplasia and breast implants, with reply by Raso, et al. [letter-reply]. Archives of Pathology and Laboratory Medicine. 1995a Feb, 119, (2): 116. CAPSULE-CONTRACTURE/silicon measurement/letter.

Raso, D. S., Greene, W. B., and Metcalf, J. S. Silicone breakdown and clinical implications of mammary and extramammary synovial metaplasia in periprosthetic capsules [letter]. Plast. Reconstr. Surg. 1995b Dec, 96, (7): 1747. CAPSULE-CONTRACTURE/local complications/letter.

Ratner, B. D. ESCA for the study of biomaterial surfaces. Chiellini, E., Guisti, P., Migharesi, C., and Nicolais, L., eds. Polymers in Medicine II. New York: Plenum Press, 1986, pp. 13-25. SILICONE CHARACTERIZATION.

Ratner, B. D., Leach-Scampavia, D., Cridon, W., Tidwell, C. D., Boland, T., and Yang, P. Surface properties of filled silicone elastomers. Transactions of the Society for Biomaterials. 1994, 17, 22. SILICON MEASUREMENT/general.

Reddick, L. P. Lack of correlation between silicone breast implants and scleroderma [letter]. Plast. Reconstr. Surg. 1992 Mar, 89, (3): 575-576. CONNECTIVE TISSUE DISEASE.

Reed, M. J. The silicone controversy [letter]. Immunology Today. 1996 Mar, 17, (3): 147. IMMUNE EFFECTS/letter.

Rees, T. D. Local and systemic response to injectable silicone fluid. in: Rubin, L. R., Ed. Biomaterials in Reconstructive Surgery. St. Louis: The C.V. Mosby Company, 1983. SILICONE INJECTION.

Reintgen, D., Berman, C., and Cox, C. et al. The Anatomy of Missed Breast Cancers. Surg. Oncol. 1993, 2, 65-75. CANCER/mammography.

Reisch, M. Dow Chemical waylaid by implants. Chemical and Engineering News. 1998, Jan 11, (6-7). GENERAL.

Rempel, J. H. On closed compression rupturing of contracted breast implant capsules [letter]. Plast. Reconstr. Surg. 1977, 59, 838-839. RUPTURE/local complications/closed capsulotomy/letter.

Reveille, J. D., Targoff, I. N., Mimori, T., Nguyen, H. C., Goldstein, R., and Arnett, F. C. MHC class II alleles associated with myositis [abstract]. Arthritis and Rheumatism. 1992, 35 (Supplement), S84. IMMUNE EFFECTS.

Riordan, J., and Auerbach, K. Breast feeding problems. in: Riordan, J., and Auerbach, K., Editors. Breastfeeding and human lactation. Boston: Jones and Bartlett, 1993. BREAST FEEDING.

Robinson, C. Case report of asymmetrical striae following breast augmentation [letter]. Plast. Reconstr. Surg. 1997 Jan, 99, (2): 274-275. LOCAL COMPLICATIONS/letter.

Robinson, Jr. O. G. Re: Analysis of explanted silicone implants: A report of 300 patients [letter-reply]. Annals of Plastic Surgery. 1995 Jun, 35, (3): 335. RUPTURE/local complications/letter/explantation.

Robinson, O. G. Rate of rupture of silicone prostheses: excerpts from a study of over 3000 personal cases and twenty-five years experience. Birmingham, AL: 1992. RUPTURE/local complications.

Robinson, O. G. Re: Invited discussion on spontaneous autoinflation of saline mammary implants [letter and reply]. Annals of Plastic Surgery. 1998 Jan, 40, (1): 101-103. RUPTURE/deflation/letter.

Rohrich, R. J., and Clark, C. P. Controversy over the silicone gel breast implant: Current status and clinical applications. Texas Med. 1993, 89, (9): 52-58. GENERAL.

Romanelli, J. N. More on breast implants and connective tissue diseases [letter]. The New England Journal of Medicine. 1995 May 11, 332, (19): 1306. GENERAL/letter.

Romano, R. J., Stiller, J. W., Vasey, F. B., and Bradley, P. J. The development of fibromyalgia after silicone breast implants. The Korean experience. Arthritis and Rheumatism. 1995 Sep, 38, (9 (Supplement)): S325. CONNECTIVE TISSUE DISEASE.

Romano, T. J. Breast implants and connective-tissue disease [letter]. J. Amer. Med. Assoc. 1996 Jul 10, 276, (2): 102. CONNECTIVE TISSUE DISEASE/letter.

Rose, N. R. Letter to the Food and Drug Administration. European Journal of Plastic Surgery. 1992, 15, 6-8. IMMUNE EFFECTS.

Rose, N. R. Silicone implants and immune disease [invited comment]. Annals of Plastic Surgery. 1992 May, 28, (5): 499-501. SILICONE INJECTION/immune effects/connective tissue disease.

Rose, N. R., Landavere, M., and Kuppers, R. C. Silicone binding immunoglobulins in human sera. Current Topics in Immunology and Microbiology. 1996, 210, 269-282. IMMUNE EFFECTS.

Rosenau, B., Schneebaun, A. B., and et al. Development of an ELISA method for the detection of "antibodies" to silicone. Current Topics in Microbiology and Immunology: Immunology of Silicones. 1996. IMMUNE EFFECTS.

Rosenbaum, J. The American College of Rheumatology statement on silicone breast implants represents a consensus [letter]. Arthritis and Rheumatism. 1996 Oct, 39, (10): 1765. GENERAL/letter.

Rosenberg, L. The relationship between breast cancer and augmentation mammaplasty: An epidemiologic study [discussion]. Plast. Reconstr. Surg. 1986 Mar, 77, (3): 368. CANCER.

Rosenberg, R., Cambron, L. D., and Williamson, M. R. Magnetic resonance imaging of the breast [letter]. Western Journal of Medicine. 1996 Jul-1996 Aug 31, 165, (1/2): 58-59. MAMMOGRAPHY/letter.

Rosner, G., and Merget, R. Allergenic potential of platinum compounds. in: Dayan, A. D., Hertel, R. F., Heseltine, E., Kazantizis, G., Smith, E. M., and Van der Venne, M. T., eds. Immunotoxicity of Metals and Immunotoxicology. New York: Plenum Press, 1990, p. 93-102. PLATINUM.

Rothfuss, S., Schumacher, R., Baker, D., and Hamas, R. S. Studies on an unusual fluid filled bursal-like sac surrounding certain silicone-gel filled breast implants [abstract]. Arthritis and Rheumatism. 1992 Sep, 35, (9 (Supplement)): S345. CAPSULE-CONTRACTURE/local complications.

Rountree, S. D., Holiday, D. B., and Pueblitz, S. Does silicon exposure from ruptured breast implants trigger production of ANA/GM1 antibodies [abstract]. Neurology. 1995 Apr, 45, ((Supplement 4)): A462-A463. IMMUNE EFFECTS.

Roven, A. N. The real cause of silicone autoimmune disease [letter]. Plast. Reconstr. Surg. 1996 May, 97, (6): 1307. IMMUNE EFFECTS/letter.

Rowley, M. J., Teuber, S. S., Cook, A., and Gershwin, M. E. Epitope mapping of antibodies to type I collagen in women with silicone breast implants. Arthritis and Rheumatoid Abstracts. 1993 Sep. IMMUNE EFFECTS.

Royce, P. C. Breast implants and connective-tissue diseases [letter]. The New England Journal of Medicine. 1994 Nov 3, 331, (18): 1232. CONNECTIVE TISSUE DISEASE/letter.

Rubin, J. M., Helvie, M. A., Adler, R. S., and Ikeda, D. US appearance of ruptured silicone breast implants [letter]. Radiology. 1994, 190, 583-584. MAMMOGRAPHY/local complications/rupture/letter.

Rubin, L. R. The deflating saline implant—facing up to complications [editorial]. Plast. Reconstr. Surg. 1980, 65, (5): 665. RUPTURE/local complications/saline.

Rubin, L. R. Degradation of the saline-filled silicone-bag breast implant. Rubin, L. R., Ed. Biomaterials in reconstructive surgery. St. Louis, MO: C.V. Mosby Company, 1983, pp. 260-271. RUPTURE/saline/local complications.

Rubin, L. R. Polyurethanes in biomedical engineering II—Proceedings of the 2nd international conference on polyurethanes in biomedical engineering, Fellback/Stuttgart, June 18-19, 1986 [book review]. Annals of Plastic Surgery. 1988 Jul, 21, (1): 89-90. POLYURETHANE.

Rudolph, R. Capsule contraction around silicone breast implants. Rubin, L. R., Ed. Biomaterials In Reconstructive Surgery. St. Louis: The C.V. Mosby Company, 1983. CAPSULE-CONTRACTURE/local complications.

Rudolph, R. Myofibroblasts and free silicon around breast implants [letter-reply]. Plast. Reconstr. Surg. 1979, 63, (5): 720. CAPSULE-CONTRACTURE/local complications/letter.

Rudolph, R. Occurrence and activity of myofibroblasts in human capsular tissue surrounding mammary implants [discussion]. Plast. Reconstr. Surg. 1981, 68, 913. CAPSULE CONTRACTURE/local complications.

Ruhr, L. P. Analysis of a two-year gel implant study of Dow Corning Q7-2159A and Dow Corning MDF-0193 in rats for endocrine effects. Midland, Mich.: Dow Corning Corporation, 1991 Jun 6. TOXICOLOGY.

Ruhr, L. P., Hoffman, R. D., Goodman, D. G., Selwyn, M. R., and Mast, R. W. Carcinogenicity bioassay in the rats of two mammary implant envelope elastomers [abstract]. Toxicologist. 1994 Mar, 14, 835. CARCINOGENICITY.

Ryan, E. H., and Moore, W. J. Silicone breast implants and atypical autoimmune disease [letter]. Annals of Internal Medicine. 1993 Nov 15, 119, (10): 1053-1054. CONNECTIVE TISSUE DISEASE/letter.

Sadowsky, N. L. Mammography and breast implants [discussion]. Plast. Reconstr. Surg. 1988 Jul, 82, (1): 7-8. MAMMOGRAPHY.

Safavi, K. H., Heyse, S. P., and Hochberg, M. C. Estimating the incidence and prevalence of rare rheumatologic diseases. A review of methodology and available data sources [editorial]. J. Rheumatol. 1990, 17, (8): 990-993. AI-CTD BACKGROUND.

Salmon, S. E., and Kyle, R. A. Re: Induction of Plasmacytomas with silicone gel in genetically susceptible strains of mice [letter]. Journal of the National Cancer Institute. 1995 Feb 15, 87, (4): 315-316. MYELOMA/letter.

Sánchez-Guerrero, J., Karlson, E. W., Colditz, G. A., Hankinson, S. E., Hunter, D. J., Speizer, F. E., and Liang, M. H. Silicone breast implants (SBI) and connective tissue disease (CTD) [abstract]. Arthritis and Rheumatism. 1994 Sep, 37, (9 (Supplement)): S282. CONNECTIVE TISSUE DISEASE.

Sánchez-Guerrero, J., Sergen, J. S., Schur, P. H., and Liang, M. H. Rheumatic disease symptoms and silicone breast implants [letter-reply]. Arthritis and Rheumatism. 1995 May, 38, (5): 721. CONNECTIVE TISSUE DISEASE.

Sanger, J. R., Kolachalam, R., Komorowski, R. A., Yousif, N. J., and Maltoub, H. S. Silicone gel extravasation into the arm: a clinical and experimental correlation of the effect on the peripheral nerve. in: Stratmeyer, M. E., Project Officer. Silicone in Medical Devices, 1998 Feb, Baltimore, Md. Rockville, Md.: U.S. Department of Health and Human Services, 1991 Dec: 69-76. NEUROLOGIC DISEASE.

Sangster, A. G., and Hodson, M. J. Silica in higher plants. In: Evered, D., and O'Connor, M., eds. Silicon Biochemistry (CIBA Foundation Symposium 121). Sussex, U.K.: John Wiley & Sons, 1986, p. 90-111. SILICA.

Santerre, J. P., and Adams, G. A. Re: The polyurethane foam covering the Même breast prosthesis: A biomedical breakthrough or a biomaterial tar baby? Annals of Plastic Surgery. 1992 Nov, 29, (5): 477-478. POLYURETHANE/local complications/letter.

Santiago-Young, O., Sessoms, S. L., and Burns, D. Rheumatic manifestations in patients with silicone gel implants. San Antonio: 57th Annual Scientific Meeting of the American College of Rheumatology, 1993 Nov. CONNECTIVE TISSUE DISEASE.

Schain, W. S. Breast reconstruction after mastectomy: Who seeks it, who refuses? [discussion]. Plast. Reconstr. Surg. 1995 Apr, 95, (5): 823. PSYCHOSOCIAL/reconstruction.

Schain, W. S. Reasons why mastectomy patients do not have breast reconstruction [discussion]. Plast. Reconstr. Surg. 1990 Dec, 86, (6): 1123-1125. PSYCHOSOCIAL.

Schmidt, G. H. Calcification bonded to saline-filled breast implants [letter]. Plast. Reconstr. Surg. 1993 Dec, 92, (7): 1423-1425. CALCIFICATION/saline/capsule-contracture/local complications/letter.

Schmidt, G. H. Re: Analysis of explanted silicone implants: A report of 300 patients [letter]. Annals of Plastic Surgery. 1995 Sep, 35, (3): 335. RUPTURE/letter.

Schmidt, G. H. Rupture and aging of silicone gel breast implants [letter]. Plast. Reconstr. Surg. 1994 Jun, 93, (7): 1535. RUPTURE/local complications/letter.

Schned, A. R., Taylor, T. H., and Groff, G. D. Complications of silicone implant [letter]. J. Amer. Med. Assoc. 1985 Feb 1: 253-256. GRANULOMAS/local complications/letter.

Schnur, P. L. Silicon tissue assay: A measurement of capsular levels from chemotherapeutic Port-a-Catheter devices [discussion]. Plast. Reconstr. Surg. 1997 Apr, 99, (5): 1359-1361. SILICON MEASUREMENT.

Schoenfeld, Y., and Isenberg, D. A. The Mosaic of Autoimmunity. Amsterdam, Holland: Elsevier Press, 1989. AI-CTD BACKGROUND.

Schottenfeld, A. D., Laing, Gillespie, B. W., Burns, C. J., and et al. A Population-Based Case Control Study of Scleroderma Among Women: Assessment of Risk From Exposure to Silicone (Abstract No. T127). 1996 Annual Conference of ISEE. 1996 Jul. CONNECTIVE TISSUE DISEASE.

Schwarz, K. Significance and functions of silicon in warm-blooded animals. Review and outlook. in: Bendz, G., and Lindquist, I., eds. Biochemistry of silicon and related problems. New York and London: Plenum Press, 1978, p. 207-230. CHILDREN'S EFFECTS/ breast feeding/silicon measurement.

Seckel, B. R., and Costas, P. D. Total versus partial muscle coverage for steroid containing double lumen breast implants in augmentation mammaplasty. Annual Meeting of the American Society of Aesthetic Plastic Surgery. 1991, American Society of Aesthetic Plastic Surgery, New York. STEROIDS.

Seitchik, M. W. Macroscopic intraductal silicone gel [letter]. Plast. Reconstr. Surg. 1996 Feb, 97, (2): 487. MIGRATION/local complications.

Semple, J. L., Narini, P. P., and Hay, J. B. Preparation techniques for silicone gel in the evaluation of its in vivo effects [letter]. Plast. Reconstr. Surg. 1993 Oct, 92, (5): 979. SILICONE CHARACTERIZATION/letter.

Semple, J. L., Narini, P., Hay, J. B., and Szalai, J. P. Silicone gel and delayed hypersensitivity [letter]. Plast. Reconstr. Surg. 1998 Jan, 101, (1): 249-250. IMMUNE EFFECTS/letter.

Sendagorta, E. Sézary syndrome in association with silicone breast implant [letter]. Journal of the American Academy of Dermatology. 1995 Dec, 33, (6): 1060-1061. IMMUNE EFFECTS /letter.

Sergent, J. S., Fuchs, H., and Johnson, J. Silicone implants and rheumatic diseases. In: Kelley, W. N., Harris, E. D., Ruddy, S., and Sledge, C. B., eds. Textbook of Rheumatology: Update 4. W.B. Saunders Company, 1993, p. Update 1-13. GENERAL/connective tissue disease.

Shankar, R., and Greisler, H. P. Inflammation and biomaterials. Greco, R. S. Implantation Biology: The Host Response and Biomedical Devices. Boca Raton, Fla.: CRC Pr., 1994, p. 68-80. IMMUNE EFFECTS.

Shanklin, D. R. Late tissue reactions to silicone and silica. Stratmey, M. E, editor. Silicone in Medical Devices: Conference Proceedings. Baltimore, Md.: U.S. Department of Health and Human Services, Food and Drug Administration, 1991, p. 103-105. IMMUNE EFFECTS.

Shanklin, D. R. Silicone-associated diseases: Tissue findings [abstract]. Southern Medical Journal. 1993, 86, S104. CAPSULE-CONTRACTURE/local complications.

Shanklin, D. R., Dreiman, M. F., Hal, M. F., and Smalley, D. L. Anablot band frequencies and clusters in patients with silicone mammary devices, 1998. IMMUNE EFFECTS/ SILICONE CHARACTERIZATION.

Shanklin, D. R., Peterson, C., and Smalley, D. L. Enhanced urinary silicate excretion in women with implanted silicone devices [abstract]. FASEB J. 1997, 11, A548. SILICON MEASUREMENT.

Shanklin, D. R., and Smalley, D. L. Additional surgery after breast device implantation. J. Rheumatol. 1998a, 25, 2474. LOCAL COMPLICATIONS/letter.

Shanklin, D. R., and Smalley, D. L. Comparative memory T-lymphocyte response to silica: Crystalline, amorphous, fumed amorphous, and chalk [abstract]. FASEB J. 1995, 9, A1058. IMMUNE EFFECTS/silica.

Shanklin, D. R., and Smalley, D. L. Differential capsulopathy by silicone implant type [abstract]. Lab Invest. 1996, 74, 24A. CAPSULE-CONTRACTURE/local complications.

Shanklin, D. R., and Smalley, D. L. Evidence for degradation of silicones in vivo with recrystallization as silica in peripheral nerve [abstract]. FASEB J. 1996a, 10, A785. NEUROLOGIC DISEASE/silica.

Shanklin, D. R., and Smalley, D. L. The immunopathology of siliconosis. Immunologic Research. 1998b, 18, (3): 125-173. IMMUNE EFFECTS/connective tissue disease.

Shanklin, D. R., and Smalley, D. L. Risk of connective tissue disease among women with breast implants: Study adds nothing to knowledge of processes of tissue injury induced by silicone [letter]. British Medical Journal. 1998c. CONNECTIVE TISSUE DISEASE/letter.

Shanklin, D. R., and Smalley, D. L. Silicone immunopathology. Science and Medicine. 1996 Sep-1996b Oct 31: 22-31. IMMUNE EFFECTS.

Shanklin, D. R., and Smalley, D. L. Silicone immunopathology [letter-reply]. Science and Medicine. 1997 Jan-1997 Feb 28, 4, (1): 3. IMMUNE EFFECTS/letter.

Shanklin, D. R., Smalley, D. L., Hall, M. F., and Stevens, M. V. T Cell-Mediated Immune Response to Silica in Silicone Breast Implant Patients. Current Topics in Microbiology and Immunology: Immunology of Silicones. 1996b, p. 227-236. IMMUNE EFFECTS/silica.

Shanklin, D. R., Smalley, D. L., and Russano, J. Second generation silicone disease [abstract]. Journal of Investigative Medicine. 1996a Jan, 44, (1): 17A. CHILDREN'S EFFECTS/immune effects.

Shepherd, M., Cooper, B., Brown, A., and Kalton, G. Psychiatric illness in general practice. Oxford University Press, 1981. PSYCHOSOCIAL.

Shermak, M. A., Chang, B. W., Soto, A., and VanderKolk, C. A. A retrospective analysis of contracture and rupture in 379 breast implants. Presented at the 74th Annual Meeting of the American Association of Plastic Surgeons. San Diego, Calif.: American Association of Plastic Surgeons, 1995 May 2. CAPSULE-CONTRACTURE/local complications/rupture.

Shiffman, M. A. Re: Breast implants and cancer [letter]. Journal of the National Cancer Institute. 1998 Feb 4, 90, (3): 248. CANCER/letter.

Siddiqui, W. H. Evaluation of the liver microsomal enzyme induction potential of decamethylcyclopentasiloxane in the rat. Midland, Mich.: Dow Corning Corporation, 1989 Sep 18. TOXICOLOGY.

Sigal, R., Naama, H., Noone, R., and Daly, J. Silicone retards murine tumor growth [abstract]. Plast. Surg. Researchives of Council 39th Annual Mtg, Scientific Session VII, 1994 Jun 7: 223-5. CARCINOGENICITY.

Silicone Implant Survivors. Symptoms Frequently Associated with Silicone Implants. http://www.Geocities.com/HotSprings/8689/symptoms.html 1999. CONNECTIVE TISSUE DISEASE.

Silicones Environmental Health and Safety Council. Siloxane Use Summary Table. Silicones Environmental Health and Safety Council, 1994 Oct 10. SILICONE CHARACTERIZATION.

Silicones Environmental Health and Safety Council. Summary of the Chemistry and Toxicology of 56 Siloxanes Described in the ITC's 30th Report. Silicones Environmental Health and Safety Council, 1995 Aug 29. SILICONE CHARACTERIZATION/toxicology.

Silman, A. J., Black, C. M., and Welsh, K. I. Epidemiology, demographics, genetics. Clements, P. J., and Furst, D. E., eds. Systemic Sclerosis. Baltimore: Williams and Wilkins, 1996, p. 23-49. AI-CTD BACKGROUND.

Silman, A. J., and Hochberg, M. C. Epidemiology of the Rheumatic Diseases. Oxford: Oxford University Press, 1993. AI-CTD BACKGROUND.

Silveira, L. H., Cuéllar, M. L., Scopelitis, E., Martínez-Osura, P., and Espinoza, L. R. Evaluation of rheumatic complaints in women with silicone breast implants [abstract]. Arthritis and Rheumatism. 1992 Sep, 35, (9 (Supplement)): S347. CONNECTIVE TISSUE DISEASE.

Silveira, L. H., Sandifer, M., Cuéllar, M. L., Martínez-Osuna, P., Scopelitis, E., and Espinoza, L. R. Serum antinuclear antibodies in women with silicone breast implants [abstract]. Arthritis and Rheumatism. 1992, 35, (9 (Supplement)): S66. IMMUNE EFFECTS.

Silver, D. S., and Silverman, S. L. Chest pain and breast implants [letter]. Southern Medical Journal. 1996 Jan, 89, (1): 97. PAIN/local complications/letter.

Silver, D. S., Silverman, S. L., and Mendoza, M. Chest wall syndrome in patients with silicone breast implants [abstract]. Arthritis and Rheumatism. 1994, 37 (Suppl), S270. PAIN/local complications.

Silverman, B. G., Brown, S. L., and Bright, R. A. Epidemiology of silicone breast implants [letter-reply]. Annals of Internal Medicine. 1997 Apr 15, 126, (8): 667-668. CONNECTIVE TISSUE DISEASE/letter.

Silverman, B. S., Brown, S. L., Bright, R. A., and Kaczmarek, R. S. A critical assessment of the relationship between silicone breast implants and connective tissue diseases [review]. Regul Toxicol Pharmacol. 1996, 23 (1 Part 1), 74-85. IMMUNE EFFECTS/connective tissue disease.

Silverman, S., Borenstein, D., Solomon, G., Espinoza, L., and Colin, M. Preliminary operational criteria for systemic silicone related disease [abstract]. Arthritis and Rheumatism. 1996c, 39, (9 (Supplement)): S51. CONNECTIVE TISSUE DISEASE.

Silverman, S., Gluck, O., Silver, D., Tesser, J., Wallace, D., Neumann, K., Metzger, A., and Morris, R. The prevalence of autoantibodies in symptomatic and asymptomatic patients with breast implants and patients with fibromyalgia. Current Topics in Microbiology and Immunology. 1996b, 210, 318-322. IMMUNE EFFECTS/connective tissue disease.

Silverman, S., Mendoza, M., Silver, D., and et al. Measurement of fatigue in patients with silicone breast implants (SBI) as compared to fibromyalgia (FM) and rheumatoid arthritis (RA) [abstract]. Arthritis and Rheumatism. 1994 Sep, 37, (9 (Supplement)): S271. CONNECTIVE TISSUE DISEASE.

Silverman, S., Vescio, R., Silver, D., Renner, S., Weiner, S., and Berenson, J. Silicone gel implants and monoclonal gammopathies: Three cases of multiple myeloma and the prevalence of multiple myeloma and monoclonal gammopathy of undetermined significance. Current Topics in Microbiology and Immunology: Immunology of Silicones. 1996a, p. 367-374. MYELOMA.

Silversmith, P. E. Ultrasound for capsular contracture of the breast [letter]. Plast. Reconstr. Surg. 1984 Mar, 73, (3): 500. MAMMOGRAPHY/capsule-contracture/letter.

Silverstein, M. J. Augmentation mammoplasty: Its effect on breast diagnosis and treatment [abstract]. In. Breast Center Foundation Newsletter. Van Nuys, Calif.: Van Nuys Breast Clinic, 1987, p. Abstract #99. MAMMOGRAPHY/cancer.

Silverstein, M. J. Breast cancer diagnosis in the augmented patient [letter-reply]. Archives of Surgery. 1989 Feb, 124, 257-258. MAMMOGRAPHY/cancer/letter.

Silverstein, M. J. Oncologic aspects of augmentation mammaplasty [letter-reply]. Plast. Reconstr. Surg. 1995 Apr, 95, (5): 936. MAMMOGRAPHY/cancer/letter.

Simpson, J. D., Khaw, K. P., Hefeneider, S. H., and Bennett, R. M. Anti-collagen type-1 antibodies, but not anti ss-dna antibodies are elevated in silicone breast implant recipients [abstract]. Arthritis and Rheumatism. 1994 Sep, 37, (9 (Supplement)): S423. IMMUNE EFFECTS.

Slavin, S. A. Breast reconstruction with contralateral rectus abdominis myocutaneous flap [discussion]. Plast. Reconstr. Surg. 1983 May, 71, (5): 676-677. RECONSTRUCTION.

Slavin, S. A. Dynamics of IL-2 receptor stimulation in T cells from patients with silicone toxicity [abstract]. FASEB J. 1997, 11, A536. IMMUNE EFFECTS.

Slavin, S. A. T-lymphocyte response to silica in fibromyalgia (FM) [abstract]. 1996 Annual Conference of ISEE, 1996 Jul: (abstract no. T130). SILICA/AI-CTD BACKGROUND.

Smalley, D. L., and Shanklin, D. R. Age range and percentile rank of Tm lymphocyte stimulation indices (si) in 1,000 silicone breast implant patients (SBIp) [abstract]. 8th Annual Conference of the International Society for Environmental Epidemiology, August 17-21, Edmonton, Alberta, Canada. 1996. IMMUNE EFFECTS.

Smalley, D. L., Talcott, T. D., and Shanklin, D. R. Response enhancement in T lymphocyte memory testing by triphasic combination of silicaceous mitogens [abstract]. FASEB Journal. 1996b, 10, A1434. IMMUNE EFFECTS/silica.

Smith, A. L. The analytical chemistry of organosilicon materials. Smith, A. L., ed. The Analytical Chemistry of Silicones. New York : Wiley & Sons, 1991, p. 23-45, Chap. 2. SILICONE CHARACTERIZATION/silicone chemistry.

Smith, A. L. Trace analysis involving silicones. Smith, A. L., ed. The Analytical Chemistry of Silicones. New York : Wiley & Sons, 1991, p. 71-95, Chap. 4. SILICONE CHARACTERIZATION/silicone chemistry.

Smith, C. A. Breast implant controversy deserves more study [letter]. Texas Medicine. 1994 Feb, 90, (2): 7. GENERAL/letter.

Smith, M. L., and Wey, P. D. Immediate breast reconstruction in patients with locally advanced disease [open discussion]. Annals of Plastic Surgery. 1997 Apr, 38, (4): 350-351. CANCER/reconstruction.

Smith, S. D., Gerber, P. C., Meade, B. J., Butterworth, L. F., Mccay, J. A., White, K. L., and Munson, A. E. Natural killer cell activity is suppressed following exposure to silicone gel [abstract]. Toxicologist. 1994 Mar, 14, 1250. IMMUNE EFFECTS.

Solomon, G. Clinical and serologic features of 639 symptomatic women with silicone gel implants: evidence for novel disease siliconosis. Arthritis Rheum. 1994b, 37, (9): S423. CONNECTIVE TISSUE DISEASE.

Solomon, G. Clinical features of a subset of symptomatic women with silicone breast implants and extreme elevations of serum IGM [abstract]. Arthritis and Rheumatism. 1996, 39. CONNECTIVE TISSUE DISEASE/immune effects/myeloma.

Solomon, G., Borenstein, D., Bridges, A. J., Colin, M., Freundlich, B., Goldsmith, F., Silverman, S., Wallace, D., and Weiner, S. Preliminary Criteria for Silicone Related Disease (SSRD). Berkeley Delphic Panel. 1995 Oct 22. CONNECTIVE TISSUE DISEASE.

Solomon, G., Espinoza, L., and Silverman, S. Breast implants and connective-tissue diseases [letter]. The New England Journal of Medicine. 1994 Nov 3, 331, (18): 1231. CONNECTIVE TISSUE DISEASE/letter.

Solomon, G., Silverman, S., and Espinoza, L. More on breast implants and connective-tissue disease [letter-reply]. The New England Journal of Medicine. 1995, 332, 1306-1307. GENERAL/letter.

Spear, S. L. Capsulotomy, capsulectomy, and implantectomy [editorial]. Plast. Reconstr. Surg. 1993 Aug, 92, (2): 323-324. CAPSULE CONTRACTURE/local complications/closed capsulotomy/explantation.

Spear, S. L., Heppe, H., and Garvey, R. C. Diffusion characteristics of Solu-Medrol across double-lumen breast implants in vivo and in vitro. Annual Meeting of the American Society for Aesthetic Plastic Surgery, 1991 Apr 29, New York, NY. STEROIDS.

Spear, S. L., and Maxwell, G. P. Discussion of Evans, G.R.D. et al. Plast. Reconstr. Surg. 1995, 96, (5): 116-118. RADIATION.

Spiera, H. Rheumatic disease in patients with silicone implants [abstract]. Arthritis and Rheumatism. 1992, 35 (Supplement), S349. CONNECTIVE TISSUE DISEASE.

Spiera, H. Scleroderma after silicone augmentation mammoplasty [letter-reply]. J. Amer. Med. Assoc. 1988 Jul 7, 260, (2): 236-238. CONNECTIVE TISSUE DISEASE.

Spiera, H., Spiera, R. F., and Gibofsky, A. Silicone breast implants and connective tissue disease [letter-reply]. J. Rheumatol. 1994, 21, (10): 1979-1980. CONNECTIVE TISSUE DISEASE/letter.

Spiera, R. F., and Gibofsky, A. Scleroderma in women with silicone breast implants: Comment on the article by Sánchez-Guerrero et al. [letter]. Arthritis and Rheumatism. 1995 May, 38, (5): 719. CONNECTIVE TISSUE DISEASE.

Spiera, R. F., Gibofsky, A., and Spiera, H. Breast implants and connective-tissue diseases [letter]. The New England Journal of Medicine. 1994 Nov 3, 331, (18): 1232. CONNECTIVE TISSUE DISEASE/letter.

Spira, M. Clinical experience with polyurethane-covered gel-filled mammary prostheses [discussion]. Plast. Reconstr. Surg. 1981 Oct, 68, (4): 519-520. POLYURETHANE/local complications/infection/capsule-contracture.

Star, V. L., Scott, J., Sherwin, R., Hochberg, M. C., Lane, N., and Nevitt, M. Validity of self-reported physician-diagnosed rheumatoid arthritis for use in epidemiologic studies. San Antonio: 57th Annual Scientific Meeting of the American College of Rheumatology, 1993 Nov. CONNECTIVE TISSUE DISEASE.

Stark, F. O., Falender J.R., and Wright, A. P. Silicones. Wilkinson, G., Stona, F. G. A., and Abel, E. W., eds. Comprehensive Organometallic Chemistry. Volume 2 ed. Oxford: Pergamon Press, 1982. SILICONE CHEMISTRY.

Stewart, M. W., and Elliott, M. Characteristics of women with and without breast implants [letter]. J. Amer. Med. Assoc. 1997 Sep 10, 278, (10): 818. GENERAL/letter.

Stott-Kendall, P. Torn Illusions. DebCar Publishing, 1994. GENERAL.

Stroman and et al. Abstract: in-vivo mr detection of silicone gel degradation. Fifth World Biomaterials Congress, Toronto, Canada. 1996 May. SILICONE CHARACTERIZATION.

Stueber, K. A complication of tissue expander breast reconstruction [letter]. Plast. Reconstr. Surg. 1997 Apr, 99, (5): 1464-1465. MAMMOGRAPHY/local complications/expander/letter.

Stump, A. S. An Inhalation Range-Finding Reproductive Toxicity Study of Decamethylcyclo-pentasiloxane (D5) in Rats. Midland, Mich.: Dow Corning Corporation, 1996b Aug 27. TOXICOLOGY.

Stump, A. S. An Inhalation Range-Finding Reproductive Toxicity Study of Octamethylcyclotetra-siloxane. Midland, Mich.: Dow Corning Corporation, 1997 Jul 29. TOXICOLOGY.

Stump, A. S. An Inhalation Range-Finding Reproductive Toxicity Study of Octamethylcyclotetra-siloxane (D4) in Rats. Midland, Mich.: Dow Corning Corporation, 1996 Aug 27. TOXICOLOGY.

Stump, A. S. An Inhalation Range-Finding Reproductive Toxicity Study of Octamethylcyclotetra-siloxane (D4) in Rats. Midland, Mich.: Dow Corning Corporation, 1996a Mar 7. TOXICOLOGY.

Sun, L., Ricci, J. L., Alexander, H., Klein, A., Lattarulo, N., and Blumenthal, N. C. Silicone in the blood and capsule of women with breast implants (abstract). Fifth World Biomaterials Congress, Toronto, Canada. 1996. SILICON MEASUREMENT.

Sunshine, J. Evaluating the health risks of breast implants [letter]. The New England Journal of Medicine. 1996, 335, (15): 1155. GENERAL/letter.

Swan, S. H. Estimating The Prevalence and Duration of Use of Silicone Breast Implants. Abstracts of Immunology. PREVALENCE.

Swan, S. H., Teuber, S. S., and Gershwin, M. E. Silicone implant controversy [letter]. The Lancet. 1995, 345, 319. CONNECTIVE TISSUE DISEASE/letter.

Swanson, A. B. Complications of silicone elastomer prostheses [letter]. J. Amer. Med. Assoc. 1977 Aug 29, 238, (9): 939. MIGRATION/general/letter.

Swanson, A. B., Maupin, K., Nalbandian, R. M., and de Groot-Swanson, G. Host reaction to silicone implants: a long term clinical and histopathological study. In: Corrosion and Degradation of Implant Materials, Fraker, A. C.//Griffin, C. C., Eds. Philadelphia, Pa: American Society for Testing and Materials, 1985, pp. 267-277. SILICONE CHARACTERIZATION/local complications.

Swedish Cancer Society and Swedish National Board of Health and Welfare. The impact of breast cancer screening with mammography in women aged 40 to 49 years, 1996 Mar 21-1996 Mar 22, Falun, Sweden. MAMMOGRAPHY.

Taylor, R. B. Nuclear magnetic resonance spectroscopy. Smith, A. L. Ed. The Analytical Chemistry of Silicones. New York: Wiley & Sons, 1991, p. 347-419, Chap. 12. SILICON MEASUREMENT.

Taylor, R. B., and Kennan, J. J. 29Si NMR and blood silicon levels in silicon levels in silicone gel breast implant recipients. Magn Reson Med. 1996, 36, (3): 498-501. SILICON MEASUREMENT.

Tebbetts. John. Transumbilical approach to breast augmentation [letter]. Plast. Reconstr. Surg. 1994 Jul, 94, (1): 215-216. GENERAL/letter.

Teel, W. B. A population-based case-control study of risk factors for connective tissue diseases. Seattle, WA: University of Washington , 1997, c1997. CONNECTIVE TISSUE DISEASE.

Teich Alasia, S., Ambroggio, G. P., Di Vittoria, S., Sismondi, P., Stani, G. F., and Blandamura, R. Autoimmune Connective Tissue Disease and Silicone Implants. In: International Confederation for Plastic and Reconstructive Surgery, 7th Congress, 1993, Berlin. CONNECTIVE TISSUE DISEASE.

Tenenbaum, S. A., Cuéllar, M. L., Garry, R. F., and Espinoza, L. R. Production of antibodies to partially cross-linked polymers in silicone breast implant recipients. Arthritis and Rheumatism. 1993a, S118, A123 (abstr). IMMUNE EFFECTS.

Tenenbaum, S. A., Cuéllar, M. L., Silveira, L. H., Garry, R. F., and Espinoza, L. R. Identification of a novel antigen recognized by breast implant recipients [abstract]. Arthritis and Rheumatism. 1993b Sep, 36, (9 (Supplement)): S118. IMMUNE EFFECTS.

Tenenbaum, S. A., and Garry, R. F. Silicone breast implants and antipolymer antibodies [letter-reply]. The Lancet. 1997b Sep 6, 350, (9079): 740-741. IMMUNE EFFECTS/ letter.

Tenenbaum, S. A., Rice, J. C., Espinoza, L. R., and Garry, R. F. Antipolymer antibodies, silicone breast implants, and fibromyalgia [letter-reply]. The Lancet. 1997 Apr 19, 349, (9059): 1171-1172. IMMUNE EFFECTS/connective tissue disease/letter.

Tenenbaum, S. A., Rice, J. C., Plymale, D. R., Sander, D. M., Wilson, R. B., Garry, R. F., Swan, S. H., Gluck, O. S., Teser, J. R. P., Weinrib, L. R., Stribrny, K. M., Bevan, J. A., Cuellar, M. L., and Espinoza, L. R. Diagnostic and clinical criteria distinguishing silicone related disorders from classical rheumatic disease. Arthritis and Rheumatism. 1995 Sep, 38, (9 (Supplement)): S325. IMMUNE EFFECTS/connective tissue disease.

Tenenbaum, S. A., Silveira, L. H., Martinez-Osuna, P., Cuéllar, M. L., Garry, R. F., and Espinoza, L. R. Identification of a novel autoantigen recognized in silicone associated connective tissue disease [abstract]. Arthritis and Rheumatism. 1992, 35, (9 (Supplement)): S73. IMMUNE EFFECTS.

Teuber, S. S., Saunders, R. L., Halpern, G. M., Brucker, R. F., Conte, V., Goldman, B. A., Winger, E. E., Wood, W. G., and Gershwin, M. E. Serum silicon levels are elevated in women with silicone gel implants. Potter and Rose, eds. Current Topics in Microbiology and Immunology: Immunology of Silicones. Heidelburg, 1996. SILICON MEASUREMENT.

Thompson, R. M., Howard. C.C., Brewer, E. J., and et al. Compositional Analysis of Silicone Prostheses. Columbus, Oh.: Columbus Laboratories, 1979 Feb 29. SILICONE CHARACTERIZATION.

Thompson, R. M., Howard, C. C., Crowley, J. P., DeRoos, F. L., and Leininger, R. I. Literature Review: Polymeric Material Leachables and their Biologic Effects and Toxicology. Columbus, Ohio: Battelle-Columbus Laboratories: 1979. TOXICOLOGY/silicone characterization.

Tinkler, J. J. B., Campbell, H. J., Senior, J. M., and Ludgate, S. M. Evidence for an Association Between the Implantation of Silicones and Connective Tissue Disease. United Kingdom: UK Department of Health, Medical Devices Directorate, 1993 Feb. GENERAL.

Titley, O. G. The breast fish [letter]. British Journal of Plastic Surgery. 1997, 50, (4): 295. LOCAL COMPLICATIONS/letter.

Tomkins, E. C. A 28-day oral toxicity study of Dow Corning 200 fluid, 10 cst in rats. Midland, Mich.: Dow Corning Corporation, 1995 May 4. TOXICOLOGY.

Tompkins, E. C. A 13-week Subchronic Toxicity Study of Dow Corning 200® Fluid, 350 cst in Rats. Midland, Mich.: Dow Corning Corporation, 1995 Nov 7. TOXICOLOGY.

Trachtman, H., Ilowite, N., and Levine, J. Increased urinary no.3 and no.2 excretion in children breast fed by mothers with silicone implants. Arthritis and Rheumatism. 1996, 37, (supplement 9): S422. CHILDREN'S EFFECTS/breast feeding.

Travis, W. E., Balogh, K., Wolf, B. C., and Abraham, J. L. Silicone-related pathology: A review [abstract]. American Journal of Clinical Pathology. 1984 Jun, 81, 806. LOCAL COMPLICATIONS.

Tricot, G. J. K, Naucke, S., Vaught, B. A., Vesole, D., Jagannath, S., and Barlogie, B. Is the risk of multiple myeloma increased in patients with silicone implants? Current Topics in Microbiology and Immunology: Immunology of Silicones. 1996, p. 357-359. MYELOMA.

Troum, O. M., Mongan, E. S., Brody, G. S., Gray, J. D., and Quismorio, Jr. F. P. Immunological function of patients with augmentation mammoplasty (AM) [abstract]. Arthrits and Rheumatism. 1987 Apr, 30, (4 (Supplement)): S107. IMMUNE EFFECTS.

Troum, O. M., and Quismorio, Jr. F. P. Rheumatoid arthritis in a male transexual [letter]. J. Rheumatol. 1985, 12, (3): 640-641. CONNECTIVE TISSUE DISEASE.

Truppman, E. S., and Ellenby, J. D. A 13-year evaluation of subpectoral augmentation mammoplasty. Symposium on Aesthetic Surgery of the Breast. St. Louis: Mosby, 1978, p. 344-352. CAPSULE CONTRACTURE.

Tugwell, P. Rheumatology: Clinical case definitions/diagnoses and clinical associations. Silicone breast implants in relation to connective tissue diseases and immunologic dysfunctrion: National Science Panel, 1998 Nov 17. CONNECTIVE TISSUE DISEASE/immune effects.

U.S. Congress House of Representatives. The FDA's Regulation of Silicone Breast Implants. A staff report prepared by the Human Resources and Intergovernmental Relations Subcommittee of the Committee on Government Operations. Washington, D.C.: U.S. Government Printing Office, 1992 Dec. GENERAL.

U.S. Congress House of Representatives. Is the FDA Protecting Patients from the Dangers of Silicone Breast Implants? Hearing before the Human Resources and Intergovernmental Relations Subcommittee of the Committee on Government Operations. Washington, D.C.: U.S.Government Printing Office, 1990 Dec 18. GENERAL.

U.S. Department of Health and Human Services, Public Health Service. Healthy People 2000: national health promotion and disease prevention objectives—full report with commentary. Washington, D.C.: Government Printing Office, 1991. GENERAL.

U.S. Environmental Protection Agency. Thirtieth Report of the Interagency Testing Committee to the Administrator, receipt of report and request for committee regarding priority testing list of chemicals. Federal Register. 1992 Jul 9, 57, (152): 30608. TOXICOLOGY.

Udkoff, R., Alim, A., Ahn, C., Shaw, W., and Bassett, L. W. MR imaging in the evaluation of breast implants [abstract]. Radiology. 1991, 181, 347. MAMMOGRAPHY.

Uretsky, B. F. Systemic illness and augmentation mammaplasty [letter-reply]. Annals of Plastic Surgery. 1980 May, 4, (5): 436. IMMUNE EFFECTS/letter.

Utell, M. J., Plotzke, K. P., Varaprath, S., Lane, T. H., and Kolesar, G. B. Clinical Studies on the Respiratory Effects of Octamethylcyclotetrasiloxane (D4): Mouthpiece and Nasal Exposures. Midland, Mich.: Dow Corning Corporation, 1997 Sep 4. TOXICOLOGY.

Vaamonde, R., Cabrera, J. M., Vaamonde-Martín, R. J., Jimena, I., and Marcos Martín, J. Silicone granulomatous lymphadenopathy and siliconomas of the breast. Histology and Histopathology. 1997 Oct, 12, (4): 1003-1011. GRANULOMAS/silica/local complications/lymphadenopathy.

Valesini, G., Bavoillot, D., and Pittoni, V. Silicone breast implants and connective-tissue diseases [editorial]. Clinical and Experimental Rheumatology. 1995, 13, 521-523. CONNECTIVE TISSUE DISEASE.

Van Der Voet, G. B. Human exposure to lithium, thalium, antimony, gold, and platinum. In: Chang, L. W., ed. Toxicology of Metals. Boca Raton: Lewis Publishers, 1996, p. 455-460, Ch. 28. PLATINUM/toxicology.

Van Dyke, M. E. Chemical Characterization of Extract Residues from Silicone Gel-Filled Mammary Implant Devices. Midland, Mich.: Dow Corning Corporation, 1994 Aug 24. SILICONE CHARACTERIZATION.

Van Dyke, M. E., and Fowler, D. G. Evaluation of Techniques for the Determination of Analytes Present in Gel Bleed from Silicone Gel-Filled Mammary Implant Devices. Midland, Mich.: Dow Corning Corporation, 1994 Aug 17. SILICONE CHARACTERIZATION.

Van Dyke, M. E., and Fowler, D. G. A Study of Inter-Laboratory Testing Consistency for Determining the Chemical Properties of Dow Corning Silicone Gel-Filled Mammary Implant Devices. Midland, Mich.: Dow Corning Corporation, 1993 Dec 9. SILICONE CHARACTERIZATION.

Van Oss, C. J., and Naim, J. O. Aspecific Immunoglobulin Binding to Hydrophobic Surfaces. Current Topics in Microbiology and Immunology: Immunology of Silicones. 1996, 210, 85-91. IMMUNE EFFECTS.

Van Vollenhoven, R. Breast implants and connective tissue diseases [letter]. The New England Journal of Medicine. 1995 Nov 23, 333, (21): 1424. CONNECTIVE TISSUE DISEASE/letter.

Varaprath, S. to LeVier, R. R.1991 Jun 19. LOCAL COMPLICATIONS/letter.

Varaprath, S. to LeVier, R. R. Dow Corning: 1992 Jan 30. LOCAL COMPLICATIONS/letter.

Varaprath, S. Non-Regulated Study: Identification of Major Metabolites of Octamethylcyclotetra-siloxane (D4) in Rat Urine. Midland, Mich.: Dow Corning Corporation, 1996 Dec 17. SILICON MEASUREMENT/toxicology.

Varaprath, S., Salyers, K. L., and Plotzke, K. P. Non-Regulated Study: Identification of Major Metabolites of Octamethylcyclotetrasiloxane (D4) in Rat Urine. Midland, Mich.: Dow Corning Corporation, 1997 Aug 26. SILICON MEASUREMENT.

Varga, J., and Jimenez, S. A. (Thomas Jefferson University). Systemic sclerosis, 'human adjuvant disease' and other chronic systemic autoimmune diseases following augmentation mammoplasty. Stratmeyer, M. E., Project Officer. Silicone in Medical Devices, 1991 Feb, Baltimore, Md. Rockville, Md.: U.S. Department of Health and Human Services, 1991 Dec. CONNECTIVE TISSUE DISEASE.

Varga, J., and Jiminez, S. A. Augmentation mammoplasty and scleroderma [editorial]. Archives of Dermatology. 1990 Sep, 126, 1220-1222. CONNECTIVE TISSUE DISEASE.

Vasey, F. B. Clinical experience with systemic illness in women with silicone breast implants: Comment on the editorial by Rose [letter]. Arthritis and Rheumatism. 1997, 40, (8): 1545. CONNECTIVE TISSUE DISEASE/letter.

Vasey, F. B., and Aziz, N. Breast implants and connective tissue diseases [letter]. The New England Journal of Medicine. 1995 Nov 23, 333, (21): 1423. CONNECTIVE TISSUE DISEASE/letter.

Vasey, F. B., Aziz, N., Havice, D., Wells, A. F., and Haley, J. A. Prospective clinical status comparison between women retaining gel breast implants vs. women removing implants, Amer. Coll. Rheum. Mtg. (abstract). Arthritis and Rheumatism. 1996, 39. CONNECTIVE TISSUE DISEASE/explantation.

Vasey, F. B., Aziz, N., and Leaverton. Silicone Breast Implant Outcome Study (Abstract No. T69). 1996 Annual Conference of ISEE, 1996 Jul. CONNECTIVE TISSUE DISEASE.

Vasey, F. B., Aziz, N., Seleznick, M. J., Wells, A. F., and Valeriano, J. Silicone gel implant explantation [letter]. Plast. Reconstr. Surg. 1995 Dec, 96, (7): 1748-1749. EXPLANTATION/connective tissue disease/letter.

Vasey, F. B., Bocanegra, T. S., Havice, D. L., Seleznick, M. J., Bridgeford, P. H., and Germain, B. F. Silicone associated connective tissue disease: Onset of systemic signs and symptoms after traumatic rupture of silicone gel filled breast implants [abstract]. Arthritis and Rheumatism. 1992a, 24, (Supplement): S212. CONNECTIVE TISSUE DISEASE/local complications/rupture.

Vasey, F. B., Espinoza, L. R., Martinez-Osuna, P., Seleznik, M. J., Brozena, S. J., and Penske, N. A. Silicone and rheumatic disease: Replace implants or not? [letter]. Archives of Dermatology. 1991 Jun, 127, 907. CONNECTIVE TISSUE DISEASE/immune effects/explantation.

Vasey, F. B., Havice, D., Sileznick, M. T., and et al. Clinical manifestations of fifty consecutive women with silicone breast implants and connective tissue disease. Arthritis and Rheumatism. 1992b Sep, 35, (9 (Supplement)): S212. CONNECTIVE TISSUE DISEASE.

Vasey, F. B., Seleznick, M., and Wells, A. F. Rheumatic disease symptoms and silicone breast implants: Comment on the article by Cook et al. and the article by Sánchez-Guerrero et al. Arthritis and Rheumatism. 1995 May, 38, (5): 719-721. CONNECTIVE TISSUE DISEASE.

Vecchione, T. R. On closed compression to rupture capsules around breast implants [letter]. Plast. Reconstr. Surg. 1977 Jun, 59, (6): 840. CLOSED CAPSULOTOMY/rupture/letter/local complications.

Venanzi, W. E. The positive ANA by HEp-2 cell line assay in a normal population [abstract]. Arthritis and Rheumatism. 1994 Jun, 37, (6 (Supplement)): R19. IMMUNE EFFECTS.

Versaci, A. D. Refinements in reconstruction of congenital breast deformities [discussion]. Plast. Reconstr. Surg. 1985 Jul, 76, (1): 81-82. EXPANDER/reconstruction.

Vessman, J., Hammar, C., Lindeke, B., Stromberg, S., LeVier, R., Robinson, R., Spielvogel, D., and Hanneman, L. Analysis of some organosilicone compounds in biological material. Bendz, G., and Lindqvist, I., eds. Biochemistry of Silicon and Related Problems. New York and London: Plenum Press, 1978, p. 535-558. SILICONE CHARACTERIZATION/silicon measurement.

Vinnik, C. A. The hazards of silicone injections [editorial]. J. Amer. Med. Assoc. 1976a Aug 23, 959. SILICONE INJECTION.

Vinnik, C. A. Migratory silicone-clinical aspects of silicone in medical devices. in. Silicone in Medical Devices, Proceedings of a Conference, 1991: DHHS, 1991. MIGRATION.

Vinnik, C. A. Silicone mastopathy. In: Owsley Jr., JQ and Peterson, RA, Editors. Symposium on Aesthetic Surgery of the Breast : proceedings of the symposium of the Educational Foundation of the American Society of Plastic and Reconstructive Surgeons, inc., and the American Society for Aesthetic Plastic Surgery, Inc., held at Scottsdale, Arizona, November 23-26, 1975. St. Louis, MO: C.V. Mosby Company, 1978. SILICONE INJECTION.

Vistnes, L. M. Tissue expansion in soft-tissue reconstruction [discussion]. Plast. Reconstr. Surg. 1984 Oct, 74, (4): 491-492. EXPANDER/reconstruction.

Vistnes, L. M., and Ksander, G. A. Tissue response to soft silicone prostheses: Capsule formation and other sequelae. Rubin, L. R., Ed. Biomaterials in Reconstructive Surgery. St. Louis: The C.V. Mosby Company, 1983, p. 318-328. CAPSULE-CONTRACTURE/local complications.

Vogel, G. E. Analysis of excreted Dow Corning® 360 fluid from oral dosing of rhesus monkey. Midland, Mich.: Dow Corning Corporation, 1972 Feb 25. TOXICOLOGY.

Vogel, H., and Edmondson, E. Pathological findings in nerve and muscle biopsies from 55 women with silicone breast implants [abstract]. Neurology. 1996 Apr: A54, Abstract No. P01.137. NEUROLOGIC DISEASE.

Volpe, R. Thyrotropin receptor autoantibodies. Peter, J. B., and Shoenfeld, Y., eds. Autoantibodies. Amsterdam: Elsevier, 1996, pp. 822-829. CHILDREN'S EFFECTS/breast feeding.

Von Heiser, F. W., von Finckenstein, J., and Bohmnert, R. Are There Systemic Side Effects after Silicone Gel Breast Implants? Presented at the Plastic Surgery Berlin Congress, 1993. CONNECTIVE TISSUE DISEASE.

Wallace, D. J., and Schwart, E. Breast implants and connective-tissue diseases [letter]. The New England Journal of Medicine. 1994 Nov 3, 331, (18): 1232-1233. CONNECTIVE TISSUE DISEASE/letter.

Watts, G. T., Caruso, F., and Waterhouse, J. A. Mastectomy with primary reconstruction [letter]. The Lancet. 1980 Nov 1, 2, 967. RECONSTRUCTION/letter.

Weiner, S. R., Bulpitt, K. J., Myers, B. L., and et al. Chronic arthropathy after silicone augmentation mammaplasty (CSA) [abstract]. Arthritis and Rheumatism. 1992, 35, (9 (Supplement)): S212. CONNECTIVE TISSUE DISEASE.

Weiner, S. R., Clements, P. J., and Paulus, H. H. Connective tissue disease after augmentation mammaplasty. Arthritis and Rheumatism. 1988, 23, R23. CONNECTIVE TISSUE DISEASE.

Weiner, S. R., Suzuki, S. M., Clements, P. J., and Paulus, H. E. Scleroderma (PSS) after augmentation mammoplasty (AM) [abstract]. Arthritis and Rheumatism. 1989, 32, (4 (Supplement)): S79. CONNECTIVE TISSUE DISEASE.

Wellisch, D. K. Psychosocial aspects of breast implantation. Gorczyca, D. P., and Brenner, R. J., eds. The Augmented Breast: Radiologic and Clinical Perspectives. New York, Stuttgart: Thieme, 1997, p. 6-15. PSYCHOSOCIAL.

Wells, R. L. Treatment of capsular contracture around retromammary implant [letter]. Plast. Reconstr. Surg. 1990 Oct, 86, (4): 811. CAPSULE-CONTRACTURE/local complications/letter.

Wexler, A. M. Scleroderma after silicone augmentation mammoplasty [letter]. J. Amer. Med. Assoc. 1988 Nov 25, 260, (20): 236-238. CONNECTIVE TISSUE DISEASE/letter.

Whidden, P. G. Augmentation mammoplasty. Transplant/Reconstr Today. 1986, 3, 43. GENERAL.

White, Jr. K. L., McDaniel, C. W., Butterworth, F., and Klykken, P. C. Non-specific binding of IgG immunoglobulins to silicone mammary implant elastomer [abstract]. FASEB Journal. 1995 Mar 9, 9, (3): 2986. IMMUNE EFFECTS.

White, K. L. Jr., Butterworth, L. F., David, D. W., and Klykken, P. C. Failure of silicone gel to exacerbate autoimmune responses in female NZB/W mice [abstract]. SOT 1997 Annual Meeting. 1997: 265. IMMUNE EFFECTS/toxicology.

Whitmore, S. E. Breast implants and connective-tissue disease [letter]. J. Amer. Med. Assoc. 1996 Jul 10, 276, (2): 102. CONNECTIVE TISSUE DISEASE/letter.

Whysner, J. Epidemiology of silicone breast implants [letter]. Annals of Internal Medicine. 1997 Apr 15, 126, (8): 667. CONNECTIVE TISSUE DISEASE/letter.

Wick, G., Wagner, R., Klima, G., and Wilflingseder, P. Immunohistochemical analysis of the connective tissue capsule formation and constriction around mammary silicone prostheses. Cellular, Molecular and Genetic Approaches to Immunodiagnosis and Immunotherapy. University of Tokyo Press, 1987, p. 231-241. IMMUNE EFFECTS/capsule contracture/local complications.

Wigley, F. M., Miller, R., Hochberg, M. C., and Steen, V. Augmentation mammoplasty in patients with systemic sclerosis: Data from the Baltimore Scleroderma Research Center and Pittsburgh Scleroderma Data Bank [abstract]. Arthritis and Rheumatism. 1992, 35, (9 (Supplement)): S46. CONNECTIVE TISSUE DISEASE.

Wilhelm, K. Silicone and autoimmunity [letter]. Autoimmunity. 1993, 14, 341-342. CONNECTIVE TISSUE DISEASE/immune effects.

Wilkinson, S. Seeking Clarity on Breast Implants. C&EN Washington. 1998 Aug 10: 53-54. GENERAL.

Williams, A. F. Silicone breast implants, breastfeeding, and scleroderma [letter]. The Lancet. 1994 Apr 23, 343, 1043-1044. CHILDREN'S EFFECTS/breast feeding/connective tissue disease/letter.

Williams, H. J., and Weisman, M. H. Silicone breast implants in patients with undifferentiated connective tissue disease [abstract]. Arthritis and Rheumatism. 1994 Sep, 37, (9 (Supplement)): S422. CONNECTIVE TISSUE DISEASE.

Williams, J. E. Augmentation mammaplasty—Inframammary approach. In: Georgiade, N. G., ed. Reconstructive Breast Surgery. St. Louis, Mo.: The C.V. Mosby Company, 1976, p. 50-67. GENERAL.

Williams, J., Jackson, I., Hoberman, L., and et al. Outcome study following removal of breast implants [abstract]. Presented At 75th Meeting of American Association of Plastic Surgeons, 1996 May. EXPLANTATION.

Williams, T. L., Naito, H. K., Chan, S. C., Homburger, H. A., and Myers, G. College of American Pathologists Position Statement: Laboratory Testing for Monitoring Patients with Silicone Breast Implants [position paper]. College of American Pathologists, 1993 Fall. GENERAL.

Wilson, M. R., and Nitsche, J. F. Immunodiffusion assays for antibodies to nonhistone nuclear antigens. Rose, N. R., Friedman, H., and Fahey, J. L., Editors. Manual of Clinical Laboratory Immunology. Washington, D.C.: American Society for Microbiology, 1986, p. 41. IMMUNE EFFECTS.

Wilson, S. D., Levier, D., Butterworth, L., and Munson, A. Natural killer cell activity is enhanced following exposure to D4 [abstract]. Society of Toxicology 35th Annual Mtg. 1966 Mar: Abstract No. 1758. IMMUNE EFFECTS.

Wilson, S. D., and Munson, A. E. Serum corticosterone levels are elevated after exposure to octamethylcyclotetrasiloxane [abstract]. Society of Toxicology 1997 Annual Meeting. 1997: 265. TOXICOLOGY.

Wilson, S. D., and Munson, A. E. Silicone-induced modulation of natural killer cell activity. Current Topics in Microbiology and Immunology: Immunology of Silicones. 1996, p. 199-208. IMMUNE EFFECTS/toxicology.

Wise, D. M. Breast implants and trauma [letter]. Plast. Reconstr. Surg. 1994a Apr, 93, (5): 1104-1105. RUPTURE/local complications/letter.

Wise, D. M. Silicone gel breast implants [letter]. J. Amer. Med. Assoc. 1994b Jul 27, 272, (4): 272-273. GENERAL.

Wolf, C. J., Brandon, H., Jerina, K., and Young, L. Long Term Aging of Implanted Silcone/ Silica Composite Breast Implants. 1997 Jul. RUPTURE.

Wolf, C. J., Srivastava, A. P., Brandon, H. J., Jerina, K. L., and Young, V. L. Chemical, physical, and mechanical analysis of explanted breast implants. Potter, M., and Rose, N., eds. Current Topics in Microbiology and Immunology: Immunology of Silicones. 1996, pp. 25-37. EXPLANTATION/rupture/local complications.

Wolfe, F. Silicone breast implants and the risk of fibromyalgia and rheumatoid arthritis [abstract]. Arthritis and Rheumatism. 1995a Sep, 38, (9 (Supplement)): S265. CONNECTIVE TISSUE DISEASE.

Wolfe, J. N. On mammography in the presence of breast implants [letter]. Plast. Reconstr. Surg. 1978 Aug, 62, (2): 286. MAMMOGRAPHY/saline/letter.

Wolfe, S. M. Breast Implants: The Debate Continues. Public Citizen's Health Research Group: *Health Letter*. 1998 Sep, 2, 2-3. GENERAL.

Wong, O. Breast implants and connective-tissue diseases [letter]. The New England Journal of Medicine. 1994 Nov 3, 331, (18): 1233. CONNECTIVE TISSUE DISEASE/letter.

Wrona, N., Koeger, A. Lefranc J. P., Rozenberg, S., Meyer, O., Blondon, J., and Bourgeois, P. Systemic clinical and immunological manifestations following silicone mammoplasty [abstract]. Arthritis and Rheumatism. 1993 Sep, 36, (9 (Supplement)): S144. CONNECTIVE TISSUE DISEASE.

York, R., and Schardien, J. L. Developmental toxicity studies with octamethylcyclotetrasiloxane (D4) in cd rats and rabbits [abstract]. Toxicologist. 1994 Mar, 14, 572. TOXICOLOGY.

Yoshida, S. H., Teuber, S. S., Gershwin, M. E., and Swan, S. H. Letters to the Editor [letter]. Life Sciences. 1995, 57, (19): 1740. CONNECTIVE TISSUE DISEASE/letter.

Young, J. F. Disposition, storage, degradation, removal and excretion of the different silicones. Silicone in Medical Devices, Proceedings of a Conference, 1991: DHHS, 1991. TOXICOLOGY.

Young, V. L. Increase of immunologically relevant parameters in correlation with Baker classification in breast implant recipients [discussion]. Annals of Plastic Surgery. 1996a May, 36, (5): 518-521. IMMUNE EFFECTS/local complications/capsule-contracture/ connective tissue disease.

Young, V. L. Testing the test: An analysis of the reliability of the silicone sensitivity test (SILS) in detecting immune-mediated responses to silicone breast implants [letter]. Plast. Reconstr. Surg. 1996b Mar, 97, (3): 681-683. IMMUNE EFFECTS/letter.

Young, V. L., Brandon, H. J., Jerina, K. L., Wolf, C., and Schorr, M. W. Failure characteristics of explanted breast implants. Fifth World Biomaterials Congress, Toronto, Canada. 1996a May. EXPLANTATION/rupture.

Young, V. L., Nemecek, J. R., Schwartz, B. D., and Phelan, D. L. HLA typing in women with and without silicone gel-filled breast implants. Current Topics in Microbiology and Immunology: Immunology of Silicones. 1996, p. 209-225. IMMUNE EFFECTS.

Young, V. L., Peters, W., Brandon, H. J., Jerina, K. L., and Wolf, C. J. Determining the Frequency of Breast Implant Failure Requires Sound Scientific Principles. Plast. Reconstr. Surg. 1998 Sep, 102, (4): 1295-1299. RUPTURE/local complications.

Young, V. L., and Schorr, M. W. Analysis of 100+ consecutive breast implants for integrity and mechanism of failure. Presentation at the 74th Annual Meeting of the American Association of Plastic Surgeons. San Diego, Calif.: American Association of Plastic Surgeons, 1995 May 2. RUPTURE/local complications.

Yuen, J. C., Klitzman, B., and Serafin, D. Biomaterials used in plastic surgery. Grecoi, R. S. Implantation Biology: The Host Response and Biomedical Devices. Boca Raton, Fla.: CRC Press, 1994, p. 192-228. GENERAL.

Zandman-Goddard, G., Blank, M., Ehrenfeld, M., Gilburd, B., Gershwin, P. J., Gershwin, M. E., and Shoenfeld, Y. A comparison of autoantibody production in asymptomatic and symptomatic women with silicone breast implants. Arthr. Rheum. 1996, 39, S149. IMMUNE EFFECTS.

Zenick, H. et al. Chapter 27. in: Hayes, A. W. Ed. Principles and Methods of Toxicology. New York: Raven Press, 1994. TOXICOLOGY.

Zide, B. Complications of closed capsulotomy after augmentation [letter]. Plast. Reconstr. Surg. 1981 May, 67, (5): 697. CAPSULE CONTRACTURE/lymphadenopathy/local complications/letter.

Zuckerman, D. The Safety of Silicone Breast Implants. 1998, briefing paper. GENERAL.

Appendixes

APPENDIX A
Brief Description of the Scientific Workshop

At the request of the National Institutes of Health (NIH), the Institute of Medicine (IOM) established a Committee on the Safety of Silicone Breast Implants to provide an independent assessment of the health effects of silicone breast implants and prepare recommendations for a research agenda. As part of its contractual obligation to NIH, the committee held a Scientific Workshop in Washington, D.C. on July 22, 1998. The workshop was intended to provide members of the committee with an opportunity to hear presentations of recent work from industry, federal government, and academic physicians and scientists investigating silicone implants and to pose questions and clarify issues with these experts. Although the committee focused on peer-reviewed, published scientific reports for this project, listening to scientific presentations and engaging in conversations with working physicians and scientists familiarized the committee with a range of relevant and useful information.

OVERVIEW OF THE WORKSHOP

Eighteen physicians and scientists made presentations at the workshop. Among these were epidemiologists, immunologists, toxicologists, silicone chemists, pathologists, plastic surgeons, radiologists, and implant manufacturer officials responsible for studies of women with implants. The committee made a decision to invite representatives from the two U.S. manufacturers currently making and selling breast implants (McGhan Medical and Mentor Corporations) and also to include a representative from the Dow Corning Corporation, as the original implant manufacturer and silicone supplier that had carried out an extensive research program. Other invited investigators were identified in conversations with federal officials, and with U.S. and Canadian scientists, by review of the scientific literature, or on the recommendation of committee members. The committee's intent was to obtain available information on current studies of women carried out in preparation for manufacturer's pre market approval (PMA) applications and also to hear presentations on major NIH-funded epidemiological and basic science work that is in progress and on scientific and clinical work from a representative sample of different disciplines, specialties, and perspectives. Two and a half hours were reserved for manufacturers, two hours for federal scientists and two and a half hours for academic physicians and scientists. The committee added a total of 45 minutes for questions, divided into three separate periods during the day. The committee was impressed by the presentations and learned much from them and from the question-and-answer periods throughout the day. Although the information imparted was somewhat informal and most of it was not published or peer reviewed, it provided a useful context and overview to familiarize the Committee with a number of issues. The agenda for the workshop follows.

WORKSHOP AGENDA

INSTITUTE OF MEDICINE
National Academy of Sciences

Committee on the Safety of Silicone Breast Implants

Second Meeting of the Committee on the Safety of Silicone Breast Implants
Scientific Workshop
July 22, 1998

Leavey Conference Center, Georgetown University,
3800 Reservoir Road, N.W., Washington D.C.

8:15 a.m.	Welcome and Introductions	Stuart Bondurant, M.D., Chair
	Epidemiology and Observational Studies	
8:30 a.m.	Update on NCI's Follow-up of Women with Augmentation Mammoplasty	Louise Brinton, Ph.D. National Cancer Institute
		Lori Brown, Ph.D. Food and Drug Administration
9:00 a.m.	Clinical Results with McGhan Breast Implants	Raymond C. Duhamel, Ph.D. McGhan Medical Corporation
9:30 a.m.	Detection of Silica and NMR in Breast Implant Capsules	V. LeRoy Young, M.D. Washington University School of Medicine
10:00 a.m.	Committee Questions	
10:15 a.m.	*Break*	
	Immunology	
10:30 a.m.	Silicones as Immunological Adjuvants	John Naim, Ph.D. Rochester General Hospital

11:00 a.m.	Peritoneal Silicone Granulomas and Plasmacytoma Genesis in Mice	Michael Potter, M.D. National Cancer Institute
11:30 a.m.	Immunopathology and T-Cell Receptor Gene Expression in Capsules Surrounding Breast Implants	Fred Miller, M.D., Ph.D. Food and Drug Administration
12:00 p.m.	Committee Questions	
12:15 p.m.	*Lunch*	

Company Data (Mentor and Dow Corning)

1:00 p.m.	Potential Extractables (quantification, exposure, and toxicology)	Roger Wixtrom, Ph.D. Environ
	Silicone in Animal Models of Autoimmunity, Unpublished Immunotoxicity Testing Results	Kimber White, M.D. Medical College of Virginia
	"Antibodies" to Silicone, Further Findings Regarding Adjuvancy of Silicone Elastomer and Gel	Noel Rose, M.D. Johns Hopkins University
	Results from Five-Year Prospective Clinical Study of >21,000 Women with Silicone Gel-Filled Breast Implants, Clinical Data for Saline-Filled Breast Implants	Bobby Purkait, Ph.D. Mentor Corporation
2:00 p.m.	Summary and Overview of the Safety of Major Components of Breast Implants	Robert Meeks, Ph.D. Dow Corning Corporation

	Compositional Studies of Silicone Breast Implants	Thomas Lane, Ph.D. Dow Corning Corporation
	An Update on Silicone–Immune System Interactions	Paal Klykken, Ph.D. Dow Corning Corporation
3:00 p.m.	Committee Questions	

Surgery, Pathology, Radiology

3:30 p.m.	Work of the University of Florida Interdisciplinary Group on Silicone	Nancy Hardt, M.D. University of Florida
4:00 p.m.	Significant Findings on Breast Implant Rupture from a Seven-Year Study of 1,619 Explants	Lu-Jean Feng, M.D. Case Western Reserve School of Medicine and Mt. Sinai Medical Center
4:30 p.m.	MR Evaluation of Breast Implant Rupture	Michael S. Middleton, Ph.D., M.D. University of California, San Diego
5:00 p.m.	Immunological Effects Associated with Silicone Breast Implants	Marilyn M. Lightfoote, M.D. Food and Drug Administration
5:30 p.m.	Committee Questions	
5:45 p.m.	Adjourn	

APPENDIX B

Description of the Public Meeting

As part of its contractual obligation to the National Institutes of Health, the committee held a public meeting in Washington, D.C. following the one-day scientific workshop and a day of deliberations. The public meeting was held to gather a broad range of views, both objective and subjective, from lay, academic, advocacy, industry, and public policy groups. The committee considered the human dimension especially necessary and appropriate. The public meeting particularly encouraged women and their families to share their accounts and experiences with silicone breast implants. Although the committee focused on the peer-reviewed, published scientific literature for this report, the personal stories of women with implants provided a valuable context for its deliberations.

PREPARATIONS FOR THE PUBLIC MEETING

The public meeting was held on Friday, July 24, 1998, at the National Academy of Sciences (NAS) Building in Washington, D.C. The originally planned location was a 130-person-capacity meeting room in the Cecil and Ida Green Building at the Institute of Medicine's (IOM's) Georgetown facility. This space was oversubscribed by the large number of individuals who wished to attend the meeting. In response, the committee secured the 674-person-capacity auditorium in the NAS building. The committee thought that the principle that no person would be turned away from the public meeting was important and justified the effort to ensure ample space to accommodate all who wanted to attend.

Public Announcement of the Meeting

The IOM prepared a public announcement of the meeting that was posted on the IOM website and mailed on May 1, 1998, to approximately 300 individuals and organizations. These included consumer groups identified from the Food and Drug Administration's (FDA's) mailing list, as well as professional organizations, industry contacts, clinicians, academicians, scientists, and legal contacts identified through review of the literature, Internet searches, and other sources. The public meeting announcement provided background on the IOM study and requested that those who wanted to give an oral statement, provide a written statement, or simply attend the public meeting as observers, register and submit certain information prior to specified deadlines. Reporters who wanted to attend were asked to register with the Office of News and Public Information.

Written Statements

This public participatory event was an opportunity for those with relevant information about the safety of silicone breast implants to advise and inform the committee. The IOM defined relevant information to include evidence on the strengths or validity of the science associating silicone breast implants with local or systemic health effects. Seven questions were included in the notice to provide a common framework for the oral and written statements. However, the IOM did not require that statements be limited to scientific evidence alone, since one of the primary intentions was to provide a forum for women with implants to share their personal stories. This inclusive effort resulted in many individuals providing both oral and written testimony on their own behalf or on behalf of special interest groups and organizations. All of those who presented written or oral statements were advised that the information presented at or submitted for the meeting would become part of the public record and be accessible through the NAS Public Access Records Office.

There were approximately 175 written statements from the various individuals and organizations, including those submitted to the committee before, at the time of, or subsequent to the public meeting. As specified in the notice, these statements were limited to five pages or less via electronic mail, telefax, or regular postal mail, submitted by the August 28, 1998, deadline. Some statements were submitted after August 28; they also were accepted. The written statements were distributed to each of the committee members at three separate meetings.

Oral Statements

Fifty-five individuals and/or organizations made oral statements to the committee (eight of those listed on the official meeting agenda did not attend). In order to give an oral statement, a request had to be submitted by June 1, 1998. All travel arrangements and expenses were the responsibility of the individual presenter or organization. Oral presentations were limited to five minutes or less. Due to time constraints, originally only 51 presenters were selected based on those best representing the array of topics. In mid June, IOM staff notified all individuals who wanted to provide oral statements of the date, location, contact information, and preliminary agenda for the meeting. Information about the number of requests submitted, the number accepted, and a description of whose request was denied and for what reasons was also included. At that time the chairman of the committee decided to extend the scheduled meeting time from 5:15 p.m. to 7:00 p.m. in order to accommodate all those asking to speak who had met the June 1, 1998, deadline.

OVERVIEW OF THE MEETING

The public meeting was organized into twelve panels of five presenters each and one panel with two presenters. The speakers were grouped primarily by topic, but each panel included a woman with a personal implant history, an investigator, a clinician, and a person from a consumer group, if possible. Approximately half of the presenters were women who shared their personal stories. The other half consisted of consumers, academicians and other scientists, physicians, and professional groups. Although statements were limited to five minutes, additional time was provided at the end of each panel for the committee's questions. At the end of all the presentations, a general question-and-answer session was held with additional questions and some statements entertained from the day's presenters and from those in the audience.

AGENDA

INSTITUTE OF MEDICINE
National Academy of Sciences

Committee on the Safety of Silicone Breast Implants

PUBLIC MEETING
July 24, 1998

Auditorium
National Academy of Sciences
2101 Constitution Avenue, N.W., Washington, D.C.

8:45 a.m.	Welcome and Introductions	Dr. Kenneth I. Shine, IOM President Stuart Bondurant, M.D., Chair
	Panel I	
9:00 a.m.	Sidney Wolfe Public Citizen's Health Research Group	
	Susan Scherr National Coalition for Cancer Survivorship	
	C. Lin Puckett American Society of Plastic and Reconstructive Surgeons (ASPRS)	
	Elizabeth Connell Emory University	
	Martha Murdock National Silicone Implant Foundation	
9:25 a.m.	Committee Questions	

Panel II

9:40 a.m. Bruce L. Cunningham
American Society for Aesthetic
Plastic Surgery (ASAPS)

Anne M. Adams
Cocoa Beach, Florida

Robert A. Ersek
Austin, Texas

Eugene P. Goldberg
University of Florida

Kim Hoffman
Niangua, Missouri

10:05 a.m. Committee Questions

Panel III

10:20 a.m. Marie Pletsch, Plastic Surgeon
Santa Cruz, California

Mary McGrath
Aesthetic Surgery Education and
Research Foundation (ASERF)

Pat Wingate
Garden of Eden, South Carolina

Kathleen M. Price
Mission of Love

Jack Fisher
University of California, San Diego

10:45 a.m. Committee Questions

Panel IV

11:00 a.m. James J. Schlesselman
University of Miami School of Medicine

Marlene Keeling
Chemically Associated Neurological DisOrders (CANDO)

Leslie J. Dorfman
Stanford University School of Medicine

Arden R. Moulin
Flower Mound, Texas

Kathy Keithley-Johnston
Toxic Discovery Network

11:25 a.m. Committee Questions

Panel V

11:40 a.m. Donald Uhlmann
University of Arizona

Michael Raymond Harbut
Wayne State University

Jeffrey Brent
University of Colorado Health Sciences Center/Toxicology Associates

Douglas R. Shanklin
University of Tennessee

Thomas D. Talcott
Talcott Development, Inc.

12:05 p.m. Committee Questions

12:20 p.m. *Lunch Break*

Panel VI

1:15 p.m. Robert F. Garry
Tulane University Medical School

Merry Grant
Victims of Induced Chemical Exposure (VOICE) and Women Injured by Medical Devices Outreach (WIMDO)

Russell B. Wilson
Autoimmune Technologies

Paul H. Wooley
Wayne State University Medical School

James M. Anderson
Case Western Reserve University

1:40 p.m. Committee Questions

Panel VII

1:55 p.m. Pierre Blais
Innoval, Canada

Sherry Henderson
Silicone Solution Outreach of North Louisiana

Jackie A. Strange
Arlington, Virginia

Suzanne Kreger
Women Injured by Medical Devices Outreach (WIMDO)

Josey Vanderpas
Women Helping Women

2:20 p.m. Committee Questions

Panel VIII

2:35 p.m. Cheston M. Berlin, Jr.
Pennsylvania State University
College of Medicine and
Penn State Geisinger Health System

Jeremiah Levine
Schneider Children's Hospital

Jama K. Russano
Children Afflicted by Toxic
Substances (CATS)

Wendy Anne Epstein
New York University School of Medicine

Nikki Kaufman
Victims of Induced Chemical
Exposure (VOICE)

3:00 p.m. Committee Questions

Panel IX

3:15 p.m. Dennis Deapen
University of Southern California

Catherine Dlugopolski
Breast Implant Information Exchange

Pamela G. Dowd
Magic Valley Breast Implant Survivors

Brenda Glenn
Mabelvale, Arkansas

Steven E. Harms
University of Arkansas for
Medical Sciences and John L.
McClellan Memorial Veterans Hospital

3:40 p.m. Committee Questions

Panel X

3:55 p.m. Beth West
United Silicone Survivors of the World, Oregon

Lisa B. Hickey
Integrity

Diana Zuckerman
Institute for Women's Policy Research

Janice Ferriell
National Breast Implant Task Force

Barbara A. Capodanno
Reach and Inform

Bernard Patten
Seabrook, Texas

4:25 p.m. Committee Questions

Panel XI

4:40 p.m. Walter Spitzer
Methods in Epidemiology Center

Barbara L. Hasenour
Kentucky Women's Health Network

V. Leroy Young
Plastic Surgery Educational Foundation

Steve Hoffman
Niangua, Missouri

Saul Puszkin
Columbia University Medical Center

5:05 p.m. Committee Questions

Panel XII

5:20 p.m. Jamey S. Lacy
Houston, Texas

Diane Stevens
Impart, Inc.

Vesta Petersen
Louisville, Kentucky

Noreen Aziz
National Cancer Institute,
National Institutes of Health

Peggy Pardo
Breast Implant Information Exchange

5:45 p.m. Committee Questions

Panel XIII

6:00 p.m. Wanda Berry
Midland, Texas

Gayle Morton
Jacksonville, Arkansas

Sybil Niden
Goldrich Command Trust Network

6:15 p.m. Committee Questions

6:30 p.m. Audience Comments and Questions

7:00 p.m. Adjourn

SUMMARIES OF STATEMENTS

Since the IOM accepted all speakers who wished to address the committee and did not invite or seek to attract any individual or category of speaker, it is unlikely that these statements reflect a representative cross section of views and information on silicone breast implants, or that the speakers are a representative cross section of individuals with interests in, these implants.

Professional Organization Statements

Statements were submitted by seven professional medical organizations: the Academy of Cosmetic Surgery, the Aesthetic Surgery Education Research Foundation, the American Academy of Clinical Toxicology, the American Association of Electrodiagnostic Medicine, the American Society for Aesthetic Plastic Surgery, the American Society of Plastic and Reconstructive Surgeons, and the Plastic Surgery Educational Foundation. All of these organizations concluded that there is no association between silicone breast implants and systemic disease based on epidemiologic and other evidence. They expressed concern about women's increasing fear and anxiety caused by misinformation or sensationalism about complications, systemic and otherwise, of breast implantation. They affirmed their commitment to high-quality patient care and noted the benefits of silicone breast implants on quality of life and their positive influence on self image and level of functioning, particularly when used for reconstructive needs.

Scientists, Physicians and Others

Scientists, physicians, and others made presentations from a number of perspectives in support of, or in opposition to, systemic or other untoward effects of silicone gel-filled and saline-filled breast implants. Some reviewed the epidemiological evidence and discussed their own epidemiological work. Some cited clinical experience with implantation and caring for large numbers of breast implant patients with little in the way of serious problems or complaints. Others related experiences they ascribed to toxic reactions and discussed silicone chemistry. The evidence for or against effects on breast feeding or on children born to women with implants was discussed. A number of presentations on rupture prevalence or rupture rates were made, of both gel and saline implants, and the pathology of breast implants was reviewed. Scientists attempting to develop tests for a potential silicone-associated disease presented their work, and those who were looking into implant problems related their findings.

This diversity of subject matter generated a number of questions from the committee. The issues covered are reviewed and discussed in the body of this report.

Consumer Groups and Personal Statements

Consumer group representatives described the history of breast implantation and problems that have arisen over time. Those who participated in FDA regulatory activities described their experiences. Personal experiences with silicone breast implants and consumer group accounts of women with breast implants comprised the majority of statements. These were not solely from sick women with breast implants. A statement was received from a child whose mother was ill and from a spouse who stated, "it is not a women's issue, but one that affects husbands, families, taxpayers, and society."

Silicone gel implants were most commonly involved, but a significant number of women had saline implants, and a few had polyurethane-coated gel implants. Women with silicone gel implants had implants of longer duration from the 1970s and 1980s. Saline implants were used in the late 1980s and early 1990s, particularly after the FDA moratorium. About half of the women reported having breast implants to increase their breast size or after pregnancy and breast feeding. Others reported having implants for reconstructive purposes after mastectomy for fibrocystic or cancerous breasts and to correct congenital abnormalities such as tuberous breasts. According to these presentations, women who received breast implants during reconstructive surgery often reported that they were given other options, but alloplastic reconstruction was encouraged as part of the recovery process and the best route to a normal appearance. Consumer group and personal statements described silicone breast implants as the best alternative available for many reconstruction patients. Some statements stressed the value to women of having a choice and made a strong argument that such products should remain available to all patients.

A preponderance of the statements, however, from women with implants for augmentation or reconstruction reflected the conviction that the silicone in these implants was responsible for illness and disability. Most of the women described themselves as living healthy and active lives prior to implantation. Breast cancer patients reported full remission and good health prior to their implants. Many reported not smoking or abusing substances such as drugs or alcohol and having no family history of diseases such as cancers, lupus, and other immune diseases. A number had been successfully employed outside the home prior to implantation, as nurses, managers, secretaries, educators, a radiology technician, a realtor, a fitness consultant, and independent business women. They were women with families and friends, and reported being very outgoing people who enjoyed activities such as walking and running, aerobics, traveling, horseback riding, sewing, and gardening. They said their lives and health took a major turn for the worse after having breast implants.

Some women expressed great satisfaction with their physical appearance immediately after receiving their implants and, at the same time, improvement in their personal and professional lives. Others, however, reported immediate procedural and local complications such as extreme pain, swelling, discoloration, discharge, infection, displacement or extrusion of the implant, and nipple necrosis. Capsular contracture and severe breast pain were reported in many cases. Pain was said by some to be so intense that it was no longer possible to sleep prone or on the side, and some reported sleeping sitting upright to find comfort. These women also commonly described implants that decreased in volume over time or ruptured. In some women, symptoms occurred within a year or two of implantation; in others, symptoms occurred after a much longer period of time.

Many women reported multiple surgeries including many unexpected operations to correct local complications, to replace ruptured or extruding implants, or to totally remove the prosthesis, which in many cases required complete mastectomies. Many reported having closed capsulotomies to relieve some of the symptoms from Class III or IV capsular contractures. In women with multiple sets of implants, a number reported having single-lumen silicone gel implants originally, replaced later by saline implants mainly because of the FDA moratorium. In one particular statement, the original implants were saline, but due to the "sloshing" that is sometimes audible with these implants, they were later changed to silicone gel prostheses.

Prior to explantation, many of these women described living with a multitude of systemic symptoms and illnesses, which were often the primary reason for implant removal since they were more debilitating than the local complications. These women said they went from feeling "young and vibrant" to feeling prematurely aged, forced to use canes for support or, sometimes, even wheelchairs. Commonly reported symptoms are listed in Table B-1.

Numerous clinical laboratory findings were reported, such as positive antinuclear antibodies and rheumatoid factor; decreased T-cells, natural killer cells, and white blood cells; and elevated immunoglobulin G (IgG) levels. Abnormal nerve conduction tests, abnormal single-phase proton emission computed tomography (SPECT) scans, electroencephalograms (EEGs), and electromyograms (EMGs) were also reported.

Women described visiting an array of specialists and experiencing

TABLE B-1 Symptoms Reported by Individual Women or Consumer Groups (not in order of prevalence or severity)

Chronic fatigue	Allergic reactions
Sleep deprivation and disturbances	Chemical and environmental sensitivities
Night sweats	Swallowing difficulty
Painful and weak muscles and joints	Burning or dry eyes
Swollen and tender glands	Blurred vision
Itching and burning skin	Low blood pressure
Photosensitivity	Cardiac arrhythmia and palpitations
Numbness and tingling in the extremities	Cold and flu like symptoms
	Generalized pain and stiffness
Migraine or severe headaches	Seizures
Memory loss and disorientation	Skin tightening and discoloration
Cognitive disturbances	High blood pressure
Neuropathy	Heart attacks
Vertigo and dizziness	Shingles
Chest pain and tightening	Drooling
Breathing difficulties	Pleuritis
Weight loss	Candida and yeast infections
Rashes	Other fungal infections
Sicca syndrome	Ringing in ears
Menstrual dysfunction	Liver problems
Incontinence	Asthma
Diarrhea or bowel irritation	Keratoconjunctivitis
Low-grade fevers	Anemia
Tremors or twitches	Interstitial cystitis
Hair loss	Systemic sclerosis
General and morning stiffness	Bone cysts
Xerostomia	Chronic pancreatitis
Oral ulcer	Back pain

years of pain while undergoing a variety of medical treatments for a number of diagnoses such as rheumatoid arthritis, lupus erythematosus, multiple sclerosis, scleroderma, fibromyalgia-like syndrome, connective tissue disease, autoimmune disease, human adjuvant disease, Hashimoto's thyroiditis, Raynaud's phenomenon, Sjögren's syndrome, chronic inflammatory demyelinating polyneuropathy, organic brain disease, systemic chronic inflammatory disorder, cardiovascular disease, breast cancer, carpal tunnel syndrome, stroke, endometriosis, Graves' disease, lung cancer, "neuromuscular disease of the gastrointestinal tract," degenerative joint disease (including temporomandibular joint), hernia, and "restrictive pulmonary defect."

As a result of their physical symptoms, many women underwent a variety of procedures and medical treatments. Explantation, mastectomy after explantation, complete hysterectomy, or salpingo-oophorectomy, and lymph node removal were common. Some women described great difficulty in getting to the source of their problems, some with physicians unconvinced of a possible connection of their illness with implants, or physicians who would not treat them when they learned they had implants. Some women said that their physicians asked, "Are you involved in a lawsuit?" rather than, "How can I help?" Many women were told they were suffering from depression or stress, and many felt they were scorned and patronized. Others thought they were considered "hysterical" or fakers, claiming illness for purposes of litigation. Many of those making statements felt that the medical community turned them away in order to protect financial interests or avoid criticism. Their medical care needs were expensive, and several described loss of health insurance as a result of loss of employment.

Women made the association of silicone implants with their health problems primarily because of the temporal sequence of events or because of media coverage and articles that emerged in the early 1990s. Many used the Internet to locate information and reported finding other women who had strikingly similar experiences. In cases where there was no standard clinical diagnosis for the signs and symptoms they were experiencing, many of these women believed they were suffering from "siliconosis" due to exposure to the silicone in the implants. They understood that this condition might not have an accepted name in the medical community, but some believed it could be a new disease that the scientific community had yet to discover because research was funded by parties with biased and ulterior motives.

Only a small number of women reported doing intensive research about silicone breast implants before implantation—using information available from physicians, articles, and other women that had received implants. Most of the women relied solely on the information provided by their physicians regarding possible health risks. Many women felt that their physicians did not really obtain informed consent, since at best they recalled being told only of very small risks of complications associated with breast implants and most often being told that the implants were completely safe. The extent to which local complications were actually discussed is unclear based on the statements, but many women asserted that they were advised of few health risks associated with silicone gel or silicone shell implants by their physicians. They were often surprised by the fact that the implants ruptured or bled and that the contents of the shell were in the body. Many believed they were sick or dying because the silicone had migrated out of the shell. Many women said their physicians had told them that the implants would " last their lifetime," never mentioning the possibility of implant leakage or rupture with silicone migration. They believed that the implant would not rupture unless it sustained a severe impact (e.g., in a car accident) and did not know that it might have to be replaced because the product was not actually designed to last a lifetime.

Some women told of having laboratory tests performed that were reported to give positive results for the presence of silicone in their extremities, spine, lymphatic system, blood, or organs such as liver, spleen, gall bladder, and brain. Some women who were encouraged to breastfeed expressed the belief that their children had become ill from ingesting the silicone and other chemicals in implants that were presumed to be present in their breast milk. They reported that their children suffered with many of the same symptoms they themselves experienced, such as chronic fatigue and pain, and that these children were diagnosed with scleroderma, esophageal dysmotility, renal infection, rash, allergy, abnormal bone growth, upper respiratory tract infections, muscle weakness, leukemia, and precocious puberty. A consumer also reported that the milk bank would not accept breast milk donations from women with implants. She wondered why, if the milk is supposedly safe for the children of mothers with implants, it isn't safe for others.

Great mistrust of manufacturers such as Dow Corning and others was repeatedly expressed. Claims were made that the manufacturers will not fully disclose all of the chemicals used in implant, or the harmful effects discovered in some animal studies. These women believe that the "chemical cocktail" in the implants is toxic to living things and does not belong in their bodies. Many women reported being totally unaware that implants were not specifically FDA approved but used under a "grandfather clause" instead. They questioned how a product could be used that had not been tested for its long-term effects on humans, noting that warning labels are placed on products such as cigarettes and alcohol. Instead of manufacturers conducting appropriate studies to test product safety before use, these women speculated that they had been the "lab rats" and "guinea pigs" that were experimented on.

Some expressed concern that the observational studies being conducted by manufacturers are not following the FDA-approved protocol and that these studies are inherently biased. Women cited what they believed to be specific violations in the studies they were involved in and accused manufacturers of putting money above safety and selling a product that could potentially be deadly. At the same time, women also felt that some members of the medical community were negligent in using a product that was not properly approved by the FDA and that physicians who allegedly knew of the illnesses being experienced by other women had failed to inform them of the possible risks.

After having their implants removed, many women reported that most of their symptoms subsided, thereby confirming their belief that the implants were the cause of their suffering. Many had hopes of recovering their health and lives again. One breast implant patient reported that she was still suffering local complications after explantation, but the majority reported relief and peace of mind after their implants were removed.

Most women suspected that breast implants might hinder the detection of breast cancer. Some women reported getting regular mammograms for cancer detection, but others expressed fear of the pain of compression and of possibly rupturing the implant. The women made a number of recommendations to the committee which included the following:

- unbiased research conducted without the involvement of the manufacturers, plastic surgeons, or any other groups with possible financial interests;
- federal government oversight of the scientific research through a task force or special committee;
- clinical research on the sick women, using not just their medical records, but performing physical examinations and laboratory tests to determine if they have classical diseases or commonalties that may suggest "a man-made disease by the manufacturers that only mimics others";
- revising informed consent forms to disclose the true incidence of local and systemic complications, and mandatory provision of a handbook or reference book for women considering implantation;
- a national implant registry for data on types of implants, complications and complaints;
- labels on implants that list all ingredients;
- standardized medical implant manufacturing; and
- screening for individual sensitivity to the chemicals in the implants.

Many women said that they were pleased to have had the opportunity to be heard. They wanted their stories to be told, with the hope that one day they could be well again and that others would not suffer the same physical and emotional pain. They expressed considerable enthusiasm for participating in research. The committee was impressed by this testimony and learned much during the day. The committee also thought that many of their recommendations had merit and might well be considered by the sponsors of this report. In fact, the committee did subsequently propose attention to informed consent and long-term surveillance and investigation of women with implants, among its other recommendations (see Executive Summary). This description of the public meeting is intended to further the intent of that meeting as an opportunity for women to be heard.

APPENDIX C
Review of the Reports of the Independent Review Group and the National Science Panel

Two comprehensive reviews relevant to the charge of the Institute of Medicine (IOM) Committee on the Safety of Silicone Breast Implants were released by distinguished groups of scientists and physicians (the Independent Review Group [IRG] and the National Science Panel [NSP]) while this report was being prepared. The reports of the IRG, NSP, and the IOM committee each contain information and analysis not found in the others, and each contains information, analysis, and conclusions which overlap with the others. These reports also differ to some extent in emphasis and in stating conclusions with or without qualifications. Although the reports reviewed somewhat different data from somewhat different perspectives, they are in substantial agreement. Together they form a mutually consistent body of current informed scientific work on the subject of health and silicone breast implants.

The IRG was established in response to concerns expressed by women in relation to silicone gel breast implants. This body was organized in the United Kingdom by the Chief Medical Officer at the request of the Minister of Health, Baroness Jay. The report of the IRG was available to the IOM Committee on the Safety of Silicone Breast Implants in July 1998. The NSP was established to review and critique the scientific literature on the possibility of a causal association between silicone breast implants and connective tissue diseases, related signs and symptoms, and immune system dysfunction. The panel was appointed by the Honorable Sam C. Pointer, Jr., coordinating judge for the federal breast implant multi-district litigation. Its purpose was to provide the court with an independent assessment of the science at issue in litigation brought by women with implants against the U.S. corporations that had made and sold silicone breast implants of all major types. The report of the NSP was available to the IOM committee in December 1998. The committee reviewed the scope, process and conclusions of the IRG and NSP reports and compared them to the same aspects of its own report.

The task of the IRG was "to review the evidence relating to the possible health risks associated with silicone gel breast implants, to examine the issues relating to pre-operative patient information, and to report to the Chief Medical Officer on its conclusions. Silicone injections, hydrogel filled implants, or other filling materials such as oil or saline were excluded from the remit given to the IRG." The breadth of this scope of work is similar to that defined by the statement of task for the IOM committee's study (see Chapter 1 of this report). Both projects addressed the full array of associations between breast implants and various diseases or health conditions, including local effects, neurological effects, and effects on children, toxicology, cancer, and autoimmune systemic disease. In addition, the IOM committee considered implant-related effects on screening and diagnostic mammography, reviewed research needs and made specific research recommendations, and included all silicone-shelled implants, not just those with silicone gel fill. The IRG also examined whether patient information was satisfactory and considered how good clinical practice could be ensured. A number of recommendations in these areas were made, as well as several suggestions for research programs.

The NSP was asked by the court, "to what extent, if any and with what limitations and caveats do existing studies, research, and reported observations provide a reliable and reasonable scientific basis for one to conclude that silicone-gel breast implants cause or exacerbate . . .'classic' connective tissue diseases, such as systemic lupus erythematosus, Sjogren's syndrome, etc., 'atypical' presentations of connective tissue diseases or symptoms of immune system dysfunctions, . . . and various diseases, symptoms, conditions, or complaints that have sometimes been asserted as possibly associated with silicone-gel implants." Local and perioperative complications were explicitly excluded from this charge. The NSP was also asked to exercise judgment regarding related issues that might require inclusion, the possible scientific basis for any claimed linkages, and whether others generally qualified in the panel's fields of expertise might legitimately disagree with its findings. The panel's work resulted in the examination of silicone toxicology, silicone immunology, and the epidemiology and rheumatology of possible systemic disease in women with silicone gel-filled implants, including silicone elastomer, gel, and fluid compounds that might be present in silicone gel-filled implants, with some attention also to low molecular weight cyclics, silica, and platinum catalysts.

This scope of work excludes most of the items defined by the statement of task for the IOM study. The NSP report did not cover breast implants other than silicone gel-filled implants, although the epidemiological studies reviewed and analyzed often either included other than gel implants or did not specify the type of implant involved. The panel report also did not examine carcinogenesis and cancer (multiple myeloma was discussed, but in the context of monoclonal gammopathy and immunology), effects on children, on mammography, pre operative patient information, or standards for clinical practice.

Although local and perioperative complications were excluded from the panel's charge, and no analysis of rupture, contracture, or other local complications was performed, a few comments on infection were made. Likewise, although the NSP did not discuss the associations of silicone gel breast implants with neurologic disease, multiple sclerosis was among the connective tissue diseases examined in the report, neurologic symptoms were among the symptoms and complaints reviewed because they are sometimes asserted to be associated with silicone-gel implants, and results from a few epidemiologic studies of neurologic diseases in women with implants were reported. Finally, although the panel report pointed out problems with existing information and identified areas in which knowledge was lacking, no research recommendations were made.

The Independent Review Group and the IOM were constituted differently. The seven-member IRG included expertise in law and pathology. The 13-member IOM committee included expertise in radiology, women's health, neurology, oncology, and silicone chemistry. Both groups included expertise in rheumatology and immunology, epidemiology, internal medicine, and plastic surgery. The committee's plastic surgeon limited her practice to pediatric plastic surgery and did not perform breast implantations; the IRG's plastic surgeon included silicone gel breast implantation in his practice. Efforts were made in both instances to enlist members who did not have previously expressed public views on the issues being considered, financial interests in breast implants, connections to manufacturers, or involvement in any ongoing litigation. One IRG member was, as noted, involved in breast implantation, and another had previously summarized the findings of pertinent epidemiological studies in scientific publications. The IRG was more closely tied to the the national government. It was housed and staffed by the British Medical Devices Agency (MDA), its website has a "gov.uk" address, and some information submitted to it is kept in confidence by the MDA (as noted below). The IOM committee was under the charter of the U.S. National Academy of Sciences (NAS), an independent, private, not-for-profit organization.

The committee met in private venues, was staffed by the IOM, and made information available to the public through its "nas.edu" website and the NAS Public Access Office.

The four-member National Science Panel included expertise in toxicology, immunology, epidemiology, rheumatology, and internal medicine. The NSP membership was reviewed for any financial conflicts of interest, involvement with breast implantation or with litigation of implant matters, or previously expressed public views on the issues at hand. The panel was an ad hoc body of the court; its support came from the Federal Judicial Center, its website has a "fjc.gov" address, and its members were questioned before and after the preparation of the NSP report in a process that was videotaped and made available as testimony in breast implant litigation where relevant (Kolata, N.Y. Times, 1998).

The IRG reviewed an extensive body of scientific literature. Its website reference list cites 1,026 references. The IRG relied on this body of peer-reviewed scientific reports, although only a limited number of references are actually cited in either the published or Internet version of its report. However, the IRG heard from, reviewed, and discussed publications of both those who support and those who do not support associations between silicone breast implants and the human health conditions considered. The IRG also gathered new evidence and actually commissioned investigations of some of the evidence. Plaintiff and defense submissions were reviewed, and data submitted by manufacturers, which included confidential business information, were used. Some oral evidence from patient groups, physicians, industry, and other parties at interest was heard. The IOM committee relied on its reference list of about 2,200–2,300 published, peer-reviewed scientific reports; used 1,000–1,100 selected industry technical reports, books, letters, opinion pieces, written statements, and abstracts as sources of secondary importance; and heard representations from scientists, women with implants, and other parties at interest. About 1,200 references are cited in the text of the IOM report. The committee carried out no independent scientific research investigations, and was not in a position to accept or keep proprietary information. Informational material submitted to the committee was made public.

Presumably all information used by the NSP was from publicly available sources. The panel was provided with more than 3,600 documents by counsel for both parties, of which 2,000 were said to be references (Kolata, N.Y. Times, 1998), and carried out its own searches of the literature, which identified 1,600 articles, some of which were duplicates. The panel also heard multiple presentations from various invited expert scientists and physicians on three occasions over a 13-month period. The panel heard from, reviewed, and discussed the publications of both those who supported and those who did not support associations between silicone gel breast implants and the human health conditions the panel was asked to evaluate.

The NSP noted in its report that it relied on the peer-reviewed scientific literature, often giving secondary or no importance to abstracts. However, the report also cites, when appropriate (though seldom), textbooks and other scientific books, a presentation from an expert, and industry technical reports. The different chapters of its report cite from approximately 60 to 110 references, each. In addition, the panel did original work and made independent calculations, such as meta-analyses and recombinations of the epidemiological data and studies. The NSP report was at the request of, was prepared for, and was delivered to, the court, but it was also quickly made available to the media and, through the Internet, to interested women, scientists, physicians, and the general public.

Although the IRG was funded by government and responded to the requirements of, and delivered reports to, its sponsor, the group intended the report for a wider audience, including women who had or were considering breast implants and their families; plastic surgeons and other clinicians; manufacturers; lawyers; health care policy makers; and scientists. The IOM report was originally ordered by the U.S. House of Representatives Committee on Appropriations. In addition to the National Institutes of Health, specifically the National Institute of Arthritis, Musculoskeletal and Skin Disease, the IOM report was intended to respond to the needs of other agencies of the U.S. Department of Health and Human Services; the U.S. Congress; women who had had implants, had them currently, or were considering them; their loved ones; physicians; scientists; implant manufacturers; and the general public. The preparation of an accompanying short lay version of the IOM report is emblematic of this interest. Legal issues were not addressed by the committee.

The IRG and IOM reports cover essentially the same subject matter. Subjects examined included a brief history of gel implants and regulatory actions; a description of gel implants; and a review of local and perioperative effects, including contracture, infection, gel fluid diffusion, and the consequences, frequency, and detection by imaging of implant rupture. In general, the IRG report contains less detail and less extensive citation. It is focused and friendly to the lay reader. The two reports are in agreement on many points in the background and descriptions of local effects. However, the IOM committee's review of the available evidence did not support the categorical conclusion of the IRG that the type of filling in an implant has not been shown to have any effect on contracture. The committee also found the evidence for exacerbation of contracture by infection still limited, whereas the IRG concluded that infection might, on occasion, exacerbate contracture. Lastly, the description of rupture, its frequency, and its consequences, by the IRG did not emphasize safety concerns as did the committee's review of the available data. The committee expressed considerably more concerns about reoperations and local complications.

The IRG report also analyzed and discussed systemic effects including immunological and pathological effects, among them inflammation and pathological signs of immune activity such as vasculitis; the presence of substances potentially capable of inciting immune disease such as silica; the prevalence of autoantibodies, antibodies to silicone, and T-cell responses to silica; silicone adjuvant activity; and the correlation of signs and symptoms of health conditions in women with implants with specific HLA (human lymphocyte antigen) types. The IRG report's findings of the lack of evidence or plausibility for the presence of silica in tissues of women with gel breast implants, the lack of credible evidence for specific silicone antibodies or adaptive immune responses to silica, and the failure to discover reliable biomarkers for a particular silicone associated systemic condition are generally consistent with the committee's views. Existing data do not allow the definite exclusion of systemic or local immune responses associated with silicone breast implants, but no valid scientific evidence currently establishes any such association. In fact, the nature of science is such that no scientific data can ever allow the definite and unexceptional exclusion of this possibility. The IRG commissioned an independent investigation that came to different conclusions than a report by one U.S. investigator of silica and the diagnosis of vasculitis in tissue of women with silicone implants.

The IRG report reviewed epidemiological studies of defined connective tissue disease or a new systemic silicone-related disease associated with silicone gel-filled breast implants. Neurological disease, effects on children born to women with implants, toxicology, and cancer were also discussed. The IRG did not find evidence to establish an association of these conditions with silicone gel breast implants. The IOM committee also found no convincing, valid scientific evidence of such associations with gel- or saline-filled breast implants. An evaluation of the effects of silicone breast implants on mammography was not part of the IRG report. Coverage of ways of ensuring quality clinical care for women undergoing breast implantation and adequate provision of preoperative information for such women was not part of the IOM committee's charge (except insofar as the committee called for adequate informed consent) and thus was not part of its review.

The body of the National Science Panel report consists of four chapters. The first chapter, "Review of Animal Studies Relevant to Silicone Toxicity," focuses on poly(dimethylsiloxane) and related silicones that are present in implants and are known to have similar chemical reactivities. Other silicones were not examined. Minimal effects by minor silicone species that are seen in animals only at high levels of exposure also were not considered, nor were studies involving silicones that were administered orally or injected in relatively large doses into tissues not accessible to breast implant silicone. The panel did not find credible evidence that silicone could be degraded to silicon or silica in the body, so studies that require this result were not reviewed (e.g., studies on the toxicology of silica).

The NSP examined historical studies of silicone toxicity, studies of silicones as adjuvants; a number of studies of silicones in animal models of autoimmune diseases (in great detail); and the immunotoxicology, inflammatory, and macrophage-activating effects of silicone. There was a brief examination of low molecular weight cyclic silicones, silanols, and platinum, which concluded that they have no toxicological implications for women with implants. In summary, the panel concluded that silicone is of low toxicity and that the local reaction to silicone is similar to other foreign-body reactions. Evidence of phagocytosis and transport of silicone by macrophages has not included evidence of systemic effects or adaptive T-cell activation. Adjuvant effects were not deemed by the NSP to have been shown to have biological significance, and the only immune effect was a suppression of natural killer (NK) cell activity insufficient to affect disease models. In 17 animal models of autoimmune disease, only 2 showed any effects of silicone, and these provided weak, preliminary evidence of a promotional effect. The panel concluded that the preponderance of the evidence indicated little probability that silicone induces or exacerbates systemic disease in humans.

The second chapter of the NSP report, "Clinical Immunology," summarizes the clinical evidence for silicone induced immune alterations in women with silicone gel breast implants. The panel introduced the discussion in this chapter by examining again what it believed to be the weak adjuvant effect, the NK-cell effects, and the effects in animal autoimmune models of some silicones noting that in general, these effects are of uncertain biological significance. The panel then reviewed relevant studies on cytokines, NK-cell function, superantigen activity, HLA types, and T-cell activation in women with silicone breast implants; antinuclear antibodies, specific autoantibodies—including anti-collagen, antimicrosomal, anti-silicone, and antipolymer antibodies; and monoclonal gammopathy and multiple myeloma. The NSP concluded that, overall, the data do not demonstrate adaptive antigenicity of silicone, immune system activation in women with silicone breast implants, or the presence of autoreactivity in women with breast implants. Absent immune system activation, it seems unlikely that there is sufficient local inflammation to account for reported symptoms in women with silicone gel breast implants. In summary, the panel concluded that there were a number of design flaws in studies of the immune system of women with breast implants and that, at the time its report was published, there were no consistent data supporting the hypothesis that silicone gel breast implants cause an alteration in systemic immune responses in women.

In the third chapter of the NSP report, "Epidemiological Analysis of Silicone Breast Implants and Connective Tissue Disease," the panel discussed descriptive epidemiology and diagnostic criteria for specific connective tissue diseases; it also carried out and discussed meta-analyses of 20 epidemiological studies of silicone breast implants, including unadjusted and adjusted effect estimates and studies of "all breast implants" and "gel-only" implants. The panel calculated the power of these analyses under various circumstances and the population attributable fractions for five connective tissue diseases. Even though this was slightly inconsistent with the approach in the rest of its report, the panel concluded that analyses using all breast implants were preferable, given the problems of identification of implant type by self-reporting and the likelihood that, in the periods of time covered by currently published epidemiological studies, more than 90% of implants were gel filled (including polyurethane-coated, double-lumen, and single-lumen gel implants). The NSP's analyses were complex, and a substantial amount of data with various studies from the literature included or excluded and with various adjustments was presented. The summary relative risk estimates varied among the meta-analyses that were adjusted or unadjusted for confounding variables, those that included or did not include various studies (e.g., Hennekens et al., 1996), and those that involved all breast implants or were limited to gel implants. The panel found that these relative risk estimates demonstrated, and the most likely conclusion from these several analyses was, that there is no meaningful or consistent association between breast implants or silicone gel-filled breast implants and connective tissue diseases or other autoimmune or rheumatic conditions. The power of the analyses was adequate to detect a small increase in relative risk, on the order of 1.2–1.8 for different conditions.

The fourth and concluding chapter of the NSP report, "Rheumatology: Clinical Case Definitions/Diagnoses and Clinical Associations," reviews studies of women with silicone gel breast implants that met clinical case definitions or classic, accepted diagnoses of connective tissue diseases or of atypical presentations of connective tissue disease, along with symptoms and signs for the strength of an association with silicone gel breast implants. The panel included 24 classic, accepted connective tissue diseases, as defined by explicit criteria or described in a reasonably consistent fashion in standard textbooks, in its review of the strength of association with breast implants. With one or two exceptions, the studies reviewed were the same as those used for the meta-analyses in the third chapter of its report. The panel also reviewed the association between undifferentiated connective tissue disease and silicone breast implants. The one applicable study had a confidence interval with a lower limit less than one (described in the report as greater than one, but the actual result reported was less than one). The panel examined the information and reports available on novel disease associated with silicone implants as an example of the atypical presentation of connective tissue disease and decided that evidence for such a condition was insufficient.

Available studies were examined for information on an association between breast implants and 48 symptoms and signs attributed to women who had had silicone breast implants. For 25 of these symptoms or signs there were no studies that contained data to review, for 17 there were no studies reporting a relative risk point estimate with a lower confidence limit greater than one, and for 6 there were discordant results (at least one, but not all studies reporting a lower limit less than one). The panel concluded that there was no appreciable association of silicone breast implants with any of the classic or accepted diagnoses, with undifferentiated connective tissue disease, or with the signs and symptoms asserted to be associated with silicone breast implants. In the case of an atypical presentation, inclusion of the exposure (silicone breast implant) in the case definition precluded evaluation since there was no possibility of comparing women with and without implants to arrive at an estimate of frequency. Furthermore, many of the signs and symptoms of the proposed condition are common and shared with a number of other conditions. No data were found and no conclusions could be reached from the literature available on the course of connective tissue disease in women with implants compared to women without implants.

The IRG also reached summary conclusions that there was no conclusive evidence for an abnormal immune response to silicone from breast implants; that there was no epidemiological evidence for any link between silicone gel breast implants and any established connective tissue disease; and that there was no good evidence for the existence of atypical connective tissue disease or undefined conditions such as "silicone poisoning." The IRG also concluded that there was no evidence that children of women with silicone gel-filled breast implants are at increased risk of connective tissue disease and that the overall biological response to silicone is consistent with conventional forms of response to foreign materials, rather that an unusual toxic reaction. In the section on toxicology, it might have been preferable to have relied on information that is available to and reviewable by others, rather than citing data that are confidential. The IRG also recommended research into the incidence of rupture and research into the nature of the symptoms of women with implants to elucidate the possible role of subclinical infection. Research to validate (or not) the work of certain other investigators was suggested.

The IOM committee found the IRG and NSP reports useful documents and is in general agreement with their findings. The NSP's thorough compilation and detailed descriptions and analyses of the epidemiological and immunological studies, and the insights from the careful meta-analyses, are particularly useful. The conclusions of each chapter of the NSP report were well supported by data and analysis and were conservatively stated. Although the report was focused, this was by design, and it had the advantage, as noted earlier, of allowing an in-depth approach.

The IOM committee agrees with the NSP's general conclusions regarding the formation of silica from silicone in the tissue of women with implants, although a discussion of the availability and biological significance, or lack thereof, of amorphous silica from implant silicone elastomer shells would have been interesting. Also, the panel cites a "fairly high estimate" of the frequency of U.S. women with breast implants (1%) and uses this value in calculating population attributable fractions. The IOM committee's estimate is approximately 1.5% of U.S. women with silicone breast implants of all kinds (1.5 million to 1.8 million U.S. women in 1997), so the source of the NSP's estimate would be of interest. The effect of this difference on the numbers of cases of connective tissue disease theoretically attributable to implants would not be significant, however. The committee's recommendations for research differed from those of the IRG. This difference may reflect the committee's and the IRG's responses to the situation and needs in their respective countries.

APPENDIX D

Glossary

Abstract Condensation or summary of a scientific article.

Achalasia Failure of the sphincter between the esophagus and stomach to relax during swallowing.

Adaptive immunity Resistance or sensitization to infection or to a foreign substance that is acquired, not innate; depends on experience with the infection or foreign substance; and leads to an ability to react to the infection or substance in the future.

Adenopathy Enlargement of glands; see Lymphadenopathy.

Adipose Pertaining to fat or fatty (e.g., adipose tissue).

Adjuvant Substance that enhances the immune response to an antigen.

Adrenal steroid Hormone of the cortex of the adrenal gland with anti-inflammatory and immunosuppressive activities, among others; a corticosteroid.

Aerobic Requiring oxygen, growing in the presence of oxygen.

Allele Any of different genes at the same location on the chromosome; different genes or alleles are referred to as heterozygous; the same genes or alleles, homozygous, for the gene product or trait.

Alloplastic Pertaining to an inert foreign body used for implantation into tissue.

Anaerobic Growing in the absence of oxygen.

Antibody Immune protein (immunoglobulin) formed in response to, and reacting specifically with, an antigen, or occurring naturally (e.g., immunoglobulin [Ig], IgA, IgD, IgE, IgG, or IgM).

Antigen Any substance capable of inducing a specific or adaptive immune response and of reacting with the products (a specific antibody, specific T lymphocyte, or both) of that response.

Apoptosis Programmed cell death.

Arthralgia Pain in a joint.

Arthritis Inflammation of a joint.

Atomic weight Mass in grams of 1 mole (6.02×10^{23} atoms) of an atomic species.

Atrophy Wasting of tissues, organs, or the whole body.

Augmentation In this report, placement of an implant for the purpose of enlarging or changing the appearance of the breast.

Autoantibody Antibody directed against a self-antigen.

Autogenous tissue Originating within the body.

Autologous Describing a graft in which the donor and recipient is the same individual.

Axilla, axillary Armpit, of the armpit.

B lymphocyte Cell representing 1530% of circulating lymphocytes, responsible for antibody.

Bias Deviation of results or inferences from the truth, or processes leading to such deviation.

Bleed (of implant) Diffusion of silicone fluid into and through the silicone shell of a silicone gel-filled implant.

Breast augmentation classification

Class I Augmented breast feels as soft as an unoperated one.

Class II Breast is less soft and implant can be palpated, but is not visible.

Class III Breast is more firm, implant can be palpated easily, and it (or distortion from it) can be seen.

Class IV Breast is firm, hard, tender, painful, and cold; distortion is often marked.

Bursa Closed sac lined with synovium and filled with fluid found or formed in areas subject to friction (e.g., where a tendon passes over bone).

Capsule Membranous structure, usually dense collagenous connective tissue enveloping another organ, joint, or part; in this report, the capsule found around an implant.

Capsulectomy Surgical removal of a capsule.

Carcinogenesis, carcinogenicity Production of cancer; ability to cause cancer.

Carcinoma Any type of malignant tumor arising from epithelial cells such as lung, intestine, or skin.

CAS number Chemical Abstracts Service number; a method for identifying chemicals.

Case control study Epidemiological method that identifies cases of disease and compares their past history of exposure to risk factors to the exposure of similar people without the disease.

Caseation Form of necrosis in which tissue contains protein and fat that looks cheese-like.

Centimeter One-hundredth of a meter, or approximately four-tenths of an inch.

Cephalosporin Broad spectrum antibiotic.

Closed capsulotomy Creation of opening in a breast implant capsule by external compression.

Clostridia Anaerobic bacterium (e.g., tetanus).

Cohort study Epidemiological method that prospectively follows a group with a condition and compares its outcomes to those of a group without the condition.

Collagen Protein substance of the white fibers of connective tissue, cartilage, or bone.

Confidence interval (CI) Range within which the true value is most likely found (e.g., 95% CI means value is within range 95% of the time).

Connective tissue Collagenous or fibrous tissue surrounding and separating muscles, organs, and other body parts (e.g., fascia).

Connective tissue disease Chronic inflammatory disease with presumed autoimmune components involving the musculoskeletal system and multiple other organs (e.g., rheumatoid arthritis, systemic lupus erythematosus, scleroderma).

Contracture Shrinkage or reduction in size; in this report, contraction of the breast implant collagenous, fibrous tissue capsule.

Cross-sectional study Analysis of a large group at one point in time.

Cubic centimeter Unit of volume equal to one-thousandth of a liter, one milliliter, or approximately 1/30 of a fluid ounce.

Cytokine Hormone-like, low molecular weight protein secreted by many cell types that regulates cell-to-cell interactions and features of the immune response (e.g., lymphokine, monokine).

Dalton (Da) Unit of mass equal to 1.0 in the atomic mass scale.

Deflation In this report, loss of saline from a saline-filled implant with partial or complete implant collapse.

Dermatomyositis, polymyositis Chronic inflammatory disease of muscle.

Dermis Layer of skin under the epidermis, consisting of a dense bed of vascular connective tissue.

Desmosome Adhesion site between two cells with a dense attachment plaque on both sides.

Device In this report, an implant, prosthesis, or appliance designed to perform a specific function, a silicone breast implant.

Edema Accumulation of excessive fluid in tissues.

Elastomer In this report, a cross-linked solid silicone reinforced with amorphous silica, an implant shell.

Electrolyte Ionizable substance in solution (e.g., salt existing as Na^+ and Cl^- in plasma, tissue fluid, or saline-filled implants).

ELISA Enzyme-linked immunosorbent assay, an immunochemical test.

Embolus Any plug (often a clot) carried by the circulation from one blood vessel to a smaller vessel that becomes occluded, thus interrupting circulation to the tissue served by that blood vessel.

Eosinophil White cell (leukocyte) with lobed nucleus and red-yellow staining granules that is asssociated with allergic or antiparasitic functions.

Epidermolysis Loosening of the outermost layers of skin (epidermis) with the formation of blisters.

Epithelial Pertaining to cells, usually in layers, that cover internal or external body surfaces and line blood vessels and other cavities in the body.

Explant, explantation In this report, an implant removed from the body, the act of doing so.

Exudation Oozing of fluid gradually out of body tissue or structure, usually because of injury or inflammation.

Fascia Sheet or band of fibrous, connective tissue that lies under the skin or encloses muscles and other organs.

Fibroblast Connective tissue cell that can form collagen.

Fibrocystic disease Condition common in women and characterized by pain and multiple cysts in the breast.

Fibromyalgia Syndrome characterized by chronic diffuse pain and tender points that occurs predominantly in women.

Fistula Abnormal passage between organs or to the body surface.

Flora Population of microorganisms, bacteria, or fungi.

Formalin Aqueous solution of formaldehyde (37%) used as a tissue preservative or fixative.

Galoctocele Cystic enlargement in the breast that contains milk.

Galactorrhea Abnormal lactation.

Gammopathy Condition marked by disturbed immunoglobulin synthesis.

Gavage Forced feeding by stomach tube.

Gel In this report, a lightly cross-linked, spongy silicone permeated with a lower weight silicone fluid.

Gentamycin Antibiotic that is particularly effective against gram-negative aerobic bacteria.

Giant cell (foreign body) Large cell with multiple nuclei distributed throughout the cytoplasm formed by macrophages and seen around foreign bodies.

Gram Unit of weight, 1/28th of an ounce, the weight of one milliliter of water at 4°C.

Granuloma Nodular chronic inflammatory lesion, consisting of various cells such as mononuclear cells, epithelioid cells, giant cells, lymphocytes, eosinophils, and plasma cells.

Hematoma Localized collection of blood, usually clotted, in an organ, tissue, or body space.

Hemosiderin Iron-containing protein, produced by phagocytic digestion of blood iron protein.

HEp-2 cells Human epithelial tissue culture cells that provide sensitive assay for antinuclear antibodies.

Hepatomegaly Enlargement of the liver.

High temperature vulcanized (HTV) In this report, cross-linked silicone molecules producing a higher molecular weight, firmer silicone made at high temperature (115–150°C).

Histiocyte Macrophage.

Histology Microscopic anatomy.

Human adjuvant disease Rheumatic signs or symptoms presumably due to immune or adjuvant response to silicone, as in adjuvant disease in rodents; a misnomer.

Human lymphocyte antigen (HLA) Substance capable of inducing immune response and present on most human cells (HLA-A, B, and C) or only on human immune cells (HLA-D) that has been shown to have a strong influence on human transplantation and association with certain human diseases.

Immunofluorescence Tissue microscopic method using antibody labeled with a dye that glows under fluorescent light; direct, the antibody is directed against the test substance itself; indirect, the antibody is directed against an immunoglobulin that reacts with the test substance.

Inflammation Local tissue protective response to injury involving dilation of blood vessels, fluid exudation, and migration of white cells.

Innate immunity Immunity based on the genetic constitution of the individual, nonspecific and not requiring or enhanced by prior exposure.

Interstitial Relating to spaces in tissue.

Intraperitoneal Within the abdominal cavity.

In vitro In an artificial (e.g., laboratory) environment.

In vivo Within the living body.

LC_{50} Concentration that kills half of the cells.

LD_{50} Mean lethal dose.

Leakage (of implant) Loss of implant filler through a breach in the implant shell (as opposed to bleed or gel fluid diffusion).

Liter Volume equal to 1.0567 quarts, a thousand cubic centimeters or milliliters.

Low bleed In this report, an implant or implant shell fabricated to lessen bleed, or gel fluid diffusion, into and through the silicone elastomer shell.

Lumen Interior space, for example, the inside of a breast implant.

Lymphadenopathy Enlargement of lymph glands or nodes.

Macrophage Monocytic cell in tissue that is large, ingests foreign bodies, and is involved in immune and other tissue functions.

Macroscopic Visible with the unaided eye.

Mesenchymal Pertaining to tissues formed of embryonic connective tissue (e.g., connective tissue, blood and lymphatic vessels).

Meter Length equal to 39.37 inches.

Methylprednisolone Synthetic adrenal cortical steroid.

Microgram One-millionth of a gram.

Microscopic Extremely small, visible only with a microscope.

Microsurgical flap Mass of tissue, dissected free and connected to blood vessels at a new site by using low-power microscopic magnification.

Milligram One-thousandth of a gram.

Milliliter One-thousandth of a liter, or one cubic centimeter.

Millimeter One-thousandth of a meter, or 4/100 of an inch.

Modulus In this report, stiffness or hardness of silicone, adjustable by cross-linking.

Molecular Weight Sum of atomic weights of all the atoms that constitute a molecule.

Monoclonal Derived from a single cell.

Monocyte Mononuclear phagocytic cell formed in bone marrow and transported to tissues to become a macrophage.

Morphea Localized scleroderma, characterized by thickened dermal fibrous tissue plaques.

Musculocutaneous flap Compound flap of skin and muscle with adequate blood supply to permit a sufficient graft to be transferred.

Myalgia Pain in a muscle or muscles.

Mycobacteria Slow-growing bacteria with certain staining characteristics (e.g., tuberculosis).

Myeloma, multiple myeloma Plasma cell tumor or plasma cell malignancy originating in bone marrow and producing an abnormal protein, usually a monoclonal IgG.

Myositis Inflammation of a voluntary muscle.

Nanogram One-billionth of a gram.

Nanometer One-billionth of a meter.

Necrosis Pathologic death of one or more cells, a tissue, or an organ.

Neoplasia Abnormal tissue growth; benign tumor or cancer.

Neuritis Inflammation of a nerve with pain, tenderness, anesthesia, and paralysis.

Neuropathy Functional disturbance or pathological change in the peripheral nervous system, generally not inflammatory.

Odds ratio Estimate of the relative risk, usually calculated for data from case control studies.

Omentum Membrane (of peritoneum) that passes from the stomach to the intestine.

Open capsulotomy Incision or opening in a breast implant capsule made by an open surgical approach.

Osmotic pressure Pressure required to stop solvent from moving through a membrane toward the higher concentration of solute.

Parenteral Given by injection into other than the gastrointestinal tract.

Parts per million (ppm) Concentrations of vapors in air are usually expressed in ppm, a gas volume ratio, which can be converted to mass concentration (e.g., mg/m^3) by dividing molecular weight in grams × concentration in ppm by 0.0245.

Pectoral muscles (pectoralis major, pectoralis minor) Muscles from the front of the chest to the upper arm, collar bone, and shoulder blade that rotate the arm toward the midline and pull it forward and downward; when used to cover an implant, the implant is referred to as submuscular or subpectoral.

Pedicle Stalk in a flap through which the blood supply passes.

Peer reviewed Examined by those with expertise for accuracy, relevance, and other measures of scientific quality.

Periosteum Connective tissue layer covering bone.

Peritoneal cavity Abdominal cavity lined with peritoneum, a smooth thin membrane investing its organs and walls.

pH Symbol for acidity (less than 7) or alkalinity (greater than 7); pH 7 is neutral.

Phagocytic, phagocytosis Pertaining to cells that ingest microorganisms, cell fragments, or small particles, the process in which this occurs.

Pharmacokinetic Pertaining to movement of drugs within the body.

Plasma cell Cell derived from a B lymphocyte that is active in producing antibody.

Pneumonitis Inflammation of the lung.

Pneumothorax Accumulation of air in the chest cavity, inside the chest but not in the lung.

Polyclonal Derived from different cells.

Polymer Substance of high molecular weight made up of a chain of repeated units.

Polymorphism Occurrence in more than one form, varying genes, or alleles at the same chromosomal location.

Polymorphonuclear Having a deeply lobed nucleus that appears multiple, as in a polymorphonuclear leukocyte, an acute inflammatory, circulating white cell.

Popliteal Back of the knee.

Prosthesis Device or artificial substitute for a body part.

Ptosis Prolapse or drooping.

Radiolucent Relatively penetrable by x-rays.

Radiopaque Relatively impenetrable by x-rays.

Raynauds phenomenon Sudden reversible pallor of fingers, hand, toes, or tip of the nose caused by cold.

Reconstruction In this report, reforming of the breast with an alloplastic device, autogenous tissue, or both.

Relative risk Ratio of disease incidence in those with a risk factor to incidence in those without the risk factor.

Renal Pertaining to the kidney.

Rheumatoid arthritis (RA) Chronic inflammatory disease of unknown cause affecting multiple joints.

Room temperature vulcanized (RTV) In this report, cross-linked silicone molecules producing a higher molecular weight, firmer silicone made at room temperature.

Rupture In this report, a breach of any size in the integrity of a silicone breast implant shell.

Sarcoma Malignant tumor of connective tissue, formed by proliferation of mesodermal cells.

Scleroderma (Ssc) Chronic inflammatory disease characterized by thickening, tightening, nonpitting hardening of the skin of both extremities and trunk.

Sensitivity True-positive results as a proportion of the total of true-positive and false-negative results (i.e., the likelihood of detecting a condition).

Seroma Cystic accumulation of serous (similar to blood serum) fluid in tissue.

Shunt Passage or anastomosis between two natural channels; diversion of an accumulation of fluid to an absorbing or excreting system.

Sicca Dryness.

Silica, amorphous Very finely divided, noncrystalline silicon dioxide.

Silica, crystalline Silicon dioxide in organized crystalline form.

Silicon Shiny silvery element with an atomic weight of 28.

Silicone Compound or polymer of silicon, oxygen, and carbon (e.g., polydimethylsiloxane, PDMS).

Sjogrens syndrome (SS) Chronic inflammatory disease, or syndrome accompanying other diseases, and characterized by dryness of the mouth and eyes.

Specificity True-negative results as a proportion of the total of true-negative and false-positive results (i.e., the likelihood that a positive result is accurate).

Steroid See Adrenal steroid.

Subcutaneous Beneath the skin, but above the fascia and muscle.

Subglandular (retroglandular) In this report, referring to the position of a breast implant under the mammary gland, but on top of the muscles of the chest.

Submammary (retromammary) Subglandular.

Submuscular (retromuscular) In this report, referring to the position of a breast implant wholly or partially under the muscles on the front of the chest (e.g., pectoralis major, pectoralis minor, or serratus anterior).

Subpectoral (retropectoral) Submuscular.

Syndrome Aggregate of signs and symptoms that together constitute the picture of a disease.

Systemic lupus erythematosus (SLE) Chronic inflammatory disease affecting multiple organs, joints, kidney, heart, and blood vessels.

T lymphocyte Cell representing 70–85% of circulating lymphocytes that produces cytokines and is responsible for cellular immunity, delayed hypersensitivity, and graft rejection.

Teratogen Agent that causes abnormal fetal development.

Titer Amount of a substance that can be manipulated by serial dilution (e.g., 1:40, 1:80, 1:160).

Toxic shock syndrome Infection, primarily with *Staphylococcus aureus*, often around foreign bodies, characterized by diarrhea, flaking skin rash, fever, shock, and substantial mortality.

Triamcinolone Synthetic adrenal cortical steroid.

Urethra, urethral Canal from the urinary bladder to the exterior of the body, pertaining to this canal.

Vasculitis Inflammation of a blood vessel or vessels (e.g., as seen in connective tissue disease).

Visceral peritoneum Membrane lining the internal organs of the abdominal (peritoneal) cavity.

REFERENCES

Dictionary of the Rheumatic Diseases, American Rheumatism Association, 1988.

Dorlands Illustrated Medical Dictionary, W. B. Sanders Company, 1994.

Segen, J. C., The Dictionary of Modern Medicine, Parthenon Publishing Group, 1992.

Stedmans Medical Dictionary, Williams and Wilkins, 1995.

Index

A

B

C

D

G

H

I

J

K

L

M

N

O

P

R

S

T

U

V

W

X